THE WASHINGTON MANUAL®

Hematology and Oncology   Subspecialty Consult

FIFTH EDITION

THE WASHINGTON MANUAL®

Hematology and Oncology   `Subspecialty Consult`

FIFTH EDITION

Editors

Brian A. Van Tine, MD, PhD

Professor of Medicine and Pediatrics
Division of Medical Oncology
Washington University School of
   Medicine
St. Louis, Missouri

Meagan A. Jacoby, MD, PhD

Associate Professor of Medicine
Division of Oncology
Bone Marrow Transplantation &
   Leukemia
Washington University School of
   Medicine
St. Louis, Missouri

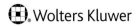 Wolters Kluwer

Philadelphia • Baltimore • New York • London
Buenos Aires • Hong Kong • Sydney • Tokyo

Acquisitions Editor: Joe Cho
Development Editor: Cindy Yoo
Editorial Coordinator: Chester Anthony Gonzalez
Editorial Assistant: Kristen Kardoley
Marketing Manager: Kirsten Watrud
Production Project Manager: Matthew West
Manager, Graphic Arts & Design: Stephen Druding
Manufacturing Coordinator: Lisa Bowling
Prepress Vendor: Aptara, Inc.

Fifth Edition

9 8 7 6 5 4 3 2 1

Printed in Mexico

Library of Congress Cataloging-in-Publication Data

Names: Van Tine, Brian A., editor. | Jacoby, Meagan A., editor.
Title: The Washington manual hematology and oncology subspecialty consult /
    editors, Brian A. Van Tine, Meagan A. Jacoby.
Other titles: Hematology and oncology subspecialty consult
Description: Fifth edition. | Philadelphia, PA : Wolters Kluwer, [2025] |
    Includes bibliographical references and index. | Summary: "Concise, portable, and user-friendly, The Washington Manual Hematology and Oncology Subspecialty Consult provides quick access to the essential information needed for the workup and treatment of hematologic diseases and cancers. Authored by WUSTL hematology-oncology fellows and junior faculty (the physicians who have the most recent experience with the issues and questions that arise while training in these subspecialties), the book is ideal for those earlier in their career, such as incoming Hem-Onc fellows, residents, and medical students rotating on hematology and oncology subspecialty services. To the point and practical (like all Washington Manuals), this book is also useful as a first-line resource for general internists and primary care providers"– Provided by publisher.
Identifiers: LCCN 2024030365 (print) | LCCN 2024030366 (ebook) |
    ISBN 9781975212841 (paperback) | ISBN 9781975212858 (epub)
Subjects: MESH: Hematologic Diseases–diagnosis | Neoplasms–diagnosis |
    Hematologic Diseases–drug therapy | Neoplasms–drug therapy |
    Diagnosis, Differential | Handbook
Classification: LCC RC280.H47 (print) | LCC RC280.H47 (ebook) | NLM WH 39
    | DDC 616.99/418–dc23/eng/20240801
LC record available at https://lccn.loc.gov/2024030365
LC ebook record available at https://lccn.loc.gov/2024030366

QUADM1024

Contributors

Favour Ayomide Akinjiyan, PhD
MD/PhD Candidate
Department of Internal Medicine
Washington University School of Medicine
St. Louis, Missouri

George Ansstas, MD
Associate professor
Department of Internal Medicine/ Oncology
Washington University School of Medicine
St. Louis, Missouri

Anthony Apicelli, MD, PhD
Associate Professor
Department of Radiation Oncology
Washington University School of Medicine
St. Louis, Missouri

Olivia Aranha, MD, PhD
Associate Professor of Medicine
Division of Medical Oncology
Washington University School of Medicine
St. Louis, Missouri

Christine Auberle, MD
Chief Fellow
Divisions of Hematology and Oncology
Washington University School of Medicine
St. Louis, Missouri

Kaiden Barozinsky
Clinical Research Coordinator
Washington University School of Medicine
St. Louis, Missouri

Michael D. Bern, MD, PhD
Clinical Fellow
Division of Medical Oncology
Washington University School of Medicine
St. Louis, Missouri

Omar Hameed Butt, MD, PhD
Assistant Professor
Washington University School of Medicine
St. Louis, Missouri

Amanda F. Cashen, MD
Professor of Medicine
Department of Oncology
Washington University School of Medicine
St. Louis, Missouri

Giordano F. Cittolin Santos, MD
Fellow
Division of Medical Oncology
Washington Universality School of Medicine
St. Louis, Missouri

Katherine Clifton, MD
Assistant Professor
Department of Medicine
Washington University School of Medicine
St. Louis, Missouri

Jared Cohen, MD
Fellow
Division on Medical Oncology
Washington University School of Medicine
St. Louis, Missouri

Oladipo Cole, MD
Fellow
Divisions of Hematology and Oncology
Washington University School of Medicine
St. Louis, Missouri

Ryan Day, MD, PhD
Instructor of Medicine
Washington University School of Medicine
St. Louis, Missouri

Nicole C. Foley, MD
Chief Fellow
Divisions of Hematology and Oncology
Washington University School of Medicine
St. Louis, Missouri

Patrick M. Grierson, MD, PhD
Assistant Professor of Medicine
Washington University School of Medicine
St. Louis, Missouri

Sasha Haarberg, PharmD, BCOP
Clinical Pharmacist
Division of Oncology
Washington University School of Medicine
St. Louis, Missouri

Andrea R. Hagemann, MD, MSCI
Professor
Department of OBGYN
Washington University School of Medicine
St. Louis, Missouri

Brett H. Herzog, MD, PhD
Assistant Professor of Medicine
Division of Medical Oncology
Washington University School of Medicine
St. Louis, Missouri

Angela C. Hirbe, MD, PhD
Associate Professor of Medicine
Division of Medical Oncology
Washington University School of Medicine
St. Louis, Missouri

Michael D. Iglesia, MD, PhD
Instructor of Medicine
Division of Medical Oncology
Washington University School of Medicine
St. Louis, Missouri

Ronald Jackups Jr, MD, PhD
Professor, Pathology and Immunology
Division of Laboratory and Genomic
    Medicine
Washington University School of Medicine
St. Louis, Missouri

Tanner M. Johanns, MD, PhD
Assistant Professor of Medicine
Division of Medical Oncology
Washington University School of Medicine
St. Louis, Missouri

Brendan Knapp, MD
Clinical Fellow
Division of Medical Oncology
Washington University School of Medicine
St. Louis, Missouri

Constantine N. Logothetis, MD
Fellow
Divisions of Hematology and Oncology
Washington University School of Medicine
St. Louis, Missouri

Mustafaa Mahmood, MD
Resident
Department of Radiation Oncology
Washington University School of Medicine
St. Louis, Missouri

Nathan B. McLamb, MD
Assistant Professor, Pathology and Immunology
Department of Pathology and Immunology
Washington University School of Medicine
St. Louis, Missouri

Renee Morecroft, MBBS
Physician
Department of Oncology
Washington University School of Medicine
St. Louis, Missouri

Daniel Morgensztern, MD
Professor
Division of Medical Oncology
Washington Universality School of Medicine
St. Louis, Missouri

Imran Nizamuddin, MD
Fellow
Divisions of Hematology and Oncology
Washington University School of Medicine
St. Louis, Missouri

Thomas A. Odeny, MD, MPH, PhD
Assistant Professor of Medicine
Division of Medical Oncology
Washington University School of Medicine
St. Louis, Missouri

Peter Oppelt, MD
Associate Professor of Medicine
Washington University School of Medicine
St. Louis, Missouri

Giulia Petrone, MD
Fellow
Department of Hematology and Oncology
Washington University School of Medicine
St. Louis, Missouri

Sana Saif Ur Rehman, MD
Assistant Professor of Medicine
Division of Hematology
Washington University School of Medicine,
St. Louis, Missouri

Melissa A. Reimers, MD
Associate Professor of Medicine
Washington University School of Medicine
St. Louis, Missouri

Kaleigh Roberts, MD, PhD
Clinical Fellow Associate in Neuropathology
Washington University School of Medicine
St. Louis, Missouri

Kristen M. Sanfilippo, MD, MPHS
Associate Professor of Medicine
Division of Hematology
Washington University School of Medicine
Staff Physician
Hematology/Oncology
St. Louis Veterans Administration Medical
   Center
St. Louis, Missouri

Joshua I. Siner, MD
Fellow
Divisions of Hematology and Medical
   Oncology
Washington University School of Medicine
St. Louis, Missouri

Michael J. Slade, MD, MSCI
Assistant Professor of Medicine
Division of Oncology
Washington University School of Medicine
St. Louis, Missouri

Nicholas C. Spies, MD
Chief Resident, Clinical Pathology
Department of Pathology and Immunology
Washington University School of Medicine
St. Louis, Missouri

Stefan P. Tarnawsky, MD, PhD
Fellow
Divisions of Hematology and Oncology
Washington University School of Medicine
St. Louis, Missouri

Suzanne R. Thibodeaux, MD, PhD
Associate Professor, Pathology and Immunology
Department of Pathology and Immunology
Washington University School of Medicine
St. Louis, Missouri

Nikolaos A. Trikalinos, MD
Associate Professor of Medicine
Washington University School of Medicine
St. Louis, Missouri

Saiama N. Waqar, MD
Professor of Medicine
Division of Medical Oncology
Washington University School of Medicine
St. Louis, Missouri

Jeffrey P. Ward, MD, PhD
Assistant Professor of Medicine
Division of Medical Oncology
Washington University School of Medicine
St. Louis, Missouri

Mia C. Weiss, MD
Assistant Professor of Medicine
Washington University School of Medicine
St. Louis, Missouri

Joanna C. Yang, MD, MPH
Associate Professor of Radiation Oncology
Department of Radiation Oncology
Washington University School of Medicine
St. Louis, Missouri

Amy W. Zhou, MD
Associate Professor of Medicine
Division of Hematology
Washington University School of Medicine,
St. Louis, Missouri

Alice Zhou, MD, PhD
Assistant Professor
Department of Medicine
Washington University School of Medicine
St. Louis, Missouri

Imran Zoberi, MD
Professor of Radiation Oncology
Department of Radiation Oncology
Washington University School of Medicine
St. Louis, Missouri

Department Chair's Note

I t is a pleasure to present the new of edition of the *Hematology and Oncology Subspecialty Consult*, which is part of The *Washington Manual® Subspecialty Consult* series. This pocket-size book focused on hematology and oncology continues to be an excellent medical reference for students, residents, interns, and other practitioners who need access to practical clinical subspecialty information to diagnose and treat patients with bleeding and clotting problems, hematology disorders, and malignancies. Medical knowledge continues to increase at an astounding rate, which creates a challenge for physicians to keep with up the biomedical discoveries, genetic and genomic information, and novel therapeutics that can positively impact patients with hematology disorders and cancer. *The Hematology and Oncology Subspecialty Consult* addresses this challenge by concisely and practically providing current scientific information for clinicians to aid them in the diagnosis, investigation, and treatment of hematologic disorders, hematologic malignancies, and solid tumors.

I want to personally thank the authors, who include house officers, fellows, and attendings at Washington University School of Medicine and Barnes-Jewish Hospital. Their commitment to patient care and education is unsurpassed, and their efforts and skill in compiling this subspecialty manual are evident in the quality of the final product. In particular, I would like to acknowledge our editors, Drs. Brian A. Van Tine and Meagan A. Jacoby, who have worked tirelessly to produce another outstanding edition of this manual. The *Hematology and Oncology Subspecialty Consult* will provide practical knowledge that can be directly applied at the bedside and in outpatient settings to improve patient care.

Sincerely,

Victoria Fraser, MD
Adolphus Busch Professor and Chairman
Department of Medicine
Washington University School of Medicine
St. Louis, Missouri

Preface

We are pleased to present the fifth edition of *The Washington Manual® Hematology and Oncology Subspecialty Consult*. Since the fourth edition was published in 2016, the fields of medical oncology and hematology has rapidly evolved with many new classes of agents including CART cell therapies and Antibody Drug Conjugates (ADCs). This had led to the approval of numerous anticancer drugs and the discovery of new biomarkers and therapeutic targets. Nonetheless, in the midst of rapidly evolving treatment paradigms, a firm grounding in the fundamentals of diagnosing and caring for patients with hematologic and oncologic disorders remains critical for those training and working in these fields.

This edition has been updated to include new standards in the treatment of malignancies and hematologic disorders, mechanisms of action of new therapeutic agents, and the current use of molecular prognostic factors. The information in each chapter is presented in a consistent format, with important references cited. Our goal is to provide a concise, practical reference for fellows, residents, and medical students rotating on hematology and oncology subspecialty services. The authors are hematology–oncology fellows or the subspecialty faculty, the physicians who have recent experience with the issues and questions that arise in these subspecialties. Primary care practitioners and other health care professionals also will find this manual useful as a quick reference source in hematology and oncology.

As the practice of hematology and oncology continues to evolve, changes in dosing and indications for chemotherapy, cellular therapies, and targeted therapies will occur, and staging systems will be modified. We recommend a handbook of chemotherapy regimens and an oncology staging manual to complement the information in this book. And of course, clinical judgment is imperative when applying the principles presented here to the care of individual patients.

We appreciate the effort and expertise of everyone who contributed to this edition of the *Hematology and Oncology Subspecialty Consult*. In particular, we would like to thank the authors for their enthusiastic efforts to distill volumes of medical advances into a concise, usable format. We also recognize the faculty in the divisions of hematology, oncology, bone marrow transplantation, radiation oncology, pathology, and gynecologic oncology at Washington University for their mentorship and commitment to education.

—B.V.T. and M.J.

Contents

PART I. HEMATOLOGY

PART II. ONCOLOGY

Hematology

Introduction and Approach to Hematology

Christine Auberle

Approach to the Hematology Patient

GENERAL PRINCIPLES

Definition

Hematology is a heterogeneous subspecialty that includes the diagnosis and treatment of thrombotic disease, bleeding disorders, benign quantitative and qualitative cellular disorders which may be inherited or acquired, as well as various malignant conditions. The clinical hematologist utilizes the patient's history, physical examination, labs, peripheral smear, and bone marrow biopsy to make the correct diagnosis and to make accurate recommendations. This chapter introduces the basic tools and approach available to the hematologist, while the workup and treatment of specific hematologic diseases will be detailed in the following chapters.

DIAGNOSIS

Clinical Presentation

History

The medical history is the first step in hematology diagnostic assessment. Table 1-1 offers some general questions for evaluating hematologic disorders.

Physical Examination

The physical examination is also an important part of the diagnostic process. Along with the history, it can suggest a diagnosis, guide laboratory testing, and aid in the differential diagnosis. Table 1-2 offers some general physical examination findings that are useful in the hematology patient.

Diagnostic Testing

Laboratories

The clinician should be comfortable using the complete blood count (CBC) and peripheral smear to evaluate patients for possible hematologic disorders. Patients may be referred to a hematologist based on a laboratory abnormality that is drawn for a reason other than the diagnosis of a primary hematologic disorder. There are certain limiting values in hematology that can help exclude or confirm the need for further testing or signal possible serious physiologic consequences (Table 1-3).

- **The peripheral smear.** The visual study of peripheral blood is often necessary to diagnose hematologic and nonhematologic diseases. In some cases, automated hematology analyzers are able to provide a large number of data regarding all the blood cells but will not be able to detect subtle anomalies critical in the diagnosis; for example, the finding of schistocytes in thrombotic thrombocytopenic purpura.

  Slides for a peripheral smear are typically prepared either by automated methods or by qualified technicians in a specialized laboratory. This step is critical since poorly processed

TABLE 1-1   HISTORY OF THE HEMATOLOGY PATIENT

Pertinent Medical History	Hematologic Differential Diagnosis
History of present illness	
Recent infections	
Fever, chills, and rigors	Leukemias, lymphomas, and multiple myeloma
Antibiotic use	Hemolysis
Bleeding	
Hemorrhage, epistaxis, bleeding gums, petechiae, ecchymosis, and menorrhagia	Thrombocytopenia, leukemias, and coagulation disorder
Hemarthrosis	Clotting factor deficiency
Skin coloration	
Pallor	Anemia
Jaundice	Hemolysis
Dyspnea, chest pain, and orthostasis	Anemia
Pica	Iron deficiency
Abdominal fullness, early satiety	Splenomegaly
Alcoholism, poor nutrition, and vegetarianism	Megaloblastic anemia
Headache, neurologic deficits	Leukostasis, thrombocytopenia, thrombosis, and Waldenström macroglobulinemia
Pruritus	Polycythemia, Hodgkin lymphoma
Past medical history	
Prior malignancies, chemotherapy	Secondary malignancies (leukemia), myelodysplasia
HIV risk factors	Anemia, thrombocytopenia
Previous hepatitis	Anemia, cryoglobulinemia
Pregnancy	Anemia, HELLP syndrome
Venous thrombosis	Thrombophilia
Family history	
Bleeding disorders	Hemophilias, von Willebrand disease
Anemia (African American, Mediterranean, and Asian)	Hemoglobinopathies

HELLP, hemolysis, elevated liver enzymes, and low platelet count.

samples can lead to incorrect diagnoses. Smears may be prepared on glass slides or coverslips. Ideally, **blood smears should be prepared from uncoagulated blood** and from a sample collected from a finger stick. In practice, most slides are prepared from blood samples containing anticoagulants and are thus prone to the introduction of morphologic artifacts. Blood smears are normally stained using Wright or May–Grünwald–Giemsa stain.

○ **Examination of the peripheral smear.** Examination of the smear should proceed systematically and begin under low power to identify a portion of the slide with optimal cellular distribution and staining, which normally corresponds to the thinner edge of the sample. As a general rule, the **analysis starts with RBCs, continues with leukocytes, and finishes with platelets**. Under **low power** (×10–×20), it is possible to

TABLE 1-2	PHYSICAL EXAMINATION IN THE HEMATOLOGY PATIENT
Pertinent Examination Findings	**Hematologic Differential Diagnosis**
HEENT	
Conjunctival or mucosal pallor	Anemia
Jaundice	Hemolysis, hyperbilirubinemia
Conjunctival or mucosal petechiae	Thrombocytopenia
Glossitis	Iron deficiency, vitamin B12 deficiency
Lymphadenopathy	Lymphoma
Skin/nails	
Pallor	Anemia
Jaundice	Hyperbilirubinemia
Bronze appearance	Hemochromatosis
Spoon nails (koilonychia)	Iron deficiency
Ecchymosis, petechiae	Thrombocytopenia
Erythematous, indurated plaques	Mycosis fungoides
Cardiovascular	
Tachycardia, S4	Severe anemia with high-output cardiac failure
Abdominal	
Splenomegaly	Hairy cell or other leukemias, polycythemia, and lymphomas
Neurologic	
Loss of vibratory sense and proprioception (dorsal and lateral columns)	Megaloblastic anemia
Musculoskeletal	
Bone pain/tenderness	Multiple myeloma

HEENT, head, ears, eyes, nose, and throat.

analyze general characteristics of RBCs to discover, for example, the presence of rouleaux associated with multiple myeloma, estimate the WBC and platelet counts, and determine the presence of abnormal populations of cells, such as blasts, by scanning over the entire smear. Under **high power** ($\times 100$), each of the cell lineages is examined for abnormalities in number or morphology.

○ **Red blood cells.** Quantitative analysis of RBCs is difficult on a peripheral smear. Automated analyzers are used to calculate:

MCHC, the mean corpuscular Hgb concentration, expressed as grams per deciliter;

MCH, the mean corpuscular Hgb, expressed as picograms; and

MCV, the mean corpuscular volume, expressed as femtoliters (10^{-15} L).

Qualitative analysis of RBCs should demonstrate uniform round cells with smooth membranes and a pale central area with a round rim of red Hgb. Variations in size are called anisocytosis, and variations in shape are called poikilocytosis. The following abnormalities may be observed:

■ **Erythrocyte size and shape:**

□ **Hypochromia** corresponds to a very thin rim of Hgb and a larger central pale area. These red cells are often microcytic and are seen in iron deficiency, thalassemias, and sideroblastic anemia.

TABLE 1-3	DECISION LIMITING VALUES FOR COMMON HEMATOLOGIC TESTS	

Diagnostic Test	Limiting Value	Comment
Hgb	<5 g/dL	Transfusion indicated, even in the absence of symptoms
	<10 g/dL	Anemia workup indicated
Hct	>70%	Urgent phlebotomy indicated
Platelet count	<10,000/μL	Risk of spontaneous bleeding
	<50,000/μL	Risk of bleeding increased with surgery/trauma
	>500,000–1,000,000/μL	Risk of thrombosis
	>2,000,000/μL	Risk of bleeding
Neutrophil count	<500/μL	Greatest risk of infection
Blast count (acute leukemia)	>100,000/μL	Risk of leukostasis—urgent treatment indicated
Prothrombin time	<1.5 × control	No increased bleeding risk
	>2.5 × control	Risk of spontaneous bleeding
Partial prothrombin time	<1.5 × control	No increased bleeding risk
	>2.5 × control (>90 s)	Risk of spontaneous bleeding
Bleeding time	>20 min	Possible risk of spontaneous bleeding
Antithrombin	<50% normal level	Risk of spontaneous thrombosis

□ **Polychromasia** (blue hue of cytoplasm) is due to the presence of RNA and ribosomes in reticulocytes.

□ **Microcytosis** (<6 μm): Differential diagnosis includes iron-deficiency anemia, anemia of chronic disease/anemia of inflammation, thalassemias, and sideroblastic anemia. These cells are usually hypochromic and have prominent central pallor.

□ **Macrocytosis** (>9 μm in diameter): Differential diagnosis includes liver disease, alcoholism, aplastic anemia, and myelodysplasia. Megaloblastic anemias (B_{12} and folate deficiencies) have macro-ovalocytes (large oval cells). *Reticulocytes* are large immature red cells with polychromatophilia.

□ **Schistocytes** (fragmented cells) are caused by mechanical disruption of cells in the microvasculature. Differential diagnosis includes thrombotic thrombocytopenic purpura/hemolytic–uremic syndrome, disseminated intravascular coagulation, hemolysis, elevated liver enzymes, and low platelet count (HELLP) syndrome, mechanical fragmentation by malfunctioning cardiac valves or cardiac assist devices, and malignant hypertension.

□ **Acanthocytes (Spur cells)** are spiculated cells with irregular projections of varying length seen in liver disease.

□ **Echinocyte (Burr cells)** appear as cells with short, evenly spaced cytoplasmic projections and may be an artifact of slide preparation or found in renal failure and uremia.

□ **Bite cells** (cells with a smooth semicircle extracted) are due to spleen phagocytes that have removed Heinz bodies consisting of denatured Hgb. They are found in hemolytic anemia due to glucose-6-phosphate dehydrogenase deficiency.

□ **Spherocytes** (round, dense cells with absent central pallor) are seen in immune hemolytic anemia and hereditary spherocytosis.

□ **Sickle cells** (sickle-shaped cells) are due to polymerization of Hgb S. They are found in sickle cell disease but not in sickle cell trait.

□ **Target cells** (cells with extra Hgb in the center surrounded by a rim of pallor—bull's-eye appearance) are due to an increase in the ratio of cell membrane surface area to Hgb volume within the cell. They have a central spot of Hgb surrounded by a ring of pallor from the redundancy in cell membrane. They are found in liver disease, postsplenectomy, hemoglobinopathies, and thalassemia.

□ **Teardrop cells/dacryocytes** (teardrop-shaped cells) are found in myelofibrosis and myelophthisic states of marrow infiltration.

□ **Ovalocytes** (elliptical cells) are due to the abnormal membrane cytoskeleton found in hereditary elliptocytosis.

□ **Leukoerythroblastic smear** (teardrop cells, nucleated red cells, and immature white cells) is found in marrow infiltration or fibrosis (myelophthisic conditions).

■ **Erythrocyte inclusions:**

□ **Howell–Jolly bodies** (small, single, and purple cytoplasmic inclusions) represent nuclear remnant DNA and are found after splenectomy or with functional asplenism.

□ **Basophilic stippling** (dark-purple inclusions, usually multiple) arises from precipitated RNA found in lead poisoning and thalassemia.

□ **Pappenheimer bodies** consist of iron-containing granules that appear in clusters on the periphery found in sideroblastic anemias, thalassemia, and postsplenectomy.

□ **Nucleated red cells** are not normally found in peripheral blood. They appear in hypoxemia and myelofibrosis or other myelophthisic conditions, as well as with severe hemolysis.

□ **Heinz bodies** (inclusions seen only on staining with crystal violet) represent denatured Hgb and are found in glucose-6-phosphate dehydrogenase deficiency after oxidative stress.

□ **Parasites**, including malaria and babesiosis, may be seen within red cells.

■ **Erythrocyte distribution:**

□ **Rouleaux** (red cell aggregates resembling a stack of coins) is due to the loss of normal, repelling electrostatic charge, due to coating with abnormal paraprotein, such as in multiple myeloma.

□ **Agglutination** results from antibody-mediated clumping and can be temperature dependent such as in cold-agglutinin disease.

□ **Erythrophagocytosis** occurs when macrophages or neutrophils ingest red cells and is rarely seen in peripheral blood.

○ **White blood cells.** WBCs normally seen on the peripheral smear include mature granulocytes (neutrophils, eosinophils, and basophils), lymphocytes and monocytes. Under normal conditions, immature myeloid and lymphoid cells are not seen, and their presence is related to conditions such as infections and hematologic malignancies.

■ **Neutrophils** comprise 55–60% of total WBCs (1.8–6.6 × 10^9/L). They have nuclei containing three or four lobes and granular cytoplasm. The normal size is 10–15 μm. The cytoplasmic granules correspond to enzymes that are used during the acute phase of inflammation. Increased prominence of cytoplasmic granules is indicative of systemic infection or therapy with growth factors and is known as *toxic granulation*. Neutrophil development progresses through the following forms: myeloblast, promyelocyte, myelocyte, metamyelocyte, band, and then mature neutrophil. Only mature neutrophils and bands are normally found in peripheral blood. Metamyelocytes and myelocytes may be found in pregnancy, infections, and leukemoid reactions. The presence of less mature forms in the peripheral blood is indicative of hematologic malignancy or myelophthisis.

■ **Lymphocytes** comprise 25–35% of total WBCs (1.2–3.3 × 10^9/L). They contain a dark, clumped nucleus and a scant rim of blue cytoplasm. The differentiation of T and B cells using light microscopy is very difficult. The normal size is 7–18 μm.

Atypical (or reactive) lymphocytes, as seen in viral infections, contain more extensive, malleable cytoplasm that may encompass surrounding red cells.

- **Eosinophils** comprise 0.5–4% of total WBCs (0–0.5 × 10^9/L). These are large cells containing prominent red/orange granules and a bilobed nucleus. The normal size is 10–15 μm. Increased numbers can be found in parasitic infections, allergic disorders, neoplastic disorders, connective tissue diseases, and drug reactions.

- **Monocytes** comprise 4–8% of total WBCs (0.2–1.2 × 10^9/L). These larger cells have an eccentric U-shaped nucleus. They contain blue cytoplasm and are the precursors of the mononuclear phagocyte system (macrophages, osteoclasts, alveolar macrophages, Kupffer cells, and microglia). The usual size is 12–20 μm.

- **Basophils** comprise 0.01–0.3% of total WBCs (0–0.2 × 10^9/L). Their cytoplasm contains large dark-blue granules and a bilobed nucleus. They are involved in inflammatory reactions, and increased numbers are also seen in chronic myeloid leukemia. As for eosinophils, the normal size is 10–15 μm.

- **WBC abnormalities** on peripheral smear:
  - **Pelger–Huët anomaly** (neutrophils have a bilobed nucleus connected by a thin strand and decreased granulation) is seen as an autosomal dominant inherited condition. Pseudo-Pelger–Huët cells can be seen in myelodysplastic neoplasms (MDS).
  - **Hypersegmented neutrophils** (more than four nuclear lobes) are found in megaloblastic anemias (vitamin B$_{12}$ and folate deficiencies).
  - **Blast cells** (myeloblasts or lymphoblasts [large cells with large nuclei and prominent nucleoli]) are seen in acute leukemia.
  - **Auer rods** (rodlike granules in blast cytoplasm) are pathognomonic for myeloblasts, and raise concern for acute myeloid leukemia, especially acute promyelocytic leukemia (M3), or MDS with increased blasts.
  - **Dohle bodies** are pale blue areas in neutrophil cytoplasm seen in infection and pregnancy.
  - **Hairy cells** (lymphoid cells with ragged cytoplasm) are seen in hairy cell leukemia.
  - **Sézary cells** (atypical lymphoid cells with cerebriform nuclei) are seen in cutaneous T-cell lymphoma.

○ **Platelets.** Platelets appear as small (1–2 μm in diameter), purplish cytoplasmic fragments without a nucleus, containing red/blue granules. Derived from bone marrow giant cells called megakaryocytes, they are involved in the cellular mechanisms of primary hemostasis leading to the formation of blood clots. Normal counts are 150,000–400,000/μL of peripheral blood. The number of platelets per high-power field multiplied by 20,000 usually estimates the platelet count per microliter. Alternatively, one should find one platelet for every 10–20 red cells.

- **Pseudothrombocytopenia** represents clumping of platelets in blood samples collected in EDTA, resulting in spuriously low platelet counts. This phenomenon can be avoided by using citrate to anticoagulate blood samples sent for blood counts.

Diagnostic Procedures

Bone marrow evaluation. For many hematologic diseases that affect the bone marrow, evaluation of the peripheral blood smear does not provide sufficient information, and a direct examination of the bone marrow is required to establish the diagnosis.

- **Indications and contraindications.** The most common indications for bone marrow evaluation are workup of bone marrow malignancies; staging of marrow involvement by metastatic tumors; assessment of infectious diseases that may involve the bone marrow (i.e., HIV, tuberculosis); determination of marrow damage in patients exposed to radiation, drugs, and chemicals; and workup of metabolic storage diseases. There are a few absolute contraindications for the procedure, including infection, previous radiation therapy at the site of biopsy, and poor patient cooperation. Thrombocytopenia is not a contraindication to bone marrow biopsy, although it may be associated with more procedure-related bleeding. Patients who have a coagulopathy require factor replacement or withholding of anticoagulation to minimize bleeding complications.

- **Technique.** In adults, the most common place to do the procedure is the posterior superior iliac crest, as it allows collection of both aspirate and biopsy specimens and is associated with minimal morbidity or complications. Another potential biopsy site is the anterior iliac crest. For other biopsy sites in adults, or open bone biopsies, surgical consultation is recommended. Usually, a *Jamshidi* bone marrow aspiration and biopsy needle is used. Additional aspirate is often obtained for studies such as flow cytometry, cytogenetics, next-generation sequencing, and cultures. In some instances, marrow cannot be aspirated and only a biopsy is obtained (a "dry tap"). This can be due to the technique, or may signal myelofibrosis or previous local radiotherapy. In such cases, touch preparations of the biopsy can be made to allow for a cytologic examination. The biopsy specimen is embedded in a buffered formaldehyde-based fixation for further processing.
- **Complications.** Bleeding at the site of puncture is the most common complication. It is usually well controlled with compression, but some thrombocytopenic patients will require platelet transfusions. Other uncommon complications are infections, tumor seeding in the needle track, and needle breakage.
- **Bone marrow examination**
  ○ The examination of the bone marrow aspirate begins under **low power** to obtain an impression of overall cellularity, an initial scan for any abnormal populations of cells or clumps of cells, and an evaluation of the presence or absence of bone marrow spicules. Megakaryocytes are normally seen under low power as large multinucleated cells. The overall cellularity of the marrow is difficult to estimate from the aspirate because of contamination with peripheral blood.
  ○ The **myeloid-to-erythroid (M:E) ratio** is also determined under low power and is normally 3:1–4:1. The ratio is increased in chronic myeloid leukemia due to an increase in granulocyte precursors and is increased in pure red cell aplasia due to a decrease in red cell precursors. The ratio is decreased in hemolytic disorders in which increased erythroid precursors are present or in agranulocytic conditions secondary to chemotherapeutic agents or other drugs.
  ○ Under **high power**, the aspirate should contain a variety of cells representative of various stages of myeloid and erythroid maturation. Myeloid cells progress from myeloblasts to promyelocytes, myelocytes, metamyelocytes, band forms, and then mature neutrophils. As these cells mature, their nuclear chromatin condenses, with a resultant decrease in the nuclear-to-cytoplasmic ratio. Their cytoplasm gradually develops granules seen in mature neutrophils.
  ○ **Erythroid precursors** progress from proerythroblasts through varying stages of normoblasts known as *basophilic, chromatophilic,* and *orthochromic.* The nucleus gradually condenses, and the cytoplasm gradually takes on the pinkish hue of Hgb found in mature red cells.
  ○ **Bone marrow core biopsies** are fixed in a buffered formaldehyde-based solution and then embedded in paraffin or plastic. Biopsies are used to assess the cellularity of the bone marrow and the presence of neoplasias, infections, or fibrosis. Cellularity is estimated by observing the ratio of hematopoietic cells to fat cells. Cellularity is usually 40–60% in adults, typically declines with advancing age and can be estimated as follows: Cellularity (%) = 100 – age (years).
- **Pancytopenia** occurs when all three cell lines, WBCs, RBCs, and platelets are low. The initial workup should include a thorough history and physical and CBC, comprehensive metabolic panel, peripheral smear, iron studies, B_{12} level, folate level, reticulocyte count, prothrombin time, partial thromboplastin time, lactate dehydrogenase, haptoglobin, hepatitis serologies and HIV. Additional workup can include copper, zinc, serum protein

electrophoresis, antinuclear antibody test, erythrocyte sedimentation rate, c-reactive protein, Coomb's test, bone marrow biopsy, and an ultrasound of the spleen. Etiologies can include but are not limited to:

- Poor production by the bone marrow including nutritional deficiencies, bone marrow infiltration from malignancy, myelofibrosis, infection, medications, and congenital bone marrow failure disorders.
- Increased destruction or consumption of cells through DIC, paroxysmal nocturnal hemoglobinuria, hemophagocytic lymphohistiocytosis, autoimmune disorders, or hypersplenism from conditions such as congestive heart disease, storage diseases, and cirrhosis.

- **Cytosis** occurs when one or more cell lines are increased above the upper limit of normal. While each of the cell lines will be addressed in their respective chapters, common etiologies for elevation in each include:
  - **Erythrocytosis** can result from relative polycythemia from decreased plasma volume, polycythemia vera, secondary causes such as obstructive sleep apnea, smoking, androgens, anabolic steroids, carbon monoxide poisoning, and inherited conditions such as familial polycthemia, Chuvash polycythemia, or congenital methemoglobinemias.
  - **Leukocytosis** depends largely on the subset of cells increased (e.g., neutrophils, lymphocytes, eosinophils). The most common etiologies include infections, malignancy, allergic reactions, or inflammation.
  - **Thrombocytosis** may due to a clonal process as in a myeloid neoplasm or reactive process such as in iron deficiency, infection, inflammation, drug-induced or from splenectomy.

White Blood Cell Disorders: Leukopenia and Leukocytosis

2

Nicole C. Foley

Leukopenia

GENERAL PRINCIPLES

- The normal white blood cell (WBC) count varies, but in general it ranges from 4×10^9 to 11×10^9 cells/L (Table 2-1). It is composed of those cells committed to the leukocyte lineage: granulocytes (neutrophils, eosinophils, basophils), monocytes, and lymphocytes. Neutrophils make up about 60% of the peripheral blood nucleated cells. A person's age, sex, and ethnic background should be taken into consideration when determining normal ranges.
- **Leukopenia is defined as a WBC count $<3.8 \times 10^9$ cells/L.** This lower limit of normal varies with age and race. The absolute neutrophil count (ANC) is highest at birth and slowly declines; older adults may experience a decline in lymphocyte count with normal aging. While of no pathologic significance, neutrophil counts are lower in persons of African ancestry and in some Middle Eastern populations as compared to persons of European decent.[1] Additionally, 5% of the normal population will fall outside of the normal reference range. Leukopenias can be divided according to clinically relevant cell lineages: neutrophils and lymphocytes. While monocytopenia (absolute monocyte count $<0.2 \times 10^9$/L) occurs rarely outside of general pancytopenia, it can be a notable feature of aplastic anemia and hairy cell leukemia in which it contributes a predisposition to infection.

Neutropenia

GENERAL PRINCIPLES

Definition

The ANC is obtained by taking the percentage of neutrophils identified on a 100-cell differential or by the Coulter counter and multiplying by the total WBC count. Neutropenia

TABLE 2-1	AVERAGE ADULT WBC COUNT	
Cell	Percentage	Absolute Count ($\times 10^9$/L)
Leukocytes		3.8–9.9
Neutrophils	40–75	1.7–6.5
Monocytes	4–13	0.2–0.8
Eosinophils	0–6	0–0.5
Basophils	0–3	0–0.1
Lymphocytes	20–54	0.8–3.3

Data from Barnes-Jewish Hospital Laboratory References, Barnes-Jewish Hospital, St. Louis, MO.

is classified as **mild** (ANC 1–1.5 × 10^9/L), **moderate** (ANC 0.5–1 × 10^9/L), or **severe** (ANC <0.5 × 10^9/L). **Agranulocytosis** is the total absence of granulocytes.

Epidemiology

In the United States, low neutrophil counts are five times more prevalent in African Americans than non-Hispanic Whites or American Mexicans.[2] This discrepancy is primarily accounted for by normal variants in ANC associated with genetic polymorphisms and is discussed in more detail below.

Etiology

Causes of neutropenia are reported in Table 2-2. Severe neutropenia can be congenital or acquired. Congenital causes can be suggested by family history or associated syndromic defects and are typically diagnosed in childhood.[3] Most cases of neutropenia are acquired and related to decreased granulocyte production and, less often, increased destruction. Pseudo-neutropenia may be found when analyzing blood several hours old or in the presence of paraproteinemia and certain anticoagulants that can cause clumping. Some individuals (most commonly persons of African descent, Sephardic Jews, West Indians, Yemenites, Greeks, and Arabs) have an ANC <1.5 × 10^9/L with no history of recurrent or severe infections, other cytopenias or associated illnesses. One cause for this inherited finding

TABLE 2-2	CAUSE OF NEUTROPENIA
Primary hematologic disorders	*Congenital/Inherited* Reticular dysgenesis Severe congenital neutropenia (Kostmann syndrome) Cyclic neutropenia Dyskeratosis congenita Shwachman–Diamond syndrome Chédiak–Higashi syndrome Glycogen storage disease, Type Ib Hermansky–Pudlak syndrome, Type II *Acquired* Acute and chronic leukemias Aplastic anemia and pure white cell aplasia Chronic idiopathic neutropenia Nutritional: copper, vitamin B_{12}, and/or folate deficiency; alcoholism
Secondary disorders	Isoimmune neutropenia of the neonate (transplacental IgG specific for paternal neutrophil antigens) Autoimmune neutropenia Neutropenia with autoimmune diseases Systemic lupus erythematosus Rheumatoid arthritis Felty syndrome Sjögren syndrome Neutropenia with clonal large granular lymphocytosis Marrow infiltrative process Drug induced (Table 2-3) Neutropenia with infectious diseases Viral: EBV, parvovirus, and HIV Hypersplenism

is designated "Duffy-null associated neutrophil count (DANC)" due to its association with the Duffy null [Fy(a-b-)] red blood cell (RBC) phenotype which is protective against malaria.[4] DANC was formerly called "benign ethnic neutropenia," however this term has been abandoned as it erroneously implied a pathologic condition or risk for infection.

Pathophysiology

Neutropenia results from decreased production, ineffective granulopoiesis, increased margination to peripheral pools, or increased peripheral destruction. Acquired neutropenias are usually a result of infection, toxins/drugs, or immune disorders. As with all neutropenias, the propensity to infection from neutropenia depends on the adequacy of the bone marrow reserve pool. Viral, parasitic, or bacterial infections may cause transient neutropenia, with the specific time to onset and resolution dependent on the pathogen involved. The underlying mechanism involves increased margination, sequestration, and destruction by circulating antibodies. Drug and toxin exposure usually follows a temporal course, with neutropenia developing after continued drug exposure of days to months. The mechanism of drug-induced neutropenia can be antibody-mediated or occur via direct toxic effects on the marrow. Drugs at higher risk of causing neutropenia are highlighted in Table 2-3. Primary immune disorders mediate neutropenia through antibody-mediated neutrophil destruction.

DIAGNOSIS

Clinical Presentation

- Neutropenia is often incidentally discovered on a complete blood count (CBC) but patients may present with fever or other signs of infection. Individuals with ANC >1 × 10^9/L are at low risk of infection. Those with ANC 0.5–1 × 10^9/L have only a slight increased risk of infection unless other contributing factors are present. With ANC <0.5 × 10^9/L, individuals are at significantly higher risk of infection which also depends on the cause and duration of neutropenia. Severe neutropenia predisposes patients to infections by organisms normally found on the skin, in the nasopharynx, and as part of the intestinal flora. **Signs of infection**, such as purulence, may be less evident, given the low neutrophil count.
- The initial evaluation should include a complete history and physical examination. The **history** should inquire about systemic symptoms of infection, recent exposures, new medications, and personal and family history of neutropenia. Abnormal vital signs may indicate sepsis or septic shock and are critical to triage the patient appropriately. **Physical examination** should evaluate for subtle clues of infection and investigate signs that would suggest the cause of neutropenia—macroglossia (vitamin deficiency), lymphadenopathy (malignancy, infection), skin and joint changes (rheumatologic disorder), and splenomegaly (sequestration, Felty syndrome).

Diagnostic Testing

Initial laboratory evaluation starts with a **CBC** with complete differential and review of the peripheral blood smear. In cases of asymptomatic mild neutropenia, serial CBC examination to rule out cyclic neutropenia may be considered. Additional studies should be guided by the history and physical examination, in conjunction with any concurrent abnormalities identified on the CBC with differential. Further testing for nutritional deficiencies should include vitamin B_{12}, folate, and copper. For patients suspected of an autoimmune disorder, antinuclear antibody and rheumatoid factor titers can be sent to evaluate for immune-mediated neutropenia. Antineutrophil antibodies can be detected in most cases of autoimmune neutropenia (AIN), however the false negative is high unless several methods are used in conjunction.[5,6] HIV, hepatitis, and Epstein–Barr virus (EBV) serologies start the initial infectious workup. If anemia or thrombocytopenia occurs in combination with neutropenia, direct examination of the bone marrow via bone marrow biopsy is usually

TABLE 2-3   DRUGS CAUSING NEUTROPENIA

Drug Class	Common Examples
Analgesics and anti-inflammatory agents	Indomethacin, para-aminophenol derivatives, e.g., acetaminophen Pyrazolone derivatives, e.g., phenylbutazone
Antibiotics	Cephalosporins Chloramphenicol Penicillins Sulfonamides Trimethoprim-sulfamethoxazole Vancomycin
Anticonvulsants	Phenytonin Carbamazepine
Antidepressants	Amitriptyline Imipramine
Antihistamines, H_2-blockers	Cimetidine Ranitidine
Antimalarials	Dapsone Quinine Chloroquine
Antithyroid drugs	Carbimazole Methimazole Propylthiouracil
Cardiovascular drugs	Captopril Hydralazine Propranolol
Diuretics	Hydrochlorothiazide Acetazolamide
Hypnotics and sedatives	Chlordiazepoxide Benzodiazepines
Atypical antipsychotics	Chlorpromazine Olanzapine Clozapine
Other drugs	Allopurinol Colchicine Penicillamine Ticlopidine

warranted, unless a cause is obvious. Bone marrow examination with cytogenetic and molecular testing is most useful for ruling out leukemia and myelodysplastic syndromes, as well as assessing the severity of the marrow defect.

TREATMENT

- Treatment is guided by the underlying etiology and severity of neutropenia. The major complication associated with neutropenia is infection. Treatment can range from close

observation in patients with benign neutropenia to antibiotics and growth factor support in patients with neutropenic fevers.
- **Supportive care** with broad-spectrum antibiotics and IV fluids for febrile or septic patients is essential while an investigation into the cause of neutropenia is underway. Common sites of infection include mucous membranes, skin, perirectal and genital areas, bloodstream, and lungs. Most commonly, endogenous bacterial flora becomes pathogenic (*Staphylococcus* from skin or gram-negative organisms from the gut). Antibiotics should be continued until the ANC is >500/L for 2 days and the fever subsides. If fever and neutropenia persist, empiric antifungal coverage should be considered.
- **Growth factors,** such as granulocyte colony-stimulating factor (G-CSF), can be used to speed count recovery in drug-induced neutropenia, including in patients receiving myelosuppressive chemotherapy with >20% risk of neutropenic fever. Patients with severe chronic neutropenia and other inherited, and sometimes acquired, bone marrow failure syndromes may also benefit from G-CSF administration.
- Cases caused by drug toxicity should improve with removal of the drug within 1–3 weeks. Infectious etiologies resolve with treatment of the infection or shortly after a viral infection has subsided. Autoimmune forms of neutropenia may warrant treatment with immunosuppressive agents.

Lymphocytopenia

GENERAL PRINCIPLES

Definition

Lymphocytopenia is defined as an **absolute lymphocyte count $<1.0 \times 10^9$/L.** The absolute lymphocyte count is comprised of approximately 60–80% T cells, 10–20% B cells, and 5–10% NK cells. Normally T cell subtypes in the peripheral blood are 60–70% CD4+ helper T cells and 30–40% cytotoxic CD8+ T cells.

Etiology

- Lymphocytopenia is most often acquired, but congenital causes should also be considered in children and young adults. Etiologies of lymphocytopenia are listed in Table 2-4. Causes of acquired lymphocytopenia can generally be categorized as infectious diseases, iatrogenic, nutritional, and systemic diseases associated with lymphocytopenia.
- The most common infectious disease associated with lymphopenia is acquired immunodeficiency syndrome (AIDS) caused by HIV. In patients with AIDS, lymphopenia is mediated by increased destruction and clearance of CD4+ T cells infected with HIV-1 or HIV-2. Several other viral illnesses are associated with transient lymphopenia during the acute phase of infection, which is thought to contribute to a disease course–related immunodeficiency that increases the risk for opportunistic infections. In patients with COVID-19, lower numbers of circulating lymphocytes have been associated with increased disease severity and worse prognosis.[7]
- Patients who appear to have low or absent CD4 cells, in the absence of significant illness, should be evaluated for OKT4 epitope deficiency. The OKT4 antigen is standardly used to detect CD4 cells by flow cytometry, therefore individuals with this phenotype have falsely low/absent CD4 cells by routine testing but do not develop infections.[8]

TREATMENT

Most causes of lymphocytopenia are acquired, and the management focuses on treating the underlying illness. As infectious etiologies are appropriately treated with antimicrobial therapy, the associated lymphocytopenia usually resolves within a couple of weeks. Zinc

TABLE 2-4 CAUSES OF LYMPHOCYTOPENIA

Congenital	Severe combined immunodeficiency Common variable immune deficiency Congenital thymic aplasia (DiGeorge syndrome) X-linked agammaglobulinemia (Bruton agammaglobulinemia) Wiskott–Aldrich syndrome Purine nucleoside phosphorylase deficiency Ataxia-telangiectasia
Acquired	Aplastic anemia Viral infection: HIV/AIDS, coronavirus (severe acute respiratory syndrome [SARS], COVID-19), hepatitis, influenza, herpes simplex virus Bacterial infection: tuberculosis, rickettsiosis, ehrlichiosis Immunosuppressive agents: antilymphocyte globulin, alemtuzumab, glucocorticoids Extracorporeal bypass circulation Chemotherapy Radiation Renal or hematopoietic stem cell transplantation Hemodialysis Major surgery
Systemic diseases	Autoimmune diseases: systemic lupus erythematosus, Sjögren syndrome, myasthenia gravis, systemic vasculitis Hodgkin lymphoma Carcinoma Sarcoidosis Heart failure Thermal injury Strenuous exercise
Nutritional	Ethanol abuse Zinc deficiency

deficiency responds to repletion of zinc and should be part of the initial screen, along with examination of the peripheral blood smear. Inherited causes predispose to recurrent and opportunistic infections. In general, prophylactic antibiotics strategies similar to those used with patients with HIV can be applied to patients with CD4 counts ≤200 cells/μL.

Leukocytosis

GENERAL PRINCIPLES

Leukocytosis is a broad term referring to an elevated WBC count in the peripheral blood. While most often caused by neutrophilia, leukocytosis can also be the result of increased monocytes, eosinophils, basophils, and/or lymphocytes. Leukocytosis commonly reflects a normal bone marrow response to inflammation or infection, or can be caused by leukemia or myeloproliferative disorders. The maturation of WBCs is influenced by G-CSFs, interleukins (ILs), tumor necrosis factor, and complement components.

Definition

Leukocytosis is defined as a WBC count >11 × 10^9 cells/L in most clinical laboratories.

Classification

The evaluation and differential diagnosis of leukocytosis should be principally guided by the WBC component specifically elevated: neutrophils, eosinophils, basophils, monocytes, or lymphocytes.

Etiology

Most cases of leukocytosis are a result of the bone marrow reacting to inflammation or infection. A **leukemoid reaction** refers to an excessive WBC elevation (>50,000/μL) that is not due to a primary bone marrow disorder such as leukemia. Predominately mature neutrophils are elevated, often accompanied by an increase in bands in the peripheral blood. Leukemoid reactions can be associated with infections (especially in patients with asplenia), as well as with the use of certain medications such as growth factors and all-trans retinoid acid (ATRA). Vigorous exercise and acute physical or emotional stress can cause leukocytosis, and usually resolves in hours once the stress is eliminated. In patients with surgical or functional asplenia/hyposplenia, chronic leukocytosis can occur related to demargination of leukocytes typically stored in the spleen, and is sometimes associated with thrombocytosis. In addition to ATRA and growth factors, medications such as glucocorticoids, catecholamines, and lithium can increase the WBC count. In patients with hemolytic anemias (sickle cell and autoimmune types) leukocytosis is related to nonspecific effects of increased erythropoiesis and inflammation. Nonhematologic malignancies can also cause a leukocytosis that is multifactorial in etiology, but can be related to a paraneoplastic process. Cigarette smoking is a common cause of mild leukocytosis that is possibly related to inflammation, although the specific mechanism is unknown. Finally, acute and chronic leukemias and myeloproliferative disorders can also present with leukocytosis.

Pathophysiology

In the bone marrow, stem cells differentiate into megakaryoblasts (precursors to megakaryocytes, which will produce platelets), erythroblasts (precursors of RBCs), myeloblasts (will differentiate into neutrophils, eosinophils, and basophils), monoblasts (precursors to monocytes), and lymphoid progenitor cells (precursors to B and T lymphocytes). All cells originating from myeloblasts, monoblasts, and lymphoblasts are considered "leukocytes." The mechanism of leukocytosis is best described from the perspective of which cell line is elevated.

DIAGNOSIS

The differential diagnosis of leukocytosis is extensive, and common causes are listed in Table 2-5. Increases in the absolute numbers of lymphocytes, eosinophils, monocytes, or basophils occur less commonly in leukocytosis than neutrophilia and help to direct the workup and management.

Neutrophilia

GENERAL PRINCIPLES

Definition

Neutrophilia refers to an increase in peripheral blood neutrophils at least two standard deviations above the mean, generally corresponding to **ANC >7.7 × 10^9/L** in adults. The neutrophil count is influenced by shifts in neutrophils among four major compartments:

TABLE 2-5 CAUSES OF LEUKOCYTOSIS

Normally responding bone marrow
  Infection
  Inflammation
  Tissue necrosis, infarction, burns
  Stress, overexertion, seizures, anxiety, anesthesia
Drugs
  Corticosteroids, lithium, β-agonists
Trauma
Splenectomy
Hemolytic anemia
Malignancy
Leukocytosis of pregnancy
Abnormal bone marrow
  Acute and chronic leukemias
  Myeloproliferative disorders

the bone marrow, the circulation, the marginated pool, and the tissues. Only about 5% of neutrophils are in circulation at any given time, with a half-life of 6–10 hours. Most neutrophils and their precursors are contained in storage pools in the bone marrow at 10–20 times their circulating numbers. About 50% of peripheral blood neutrophils are circulating and the other 50% are marginated along vessel walls and in the spleen. This pool can be rapidly increased, within hours from the bone marrow stores or within minutes from demarginating neutrophils along blood vessel walls. Neutrophils move to sites of inflammation and infection and act as phagocytes. Their trafficking depends on chemotaxins and surface molecules such as selectins to mediate rolling and integrins to mediate adhesion and transmigration of blood vessels.

Pathophysiology

The pathophysiology of **primary neutrophilia** may be related to inherited deficiencies in adhesion molecules or, in the case of myeloproliferative disorders, constitutive expression and activation of a growth-promoting receptor tyrosine kinase such as BCR/ABL or JAK2. **Secondary neutrophilia**, seen in infection and inflammation, is related to demargination from storage pools in the bone marrow and peripheral blood signaled by endotoxin and proinflammatory cytokines such as tumor necrosis factor-α, IL-6, IL-1B, IL-8, G-CSF, and granulocyte/macrophage colony–stimulating factor (GM-CSF).

DIAGNOSIS

Differential Diagnosis

- Neutrophilia can be spurious, primary (clonal), or related to secondary causes (reactive). Etiologies of neutrophilia are listed in Table 2-6. **Spurious leukocytosis** can be a result of the automated cell counter (Coulter counter) counting clumps of platelets as leukocytes and is usually associated with pseudo-thrombocytopenia. Agglutinated cryoglobulins can also be falsely counted as leukocytes when temperatures decrease below body temperature.
- **Primary causes** of neutrophilia may be inherited as germline mutations and associated with specific syndromes (i.e., leukocyte adhesion deficiency, Down syndrome). Myeloproliferative neoplasms are acquired forms of primary neutrophilia and include chronic

TABLE 2-6	CAUSES OF NEUTROPHILIA
Spurious causes	Cryoglobulinemia Platelet clumping
Primary causes	Hereditary neutrophilia Chronic idiopathic neutrophilia Chronic myeloid leukemia Myeloproliferative disorders (polycythemia vera, myelofibrosis) Leukocyte adhesion deficiency Down syndrome
Secondary causes	Infection Smoking Medications: glucocorticoids, β-agonists, lithium, granulocyte colony–stimulating factor (G-CSF)/granulocyte-macrophage CSF (GM-CSF), all-trans retinoic acid (ATRA) Nonhematologic malignancy: large cell lung cancer Stress, exercise Hemolytic anemia, sickle cell disease Leukoerythroblastic reaction: marrow invasion by tumor, fibrosis, and granulomatous reaction Asplenia

myeloid leukemia (CML), chronic neutrophilic leukemia, polycythemia vera, and essential thrombocythemia, among others.

• **Secondary causes** are the more common underlying etiology of neutrophilia. These include infection, cigarette smoking, chronic inflammation (i.e., rheumatoid arthritis, inflammatory bowel disease), medications, chronic marrow stimulation (i.e., hemolytic anemia, idiopathic thrombocytopenic purpura), asplenia, marrow invasion, and nonhematologic malignancy.

Diagnostic Testing

Initial laboratory evaluation starts with review of the **peripheral blood smear** to confirm automated counts and rule out spurious leukocytosis. The smear may suggest a secondary cause such as infection or inflammation with increased bands, vacuolization, Döhle bodies, and toxic granulations in neutrophils. A marrow-infiltrating process is suggested by a leukoerythroblastic reaction that shows a "left shift" (increased myelocytes and metamyelocytes in the marrow and bands in the peripheral blood) and nucleated RBCs. Acute leukemia is suggested by circulating blasts, which may be incorrectly counted as monocytes or neutrophils on an automated differential. If no secondary causes of neutrophilia can be identified, genetic testing by **conventional karyotyping** or **fluorescence in situ hybridization (FISH)** to evaluate for the Philadelphia chromosome or BCR::ABL1 fusion gene, respectively, can be done to evaluate for CML. A **leukocyte alkaline phosphatase (LAP) score** is of historical importance but is no longer commonly used because of inter-operator variability and the integration of cytogenetics and molecular testing into common practice. A low LAP score can be seen in CML, and a high LAP score suggests inflammation or infection.

TREATMENT

Treatment depends on the underlying etiology. Treatment of primary etiologies such as CML and myeloproliferative disorders is discussed elsewhere in this book. Resolution of secondary neutrophilia requires treatment of the underlying cause.

Eosinophilia

GENERAL PRINCIPLES

Eosinophilia is defined as an absolute eosinophil count (AEC) $\geq 0.5 \times 10^9$/L. **Hypereosinophilia** is defined as persistent eosinophilia of $\geq 1.5 \times 10^9$/L, with or without evidence of end-organ damage. **Hypereosinophilic syndromes (HES)** are defined as AEC $\geq 1.5 \times 10^9$/L, identified on two or more CBCs performed at least 1 month apart, *plus* organ dysfunction attributable to eosinophilia. Eosinophilia can be associated with numerous conditions including allergic, infectious, inflammatory and neoplastic disorders, however is most commonly due to secondary causes. Table 2-7 reviews causes of eosinophilia.

TABLE 2-7 CAUSES OF EOSINOPHILIA

Allergic
    Asthma
    Allergic rhinitis
    Drug hypersensitivity (drug reaction with eosinophilia and systemic symptoms [DRESS])
Dermatologic
    Atopic dermatitis
Infections
    Tissue invasive parasites: strongyloidiasis, schistosomiasis, hookworm
    Fungi: coccidiomycosis, histoplasmosis, allergic bronchopulmonary aspergillosis
    Viral: HIV
Immunologic disorders
    Collagen-vascular disease
    Hyper-IgE syndrome
    Systemic lupus erythematosus
Pulmonary conditions
    Idiopathic acute or chronic eosinophilic pneumonia
Malignancies
    Non-Hodgkin lymphoma
    Hodgkin lymphoma
    Acute eosinophilic leukemia
    Myeloid/Lymphoid neoplasms with eosinophilia and tyrosine kinase gene fusions
Myeloproliferative disorders
    Chronic myeloid leukemia
    Polycythemia vera
    Myelofibrosis
Adrenal insufficiency: Addison disease
Sarcoidosis

DIAGNOSIS

The initial evaluation should include a detailed history assessing for potential exposures (travel, medications, diet, occupation) and a full review of systems focusing on constitutional, cutaneous, cardiac, respiratory, gastrointestinal, and neurologic symptoms. Physical examination is required to assess for adenopathy, splenomegaly, and skin manifestations. Initial laboratory testing should include repeat CBC with differential, chemistry panel, and review of the peripheral smear. Reviewing historical CBC data may help to connect the onset and duration of eosinophilia with the presence of symptoms. Additional lab testing should be individualized, but can include stool examination for ova and parasites, cardiac troponin, serum tryptase, vitamin B_{12}, cortisol, IgE, and IL-5 levels. If a secondary cause is not identified, additional blood and/or bone marrow studies to consider include: workup for myeloid/lymphoid neoplasms with eosinophilia and tyrosine kinase gene fusions (such as *PDGFRA*, *PDGFRB*, *FGFR1* rearrangements, among others) T-cell receptor gene rearrangement by PCR, immunophenotyping, and/or myeloid gene panel by next-generation sequencing.[9] Bone marrow evaluation with immunohistochemistry for CD117, tryptase, and CD25 may be warranted if serum tryptase is elevated.

TREATMENT

The duration and severity at which eosinophilia will cause tissue damage in individual patients is not well known. Insufficient data exist to support the initiation of therapy based on a prespecified AEC threshold in the absence of end-organ damage. In most cases, a formal diagnosis as to the cause of eosinophilia is required prior to proceeding with disease-specific therapy. However, immediate treatment may be indicated in a patient presenting with signs/symptoms attributable to blood or tissue hypereosinophilia with evidence of leukostasis, potentially life-threating complications of hypereosinophilia (e.g., acute heart failure, thromboembolic events), or in the setting of extreme eosinophilia (AEC >100 × 10^9/L). When indicated, immediate treatment with high-dose corticosteroids is the preferred option to quickly reduce peripheral blood eosinophils. In patients that do not respond adequately to high-dose corticosteroids, use of cyclophosphamide, rituximab, or hydroxyurea can be considered. Alternatively, leukopheresis can also rapidly lower the eosinophil count. For patients with myeloid malignancies associated with eosinophilia, therapy is dictated by disease-specific guidelines and discussed in more detail in subsequent chapters. The multikinase inhibitor, imatinib is considered definitive first-line therapy in patients with *FIP1L1-PDGFRA*–positive disease, as well as in rare cases of alternative *PDGFRA* fusions and rearranged *PDGFRB*.[10]

Basophilia

GENERAL PRINCIPLES

Definition

Basophils are the least frequent of the three granulocytes, typically accounting for <1% of blood leukocytes. Basophilia is defined as an **absolute basophil count >0.2 × 10^9/L**. Basophils are inflammatory mediators, and their granules contain histamine, glycosaminoglycans, major basic protein, proteases, and other inflammatory and vasoactive substances. Their primary function is to activate the type 1 hypersensitivity reaction mediated through surface receptors for IgE.

Etiology

Basophilia can be associated with hypersensitivity or inflammatory reactions (i.e., allergies, asthma, ulcerative colitis, juvenile rheumatoid arthritis), endocrinopathies (i.e., hypothyroidism, diabetes mellitus, estrogen administration), infections particularly with helminths or tuberculosis, as well as with iron deficiency and exposure to ionizing radiation. However, the most common cause of basophilia is clonal myeloid disorders, including myeloproliferative neoplasms and several forms of myeloid leukemia. An increased absolute basophil count occurs in virtually all patients with CML. A slight increase in the absolute basophil count may represent an early indicator of a myeloproliferative neoplasm.

DIAGNOSIS

Review of the peripheral smear confirms basophilia, and management focuses on the underlying etiology. Peripheral blood can be sent for **BCR/ABL** and **JAK2** to evaluate for a myeloproliferative disorder. If initial testing is negative and suspicion of a myeloproliferative disorder remains high, additional testing for **CALR** and **MPL** mutations should be performed, and a bone marrow biopsy may be necessary.

Monocytosis

GENERAL PRINCIPLES

Definition

Monocytosis is defined as an **absolute monocyte count >0.8 × 10^9/L**. Monocytes are cells in transit from the marrow to the tissues where they transform into macrophages. They play a role in acute and chronic inflammatory reactions.

Etiology

Monocytosis is most commonly associated with a hematologic disorder, which can be either benign or malignant. Benign etiologies of monocytosis include postsplenectomy state, immune hemolytic anemia, idiopathic thrombocytopenic purpura, and chronic or drug-induced neutropenias. Monocytosis can also be seen with myeloid neoplasms including CML, myelodysplastic neoplasms (MDS), and myelodysplastic/myeloproliferative neoplasms (MDS/MPN) such as chronic myelomonocytic leukemia (CMML), as well as in the context of lymphoid malignancies. Other causes include inflammatory disorders (sarcoidosis, lupus), bacterial infections, alcoholic liver disease, and myocardial infarction, among others.

DIAGNOSIS

Review of the peripheral smear confirms monocytosis, and treatment is focused on the underlying etiology. After excluding secondary causes, peripheral blood can be sent for **BCR/ABL** and **JAK2** to evaluate for a myeloproliferative disorder. If initial testing is negative and suspicion of a myeloproliferative disorder remains high, additional testing for **CALR** and **MPL** mutations should be performed, as well as a bone marrow biopsy.

Lymphocytosis

GENERAL PRINCIPLES

Lymphocytosis is defined as an **absolute lymphocyte count >4.0 × 10^9/L**. Lymphocytosis can be categorized as polyclonal or monoclonal. Polyclonal, or reactive, lymphocytosis results from factors extrinsic to lymphocytes, such as infections and/or inflammation.

TABLE 2-8   CAUSES OF LYMPHOCYTOSIS

Primary lymphocytosis	Acute lymphocytic leukemia
	Chronic lymphocytic leukemia
	Prolymphocytic leukemia
	Hairy cell leukemia
	Adult T-cell leukemia
	Large granular lymphocytic leukemia
	Monoclonal B-cell lymphocytosis
Reactive lymphocytosis	Infectious mononucleosis
	Epstein–Barr virus
	Cytomegalovirus
	Herpes simplex virus (and other herpes viruses)
	Toxoplasma *gondii*
	Adenovirus
	Bordetella pertussis
	Stress
	Post-trauma
	Postsplenectomy
	Cigarette smoking
	Hypersensitivity reactions
	Drug-induced
	Serum sickness
	Autoimmune
	Lymphocytosis of large granular lymphocytes
	Rheumatoid arthritis
	Malignant thymoma
	Hyperthyroidism

Monoclonal, or primary, lymphocytosis results from the acquisition of somatic mutations resulting in the clonal expansion of lymphoid progenitors. Table 2-8 reviews causes of lymphocytosis. Cell surface markers are important in distinguishing polyclonal and monoclonal lymphocytosis.

DIAGNOSIS

A peripheral blood smear should be reviewed for evidence of reactive lymphocytes associated with infection, large granular lymphocytes associated with large granular lymphocytic leukemia, smudge cells associated with chronic lymphocytic leukemia (CLL), or blasts associated with acute leukemia. **Peripheral blood flow cytometry immunophenotyping** is useful for differentiating benign from neoplastic lymphocytic proliferations. Analysis for immunoglobulin or T-cell receptor gene rearrangements would further support a monoclonal B-cell or T-cell lymphoproliferative disorder, respectively.

TREATMENT

Management of hematologic malignancies including CLL is discussed in subsequent chapters. Resolution of infectious etiologies results in resolution of the lymphocytosis. Finally, removal of allergens such as drugs or venom results in resolution of the lymphocytosis associated with hypersensitivity reactions.

REFERENCES

1. Lim EM, Cembrowski G, Cembrowski M, Clarke G. Race-specific WBC and neutrophil count reference intervals. *Int J Lab Hematol*. 2010;32(6 Pt 2):590–597.
2. Zhou J, Zhou N, Liu Q, et al. Prevalence of neutropenia in US residents: a population based analysis of NHANES 2011–2018. *BMC Public Health*. 2023;23(1):1254.
3. Boxer LA, Newburger PE. A molecular classification of congenital neutropenia syndromes. *Pediatr Blood Cancer*. 2007;49(5):609–614.
4. Atallah-Yunes SA, Ready A, Newburger PE. Benign ethnic neutropenia. *Blood Rev*. 2019;37: S0268-960X(19)30024-4.
5. Farruggia P. Immune neutropenias of infancy and childhood. *World J Pediatr*. 2016;12(2):142–148.
6. Farruggia P, Fioredda F, Puccio G, et al. Autoimmune neutropenia of infancy: Data from the Italian neutropenia registry. *Am J Hematol*. 2015;90(12):E221–E222.
7. Liao D, Zhou F, Luo L, et al. Haematological characteristics and risk factors in the classification and prognosis evaluation of COVID-19: a retrospective cohort study. *Lancet Haematol*. 2020;7(9):e671–e678.
8. Bach MA, Phan-Dinh-Tuy F, Bach JF, et al. Unusual phenotypes of human inducer T cells as measured by OKT4 and related monoclonal antibodies. *J Immunol*. 1981;127(3):980–982.
9. Shomali W, Gotlib J. World Health Organization-defined eosinophilic disorders: 2022 update on diagnosis, risk stratification, and management. *Am J Hematol*. 2022;97(1):129–148.
10. Jovanovic JV, Score J, Waghorn K, et al. Low-dose imatinib mesylate leads to rapid induction of major molecular responses and achievement of complete molecular remission in FIP1L1-PDGFRA–positive chronic eosinophilic leukemia. *Blood*. 2007;109(11):4635–4640.

Red Blood Cell Disorders

3

Sana Saif Ur Rehman

Anemia

GENERAL PRINCIPLES

Definition

Anemia is defined as a decrease in circulating RBC mass, the usual criteria being a hemoglobin (Hgb) <12 g/dL or hematocrit (Hct) <36% for women, and an Hgb <14 g/dL or Hct <41% for men. Anemia is commonly encountered in inpatient medicine and thus a frequent reason for hematology consults. A systematic approach to anemia is best for narrowing down the diagnosis and guiding the subsequent workup.

Etiology

While there can be some overlap, anemia can be divided into three broad categories: **blood loss (acute or chronic), increased destruction of RBCs (hemolysis)**, and **decreased production of RBCs**. Blood loss can be evaluated by a careful evaluation of the patient, including volume status. The reticulocyte count will usually help differentiate between states with decreased production (reticulocyte index [RI] <2%; see Diagnostic Testing for description of RI) and those associated with increased destruction (implied when the RI is >2%).

DIAGNOSIS

Clinical Presentation

History

As with any other medical condition, the history and physical examinations play key roles in approaching anemia. Based on symptomatology, one can discern the timeline (acute, subacute, or chronic), the severity, and even the underlying etiology. Patients can be asymptomatic, but those patients with an Hgb <7 g/dL will usually have symptoms. Acute clinical manifestations include those typical of hypovolemia (pallor, visual impairment, syncope, hypotension, and tachycardia) and require immediate attention. Chronic symptoms will reflect tissue hypoxia (fatigue, headache, dyspnea, lightheadedness, and angina). In addition to the usual symptoms of anemia, iron deficiency is often associated with **pica** (consumption of nonfood substances such as corn starch or ice). A history of the clinical manifestations, including initial presentation, time of onset, potential source of blood loss, family history, and medication history must be evaluated carefully.

Physical Examination

On examination, one can note pallor, alopecia, atrophic glossitis, angular cheilosis, congestive heart failure (with severe and chronic anemia), koilonychias (spoon nails), Plummer–Vinson or Patterson–Kelly syndrome (dysphagia, esophageal web, and atrophic glossitis with iron-deficiency anemia), blue sclera, and brittle nails, as well as hypotension and tachycardia.

Diagnostic Testing

- The **complete blood count** (CBC) measures WBCs, Hgb, Hct, platelets, as well as measures of the *red cell indices*. The Hgb is a measurement of mass of Hgb in blood (grams per deciliter), whereas the Hct is the physical amount of space that the Hgb occupies as a percentage of the whole that the red cells occupy. Remember that the Hgb and Hct are unreliable indicators of red cell volume in the setting of rapid shifts of intravascular volume (i.e., acute bleeding).
- The most useful red cell indices include the **mean corpuscular volume** (MCV), **red cell distribution width** (RDW), and **mean cell Hgb concentration** (MCHC). MCV is the mean size of the red cells; the normal range is 80–100 fL. RBCs can be classified as microcytic when the MCV is <80 fL and as macrocytic when it is >100 fL. RDW is a measure of variability in the size of the red cells and is calculated as: RDW = (standard deviation of red cell volume ÷ mean cell volume) × 100. An elevated RDW indicates increased variability in RBC size. The MCHC describes the concentration of Hgb in each cell.
- The **reticulocyte count** measures the immature red cells in the blood as a percentage of the whole and reflects the bone marrow's (BM's) response to anemia (i.e., a normal BM response is to increase the production of red cells in anemia so that the observed reticulocyte count goes up). A nascent RBC lives on average for 120 days, and the BM is constantly replenishing the bloodstream with new RBCs, with the normal reticulocyte count being ~1%. In the setting of anemia or blood loss, the BM should increase its production of RBC in proportion to loss of RBC, and thus a 1% reticulocyte count in the setting of anemia is inappropriate. The RI is calculated as percentage reticulocytes × (actual Hct/normal Hct) and is important in determining if a patient's BM is responding appropriately to the level of anemia. In normal individuals, an RI of 1–2 is acceptable; however, an RI of <2 with anemia indicates decreased production of RBCs. An RI of >2 with anemia may indicate hemolysis or loss of RBC, leading to increased compensatory production of reticulocytes.
- The **peripheral smear** is a required part of the initial hematologic evaluation. The shape, size, and orientation of cells in relation to each other are important factors to look for in a smear. RBCs can appear in many abnormal forms, such as acanthocytes, schistocytes, spherocytes, and teardrop cells, and abnormal orientations such as rouleaux formation.
- A **BM biopsy** may be indicated in cases of normocytic anemias with a low RI without an identifiable cause or anemia associated with other cytopenias. The biopsy may confirm myelophthisic process (i.e., presence of teardrop or fragmented cells, normoblasts, or immature WBCs on peripheral blood smear) in the setting of pancytopenias.

ANEMIAS ASSOCIATED WITH DECREASED PRODUCTION

The approach to an anemia associated with decreased production of red cells is to divide them into categories based on red cell size with the MCV. Depending on the MCV, **microcytic** (<80 fL), **normocytic** (80–100 fL), and **macrocytic** (>100 fL) anemias have distinct differential diagnoses.

Microcytic Anemias

Iron-deficiency anemia, sideroblastic anemia, and anemia of chronic disease make up the bulk of the microcytic anemias. The degree of microcytosis may give a clue to the possible underlying diagnoses. A very low MCV typically does not represent anemia of chronic disease or sideroblastic anemia (Table 3-1).

TABLE 3-1	CAUSES OF MICROCYTIC ANEMIAS BY MEAN CORPUSCULAR VOLUME (MCV)

MCV, 70–80	MCV, <70
Iron deficiency	Thalassemia
Anemia of chronic disease	Iron deficiency
Thalassemia	
Sideroblastic anemia	

Iron-Deficiency Anemia

GENERAL PRINCIPLES

Etiology

- Iron-deficiency anemia can be caused by decreased intake/absorption of iron or loss of iron from chronic blood loss. **Dietary deficiency** is usually seen in infants who are milk-fed. In early childhood, it can be seen in meat-deficient diets. It can also occur in the setting of increased requirements, such as pregnancy and early childhood. **Malabsorption** of iron can occur in the setting of partial gastrectomy, as hypochlorhydria/achlorhydria impairs iron absorption. Iron is most actively absorbed in the duodenum. Decreased transit time through the duodenum, as seen in chronic diarrhea, may result in iron deficiency. Gastrointestinal causes for iron deficiency (e.g., atrophic gastritis, *Helicobacter pylori* gastritis, and celiac disease) should be considered in patients with otherwise unexplained iron deficiency, especially when a patient is refractory to oral iron therapy.[1]
- **Chronic blood loss** is the most common cause of iron deficiency in adults. It is usually lost via the GI tract by ulcerative disease, gastritis, cancer, hemorrhoids, or arteriovenous malformation, with ulcers and colon malignancies being the most common. Menorrhagia/menstruation, hematuria due to genitourinary cancer, frequent blood donation, and frequent phlebotomy in hospitalized patients are additional causes of chronic blood loss. **It should be noted that the diagnosis of iron deficiency in an adult mandates evaluation for GI malignancy.**

DIAGNOSIS

Diagnosis involves serum testing of iron with an iron panel and ferritin level. The iron panel includes **serum iron level, total iron binding capacity** (TIBC), **unsaturated iron binding capacity** (UIBC), and **transferrin saturation** (Tsat).

- Serum iron levels reflect the level of iron immediately available for blood production. TIBC is an indirect method of determining the transferrin level in serum. Transferrin is an iron-transporting protein that is capable of associating with up to 1.254 g of iron per 1 g of protein. In one series, a Tsat <15% was 80% sensitive as an indicator of iron deficiency, but only 50–65% specific.
- Serum **ferritin** (intracellular iron storage protein) should also be checked and, when low, almost always signifies iron deficiency. Virtually all patients with serum ferritin concentrations <10–15 ng/mL are iron deficient, with a sensitivity of 59% and a specificity of 99%.[2] However, it is an acute phase reactant and can be falsely elevated in inflammatory states. The effect of inflammation is to elevate serum ferritin approximately threefold. A useful rule of thumb in such patients is to divide the patient's serum ferritin concentration by 3; a resulting value of 20 or less suggests concomitant iron deficiency.

- Serum transferrin receptor (sTfR) provides a quantitative measure of total erythropoietic activity, since its concentration in serum is directly proportional to erythropoietic rate and inversely proportional to tissue iron availability. Typically, in iron-deficiency anemia, the iron level is low, the TIBC is in the normal to high range, sTfR is high, and ferritin is depleted. The Tsat, the percentage of transferrin that is bound to iron, can be a somewhat less reliable measure of iron. Low Tsat is associated with iron-deficiency states, while high saturation is associated with excess iron. The gold standard for diagnosis of an iron-deficiency anemia is a BM biopsy with iron staining; however, this is rarely necessary.
- Of note, patients can have microcytic normochromic (concentration of Hgb in the erythrocytes is within the normal range of 32–36%) anemia that eventually progresses to microcytic hypochromic as the anemia progresses. With worsening iron-deficiency anemia, there is a gradual increase in anisocytosis and poikilocytosis (abnormally shaped cells).

TREATMENT

- In addition to diagnosing the patient with iron-deficiency anemia, it is important to discover and treat the underlying cause of the iron deficiency, if possible. **Iron replacement** may be given by oral iron salts, which should be given between meals because food or antacids may decrease absorption. Ascorbic acid given with iron sulfate may increase absorption. Earlier replacement regimens recommended TID dosing (e.g., ferrous sulfate, 325 mg PO tid (equivalent of 65 mg elemental iron). However, data suggest that iron absorption from supplements is greater with alternate day than with consecutive day dosing, in iron-deficient anemic women.[3] Enteric-coated forms are not well absorbed and should not be used.
- **Parenteral iron** is given when the patient is intolerant of oral iron, when iron losses exceed the capacity to replete orally, or in the setting of malabsorption. There is about a 1 in 300 risk of a serious reaction including anaphylaxis. The absolute risk for life-threatening adverse reactions for iron sucrose, ferric gluconate complex, low-MW dextran, and high-MW dextran is 0.6, 0.9, 3.3, and 11.3 per million doses, respectively.
- The amount of iron needed can be calculated as the amount of iron needed to replace the missing Hgb added to the amount necessary to replete the total body iron stores (usually estimated as approximately 1000 mg) by the formula: Total dose (mg) = {[normal Hgb (g/dL) − patient Hgb (g/dL)] × body weight [kg] × 2.2} + 1000 mg. However, in practice, iron is often infused at a dose of 1–1.2 g without formal calculation of iron repletion.
- One can expect an increase in the reticulocyte count within 7–10 days, and correction of anemia usually occurs within 6–8 weeks if ongoing blood loss is stopped. Treatment should continue for approximately 6 months (on PO iron) to fully restore tissue stores.

Sideroblastic Anemias

Sideroblastic anemias are characterized by ineffective erythropoiesis and the presence of ringed sideroblasts in the BM. The term *ringed* refers to the accumulation of iron in the mitochondria that surrounds the periphery of the nucleus. There are hereditary and idiopathic forms, as well as forms associated with drugs or toxins such as alcohol, lead, isoniazid (INH), zinc toxicity with resulting copper deficiency, and chloramphenicol. There is no cure for hereditary sideroblastic anemia, and treatment is aimed at preventing end-organ damage from iron overload (chelation therapy). Drug-induced sideroblastic anemias are commonly reversible when the offending agent is discontinued. For sideroblastic anemia caused by isoniazid treatment, high-dose pyridoxine supplementation (up to 200 mg/d PO) often reverses the anemia and allows for continuation of the drug.

Lead Poisoning

An additional diagnosis to consider in cases of microcytic, hypochromic anemias is lead poisoning. This is a rare but treatable form of microcytic anemia in adults and usually results from a work or an environmental exposure. The diagnosis is suggested by finding basophilic stippling on the peripheral smear.

Anemia of Chronic Disease

Anemia of chronic disease usually presents as a normocytic anemia; however, it can be microcytic (usually mild) in a minority of cases.

Thalassemias

GENERAL PRINCIPLES

Epidemiology

β-Thalassemia is more common in Mediterranean, African, and Southeast Asian populations and is thought to offer resistance to falciparum malaria.

Pathophysiology

- The major Hgb in adults is Hgb A, a tetramer consisting of one pair of α-globin chains and one pair of β-globin chains.[4] In normal subjects, globin chain synthesis is very tightly controlled, such that the ratio of production of α to non-α chains is 1 ± 0.05. Thalassemia refers to a spectrum of diseases characterized by reduced or absent production of one or more globin chains, thus disrupting this closely regulated ratio.
- β-**Thalassemia major** results from a total lack of production of β-globin chain. It causes lack of adequate Hgb A formation, leading to microcytic, hypochromic cells. Complications of severe β-thalassemia include skeletal deformities resulting from erythropoietin-stimulated expansion of BM, hepatosplenomegaly from extramedullary hematopoiesis, and secondary hemochromatosis from repeat blood transfusions and increased dietary absorption of iron.
- β-**Thalassemia minor** is loss of only one of the two alleles coding for the β-globulin gene. It is usually an asymptomatic condition manifested by microcytosis and a normal RDW. It is accompanied by a mild anemia (if any). On electrophoresis in patients with β-thalassemia minor, over 90% of the Hgb will be Hgb A along with an elevation in the Hgb A2 value, sometimes as high as 7% or 8%, and an increase in Hgb F in about 50% of patients.
- α-**Thalassemia** results from decreased production of α-globin chains, of which there are four in total. The severity of anemia depends on the number of defective α-genes. Hgb H disease is due to the loss of three of the four α-globin loci. Adult patients have a moderate degree of anemia, and their Hgb electrophoresis pattern shows 5–30% Hgb H (β-4 tetramers). Hydrops fetalis with Hgb Barts (γ-4 tetramers) is due to loss of all four α-globin loci. This condition is incompatible with extrauterine life. Diagnosis is by Hgb electrophoresis for β-thalassemia and severe α-thalassemia. Mild α-thalassemia may be detected by α:β ratio or by molecular testing, although neither is widely available.

TREATMENT

The treatment of thalassemias usually depends on the severity of the genetic defect and resultant clinical sequelae. The minor thalassemias are commonly asymptomatic and

TABLE 3-2	CAUSES OF NORMOCYTIC ANEMIA ASSOCIATED WITH A DECREASED RETICULOCYTE COUNT

Malignancies and other marrow infiltrative diseases
    Leukemia, myelodysplastic neoplasms (MDS), lymphoma
    Metastatic cancer
    Plasma cell disorders
    Granulomatous disease

Stem cell disorders
    Myelofibrosis
    Aplastic anemia
    Pure red cell aplasia

Due to other medical conditions
    Anemia of renal disease
    Anemia of chronic disease
    Endocrine disorders

require no therapy. The major thalassemias may be treated by chronic transfusions, chelation therapy to avoid iron overload (due to transfusions), and splenectomy. For ferritin concentrations >1000 ng/mL, chelation therapy may reduce the long-term complications of iron overload. Options for chelation include the intramuscular or subcutaneous iron chelator deferoxamine and oral iron chelator deferasirox.

Normocytic Anemias

Normocytic anemias can be associated with an elevated reticulocyte count, which represents hemolytic anemia (HA) or bleeding, or a decreased reticulocyte count, which typically represents a hypoproliferative disorder (Table 3-2). Normocytic anemia may be an early finding in BM failure. Aplastic anemia is actually a BM failure syndrome and is discussed in Chapter 8. Pure RBC aplasia involves a selective destruction of RBC precursors and can be congenital or acquired. It is often associated with viral infections (e.g., parvovirus). Symptoms are related to the anemia. Diagnosis is via BM biopsy showing absence of erythroid elements but with preservation of other cell lines. The absolute reticulocyte count is always less than 10,000/µL (reticulocyte percentage, <1%). Treatment includes supportive measures with transfusions as needed.

Anemia of Chronic Disease (Anemia of Chronic Inflammation)

This condition is often associated with malignancy, infection, and inflammatory states. It may occur in patients with chronic infections (e.g., osteomyelitis), HIV, or inflammatory diseases (e.g., lupus or rheumatoid arthritis). These disorders have in common the inhibition of normal RBC synthesis due to the underlying disorder. They may act by inadequate release of or insensitivity to erythropoietin. Other etiologies include deficiency in mobilization of iron from the reticuloendothelial system. One acute phase protein that appears to be most directly involved in iron metabolism is hepcidin. Although assays to measure serum hepcidin are not yet routinely available for clinical use, hepcidin levels may distinguish iron-deficiency anemia and anemia of chronic disease, alone or in combination with other tools.[5,6]

Anemia of chronic disease is most often a normocytic, normochromic anemia with a decreased reticulocyte count, but it may also present as a mild microcytic anemia. The serum iron concentration and TIBC are usually both low, often giving a normal Tsat (although this may be low or low-normal range). Serum ferritin, however, is an acute phase reactant and is often elevated in inflammatory diseases and infections. BM examination, if done, typically shows present iron stores. Symptoms and physical examination of the anemia of chronic disease patient are dependent on the patient's underlying condition. The anemia is typically mild and does not require blood transfusion. The more appropriate treatment is to treat the underlying condition.

Myelophthisic Anemias

Myelophthisic anemias refer to those with evidence of hematopoiesis outside the BM or infiltration of the BM by nonhematologic cells. Causes include metastatic carcinoma to the BM (e.g., breast, lung, prostate, kidney), myeloproliferative neoplasms, multiple myeloma, leukemias, and lymphoma. These are often suspected by a typical appearance of the peripheral smear (nucleated RBC, teardrop-shaped RBCs, and immature WBCs) and a "dry tap" on BM aspiration. BM biopsy results are dependent on the underlying disease. Treatment is directed toward the underlying disorder.

Anemia of Chronic Renal Failure

Anemia of chronic renal failure is due to erythropoietin deficiency. The anemia **generally starts when CrCl <45 mL/min and worsens with declining renal function**. When possible, treatment involves first treating the underlying renal dysfunction. **Erythropoietin** can be given at 50–100 U/kg IV or SC 3×/wk, with readjustments based on response. Response to erythropoietin is usually seen after 8–12 weeks of treatment.

Endocrine Disorders

Anemia due to endocrine disorders is seen in hypothyroidism, adrenal insufficiency, and gonadal dysfunction. Estrogens tend to inhibit red cell synthesis, and testosterone tends to stimulate it. Correction of the underlying endocrine disorder may improve the anemia.

Macrocytic Anemias

Anemias that have an **MCV of more than ~100 fL** are macrocytic anemias. These may be separated into two categories based on features seen on peripheral smear: megaloblastic and nonmegaloblastic. *Megaloblastic* features include the presence of oval macrocytes and hypersegmentation of the polymorphonuclear neutrophils (PMNs). They are a consequence of abnormal maturation of these cells and nuclear/cellular asynchrony. Examples of megaloblastic anemia include vitamin B_{12} deficiency, folate deficiency, and drug-induced. *Nonmegaloblastic* features include the presence of round macrocytes without hypersegmentation of the PMNs. Causes of nonmegaloblastic macrocytic anemia include liver disease, hypothyroidism, alcohol-induced reticulocytosis and reticulocytosis secondary to HA, and myelodysplastic syndrome (see Chapter 9 for further discussion).

Vitamin B$_{12}$ Deficiency

The daily requirement of vitamin B$_{12}$ is 2 μg/d, and a typical diet provides 5–15 μg/d, with the liver capable of storing ~2000–5000 μg. Thus, it takes up to 3–6 years for deficiency to develop once absorption completely ceases.

GENERAL PRINCIPLES

Etiology

Etiologies include pernicious anemia (the most common cause), gastrectomy or gastric bypass surgery, ileal disorders (sprue, inflammatory bowel disease, and lymphoma), bacterial overgrowth in the small intestine, fish tapeworms, and inadequate intake (this is very rare and only occurs in the strict vegetarian).

Clinical Presentation

Symptoms include burning sensation of the tongue, vague abdominal pain, diarrhea, numbness, paresthesia, and mental impairment. On examination, one can note glossitis, smooth tongue, dorsal column findings (decreased vibration and proprioception), and corticospinal tract findings (motor weakness, spasticity, and positive Babinski sign). Of note, patients can present with neurologic signs without overt anemia.

DIAGNOSIS

Diagnostic Testing

In cases of borderline-low B$_{12}$ values, one can measure **serum methylmalonic acid** and **homocysteine levels**, which are elevated in vitamin B$_{12}$ deficiency. Once the deficiency is established, an attempt should be made to identify the etiology. The presence of **anti-intrinsic factor antibodies** or **antiparietal cell antibodies** lends support to the diagnosis of pernicious anemia. Surgical history can reveal postsurgical etiologies. Suspicion of ileal disorder can be evaluated by endoscopy. Stool ova and parasites should be performed if suspicious of parasitic infection. A therapeutic trial of antibiotics may be given if bacterial overgrowth is suspected.

TREATMENT

Treatment usually includes vitamin B$_{12}$, 1 mg IM or SC daily for 7 days, then weekly for 1 month, followed by monthly doses thereafter. Oral vitamin B$_{12}$ at doses of 1–2 mg daily may be just as effective as IM administration.[7] Failure to correct or identify the underlying mechanism of deficiency may require lifelong therapy.

MONITORING/FOLLOW-UP

Reticulocytosis should occur in 5–7 days, with resolution of hematologic abnormalities in approximately 2 months. Resolution of neurologic abnormalities depends on their duration before treatment and may take up to 18 months. Neurologic deficits can be permanent.

Folate Deficiency

• The daily requirement of folate is 50–100 μg/d, with body stores of ~5–10 mg. Depletion can occur after about 2–4 months of persistent negative balance.

- Etiologies include inadequate intake (e.g., alcoholics), decreased absorption (e.g., sprue, bacterial overgrowth, certain drugs such as phenytoin and oral contraceptives), or states of increased requirements (HA, pregnancy, chronic dialysis, and exfoliative dermatitis). Folate deficiency can also be iatrogenic, such as treatment with folic acid antagonists (e.g., methotrexate, trimethoprim).
- Symptoms and physical examination are similar to vitamin B_{12} deficiency except that **neurologic features are not present**. Both serum and RBC folate levels must be measured. Serum folate is more labile and subject to acute rise after a folate-rich meal; RBC folate is a better indicator of tissue stores.
- It is important to **rule out vitamin B_{12} deficiency** before repletion with folate, because folate may improve the hematologic abnormalities in vitamin B_{12} deficiency but will not correct the neurologic manifestations.
- Treatment is with oral folate (1 mg/d), with resolution of hematologic abnormalities in approximately 2 months.

Drug-Induced Anemia

Several drugs can cause a macrocytic anemia by affecting DNA synthesis. Offenders include purine analogs (e.g., 6-mercaptopurine, azathioprine), pyrimidine analogs (5-fluorouracil, cytarabine), hydroxyurea, and anticonvulsants (phenytoin, phenobarbital). Reverse transcriptase inhibitors (zidovudine [AZT], etc.) may cause macrocytosis without anemia. Therapy is cessation of the offending agent or toleration of a mild anemia if the drug is therapeutically needed.

Nonmegaloblastic Anemia

Nonmegaloblastic anemias typically have round macrocytes without hypersegmentation of PMNs on peripheral smear. MCV of nonmegaloblastic anemias is rarely >110–115. A value higher than this would tend to support a megaloblastic etiology. When the reticulocyte count is elevated, it suggests an etiology such as alcohol, hypothyroidism, or liver disease. HA can produce a macrocytosis via increased production of reticulocytes. Nonmegaloblastic anemias are usually treated by identifying and treating the underlying etiology, such as discontinuation of alcohol use and thyroid hormone replacement.

ANEMIAS ASSOCIATED WITH INCREASED DESTRUCTION

Table 3-3 lists causes of anemia associated with increased RBC destruction. HAs can be classified by the location of hemolysis or the mechanism of hemolysis.

Location of Hemolysis

- **Extravascular:** Cell destruction occurs in the reticuloendothelial system, usually in the spleen.
- **Intravascular:** RBC destruction takes place within the circulation.

TABLE 3-3	CAUSES OF INCREASED RBC DESTRUCTION
Hereditary	**Acquired**

RBC membrane disorders
   Spherocytosis
   Elliptocytosis
	Immune related
	   Warm antibody
	   Cold agglutinin
	   Transfusion reaction

RBC enzyme disorders
   Pyruvate kinase deficiency
   Hexokinase deficiency
   G-6-PD deficiency
	Nonimmune
	   Microangiopathic hemolytic anemia
	   Infection
	   Hypersplenism

Disordered Hgb synthesis
   Hemoglobinopathy (i.e., sickle cell)
   Thalassemias
	Paroxysmal nocturnal hemoglobinuria

Mechanism of Hemolysis

- **Intrinsic:** Hemolysis is caused by a defect in the RBC membrane or contents.
- **Extrinsic:** Factors outside the RBC, such as serum antibody, trauma within circulation, infection, lead to RBC damage.

In general, most intrinsic causes are hereditary, and most extrinsic causes are acquired.

Hemolytic Anemias

GENERAL PRINCIPLES

HAs are disorders in which the **destruction of RBCs leads to a decrease in circulating RBC mass**. Acute hemolysis may be accompanied by a wide variety of signs and symptoms, many of which may point to the underlying etiology.

DIAGNOSIS

Patients may present with fever, chills, jaundice, back and abdominal pain, splenomegaly, and brown or red urine. Peripheral blood smear remains a useful tool both to confirm the diagnosis of hemolysis and to aid in discerning the underlying etiology. Some signs commonly found on peripheral smears include spherocytes (autoimmune HA, hereditary spherocytosis), helmet cells or schistocytes (microangiopathic HA), sickle cells and Howell–Jolly bodies (sickle cell anemia), spur cells (in liver diseases), bite cells or Heinz bodies (glucose-6-phosphate dehydrogenase [G-6-PD] deficiency), and agglutination (cold agglutinin). Laboratory abnormalities suggestive of hemolysis, though not specific, include increased lactate dehydrogenase, decreased haptoglobin, and increased unconjugated bilirubin. In addition, signs of compensatory increased RBC production such as an increase in reticulocyte count are typically present. Other useful laboratory tests include the **direct antiglobulin test (Coombs test)**, which detects antibodies (usually IgG) or complement (usually C3) bound to the surface of circulating RBCs by mixing *patient RBCs* with *anti-IgG*. Positive results occur when allo- or autoantibodies to RBC antigens are present, or when there is nonspecific adherence of other Ig or immune complexes to the RBC surface. The **indirect Coombs test**, which mixes the patient's serum with normal RBCs, is used to detect the presence of any anti-RBC antibody in the serum.

Sickle Cell Anemia

Sickle cell anemia is caused by a defect in the β-globin chain, resulting in sickling of RBC under oxidative stress. See Chapter 12 for further details.

Glucose-6-Phosphate Dehydrogenase Deficiency

- G-6-PD deficiency is an X-linked disorder that is fully expressed in males and homozygous females and variably expressed in heterozygous females. G-6-PD is the rate-limiting enzyme in the pentose phosphate pathway that helps maintain intracellular levels of glutathione, which serves to protect RBC against oxidative damage. In patients with G-6-PD deficiency, the presence of oxidative stress results in an inability to maintain Hgb in a reduced state, which, in turn, leads to Hgb precipitation within RBCs (Heinz body formation) and intravascular hemolysis. Two main variants of G-6-PD lead to clinically significant hemolysis: *G-6-PD A⁻* and *G-6-PD Mediterranean*. G-6-PD A⁻, which occurs in 10% of black individuals, has normal enzyme activity in young RBCs but a marked deficiency of enzyme activity in older cells. Therefore, when oxidatively challenged, only the older cells lyse. This form is typically milder and self-limited. The G-6-PD Mediterranean variant occurs in people of Middle Eastern and Mediterranean descent, and is characterized by a nearly complete lack of G-6-PD. Hemolysis in this form tends to be more severe compared to the A⁻ variant.
- The diagnosis of G-6-PD deficiency is suspected when hemolysis occurs after any form of oxidative stress, most commonly from starting on drugs known to precipitate hemolysis in a G-6-PD deficient patient (Table 3-4). Other triggers of hemolytic crises include certain foods, most notably fava beans, illnesses such as severe infections, and diabetic ketoacidosis. Findings on the peripheral blood smear suggestive of the diagnosis include Heinz bodies and "bite" cells. Heinz bodies are Hgb precipitants in the RBC, while bite cells are deformed RBCs that result from attempts by macrophages in the spleen to remove the Heinz bodies.
- Definitive diagnosis is made by measuring G-6-PD enzyme activity level. **In suspected G-6-PD A₂ variant, enzyme levels should not be measured during acute hemolysis.** In these patients, older RBCs containing the defective enzymes have mostly been lysed during acute hemolysis, and the normal enzyme activities in the remaining younger RBCs and reticulocytes will provide a false-negative result. It is, therefore, advisable to wait 3–4 weeks after the acute episode to get a true representation of the enzyme activity

TABLE 3-4	PRECIPITANTS OF HEMOLYSIS IN GLUCOSE-6-PHOSPHATE DEHYDROGENASE DEFICIENCY

Infection: *Escherichia coli, Salmonella, Streptococcus pneumoniae,* viral hepatitis

Drug-induced
    Antimalarials: primaquine and chloroquine
    Antibiotics: sulfonamides, dapsone (dapsone USP, DDS), and nitrofurantoin
        (macrodantin)
    Phenazopyridine (pyridium)
    Analgesics: in some cases, salicylates

Fava beans (in the Mediterranean variant only)

Naphthalene

level. The same does not apply to the Mediterranean variant, as both younger and older red cells are affected.

- Treatment is supportive, with transfusions as needed, and preventive, with avoidance of oxidative precipitant.

Hereditary Spherocytosis (Membrane Defect)

- Hereditary spherocytosis is an autosomal dominant disorder most common in patients of Northern European descent. In these patients, a defect in a membrane cytoskeletal protein leads to loss of surface area on the RBCs, resulting in spherocyte formation. Hemolysis of the spherocytic RBCs occurs primarily in the spleen.
- Clinical presentation may vary from asymptomatic to profound anemia and jaundice, depending on the severity of spherocytosis. Some patients may present with cholelithiasis. **Splenomegaly** is detected in most patients due to extravascular hemolysis. Peripheral blood smears reveal spherocytes. The MCV is normal or slightly low and is of little diagnostic value. However, considering the degree of reticulocytosis, the MCV is actually low. In unsplenectomized children, e.g., elevations in MCHC (>35 g/dL [normal 31.1–34 g/dL]) and RDW (>14 [normal mean 12.6]) have a sensitivity of 63% and specificity of 100% for the diagnosis of HS, making these combined indices a powerful screening tool.[8] The *osmotic fragility test*, which measures the RBC resistance to hemolysis when incubated in hypotonic saline, will show increased hemolysis.
- Treatment is largely supportive, with transfusions as needed and folate supplement to support increased erythropoiesis. Splenectomy, which corrects the anemia but not the underlying defect, may be considered in patients with severe anemia.

Acquired Immune Hemolytic Anemia

WARM ANTIBODY

Warm antibody is the most common form of autoimmune HA. The most common antibodies involved are IgG and they are most active at 37°C. Sixty percent of cases are *idiopathic* (or *primary*), whereas 40% are *secondary*. Secondary causes include chronic lymphocytic leukemia, non-Hodgkin lymphoma, Hodgkin lymphoma, autoimmune disorders (such as systemic lupus erythematosus), and drugs. **Drug-related antibodies** can occur by three main mechanisms:

- **Autoantibody:** Antibody against rhesus (e.g., methyldopa) is produced.
- **Hapten:** Drug binds to the RBC membrane, acting as hapten, which serves as a target for antibodies. Hemolysis typically occurs 1–2 weeks after treatment (e.g., penicillin, cephalosporins).
- **Immune complex:** Drug binds to plasma protein, evoking an antibody response. The drug–protein–antibody complex then nonspecifically coats RBCs, resulting in complement-mediated lysis (e.g., quinidine, INH, sulfonamides).

Warm antibodies usually cause extravascular hemolysis by the spleen, leading to splenomegaly. Almost all are panagglutinins (i.e., react with most donor RBCs), thus making cross-matching difficult. Treatment for drug-induced hemolysis is withdrawal of the offending agent, as hemolysis will stop with clearance of the drug. Steroids (prednisone) and immunoglobulins remain the most commonly used initial therapies. Prednisone up to 1 mg/kg/d may be used for severe hemolysis in idiopathic forms until Hgb reaches normal levels over a few weeks, and then it may be tapered. Intravenous immunoglobulins may be effective in controlling hemolysis, though its benefits tend to be short lived. Splenectomy is an option for patients who fail or relapse after steroid taper. If steroids and splenectomy both fail, other immunosuppressives such as rituximab, cyclosporine, azathioprine, and cyclophosphamide should be considered. **Transfusions should be avoided**, if possible, as they may result in more hemolysis.

COLD ANTIBODY

Most cold antibodies are IgM and active at <30°C. Acute onset is often associated with infectious causes such as mycoplasma pneumonia and infectious mononucleosis, whereas chronic forms occur with lymphoproliferative disorders or are idiopathic. The two main manifestations are acrocyanosis (ears, nose, and distal extremities) and hemolysis (complement mediated). Symptoms mainly occur in distal body parts, where the temperature often drops below 30°C. In these cold temperatures, IgM will bind to the RBCs, leading to complement fixation and hemolysis. The antibody dissociates from the RBCs as the temperature rises above 30°C. Hemolysis is not usually seen unless cold agglutinin titers are above 1 in 1000. Treatment mainly involves avoidance of cold exposure and treatment of the underlying disorder. While certain immunosuppressive agents and plasmapheresis may be effective, splenectomy and steroids are of limited therapeutic value.

Acquired Nonimmune Hemolytic Anemia

Acquired causes of nonimmune HA are often secondary to physical damage in the vasculature, chemical changes, or infections. Microangiopathic and macroangiopathic HAs represent the most common causes of physical damage. In these cases, changes in the vasculature result in the destruction of RBCs due to physical stress. Conditions associated with these forms of HAs include disseminated intravascular coagulation (DIC), thrombotic thrombocytopenic purpura (TTP), hemolytic-uremic syndrome (HUS), prosthetic heart valves, and severe aortic stenosis. DIC, TTP, and HUS are discussed in Chapter 4. Osmotic changes and certain snake and spider venom are examples of chemical damages to RBCs. HA is a characteristic feature of malarial infections. Table 3-5 lists the causes of acquired nonimmune HA.

Polycythemia

- Secondary polycythemia refers to erythrocytosis, which is defined as increased RBC mass. Chronic generalized or local hypoxia causes the body to respond by producing RBC mass to compensate. Chronic hypoxia from congenital heart disease, lung diseases, or smoking, or local hypoxia to the kidneys can increase erythropoietin production from the kidneys, which in turn increases production of RBCs. On physical examination, a ruddy complexion can be seen in patients with secondary polycythemia. In patients who are suffering from chronic hypoxia at severe levels, clubbing or even cyanosis may be found. Usually, no therapy is indicated in patients with erythrocytosis, as it is a physiologic response to hypoxia and is a compensatory mechanism.
- **Secondary polycythemia can be distinguished from primary polycythemia (polycythemia vera) by the erythropoietin level,** which is elevated in secondary polycythemia and low or normal in polycythemia vera. Polycythemia vera is a stem cell disorder leading to increased RBC mass, which is discussed further in Chapter 10.

TABLE 3-5	TYPES OF ACQUIRED NONIMMUNE HEMOLYTIC ANEMIAS

Microangiopathic hemolytic anemia
    Thrombotic thrombocytopenic purpura
    Disseminated intravascular coagulation
    Hemolytic-uremic syndrome
    Eclampsia
    Malignant hypertension
    Metastatic adenocarcinoma

Macroangiopathic hemolytic anemia
    Prosthetic valve
    Severe aortic stenosis

Physical and chemical
    Snake and spider venom
    Osmotic hemolysis from freshwater drowning
    Damage to RBC membranes from third-degree burns

Infection
    Malaria
    Clostridium difficile
    Babesiosis

Hypersplenism

Paroxysmal nocturnal hemoglobinuria

REFERENCES

1. Hershko C, Hoffbrand AV, Keret D, et al. Role of autoimmune gastritis, *Helicobacter pylori* and celiac disease in refractory or unexplained iron deficiency anemia. *Haematologica.* 2005;90(5):585–595.
2. Guyatt GH, Oxman AD, Ali M, Willan A, McIlroy W, Patterson C. Laboratory diagnosis of iron-deficiency anemia: an overview. *J Gen Intern Med.* 1992;7(2):145–153.
3. Stoffel NU, Zeder C, Brittenham GM, Moretti D, Zimmermann MB. Iron absorption from supplements is greater with alternate day than with consecutive day dosing in iron-deficient anemic women. *Haematologica.* 2020;105(5):1232–1239.
4. Olivieri NF. The beta-thalassemias. [Published erratum appears in *N Engl J Med.* 1999;341(18):1407.] *N Engl J Med.* 1999;341:99–109.
5. Nemeth E, Valore EV, Territo M, Schiller G, Lichtenstein A, Ganz T. Hepcidin, a putative mediator of anemia of inflammation, is a type II acute-phase protein. *Blood.* 2003;101(7):2461–2463.
6. Thomas C, Kobold U, Thomas L. Serum hepcidin-25 in comparison to biochemical markers and hematological indices for the differentiation of iron-restricted erythropoiesis. *Clin Chem Lab Med.* 2011;49(2):207–213.
7. Kuzminski AM, Del Giacco EJ, Allen RH, Stabler SP, Lindenbaum J. Effective treatment of cobalamin deficiency with oral cobalamin. *Blood.* 1998;92(4):1191–1198.
8. Michaels LA, Cohen AR, Zhao H, Raphael RI, Manno CS. Screening for hereditary spherocytosis by use of automated erythrocyte indexes. *J Pediatr.* 1997;130(6):957–960.

Platelets: Thrombocytopenia and Thrombocytosis

Joshua I. Siner

4

Thrombocytopenia

GENERAL PRINCIPLES

Definition

Platelets are an essential functional unit necessary for primary hemostasis, the process in which a platelet plug forms to mitigate vascular blood loss. The normal platelet range is between 150,000 and 450,000/μL. Thrombocytopenia occurs when the platelet count drops below 150,000/μL.

Classification

Causes of thrombocytopenia can be classified into pseudothrombocytopenia, impaired platelet production, consumptive thrombocytopenia, sequestration into the reticuloendothelial system, nonimmune thrombocytopenia, and drug-induced thrombocytopenia.

DIAGNOSIS

Clinical Presentation

Thrombocytopenia may be found incidentally on a routine complete blood count (CBC). The CBC is the essential first evaluation in patients presenting with evidence of bleeding, including petechiae, purpura, or overt bleeding, especially of the mucosa. All patients with thrombocytopenia should undergo a thorough history and physical examination before deciding upon further diagnostic testing, as certain conditions associated with thrombocytopenia may be obvious to the clinician.

Differential Diagnosis
- **Pseudothrombocytopenia**
  - Platelet agglutination due to EDTA-dependent autoantibodies. Counts correct upon repeat testing using citrated whole blood and does not correlate with a bleeding diathesis.
- **Impaired platelet production**
  - Acquired
    - Infectious diseases: HIV, hepatitis C, parvovirus, varicella, rubella, mumps
    - Marrow infiltration (leukemia, lymphoma, some solid tumors)
    - Radiotherapy and chemotherapy
    - Paroxysmal nocturnal hemoglobinuria
    - Myelodysplastic syndrome
    - Acquired aplastic anemia
    - Nutritional deficiencies: folate, vitamin B_{12}, copper
    - Alcohol
  - Congenital: von Willebrand disease type 2B, Wiskott–Aldrich syndrome, Alport syndrome, Fanconi syndrome, May–Hegglin anomaly, congenital amegakaryocytic thrombocytopenia, Bernard–Soulier syndrome, Gray platelet syndrome, thrombocytopenia with absent radius (TAR) syndrome, and others.

- **Increased platelet destruction**
  - Immune mediated
  - Autoimmune thrombocytopenic purpura
  - Secondary (infections, pregnancy-related, lymphoproliferative disorders, collagen vascular disease)
  - Posttransfusion purpura
    - Heparin-induced thrombocytopenia (HIT)
    - Vaccine-induced immune thrombotic thrombocytopenia (VITT)
  - Idiopathic
- **Nonimmune thrombocytopenia**
  - Thrombotic microangiopathies
    - Thrombotic thrombocytopenic purpura (TTP), hemolytic-uremic syndrome (HUS), and atypical HUS
  - Eclampsia/HELLP (hemolysis, elevated liver enzymes, and low platelets) syndrome
  - Disseminated intravascular coagulation (DIC)
  - Kasabach–Merritt syndrome (fast-growing vascular tumors sequester and destroy platelets)
- **Abnormal platelet distribution**
  - Splenomegaly or hypersplenism
  - Massive transfusion
  - Hypothermia
- **Drug-induced thrombocytopenia**

Immune-Mediated Thrombocytopenia

GENERAL PRINCIPLES

Definition

Immune (idiopathic) thrombocytopenia (ITP) is a common acquired disorder characterized by isolated thrombocytopenia[1] caused by increased platelet destruction or impaired thrombopoiesis by antiplatelet antibodies.[2]

Classification

- **Primary ITP** is an immune-mediated disorder without a clear cause.
- **Secondary ITP** is caused by an underlying disease, such as infections, lymphoproliferative disorders, autoimmune diseases, or associated with drug therapy.
- ITP can be further classified as **acute** (<3 months), **persistent** (3–12 months), or **chronic** (>12 months).

DIAGNOSIS

Clinical Presentation

Patients with severe thrombocytopenia may present incidentally in routine CBCs, but will often present with bleeding manifestations including petechiae, purpura, and mucosal bleeding (epistaxis, gingival bleeding, and menorrhagia). Less frequently, patients present with more severe bleeding from the gastrointestinal tract or intracranial hemorrhage requiring intensive care support.

History and Physical Examination

Patient history should include a focus on bleeding symptoms and causes of secondary ITP or other hematologic disorders. Of particular importance are constitutional symptoms, prior thrombocytopenia and time course of development, autoimmune diseases, hematologic diseases, liver disease, recent or chronic infections, recent transfusions, recent immunization, and medication exposures. The physical examination is usually normal except for findings associated with bleeding. Other physical findings such as splenomegaly, lymphadenopathy, or constitutional symptoms would suggest a secondary thrombocytopenia.

DIAGNOSTIC TESTING

- ITP is a **diagnosis of exclusion**, as there is no definitive diagnostic test. No antiplatelet antibody tests are sufficiently sensitive or specific to make the diagnosis.
- The CBC should reveal isolated thrombocytopenia unless bleeding is severe enough or sufficiently prolonged to produce a concurrent anemia.
- **Evans syndrome** is an autoimmune hemolytic anemia and ITP either in synchrony or in series.
- Review of the **peripheral blood smear** is essential to rule out other causes of thrombocytopenia, including pseudothrombocytopenia and microangiopathic hemolytic anemias (MAHAs). The presence of large/giant (immature) platelets is a feature of ITP.
- A **bone marrow biopsy** can be considered in patients older than 60 years of age or when the history and physical or other diagnostic data raise suspicion for an underlying hematologic disease—including refractoriness to initial ITP-directed therapies.
- **HIV, HCV,** and ***Helicobacter pylori* testing** should be considered in at-risk patients.
- Baseline thyroid function testing and quantitative serum immunoglobulin and serum protein electrophoresis testing should also be considered.

TREATMENT

The primary goal of treatment for ITP is to prevent bleeding. If the platelet count is >50 × 10^9/L, patients can be observed. Patients with platelet counts between 30 and 40 × 10^9/L usually do not require treatment but need careful follow-up. Patients with a platelet count <10 × 10^9/L require treatment due to the risk of life-threatening bleeding. Multiple therapeutic modalities exist, and treatment should be tailored for each individual patient.[3]

First-Line Therapy

- **Corticosteroids:** Dexamethasone pulse-dose of 40 mg for 4 days is equivalent to prednisone 1 mg/kg/d at inducing a sustain platelet response and avoids the prolonged taper and side effects of prednisone can be given until normalization of platelet count, at which point steroids can be tapered to avoid side effects.[4]
- **IVIg:** IVIg can be given at a dose of 1 g/kg/d × 2 days or 0.4 g/kg/d × 5 days with consideration of maintenance dosing. This is often used in conjunction with steroids in the first line when patients have critical bleeding or without an appropriate response to steroids.
- **IV anti-D:** 50–75 µg/kg/d of IV anti-D can be considered in Rh(D) positive patients who have not undergone splenectomy and who do not have history of autoimmune hemolytic anemia. Anti-Rh(D) antibodies bind Rh-positive erythrocytes and cause splenic destruction, so more antibody-coated platelets survive in the circulation.[2] Careful consideration is needed to assess hemolysis after introduction and the patient's ability to tolerate an acute anemia.

Second-Line Therapy

- **Splenectomy:** Splenectomy should be considered if platelet count remains <10 × 10^9/L after 2–3 months of appropriate therapy or in patients who only achieve transient responses.[2] Approximately two-thirds of patients achieve normal platelet counts following splenectomy and often can have durable responses.
- **Rituximab:** Rituximab is an effective therapeutic option for patients who are refractory to steroids and intravenous immune globulin (IVIg), and may be considered in patients

regardless of splenectomy status. Overall response rate is approximately 60%. Patients typically respond in 4–6 weeks after four weekly doses of 375 mg/m^2 and up to one-third may remain in remission for more than 1 year.[5]

- **Thrombopoietin (TPO) receptor agonists:** TPO mimetics trigger megakaryocyte growth and differentiation. The currently available TPO receptor agonists are romiplostim, eltrombopag, and avatrombopag. The response rate of romiplostim has been reported to be approximately 80%[6] and eltrombopag had similar results.[7] Avatrombopag was initially approved for patients with chronic liver disease and thrombocytopenia requiring increased platelet count for a procedure.

- **Other treatment options:** Multiple drugs can be considered as second-line agents including rilzabrutinib (bruton tyrosine kinase [BTK] inhibitor), fostamatinib (spleen tyrosine kinase inhibitor), steroid-sparing agents including azathioprine, cyclosporine A, mycophenolate mofetil. Additional chemotherapeutic agents with efficacy include cyclophosphamide and vinca alkaloid regimens. Finally, danazol and dapsone have been shown to produce platelet responses to a lesser degree in selected populations in conjunction with steroids.

Refractory ITP

For patients with severe refractory disease, combination chemotherapy may need to be implemented. Allogeneic stem cell transplantation has been used successfully.

Emergency Therapy

In emergent situations, such as in life-threatening bleeding or emergency surgery, combination therapies and platelet transfusions (including prolonged platelet infusions) should be considered. Aminocaproic acid may be used to reduce bleeding in persistently thrombocytopenic patients.[3]

Thrombotic Thrombocytopenic Purpura, Hemolytic-Uremic Syndrome, and Complement-Mediated (Atypical) Hemolytic-Uremic Syndrome

GENERAL PRINCIPLES

Definition

TTP, HUS, and complement-mediated (atypical) HUS are clinically similar disorders that are associated with MAHA, thrombocytopenia, and microvascular thrombosis. Clinical manifestations depend on the affected vascular bed and it is typical to observe neurologic and renal involvement. Pathophysiology distinguishes the three disorders and dictates treatment. When neurologic impairment is present, the patient is more likely to be classified as TTP, whereas acute renal failure is a hallmark of HUS. Atypical HUS tends to have no diarrhea but significant evidence of renal impairment.

Epidemiology

TTP has an incidence of approximately four cases per million persons. HUS is an uncommon disorder with two forms: a sporadic form more typical of adults, and a childhood form that is most commonly associated with shiga toxin–producing *Escherichia coli*. Both cause thrombocytopenia with evidence of MAHA, but they are distinct entities. TTP-HUS once had a 90% mortality rate, until the utility of plasma exchange was demonstrated. Six-month mortality now is <30% with prompt initiation of appropriate treatment.[8] The incidence of complement-mediated HUS is unknown as it is rare. It can result from either a primary disorder due to mutations in complement proteins, or it can result from the development of autoantibodies.[9]

Pathophysiology

- **Thrombotic thrombocytopenic purpura.** Acquired TTP is caused by autoantibodies that inhibit a disintegrin and metalloprotease thrombospondin type 1 repeats (ADAMTS) 13. Congenital TTP is due to an inherited deficiency of ADAMTS13 (Upshaw–Schulman syndrome.) Under normal circumstances, endothelial cells produce ultralarge von Willebrand Factor (ULvWF) molecules that are regulated and cleaved by ADAMTS13 into their typical-length multimers. In the setting of ADAMTS13 deficiency, ULvWF molecules persist and induce pathologic platelet aggregation in the microcirculation in areas of high shear stress. This leads to platelet consumption and RBC fragmentation and destruction. It should be noted that some patients with clinical TTP do not have decreased ADAMTS13 activity, implicating other unidentified factors.[8]
- **Hemolytic-uremic syndrome.** Although HUS has features in common with TTP, a deficiency or inhibitor of ADAMTS13 does not appear to be the cause of HUS. HUS also differs from TTP in that it is associated with preferential renal endothelial damage. Typical childhood HUS is associated with hemorrhagic diarrhea caused by shiga toxin–producing bacteria, such as *E. coli* 0157:H7. Shiga toxin–producing *E. coli* accounts for over 90% of the cases of HUS in children.[10]
- **Atypical HUS.** Atypical, or complement-mediated, HUS is the MAHA that is associated with the dysregulation of the alternative pathway of complement secondary to complement gene mutations or complement factor H (CFH) autoantibodies. The microvascular injury is due to uncontrolled complement activation.[9]

DIAGNOSIS

Differential Diagnosis

See Table 4-1.

TABLE 4-1	ETIOLOGY OF THROMBOTIC MICROANGIOPATHIES

Idiopathic
Estrogen use
Pregnancy-associated (HELLP)
Infections (*E. coli* 0157:H7, pneumococcal infection, HIV)
DIC
Stem cell and solid organ transplants
Malignancy
Autoimmune diseases (systemic lupus erythematosus, antiphospholipid syndrome, vasculitis)
High shear vasculature (aortic stenosis, prosthetic valves)
Malignant hypertension
Drug-induced
    Quinine
    Cyclosporine
    Tacrolimus
    Gemcitabine
    Mitomycin C
    Carfilzomib
Familial

TABLE 4-2   TTP: THE CLASSIC PENTAD OF FINDINGS

Thrombocytopenia
Microangiopathic hemolytic anemia
Neurologic changes
Renal dysfunction (predominates in HUS)
Fever

Clinical Presentation

The clinical features of TTP and HUS can overlap. The classic findings of TTP include a pentad of physical examination and laboratory findings as reported in Table 4-2. The complete pentad does not have to be present for the diagnosis; TTP often presents without fever or neurologic dysfunction. TTP may be preceded by a few weeks of malaise, but neurologic symptoms (including headache, confusion, vision changes, tinnitus, seizures, ischemic stroke, and coma) are frequently the first symptoms that bring a patient to medical attention. These symptoms may wax and wane over the course of the illness. Neurologic symptoms have also been described in patients with atypical HUS. Patients often have renal impairment, but acute kidney injury requiring dialysis is rare in TTP and more common in HUS and atypical HUS. Diarrhea is often the presenting symptom of HUS. Due to significant overlap of symptoms, clinical presentation alone is insufficient to differentiate these syndromes.

Diagnostic Criteria

Anemia and thrombocytopenia are universal. Hemolysis is evidenced by elevated lactate dehydrogenase (LDH), elevated indirect bilirubin, and decreased haptoglobin, but a **peripheral blood smear is mandatory** for diagnosis to identify schistocytes, which are the hallmark of all MAHAs. The reticulocyte count is usually elevated however may be falsely normalized from nutritional depletion with chronic hemolysis or low folate/vitamin B_{12} diets. Coagulation studies (Prothrombin time/international normalized ratio [PT/INR], partial thromboplastin time [PTT]) are usually within normal limits, and a DIC panel, including fibrinogen, fibrinogen degradation products (FDPs), and D-dimer, is useful to rule out DIC. The PLASMIC score is a pretest scoring system to identify patients with acquired TTP who are likely to benefit from upfront plasmapheresis.[11] A deficiency in the ADAMTS13 protease (typically <10% activity) can confirm the diagnosis of TTP, but treatment should not be delayed while waiting for test results. Further classification of thrombotic microangiopathy as either TTP or HUS is usually based upon age, past medical history, clinical presentation, and the presence or absence of renal dysfunction or neurologic symptoms—all of which factor into the PLASMIC score (see Table 4-3.) Due to complement activation in atypical HUS, there can be low levels of C3 and normal C4 levels, but these tests are neither sensitive nor specific enough to definitively make the diagnosis of atypical HUS. Complement mutational analysis should be done to confirm the diagnosis and dictate long-term treatment strategies.[9]

TREATMENT

- The primary treatment for TTP, HUS, and atypical HUS is **plasma exchange (plasmapheresis)**, with an estimated plasma volume exchanged daily. Plasma exchange can be done twice daily in severe cases or in cases that progress despite daily treatments. Because of the high mortality of untreated TTP or HUS, thrombocytopenia and MAHA

TABLE 4-3	CLINICAL SCORING SYSTEM FOR PLASMAPHERESIS IN PATIENT PRESENTING WITH A MAHA	
Category	1 Point	0 Point
Platelet count <30,000/μL	Yes	No
hemo**L**ysis (reticulocyte >2.5%, indirect bilirubin >2.0 mg/dL, or undetectable haptoglobin)	Yes	No
Active malignancy, or treated within the past 1 y	No	Yes
History of **S**olid organ or **S**tem cell transplant	No	Yes
MCV <90 fL	Yes	No
INR <1.5	Yes	No
Creatinine <2.0 mg/dL	Yes	No
PLASMIC Score	Risk Group	Risk of ADAMTS13 <15%
0–4	Low	0%
5	Intermediate	6%
6–7	High	72%

are sufficient to initiate plasma exchange, if no other certain cause can be identified. ADAMTS13 levels should not alter the decision to perform plasma exchange.[12] The goal of daily plasma exchange should be to reverse the thrombocytopenia and hemolysis. This can be monitored with LDH and CBC results. Plasma exchange can be tapered or stopped after the platelet count has been normal for 2 days. After remission, exacerbations due to discontinuing plasma exchange (<30 days) should lead to immediate resumption of plasma exchange.[12]

- For patients with no clinical evidence of HUS and normal ADAMTS13 activity, atypical HUS should be considered. Patients may initially respond to plasma exchange through addition of plasma complement proteins, but hemolysis typically returns when plasmapheresis is discontinued. Often patients have a poor response to plasmapheresis. In this case, treatment with **eculizumab**, a monoclonal antibody that blocks terminal complement activation, should be considered.[13] **Ravulizumab** is a newer monoclonal antibody targeting terminal complement with longer half-life and less frequent dosing.

- Suspected ADAMTS13 deficiency can also be treated with systemic corticosteroid therapy, in an effort to suppress inhibitors, at a dose of 1 mg/kg of prednisone or potentially higher doses in critically ill patients and should be considered in patients during which delay in plasmapheresis due to availability. **Caplacizumab** is a nanobody drug that targets von Willebrand factor and prevents binding to its platelet receptor. It is approved for the treatment of TTP with the expected side effect of mucosal bleeding, and unexpectedly increased rate of relapse on discontinuation which requires close monitoring.[14]

- Platelet transfusions are relatively contraindicated, except in cases of life-threatening bleeding.

- In patients with refractory or relapsing TTP and a demonstrated antibody to ADAMTS13, rituximab may achieve remission and decrease the need for plasma exchange.[15]

Disseminated Intravascular Coagulation

GENERAL PRINCIPLES

Definition

DIC is an acquired, systemic disorder of hemostasis which produces both thrombosis and hemorrhage.

Epidemiology

DIC is associated with an underlying illness and is thus a condition most frequently diagnosed and treated in hospitalized patients. Around 1% of hospital admissions may be complicated by DIC, although rates approaching 35% may be seen in patients with severe sepsis syndrome.[16]

Pathophysiology and Etiology

In DIC, an underlying illness leads to systemic activation of the coagulation cascade, likely mediated by widespread endothelial damage and the release of inflammatory cytokines. This coagulation activation leads to increased fibrin formation and subsequent thrombosis, most notably in small- and medium-sized vessels. The widespread thrombosis can lead to organ failure and MAHA. Notably, the excessive coagulatory activation and thrombosis can deplete clotting factors and platelets leading to bleeding.[17]

Risk Factors and Associated Conditions

See Table 4-4.

DIAGNOSIS

Clinical Presentation

DIC can manifest with symptoms related to thrombosis or bleeding. Thrombosis can lead to digit gangrene, stroke, or organ failure. Bleeding may be in the form of petechiae, oozing from venipuncture, intravenous catheters or wound sites, or more severely with overt hemorrhage.

Diagnostic Criteria

- There are a number of useful laboratory tests to assist in the diagnosis of DIC. The **CBC** may reveal anemia or thrombocytopenia, often <100,000/μL, related to thrombotic microangiopathy. **Coagulation studies**, including PT/INR and PTT, may be prolonged due to consumption of coagulation factors. "DIC panels" often measure **fibrinogen**, **FDP**, and **D-dimer**. Fibrinogen levels are low as a result of consumption, while the FDP and D-dimers are markers of clot dissolution and are usually elevated. It should be noted that fibrinogen is an acute phase reactant and may be elevated due to an initial underlying illness. In such situations, a declining fibrinogen level may provide a clue to the diagnosis of DIC. A peripheral smear often reveals schistocytes from the destruction of red cells.
- It is important to distinguish DIC from other conditions. Typical laboratory abnormalities with separate disease processes include liver disease (low platelets and prolonged PT and PTT but normal fibrinogen—except in severe liver disease, which may show

TABLE 4-4	CONDITIONS ASSOCIATED WITH DISSEMINATED INTRAVASCULAR COAGULATION

Systemic infection
  Gram-negative sepsis related to endotoxin
  Gram-positive organisms

Cancer
  Solid tumors including pancreatic, prostate, breast, and others
  Hematologic malignancy, most notably acute promyelocytic leukemia (AML-M3)

Trauma
  Head injury, usually life threatening
  Serious burns involving large parts of the body
  Serious crushing injuries with substantial tissue damage
  Serious fractures, most notably a femur fracture with fat embolism

Obstetric complications
  Amniotic fluid embolism
  Placental abruption

Vascular disorders
  Aortic aneurysm
  Hemangiomas, usually giant

Immune-mediated reactions
  Anaphylaxis, mediated by cytokine release
  Transfusion reactions
  Transplant rejection

Toxins
  Snake venom

IV drugs, possibly related to a drug affect, but IV drug abuse–associated systemic infections should be considered.

low fibrinogen), vitamin K deficiency (prolonged PT/PTT but normal platelets and fibrinogen), and TTP/HUS (MAHA and thrombocytopenia but normal PT, PTT, and fibrinogen).

TREATMENT

Management should be **focused predominantly on identifying and treating the underlying condition**. Symptomatic treatment of bleeding or thrombosis can be dictated by the clinical scenario. In patients with high bleeding risk or active bleeding, fresh-frozen plasma to replace clotting factors, cryoprecipitate to replace fibrinogen (target level >100 mg/dL), and platelet transfusions (target platelets >50,000/μL) are suggested. In patients predominantly in the thrombotic phase of DIC, low-dose heparin has been suggested, but this is controversial. Low–molecular-weight heparin (LMWH) may have less risk for bleeding and it could be considered as an alternative. In cases in which the patient has low antithrombin III (ATIII) levels and severe DIC, ATIII replacement (with FFP or ATIII concentrates) is a reasonable option.[18] A notable primary hematologic cause of DIC is acute promyelocytic leukemia wherein early mortality is driven by DIC and corrects with appropriate induction and fibrinogen support.

Heparin-Induced Thrombocytopenia

GENERAL PRINCIPLES

Definition and Classification

HIT can be classified into two separate entities: HIT I and HIT II.

HIT I is nonimmune mediated and characterized by a transient fall in platelet count. This form of HIT is not an indication for discontinuing heparin.

The remainder of this chapter focuses on HIT II, which will simply be referred to as HIT.

Epidemiology and Etiology

HIT is an acquired prothrombotic complication of heparin therapy. It is an immune-mediated disorder caused by **IgG antibodies that bind to platelet factor 4 (PF4)–heparin complexes**. The frequency in one meta-analysis was 2.6% in patients treated with unfractionated heparin (UFH) and 0.2% in those treated with LMWH.[19]

Pathophysiology

- As a primary specific immune response, HIT syndrome generally has a delayed onset of 4–5 days after administration of heparin or LMWH.
- PF4 is a heparin-neutralizing chemokine protein found within the α-granules of platelets. This protein binds exogenous heparin (UFH > LWMH) and forms multimer complexes which can provoke an IgG antibody formation. Once formed, the HIT-IgG Ab (HIT Ab)-PF4–heparin complex can activate platelets and other cells, generate immunogenic multimolecular complexes, and promote tissue factor expression and thrombin generation leading to significant risk for thrombosis. Platelets targeted by HIT-specific antibodies (including unactivated platelet complexes) are cleared from the circulation, causing thrombocytopenia.[20]

Risk Factors

HIT is more common in adult medical and surgical patients than in obstetric or pediatric patients. UFH is approximately 10 times more likely than LMWH to produce HIT. Patients receiving IV heparin are more likely to develop HIT than those receiving subcutaneous heparin.[20] Cardiothoracic patients are at unique at risk given their larger heparin exposures, specifically while on extracorporeal membrane oxygenation (ECMO) and intraoperative cardiac bypass.

DIAGNOSIS

Clinical Presentation

- Thrombocytopenia or a fall in platelet count of >50% occurs in 95% of patients diagnosed with HIT. The average platelet count is 50,000–70,000/μL.[20]
- There are three time courses of HIT: typical, rapid, and delayed-onset HIT.
  - In **typical-onset HIT**, thrombocytopenia develops 5–10 days after initiation of heparin therapy, approximately the amount of time necessary to generate a humoral immune response.
  - A subset of patients experience **rapid-onset HIT**, where thrombocytopenia occurs within 24 hours, indicating a recent exposure to heparin during the preceding weeks and preformed immunoglobulins.
  - **Delayed-onset HIT** occurs days after heparin has been stopped. This form of HIT is not well understood. These patients typically have a high-titer platelet-activating HIT antibody (Ab). It is uncommon for HIT to occur more than 2 weeks after discontinuation of heparin.

TABLE 4-5	CLINICAL SCORING SYSTEM FOR HEPARIN-INDUCED THROMBOCYTOPENIA		
Category	2 Points	1 Point	0 Point
Thrombocytopenia	>50% fall or nadir ≥20K	30–50% fall or nadir 10–19K	<30% fall or nadir <10K
Timing of thrombocytopenia	5–10 d or <1 d if recent exposure (30 d)	>10 d, timing unclear, or <1 d if heparin exposure 30–100 d ago	<4 d and no recent heparin exposure
Thrombosis	New thrombosis, skin necrosis, or systemic reaction to IV heparin	Progressive or recurrent thrombosis, nonnecrotizing skin lesions, suspected thrombosis	None
Other causes of thrombocytopenia	None apparent	Possible	Proven

- HIT can present as **thrombosis**. The most common manifestation is venous thromboembolism (deep venous thrombosis and pulmonary embolism) in the postoperative setting. Though less common, arterial thrombosis can occur and is manifested as stroke, myocardial infarction, or limb ischemia.
- A clinical scoring system using the four Ts (**T**hrombocytopenia, **T**iming of platelet fall, **T**hrombosis, and o**T**her causes) has been shown to help risk stratify patients with suspected HIT (Table 4-5).[21] A score of 0–8 points is possible. If the score is 0–3, HIT is unlikely. A score of 4–5 indicates intermediate probability, while a score of 6–8 makes HIT highly likely. Those with a high or intermediate score need to be treated with an alternative drug while more sensitive and specific tests for HIT are performed. Patients with a low score can safely continue receiving heparin, as the likelihood that they have HIT is extremely low.

Diagnostic Testing

Initial diagnosis should be made based on the clinical scenario and after other causes of thrombocytopenia have been ruled out. The most common first confirmatory assay is an **immunoassay for the presence of PF4/heparin antibodies**. This test is rapid and sensitive (>99%), though it lacks specificity (40–70%).[20] Functional assays are more specific than HIT immunoassays but are not as widely available due to the technical expertise required. Functional assays measure platelet activation at varying heparin concentrations. One such test, the **serotonin release assay**, utilizes radiolabeled serotonin to measure platelet activation. The test is considered positive when serotonin is released from donor platelets placed in patient serum upon a low concentration of heparin being added. These tests are reported to have >95% sensitivity and specificity.[20]

TREATMENT

The first step in treating HIT is the **discontinuation of all heparin products**. Return of laboratory assay results often takes several days. Therefore, products including heparin flushes and heparin-coated catheters, should be discontinued immediately if HIT is suspected. Because of cross-reactivity to the HIT Ab, LMWH should not be substituted. For patients who are strongly suspected of having HIT, **nonheparin anticoagulation** should be promptly instituted.

Agents which can treat HIT are direct thrombin inhibitors (lepirudin, argatroban, and bivalirudin), indirect factor Xa inhibitors (fondaparinux), direct factor Xa inhibitors (apixaban and rivaroxaban), and vitamin K antagonists (warfarin). In the acute setting there is no preferred agent and is instead driven by clinician preference and competing patient comorbidities.

- **Lepirudin** is a recombinant hirudin, a natural anticoagulant found in the salivary glands of medicinal leeches. This drug has been approved by the FDA for patients with HIT for the prevention and treatment of thrombosis. Lepirudin is renally cleared and should be dose adjusted in patients with chronic kidney disease.[22]
- **Argatroban** has also been approved by the FDA for the prevention and treatment of thrombosis associated with HIT. This drug is hepatically cleared and should be used with caution in patients with impaired hepatic function.[22]
- **Bivalirudin** is a direct thrombin inhibitor specifically approved for patients undergoing percutaneous coronary intervention.[22]
- **Fondaparinux** is a synthetic pentasaccharide Xa inhibitor which received a Grade 2C recommendation in the 2012 ACCP guidelines for the treatment of HIT. It has not been FDA approved for this indication, and controversy exists because several cases of HIT caused by fondaparinux have been reported.[22]
- **Apixaban** and **Rivaroxaban** are active site inhibitors for factor Xa with extensive clinical experience in the prevention of ischemic stroke in atrial fibrillation and treatment of venous thromboembolic disease. They were both added to the 2018 ASH guidelines for management of venous thromboembolism in HIT.
- **Warfarin** should not be used to treat a patient with HIT in the acute setting given the risk of venous limb gangrene and thrombosis with depletion of protein C given lack of heparin overlap at induction. Warfarin can be started for long-term anticoagulation when the patient has been anticoagulated with one of the above agents and the platelet count has reached a stable plateau of greater than 150,000. Warfarin should be started at a low dose (5–6 mg) with a standard INR goal of 2–3 and should overlap with one of the above agents for at least 5 days.[22]

Vaccine-Induced Immune Thrombotic Thrombocytopenia

GENERAL PRINCIPLES

- VITT or "thrombosis and thrombocytopenia syndrome," like HIT, is a disease of PF4 neoantigens which emerged with the development of vaccines for the SARS-CoV-2 pandemic. The epitope is unique from HIT and is not heparin dependent.[23]
- VITT is rare reported adverse event after vaccination and is difficult to quantify owing to low incidence numbers of cases during initial vaccination period and mitigation strategies for SARS-CoV-2 vaccines. Nearly all cases occurred with two adenoviral vector-based vaccines: ChAdOx1 nCoV-19 (Astrazeneca) and Ad26.COV2.S (Johnson & Johnson).[24]
- Cases typically occur 5–10 days after administration of an at-risk vaccine.
- The thrombotic phenotype is characterized by atypical distribution including cerebral venous sinus thrombosis, splanchnic vein thrombosis, and arterial thrombosis.
- Treatment is dependent on anticoagulation with nonheparinoid anticoagulants and high-dose IVIg. Additional treatment modalities that have been reported include corticosteroids, rituximab and eculizumab; however, current data are limited.[24]

Thrombocytosis

GENERAL PRINCIPLES

- A platelet count exceeding the reference range is called thrombocytosis. Thrombocytosis may be reactive or due to autonomous production of platelets by clonal megakaryocytes (essential thrombocythemia or other myeloproliferative disorders, covered in Chapter 10).
- **Reactive thrombocytosis** is thrombocytosis in the absence of a chronic myeloproliferative disorder. It can be seen in the setting of infection, surgery, malignancy, blood loss, iron deficiency, or postsplenectomy. The platelet count is expected to normalize when the underlying process is corrected.

REFERENCES

1. Provan D, Stasi R, Newland AC, et al. International consensus report on the investigation and management of primary immune thrombocytopenia. *Blood.* 2010;115(2):168–186.
2. Diz-Küçükkaya R, Chen J, Geddis A, et al. Chapter 119: Thrombocytopenia. In: Lichtman MA, Kipps TJ, Seligsohn U, et al., eds. *Williams Hematology.* 8th ed. McGraw-Hill; 2010.
3. Rodeghiero F, Stasi R, Gernsheimer T, et al. Standardization of terminology, definitions and outcome criteria in immune thrombocytopenic purpura of adults and children: report from an international working group. *Blood.* 2009;113(11):2386–2393.
4. Wei Y, Ji XB, Wang YW, et al. High-dose dexamethasone vs prednisone for treatment of adult immune thrombocytopenia: a prospective multicenter randomized trial. *Blood.* 2016;127(3):296–302.
5. Arnold DM, Dentali F, Crowther MA, et al. Systemic review: efficacy and safety of rituximab for adults with idiopathic thrombocytopenic purpura. *Ann Intern Med.* 2007;146(1):25–33.
6. Kuter DJ, Bussel JB, Lyons RM, et al. Efficacy of romiplostim in patients with chronic immune thrombocytopenic purpura: a double-blind randomised controlled trial. *Lancet.* 2008;371:395–403.
7. Saleh MN, Bussel JB, Cheng G, et al; EXTEND Study Group. Safety and efficacy of eltrombopag for the treatment of chronic immune thrombocytopenia: results of the long-term, open-label EXTEND study. *Blood.* 2013;121(3):537–545.
8. Sadler JE. Von Willebrand factor, ADAMTS13, and thrombotic thrombocytopenic purpura. *Blood.* 2008;112:11–18.
9. Cataland SR, Wu HM. Diagnosis and management of complement mediated thrombotic microangiopathies. *Blood Rev.* 2014;28:67–74.
10. Banatvala N, Griffin PM, Greene KD, et al; Hemolytic Uremic Syndrome Study Collaborators. The United States National Prospective Hemolytic Uremic Syndrome Study; microbiologic, serologic, clinical, and epidemiologic findings. *J Infect Dis.* 2001;183(7):1063–1070.
11. Bendapudi PK, Hurwitz S, Fry A, et al. Derivation and validation of the PLASMIC score for rapid assessment of adults with thrombotic microangiopathies: a cohort study. *Lancet Haematol.* 2017; 4(4):e157–e164.
12. George JN. How I treat patients with thrombotic thrombocytopenic purpura. *Blood.* 2010;116: 4060–4069.
13. Rathbone J, Kaltenthaler E, Richards A, Tappenden P, Bessey A, Cantrell A. A systematic review of eculizumab for atypical hemolytic uremic syndrome (aHUS). *BMJ Open.* 2013;3(11):e003573.
14. Scully M, Cataland SR, Peyvandi F, et al; HERCULES Investigators. Caplacizumab treatment for acquired thrombotic thrombocytopenic purpura. *N Engl J Med.* 2019;380(4):335–346.
15. Scully M, Cohen H, Cavenagh J, et al. Remission in acute refractory and relapsing thrombotic thrombocytopenic purpura following rituximab is associated with a reduction in IgG antibodies to ADAMTS-13. *Br J Haematol.* 2007;136(3):451–461.
16. Levi M. Disseminated intravascular coagulation. *Crit Care Med.* 2007;35:2191–2195.
17. Franchini M, Lippi G, Manzato F. Recent acquisitions in the pathophysiology, diagnosis and treatment of disseminated intravascular coagulation. *Thromb J.* 2006;4(4):4.
18. Bick R. Disseminated intravascular coagulation: a review of etiology, pathophysiology, diagnosis and management: guidelines for care. *Clin Appl Thromb Hemost.* 2002;8:1–31.
19. Martel N, Lee J, Wells PS. Risk for heparin-induced thrombocytopenia with unfractionated and low-molecular-weight heparin thromboprophylaxis: a meta-analysis. *Blood.* 2005;106:2710–2715.

20. Arepally GM, Ortel TL. Heparin-induced thrombocytopenia. *Annu Rev Med*. 2010;61:77–90.
21. Lo GK, Juhl D, Warkentin TE, Sigouin CS, Eichler P, Greinacher A. Evaluation of pretest clinical score (4 Ts) for the diagnosis of heparin-induced thrombocytopenia in two clinical settings. *J Thromb Haemost*. 2006;4:759–765.
22. Linkins LA, Dans AL, Moores LK, et al. Treatment and prevention of heparin-induced thrombocytopenia: Antithrombotic Therapy and Prevention of Thrombosis, 9th ed: American College of Chest Physicians evidence-based clinical practice guidelines. *Chest*. 2012;141(2 Suppl):e495S–E530S.
23. Huynh A, Kelton JG, Arnold DM, Daka M, Nazy I. Antibody epitopes in vaccine-induced immune thrombotic thrombocytopaenia. *Nature*. 2021;596:565–569.
24. Cines DB, Greinacher A. Vaccine-induced immune thrombotic thrombocytopenia. *Blood*. 2023; 141:1659–1665.

Introduction to Coagulation and Laboratory Evaluation of Coagulation

5

Nicholas C. Spies and Ronald Jackups Jr

INITIAL LABORATORY EVALUATION OF COAGULOPATHY

The hemostatic system is a complex, regulated sequence of reactions involving interactions among platelets, endothelium, and coagulation factors (Fig. 5-1; Tables 5-1 and 5-2).

Preanalytical Variables

The first step in the evaluation of abnormal coagulation test results is to consider factors in the patient and specimen that might give false test results.

- Contamination by anticoagulants
  - Heparin activates antithrombin, which then inactivates thrombin and factor Xa. Heparin can prolong activated partial thromboplastin time (aPTT) and, to a lesser extent, prothrombin time (PT).
  - Direct thrombin inhibitors and factor Xa inhibitors may prolong aPTT and PT.
- Incomplete collection tube filling and high hematocrit
  - Blue-capped tubes for coagulation testing contain a set amount of citrate that blocks the activation of coagulation factors in plasma.
  - Under-filled collection tubes have less coagulation factors relative to citrate, causing coagulation times to be falsely prolonged.
  - Patients with a hematocrit of >55% also have less plasma and, therefore, coagulation factors per tube, resulting in falsely prolonged clotting times.
- Plasma turbidity from lipids, bilirubin, or hemolysis can affect assays that measure transmission of light (chromogenic and optical end-point assays).

Complete Blood Count

- Leukocytosis or leukopenia may implicate a hematologic malignancy as the cause of a patient's coagulopathy.
- The complete blood count (CBC) can reveal clinically significant anemia or thrombocytopenia.
- The peripheral smear can reveal microangiopathy, platelet clumping, and red and white blood cell morphology.

Prothrombin Time/International Normalized Ratio

- Coagulation in vivo relies on the release of tissue factor from the vessel wall as it combines with circulating factor VIIa to catalyze the activation of factor X to Xa.
- When measuring the PT, tissue factor (along with phospholipid and $CaCl_2$, together called thromboplastin) is added to patient plasma, and the time to form a clot is measured in seconds.
- PT measures the *extrinsic* and *common* pathways and can detect deficiencies in factors **II, V, VII, X,** and **fibrinogen** (Fig. 5-1).
- The INR standardizes PT results between laboratories and is used to monitor warfarin therapy. INR is calculated with the following equation, where ISI is the International Sensitivity Index, a value that normalizes the activity of tissue factor for different manufacturers to a standard reference:

$$INR = (PT\ patient/PT\ laboratory\ mean)^{ISI}$$

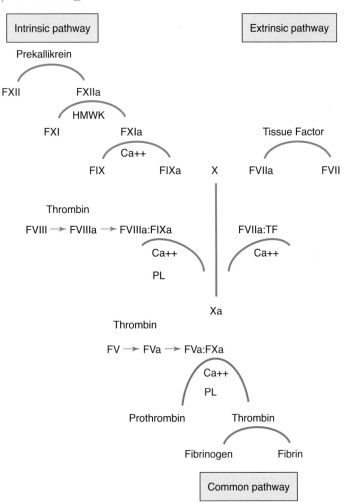

FIGURE 5-1. The normal coagulation cascade is split into the *intrinsic pathway* and the *extrinsic pathway*, either of which leads to activation of factor X to Xa. The factors after that point are referred to as the *common pathway*. Disorders of the intrinsic pathway are manifested as prolongation of the aPTT. Disorders of the extrinsic pathway are reflected by prolongation of the PT, whereas disorders of the common pathway may prolong both tests.

Activated Partial Thromboplastin Time

- The aPTT differs from the PT in that a contact activator such as silica is used in place of tissue factor to activate clotting.
- aPTT measures the *intrinsic* and *common* pathways of coagulation, and is affected by deficiencies in factors **II, V, VIII, IX, X, XI, XII,** and **fibrinogen**.

TABLE 5-1	HEMOSTASIS		
Process	Description	Abnormality	Symptoms of Dysfunction
Primary hemostasis	Platelet activation and aggregation	• Thrombocytopenia • Platelet dysfunction • von Willebrand factor (vWF) abnormalities	• Mucosal bleeding • Epistaxis • Gum bleeding • Hematochezia • Melena • Petechiae
Secondary hemostasis	Activation of the coagulation cascade and formation of a stable fibrin complex	Coagulation factor deficiency or dysfunction	• Hemarthroses • Intramuscular hemorrhage • Bleeding into deeper structures
Fibrinolysis	Lysis of fibrin plug, limiting the extent of thrombosis		

Thrombin Time

• The thrombin time (TT) measures the final step in the coagulation cascade, the ability of activated thrombin to convert fibrinogen to fibrin.
• It is often useful within the laboratory to differentiate heparin contamination from true coagulopathy.

WORKUP OF ELEVATED PT OR aPTT

The workup starts with a determination of which pathway of the coagulation cascade is defective (Table 5-2).[1]

Isolated Prolonged aPTT

• Common etiologies include factor deficiencies or inhibitors (especially VIII, IX, XI, and XII), von Willebrand disease (vWD), lupus anticoagulant (LA), heparin, and direct thrombin inhibitors (Fig. 5-2).
• The effects of heparin and direct thrombin inhibitors are ruled out with a TT.
• Further evaluation is with mixing studies and factor assays (see Advanced Coagulation Testing).

Prolonged PT

• Common etiologies include factor deficiencies or inhibitors (especially II, V, VII, and X), hypofibrinogenemia, warfarin, vitamin K deficiency, liver disease, disseminated intravascular coagulation (DIC), and factor Xa inhibitors (Fig. 5-3).
• If aPTT is also prolonged, DIC is a leading consideration. Workup should proceed as for isolated aPTT, including testing for fibrinogen and D-dimer.
• If PT is prolonged and aPTT is normal, proceed to mixing studies and factor assays.

TABLE 5-2　WORKUP OF HEMOSTASIS DISORDERS

Test	Measured Pathway	Components Added	Involved Factors	Conditions of Prolongation
PT	Extrinsic and common pathway (Fig. 5-1)	• Plasma • Thromboplastin (tissue factor and phospholipid) • Calcium	• Factor VII • Factor V • Factor X • Prothrombin • Fibrinogen	• Liver disease • Vitamin K deficiency • Warfarin • Factor Xa inhibitors • Rare congenital deficiency or inhibitor (factor VII)
aPTT	Intrinsic and common pathway (Fig. 5-1)	• Plasma • Phospholipid mixture and a surface-activating agent (e.g., silica) • Calcium	• Factor XII • Factor XI • Factor VIII • Factor IX • Factor V • Factor X • Prothrombin • Fibrinogen	• Factor deficiencies (VIII, IX, XI, and XII) • Factor inhibitors • Heparin-type products • Direct thrombin inhibitors • Lupus anticoagulant (LA) • vWD (if factor VIII is decreased)
TT	Common pathway (Fig. 5-1) Time of conversion of fibrinogen to fibrin	• Plasma • Thrombin (human or bovine)	• Fibrinogen	• Hypo- or dysfibrinogenemia • Increased fibrinogen degradation products • Monoclonal gammopathies • Heparin or heparin-like inhibitors • Direct thrombin inhibitors (lepirudin, argatroban, and bivalirudin) • Thrombin antibodies

PT, prothrombin time; aPTT, activated partial thromboplastin time; TT, thrombin time; vWF, von Willebrand factor.

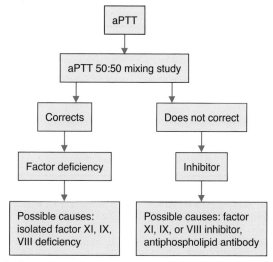

FIGURE 5-2. General workup of an elevated aPTT in the setting of a normal PT.

ADVANCED COAGULATION TESTING

Mixing Studies

A mixing study is a test of clotting performed on a mixture of patient plasma and known normal plasma to determine if a coagulation defect is due to a factor deficiency or an inhibitor (Table 5-3).

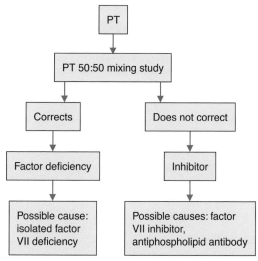

FIGURE 5-3. General workup of an elevated PT in the setting of a normal aPTT.

TABLE 5-3	MIXING STUDIES	
Result of Mixing Studies	Interpretation
Correction immediately and after 1 h	Factor deficiency
Correction (or near to correction) immediately, but no correction (PT or aPTT prolonged again) after 1 h	Factor inhibitors (specific inhibitory antibodies are time dependent, most typically factor VIII inhibitors)
No correction both immediately and after 1 h	Lupus anticoagulant

PT, prothrombin time; aPTT, activated partial thromboplastin time.

- Method: A patient's plasma is mixed with normal plasma at a 1:1 ratio and PT or aPTT tests are performed immediately and after incubation at 37°C.
- Interpretation:
  - When a patient has a factor deficiency, mixture with normal plasma will reverse the deficiency, and the *PT/aPTT will correct to normal* or near normal.
    - Because factor inhibitors are present in excess in an affected patient, they will inhibit coagulation in a mixture of patient and normal plasma. *Failure to correct* after incubation indicates an *inhibitor is present*.
    - Factor VIII inhibitors typically show more impaired correction after incubation, while LAs usually show minimal correction immediately.

Bethesda Assay

In patients with an inhibitor against a specific coagulation factor, the Bethesda assay can quantify the effect of the inhibitor.

- Method:
  - Factor activity assays are performed on serial dilutions of patient plasma mixed with normal plasma.
  - Inhibitor is quantified by Bethesda units (BU), which is the *amount of inhibitor necessary to neutralize 50% of factor activity in normal plasma.*
- Interpretation: For factor VIII inhibitors, a titer of BU <5 indicates a mild inhibitor that may be overwhelmed by larger infusions of factor VIII, whereas an inhibitor with a titer of *BU >5* will likely require infusion of a *bypass coagulation concentrate* such as recombinant factor VIIa or activated prothrombin concentrate complex to achieve hemostasis.

Factor Activity Assays

Factor assays are functional, clot-based tests of specific factors in the coagulation cascade. They can be used to diagnose a factor deficiency and to monitor therapy.

- Method: Serial dilutions are prepared with a patient's plasma and plasma known to be deficient in a specific factor. Coagulation times for these mixtures are measured and compared to a standard curve.
- Results are reported as percent activity compared to normal pooled plasma. Low values suggest factor deficiency or inhibitors.

Studies of Platelet Function
Platelet Function Analyzer-100 (PFA-100)
- The PFA-100 device initiates coagulation ex vivo and measures platelet response.[2]

- Method:
  - Citrated whole blood is aspirated through a microscopic hole (aperture) in a piece of nitrocellulose paper, which has been coated with agonists of platelet aggregation (collagen with either epinephrine [COL/EPI] or ADP [COL/ADP]).
  - Aspiration of the blood creates shear stress, promoting platelet aggregation. As platelets aggregate, they close over the hole in the nitrocellulose paper, resulting in a measured closure time.
- Interpretation:
  - The COL/EPI cartridge is sensitive to qualitative platelet disorders, especially aspirin effect and vWD.
  - The COL/ADP cartridge is less sensitive to aspirin but remains sensitive to vWD. Neither cartridge is sufficiently sensitive to ADP receptor inhibitors such as clopidogrel.
- Limitations:
  - Normal PFA-100 closure times do not rule out mild qualitative platelet disorders, and, if clinical suspicion is high, platelet aggregation studies should be performed.
  - PFA-100 has not been validated for preoperative assessment of bleeding risk in asymptomatic patients.
  - A hematocrit of <35% or a platelet count of <150,000/μL can produce falsely prolonged closure times.

Platelet Aggregation Studies
- These studies are indicated when an inherited qualitative defect in platelet function is suggested by the clinical or family history.
- Method: Various aggregating agents (arachidonic acid, collagen, ADP, epinephrine, and ristocetin) are added to the initially turbid platelet-rich plasma specimen. As platelets clump, more light passes through the plasma, and light transmission is measured and interpreted as normal or abnormal.
- Limitations:
  - This qualitative test is very labor intensive and should only be performed in highly selected cases.
  - Many prescription or over-the-counter medications can affect in vitro measurements of platelet function. Outpatients must discontinue aspirin-containing medications and clopidogrel (Plavix) for at least 7 days and NSAIDs for at least 72 hours before testing to avoid false-positive results.

LABORATORY EVALUATION OF SUSPECTED von WILLEBRAND DISEASE

Initial Diagnostic Approach
- vWD refers to a group of related disorders in which the ability of von Willebrand factor (vWF) to bind platelets or factor VIII is impaired, causing mucosal bleeding. The clinical presentation, severity, and initial laboratory findings can all vary depending on the type of vWD present. Most commonly, patients will have a normal PT and elevated or normal aPTT (Table 5-4).[3]
- Testing for vWD typically begins with measurement of vWF antigen levels, vWF activity, and factor VIII activity. No single test is adequate to diagnose vWD by itself. When abnormal tests suggest vWD, these tests should be repeated to confirm the diagnosis. See Chapter 7 for detailed discussion of vWD.

vWF Antigen Concentration (vWF:Ag)
- vWF:Ag levels are measured against a normal reference sample, and typically levels >50% of the reference are considered normal.

TABLE 5-4	LABORATORY EVALUATION OF von WILLEBRAND DISEASE				
	Factor VIII Activity	vWF Antigen	vWF Activity	RIPA	Multimer Pattern
Type 1: decrease in antigen and activity	↓	↓	↓	N/A	Decreased large multimers
Type 3: absence of vWF	↓	↓↓↓	↓↓↓	N/A	Absent
Type 2A: failure to make full length or increased cleavage	↓/−	↓	↓↓	↓↓	Absent large + intermediate multimers
Type 2B: increased binding to platelets, enhanced clearance	↓/−	↓	↓↓	↑↑	Absent large multimers
Type 2M: mutant vWF fails to bind platelets in the presence of shear stress or ristocetin	↓/−	↓	↓↓	↓↓	Normal
Type 2N: mutant vWF fails to bind factor VIII	↓↓	−	−	−	Normal
Platelet Type: GP1b defect on platelets, spontaneous vWF binding	↓/−	↓/-	↓↓	↑↑	Absent large multimers

vWF, von Willebrand factor; RIPA, ristocetin-induced platelet aggregation.

- vWF:Ag reference intervals are blood type dependent, and healthy type O subjects may have vWF concentrations as low as 40% of normal. Most laboratories do not provide blood type–specific reference intervals.
- The vWF:Ag concentration will be abnormally low in type 1, type 3, and some type 2 vWD.

vWF Activity Assays Ristocetin Cofactor Assay (vWF:RCo)

- In the ristocetin cofactor (RCo) assay, vWF activity is measured as the ability of the patient's plasma to aggregate platelets from a healthy donor in the presence of ristocetin, which promotes the binding of vWF to platelet glycoprotein (GP) Ib.
- Newer immunoassays can measure vWF activity using antibodies specific to the vWF: GPIb binding site.

TABLE 5-5 RIPA ANALYSIS RESULTS

Test Result	Type of vWD
Increased sensitivity to ristocetin; brisk platelet aggregation occurring at a low concentration of ristocetin (0.5 mg/mL)	2B
Decreased ristocetin sensitivity	2A (or 2M)

RIPA, ristocetin-induced platelet aggregation; vWF, von Willebrand factor.

- The activity result is compared to the vWF:Ag. An activity:antigen ratio of ≤0.7 suggests a qualitative defect of vWF, as found in vWD types 2A, 2B, and 2M.

Ristocetin-Induced Platelet Aggregation (RIPA)
- The aggregation of the patient's platelets is tested in the presence of different concentrations of ristocetin.
- Used for differentiating vWD type 2B from 2A or 2M (Table 5-5).
- Ristocetin-induced platelet aggregation (RIPA) is used only after the diagnosis of vWD is made and further clarification of subtype is necessary.

vWF Multimer Assay
- The multimer assay involves labor-intensive gel electrophoresis techniques to separate vWF into bands that normally range in size from 0.5 to 20 million daltons.
- Loss of large and intermediate multimers is seen in type 2A vWD. Loss of only large multimers is seen in type 2B vWD. Normal distribution of vWF multimers is seen in types 1, 2M, and 2N vWD.
- **This should not be part of initial workup for vWD**, as it is only indicated for suspected type 2.

Factor VIII Binding ELISA
- This test can aid in the diagnosis of type 2N vWD, where vWF's ability to bind factor VIII is impaired.

PFA-100
- This assay is sensitive to detect vWD but cannot differentiate between types.
- It may be used to monitor response to therapy with desmopressin acetate (DDAVP), which stimulates release of vWF from endothelial cells.

LABORATORY EVALUATION OF SUSPECTED ANTIPHOSPHOLIPID ANTIBODY SYNDROME

Antiphospholipid antibodies (LAs, anticardiolipin antibodies, and anti-β2 GP I antibodies) are acquired autoantibodies against phospholipid–protein complexes. Although these antibodies can prolong the PT and aPTT tests, they promote coagulation in vivo. They are associated with thromboembolic disease and recurrent fetal loss.

- Patients who test positive for one antiphospholipid antibody type may have multiple types, and should be tested for all antiphospholipid antibodies.
- Because transient elevations of antiphospholipid antibodies are common, *confirmatory testing is necessary after 12 weeks to establish a diagnosis.*

TABLE 5-6	**EFFECTS OF ANTICOAGULANTS ON LABORATORY TESTING AT THERAPEUTIC DOSAGES**				
Test	UFH	LMWH	DTI	DXaI	Warfarin
PT/INR	−	−	−/↑	−/↑	↑↑
aPTT	↑↑	−/↑	−/↑	−/↑	−/↑
Thrombin time	↑↑	−/↑	↑↑	−	−
Anti-Xa[a]	↑	↑	−	↑	−

[a]Anti-Xa is used to monitor therapy with UFH, LMWH, and DXaI. Ensure that your laboratory has an assay calibrated to the specific anticoagulant before ordering.
UFH, unfractionated heparin; LMWH, low–molecular-weight heparins; DTI, direct thrombin inhibitors; DXaI, direct factor Xa inhibitors.
Adapted from https://arupconsult.com/content/impacts-common-anticoagulants. See primary site for more comprehensive review.

- Anticardiolipin and anti-β2 GP I antibodies are usually detected directly by ELISA.
- There is **no specific antibody test for the diagnosis of LAs**.[4] Therefore, testing requires all of the following:
  - Demonstration of a prolonged, phospholipid-dependent clotting time (such as aPTT or common pathway clotting test).
  - Persistent prolongation of the clotting test in a mixing study.
  - Neutralization of the antiphospholipid antibody (correction of clotting time) by the addition of excess phospholipid.
  - Ruling out a specific factor inhibitor, such as an anti–factor VIII autoantibody.

INTERFERENCES OBSERVED BY COMMON ANTICOAGULANTS

Coagulation testing is often inextricably linked with pharmacologic intervention. Table 5-6 presents a set of the most common coagulation tests and the interferences that are to be expected when a patient is on therapeutic doses of popular anticoagulants.

- There is stark variation in the impact of certain therapeutics on these (and other) tests due to:
  - the laboratory's reagents[5] and testing strategy
  - the specimen's method of collection (e.g., heparinized line)
  - the assay being performed
  - the presence of other medications.

REFERENCES

1. Kamal AH, Tefferi A, Pruthi RK. How to interpret and pursue an abnormal prothrombin time, activated partial thromboplastin time, and bleeding time in adults. *Mayo Clin Proc.* 2007;82(7):864–873.
2. Hayward CP, Harrison P, Cattaneo M, Ortel TL, Rao AK; Platelet Physiology Subcommittee of the Scientific and Standardization Committee of the International Society on Thrombosis and Haemostasis. Platelet function analyzer (PFA)-100 closure time in the evaluation of platelet disorders and platelet function. *J Thromb Haemost.* 2006;4(2):312–319.
3. Sadler JE, Budde U, Eikenboom JC, et al; Working Party on von Willebrand Disease Classification. Update on the pathophysiology and classification of von Willebrand disease: a report of the Subcommittee on von Willebrand Factor. *J Thromb Haemost.* 2006;4(10):2103–2114.

4. Bonomi AB. Testing for lupus anticoagulants: all that a clinician should know. *Lupus.* 2009;18(4): 291–298.
5. Dale BJ, Ginsberg JS, Johnston M, Hirsh J, Weitz JI, Eikelboom JW. Comparison of the effects of apixaban and rivaroxaban on prothrombin and activated partial thromboplastin times using various reagents. *J Thromb Haemost.* 2014;12(11):1810–1815. Erratum in: *J Thromb Haemost.* 2015;13(3):489.
6. Moser KA, Smock KJ. Impacts of common anticoagulants on coagulation testing. ARUP Consult®. Accessed January 8, 2024. https://arupconsult.com/content/impacts-common-anticoagulants

Thrombotic Disease

6

Joshua I. Siner and Kristen M. Sanfilippo

T hrombotic disease refers to the inappropriate formation of a clot in the venous or arterial circulation. Arterial and venous thrombi classically form in the presence of **Virchow triad:** hypercoagulability, stasis, or nonphysiologic blood flow, and endothelial damage. Embolism of these clots can occur. Risk factors for venous thrombosis include immobility, surgery, increasing age, obesity, pregnancy, and an inherited or acquired hypercoagulable state (Table 6-1).[1] Thrombotic disease often results from interactions between genetic predispositions and environmental factors. Evaluation of patients presenting with thrombosis includes identification of risk factors, recommendations on appropriate anticoagulant management and duration of therapy, and in carefully selected cases, workup for thrombophilia or hypercoagulable state.

Deep Venous Thrombosis and Pulmonary Embolus

GENERAL PRINCIPLES

Definition

The term venous thromboembolism (VTE) encompasses both deep venous thrombosis (DVT) and pulmonary embolism (PE). DVT can be classified as proximal or distal, superficial, or deep. A proximal lower extremity DVT occurs in or proximal to the popliteal vein,

TABLE 6-1	CAUSES OF HYPERCOAGULABILITY LEADING TO VENOUS THROMBOEMBOLISM
Acquired Cause	**Inherited Cause**
Surgery/trauma	Factor V Leiden mutation
Malignancy	Prothrombin G20210A mutation
Myeloproliferative disorders	Hyperhomocysteinemia[a]
Pregnancy	Protein C deficiency
Oral contraceptives	Protein S deficiency
Immobilization	Antithrombin deficiency
Congestive heart failure	Increased factor VIII activity
Nephrotic syndrome	
Obesity	
Antiphospholipid antibodies[a]	
Lupus anticoagulant	
Anticardiolipin antibodies	

[a]Hyperhomocysteinemia and antiphospholipid antibodies are considered risk factors for both venous and arterial thrombosis.

whereas distal DVT occurs anywhere inferiorly. PE can be characterized as central (main pulmonary artery, lobar, or segmental arteries) or distal (subsegmental arteries). If a PE significantly impedes blood flow it can lead to pulmonary infarction.

Epidemiology

The annual incidence of DVT is approximately 1 per 1,000 persons. Prevalence of PE in patients with proximal DVT has been shown to be 40–50% in several studies, with some showing a higher prevalence of silent PE.[1-3] Mortality in PE has been estimated to be as high as 8%, even with therapy (e.g., anticoagulant therapy).[4]

Prevention

Primary prevention of VTE in high-risk patients is essential. Risk factors for VTE include, but are not limited to, infection, congestive heart failure, malignancy, stroke, acute pulmonary disease, acute rheumatic disease, inflammatory bowel disease, critical illness, pregnancy and postpartum, and surgery. Expert opinion recommends that all hospitalized medical patients older than 40 years of age, who are expected to have at least 3 days of inpatient stay, and who have one risk factor, should be provided with DVT prophylaxis. Prophylaxis can be nonpharmacologic, with compression stockings or pneumatic compression devices; however, there are no large, blinded trials proving that these interventions prevent VTE in medical patients. For patients without a contraindication, pharmacologic anticoagulant therapy is the preferred mechanism of prophylaxis. Subcutaneous unfractionated heparin three times a day, low–molecular-weight heparin (LMWH) once daily, and fondaparinux once daily have been shown to have equal efficacy in preventing VTE with minimal increased bleeding risk in hospitalized patients.[5]

DIAGNOSIS

Clinical Presentation

History

Symptoms of acute DVT and PE can be variable[6,7]; however, common symptoms include:

- DVT—acute onset of pain or cramping, swelling/edema, and/or erythema
- PE—dyspnea, pleuritic chest pain, cough, anxiety, hypoxemia, syncope, and/or hemoptysis

Physical Examination

- DVT—unilateral extremity tenderness, erythema, and edema; unequal circumference of extremities
- PE—tachypnea, tachycardia, and pleural rub

Diagnostic Testing

Laboratories

D-dimer can be used as an initial screening test, particularly in patients with low suspicion of VTE. D-dimer is the result of fibrin breakdown and is generated in many other circumstances, including infections, tumors, surgery, trauma, extensive burning, bruises, ischemic heart disease, stroke, peripheral artery disease, aneurysms, inflammatory disease, and pregnancy. The sensitivity of the D-dimer test in clinical trials ranges from 93% to 100%; however, the specificity ranges from 35% to 75%. Therefore, it is *effective for ruling out the diagnosis if negative*, but a positive D-dimer assay is not specific and additional workup is required. In cases of high clinical suspicion, additional testing should be pursued despite a negative D-dimer.

Electrocardiography

The most common finding in PE is **sinus tachycardia**. The classic ECG changes associated with PE are S wave in lead I, Q wave in lead III, and inverted T wave in lead III (**SI, QIII, TIII**). However, these findings are neither sensitive nor specific for PE (present in 13.5% of patients with PE). **New right axis deviation** can be a sign of right-sided heart strain from PE.

Imaging

- **Doppler ultrasonography** is the test of choice for diagnosing DVT.[6] The gold standard for DVT diagnosis is venography, which has sensitivity and specificity >97%.
  - A positive Doppler study should lead one to treat the patient.
  - A negative study largely rules out the diagnosis, and alternative diagnoses should be considered.
  - In cases of very high suspicion and negative Doppler study, venography, or CT (or MR) venography can be considered, especially in the case of proximal (i.e., Iliac disease)
- The most commonly used tests for the diagnosis of PE are **CT angiography** (CTA) of the lungs or **ventilation/perfusion scans** (V/Q scans). However, when clinical probability and the results of imaging are inconsistent, additional diagnostic workup is warranted.[7,8]
  - Determining a clinical pretest probability of PE is necessary before performing any diagnostic study. Objective criteria such as the **Wells Criteria** (Table 6-2) are commonly used to determine the pretest probability.
  - The **PIOPED trial** used V/Q scans in the diagnosis of acute PE (Table 6-3).[9]
  - The **PIOPED II trial** published in 2006 used CTA of the lungs and CT venography of the lower extremities to diagnose PE (Table 6-3).[10] As shown in Table 6-3, in patients with a high pretest probability and negative CTA, PE is still present in 40% of cases; therefore, these patients should undergo further testing, such as venous compression ultrasonography of the lower extremities or CT venogram of the lower extremities.
  - Based on the results of these trials, an algorithm for the diagnosis of PE has been recommended (Fig. 6-1).[11]

In special cases, such as patients with renal failure, patients with allergy to contrast dye, women of childbearing age, and pregnant women, the recommendations are guided by expert opinion. In these patients, the algorithm should begin with D-dimer testing followed by venous ultrasonography in the majority of cases. Patients with a positive D-dimer and a negative ultrasound will then need additional testing. V/Q scanning can then be used, with the realization that the testing may be nondiagnostic—and difficult to interpret in the setting of abnormal lung architecture.

TABLE 6-2	SIMPLIFIED WELLS CRITERIA FOR PRETEST PROBABILITY OF PE	
Variable		**Points**
Clinical signs and symptoms of DVT		3
Alternative diagnosis less likely than PE		3
Heart rate >100/min		1.5
Immobilization (>3 d) or surgery in previous 4 wks		1.5
Previous PE or DVT		1.5
Hemoptysis		1
Malignancy (receiving treatment, treated in the last 6 mo, or palliative)		1

Probability: ≤2 = low; 2–6 = intermediate; >6 = high.
DVT, deep venous thrombosis; PE, pulmonary embolus.

TABLE 6-3 PIOPED TRIALS

PIOPED, V/Q Scan for the Diagnosis of PE

V/Q Scan Category	80–100%	Clinical Probability of PE 20–79%	0–19%	All
High probability	96%	88%	56%	87%
Intermediate probability	66%	28%	16%	30%
Low probability	40%	16%	4%	14%
Near normal/normal	0%	6%	2%	4%

PIOPED II, CT for the Diagnosis of PE

Clinical Probability	PPV CTA	CTA + CTV	NPV CTA	CTA + CTV
High probability	96%	96%	60%	82%
Intermediate probability	92%	90%	89%	92%
Low probability	58%	57%	96%	97%

PPV, positive predictive value; NPV, negative predictive value; CTA, CT angiography; CTV, CT lower extremity venogram.

TREATMENT

Treatment of VTE with unfractionated heparin or LMWH should begin promptly after the diagnosis is established or, in situations of high clinical suspicion, while awaiting confirmatory studies.[12] Thrombolytics may be considered in selected patients with hemodynamically significant PE. Guidance for systemic or directed thrombolytics and for mechanical thrombectomy will not be reviewed here (and is reviewed in *The Washington Manual of*

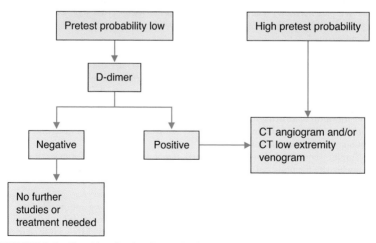

FIGURE 6-1. Algorithm for the diagnosis of PE. (Data from Writing Group for the Christopher Study Investigators. Effectiveness of managing suspected pulmonary embolism using an algorithm combining clinical probability, D-dimer testing, and computed tomography. *JAMA*. 2006;295:172–179.)

Critical Care). Individuals who are actively bleeding or at high risk for bleeding should be considered for inferior vena cava (IVC) filter placement, however IVC filters should not be considered for long-term management as they can serve as a thrombogenic nidus over time.

Medications

Most common medications used in the treatment of VTE are summarized in Table 6-4.

- **Selection of anticoagulant therapy**
  - Meta-analysis of available trials has shown that LMWH is superior to unfractionated heparin for the initial treatment (first 5–7 days) of VTE, with a lower overall mortality over the first 3–6 months and a reduced incidence of major bleeding during initial therapy.[13]
  - Common options for long-term therapy (therapy following the first 5–7 days of VTE treatment) are listed in Table 6-4. For most, direct oral anticoagulants (DOACs) are preferred over vitamin K antagonists (VKAs) for long-term therapy.[14] Some patient populations have additional considerations:
    - **Cancer:** In patients with cancer, LMWH is superior to VKAs in reducing the risk of recurrent VTE without increasing the risk of major or clinically relevant nonmajor bleeding.[15] Subsequently, the DOACs were compared to LMWH across six randomized controlled trials. A meta-analysis of these trials found that long-term treatment with DOAC versus LMWH was associated with a 33% reduction in risk of recurrent VTE with no significant increase in risk of major bleeding, but with a significant increase in the risk of clinically relevant nonmajor bleeding (risk ratio 1.63; 95% CI 1.25–2 .11).[16] It is important to note that the pooled evidence mostly consists of outcomes with the oral anti-Xa inhibitors and not dabigatran. Of note, a predominance of the bleeding events with DOACs occurs in patients with gastrointestinal and genitourinary tumors. Algorithms exist for considerations in selection of anticoagulant therapy in this population.
    - **Antiphospholipid antibody syndrome (APS):** VKAs are the treatment of choice for patients with thrombotic APS (history of arterial or venous TE). Meta-analysis of 472 patients found that treatment with DOACs versus VKAs was associated with a fivefold higher risk of subsequent arterial events. There was no difference in the risk of recurrent VTE.[17]
    - **VTE during pregnancy:** Pregnancy and postpartum increase the risk of VTE. As warfarin is teratogenic, heparins (UFH or LMWH) are the mainstay of therapy. Unfractionated or LMWH is recommended antepartum. Postpartum, the decision is based on maternal lactation status. Limited data exists regarding the safety of DOACs during lactation, thus LMWH or VKAs are recommended in this setting.
- The **duration of anticoagulant therapy** is variable and depends on a number of factors, including underlying thrombotic risk, risk of anticoagulant-related bleeding and classification of the inciting thrombotic event.[14]
  - Current recommendations[14] suggest that 3–6 months of treatment (primary treatment) is adequate for provoked DVT (i.e., an identifiable and reversible risk factor, such as surgery), while patients with chronic risk factors or unprovoked VTE should be considered for indefinite anticoagulant therapy.
  - For patients with recurrent VTE, the recommendation is lifelong anticoagulation.
    Extended dosing of anticoagulant therapy: For patients recommended indefinite anticoagulant therapy, the AMPLIFY-EXT (apixaban) and EINSTEIN-CHOICE (rivaroxaban) studies demonstrated that after completing 6–12 months of therapeutic anticoagulation dosed-reduced FXa inhibitors (apixaban 2.5 mg twice daily and rivaroxaban 10 mg once daily) were as protective as continued treatment dose (apixaban 5 mg twice daily and rivaroxaban 20 mg once daily). This strategy can be considered

TABLE 6-4 COMMON MEDICATIONS USED IN THE TREATMENT OF VTE[a]

Anticoagulant	Mechanism of Action/ Nomenclature	Initial Treatment Dose(s)	Subsequent Dose	Contraindications
Warfarin	Oral vitamin K antagonist	2–10 mg; overlapped for 4–5 d with a faster-acting anticoagulant. Goal INR 2–3 (see www.WarfarinDosing.org)	Adjusted per INR[b]	Pregnancy
Apixaban	Oral direct FXa inhibitor	10 mg PO bid × 7 d	5 mg PO bid 2.5 mg PO bid for maintenance phase	
Edoxaban	Oral direct FXa inhibitor	Initially treat with parenteral anticoagulant for 5–10 d	60 mg PO daily OR 30 mg PO daily (if CrCl 30–50 mL/min, body weight ≤60 kg, or using strong P-gp inhibitor)	
Rivaroxaban	Oral direct FXa inhibitor	15 mg PO bid × 21 d	20 mg PO daily 10 mg PO daily for maintenance phase	CrCl <30 mL/min
Dabigatran	Oral direct thrombin (FIIa) inhibitor	Initially treat with parenteral anticoagulant for 5–10 d	150 mg bid (CrCl >30 mL/min)	CrCl <15 mL/min
Dalteparin	Subcutaneous FXa > FIIa inhibition	200 IU/kg SC daily	Transition to oral agent OR for cancer patients after 30 d of initial therapy, reduce dose to 150 U/kg SC daily	HIT; hypersensitivity to pork
Enoxaparin	Subcutaneous FXa > FIIa inhibition	1 mg/kg SC q12h or 1.5 mg/kg SC q24h. Lower dose if CrCl <30 mL/min	Transition to long-term oral agent OR continue initial dosing	HIT, hypersensitivity to pork
Fondaparinux	Subcutaneous FXa inhibitor	Weight <50 kg: 5 mg SC daily Weight 50–100 kg: 7.5 mg SC daily Weight >100 kg: 10 mg SC daily	Transition to long-term oral agent OR continue initial dosing	CrCl <30 mL/min
Unfractionated heparin	Intravenous or subcutaneous binds to antithrombin	Continuous IV: Goal aPTT 2–2.5× normal range or heparin anti-Xa 0.3–0.7 units/ mL	Transition to long-term oral agent	HIT, hypersensitivity to pork

[a]Overlap therapy of warfarin and a parenteral agent should be at least 5 days until the INR is at least 2.
[b]Adapted from Bhat P, Dretler A, Gdowski M, et al. *The Washington Manual of Medical Therapeutics.* 35th ed. Wolters Kluwer Health; 2016.

for many patients on indefinite therapy. Insufficient data exists on dose-reduced therapy in patients with thrombophilia, cancer, and at extremes of body weight.

Other Nonpharmacologic Therapies

Inferior Vena Cava Filters

- The use of IVC filters has increased significantly in the past 10–20 years, even as evidence supporting their use remains insufficient.[18] Only one randomized controlled trial has compared the use of IVC filters with anticoagulation to the use of anticoagulation alone. At 2 years of follow-up, there was a mild increase in PEs (largely asymptomatic) in patients without a filter and an increase in DVT and postthrombotic syndrome (PTS) in patients with a filter. Mortality was similar between patients with and without a filter.
- The only currently recommended indication for IVC filter placement is in patients with an absolute contraindication to anticoagulation. Additional indication considerations require consideration on a patient-by-patient basis.

SPECIAL CONSIDERATIONS

- **Cerebral venous sinus thrombosis (CVST)[19]:** Although rare, CVST is important to identify because, with appropriate treatment, patients often have a good neurologic outcome. Occlusion of cerebral veins leads to localized brain edema and venous infarction, whereas occlusion of the venous sinuses leads to intracranial hypertension. About 85% of patients with CVST have an identifiable risk factor (e.g., thrombophilia, combination oral contraceptive use, recent trauma [including lumbar puncture], and infection). CVST in the setting of adenoviral-based vaccines against Sars-COV-2 vaccine-induced thrombotic thrombocytopenia (VITT) is reviewed in Chapter 4. The most common presenting symptom is unrelenting headache. The diagnosis can be difficult to make, with an average delay of 7 days from initial presentation to diagnosis. **Venography** is the current recommended diagnostic modality.

Even with the theoretical risk of causing cerebral hemorrhage, rapid initiation of anticoagulation is the treatment of choice, with therapy continuing for at least 6 months. Endovascular thrombolysis has been attempted in some patients.

- **Budd–Chiari syndrome:** Budd–Chiari syndrome encompasses various disease states that result in hepatic vein occlusion. Thrombosis of the hepatic veins leads to hepatomegaly, right-upper quadrant pain, and other sequelae of acute or chronic liver disease. The most common causes of Budd–Chiari syndrome in the Western world are the myeloproliferative neoplasms. All patients should undergo screening for thrombophilia and malignancy including myeloproliferative neoplasms and paroxysmal nocturnal hematuria. The decision to use anticoagulation should be based on the extent of liver disease and subsequent risk of bleeding. In certain cases, liver transplantation is the treatment of choice.
- **Mesenteric and portal venous thrombosis:** The main risk factors for portal vein thrombosis include local causes (cirrhosis with portal hypertension, pancreatitis, tumor, infection) as well as thrombophilic states such as myeloproliferative neoplasms. The decision to anticoagulate is complex and should be made with a multidisciplinary team (e.g., hematology, hepatology, interventional radiology, etc.). Choice of anticoagulant is supported by sparse data, with selection based on underlying hepatic function and additional patient risk factors for bleeding. Mesenteric venous thrombosis presents acutely, with a mortality rate ranging from 20% to 50%. The usual presentation is severe abdominal pain and bloody diarrhea. Risk factors include intra-abdominal inflammation and thrombophilias. Myeloproliferative neoplasms are only rarely associated with thrombosis of the mesenteric veins. Treatment includes anticoagulation and surgery if the bowel becomes necrotic.
- **Renal vein thrombosis:** Renal vein thrombosis is frequently asymptomatic and incidentally discovered. These patients should be evaluated for nephrotic syndrome as well as

other more common thrombophilias or underlying cancer. Treatment involves anticoagulation, with thrombolysis reserved for patients with an acute and marked deterioration in renal function due to thrombosis.

- **Upper extremity DVT:** Risk factors specific to upper extremity DVT include indwelling central venous catheters, local trauma, and thoracic outlet syndrome. Patients usually present with unilateral upper extremity edema. Up to one-third of upper extremity DVTs result in PE, so treatment is essential. While there are limited studies guiding treatment, it is generally recommended to fully anticoagulate patients for at least 3 months.

COMPLICATIONS

- Chronic pulmonary thromboembolic disease can result in **pulmonary hypertension**, leading to right-sided heart failure. Patients presenting with submassive or massive pulmonary emboli are at greatest risk and should be referred to a pulmonary specialist if their pulmonary pressures do no normalize after treatment. Patients with chronic thromboembolic pulmonary hypertension (CTEPH) should be managed by an interdisciplinary team including pulmonary medicine and cardiothoracic surgery. Long-term therapy generally consists of anticoagulation, pulmonary hypertension-specific therapy and evaluation for invasive treatments (i.e., pulmonary artery thromboendarterectomy or balloon angioplasty).
- **PTS** is a common complication of lower-extremity DVT.[20]
  - Symptoms vary from venous stasis pigment changes and/or slight pain and swelling to more severe manifestations such as chronic pain, intractable edema, and leg ulcers. Symptoms can be profound and affect quality of life.
  - Treatment of PTS consists of compression therapy, pharmacologic therapy (e.g., anticoagulation, horse chestnut seed extract, diosmin), wound care, and occasionally endovascular or surgical intervention.
  - Trials assessing strategies to prevent PTS are controversial, but include: prompt initiation of anticoagulant therapy at VTE diagnosis, early incorporation of compression therapy into VTE treatment, and prevention of recurrent VTE.

Inherited Thrombophilia

GENERAL PRINCIPLES

Inherited causes of thrombophilia can be either gain-of-function disorders, in which mutations lead to prothrombotic activity (activated protein C resistance/factor V Leiden, prothrombin G20210A), or loss-of-function disorders, which result in deficiencies of endogenous anticoagulants (antithrombin, protein C, and protein S). Common mutations include factor V Leiden and prothrombin G20210A mutations, while other thrombophilias, such as antithrombin, protein C, and protein S deficiencies, are rare. **When not to test**—while thrombotic diseases are frequently a diagnosis made in the setting of a hospitalization all inherited thrombophilia testing should be deferred to outpatient follow-up, with the rare exception of heparin resistance. Inpatient thrombophilia testing generates inconclusive results, has limited impact on initial anticoagulation choices, and generates high medical expenditures for patients and health systems with little benefit.

Etiology

- **Activated protein C resistance/factor V Leiden**
  - This is the most common hereditary thrombophilia in the Caucasian population (Table 6-5).[21,22] More than 90% of patients with activated protein C resistance have

TABLE 6-5	THE PREVALENCE AND THE RISK OF THROMBOSIS OF DIFFERENT CAUSES OF THROMBOPHILIA		
Causes of Thrombophilia	Prevalence	Prevalence in VTE Patients	Relative Risk of Thrombosis
Factor V Leiden	4% (in Caucasian, much less in other population)	20% (40% in patients with high risk of thrombophilia)	4–5 (heterozygous) 24–80 (homozygous)
Prothrombin G20210A mutation	2% (in Caucasian, much less in other population)	7%	2.8 (heterozygous)
Antithrombin deficiency	0.02%	2%	5
Protein C deficiency	0.2–0.4%	3.7%	3.1
Protein S deficiency	0.16–0.20%	2.3%	N/A
Elevated factor VIII levels	10%	25%	4.8

VTE, venous thromboembolism.

G1691A mutation in the factor V gene (factor V Leiden), which decreases the rate of proteolytic cleavage by activated protein C. Activated protein C resistance test should be used for screening before obtaining factor V Leiden mutation genotype. This test is performed by a clotting assay in which patient plasma is diluted in factor V–deficient plasma; in a positive test, the addition of activated protein C fails to cleave factor V, resulting in prolongation of PTT. Diagnosis is often confirmed by detection of the factor V Leiden mutation by a DNA-based assay. The risk for VTE in heterozygous patients who use combination oral contraceptives is increased 35-fold and should be avoided. Population studies have shown the presence of a heterozygous factor V Leiden mutation alone in the absence of thrombosis is insufficient to warrant prophylactic anticoagulation.[23]

- **Prothrombin G20210A mutation**
  ○ The prothrombin G20210A mutation is a substitution mutation that results in increased levels of plasma prothrombin, leading to increased generation of thrombin. Assays of prothrombin time or prothrombin antigen are neither specific nor sensitive enough for diagnosis; therefore, diagnosis is made by genotype analysis.
- **Antithrombin deficiency**
  ○ Antithrombin is a plasma protease inhibitor that irreversibly binds and neutralizes thrombin and factors Xa, IXa, and XIa, resulting in reversal of coagulation cascade. This reaction is accelerated by heparin. Therefore, antithrombin deficiency increases the risk of thrombosis. Antithrombin deficiency is relatively rare but is considered one of the more severe thrombophilias.

    Type I antithrombin deficiency is characterized by both decreased levels and decreased activity, whereas type II is characterized by decreased protease activity, with defects in either the reactive site (responsible for binding procoagulant proteases) or the heparin-binding site. Thus, resistance to the anticoagulant effects of heparin is seen in some patients. There is no difference in clinical severity between type I and type II.

Antithrombin activity assays and antigen levels are used to make the diagnosis. Acute thrombosis, heparin, liver disease, disseminated intravascular coagulation (DIC), nephrotic syndrome, and preeclampsia can all decrease antithrombin levels; therefore, diagnosis should not be made on the basis of levels obtained under these conditions.

Prospective studies indicate that the incidence of VTE in these patients is 4% per year. Nearly 70% of patients present with the first thrombotic event before the age of 35 years.

- **Protein C and S deficiency**
  - Proteins C and S are vitamin K–dependent endogenous anticoagulants. Homozygous protein C deficiency can cause neonatal purpura fulminans. Patients with either protein C or protein S deficiency can present with warfarin skin necrosis at the initiation of anticoagulation due to a transient hypercoagulable state.

    Protein C deficiency is diagnosed by an assay to detect activity, followed by immunoassays to differentiate type I (reduced antigen and activity) and type II (reduced activity) defects. Protein S binds to a plasma protein so that free protein S antigen and activity are used to screen for protein S deficiency and differentiate among type I (decreased antigen and activity), type II (decreased activity), and type III (low free protein S). DNA-based assays are not practical in both protein C and protein S deficiency, given that more than 150 mutations in the protein C gene have been described. Protein C and S levels are affected by liver disease, anticoagulation with warfarin, nephrotic syndrome, DIC, vitamin K deficiency, oral contraceptives, pregnancy, and hormone replacement therapy.

- **Elevated factor VIII levels**
  - Increased factor VIII levels have been associated with an increased risk of thrombosis (relative risk = 4.8). Elevated levels are found with increased age, obesity, pregnancy, surgery, inflammation, liver disease, hyperthyroidism, and diabetes. No gene alteration has been found, although familial clustering of increased factor VIII levels is noted. It is unclear how increased factor VIII levels lead to increased thrombotic risk and how elevated factor VIII levels may affect treatment of thromboembolism.

- **Hereditary thrombotic dysfibrinogenemia**
  - Dysfibrinogenemias are qualitative defects in the fibrin molecule. Multiple genetic defects have been described. These defects lead to VTE in 20% of patients and bleeding tendency in 25% of patients, but they are asymptomatic in 55%. Normal or low levels of fibrinogen and a prolonged thrombin time may be observed. This disorder is rare, and testing for it in patients with suspected thrombophilia is considered low priority.

DIAGNOSIS

- Screening for thrombophilia is controversial. The American Society of Hematology published guidance on thrombophilia screening in 2023, however, adoption of these guidelines is controversial. Screening should only be done only in a carefully selected population where results will inform management. Screening symptomatic and asymptomatic individuals and their family members for the presence of thrombophilia has both benefits and drawbacks. Benefits include a focus on prophylaxis with anticoagulant therapy during high-risk situations, such as surgery, immobilization, and pregnancy to prevent a first-time event, as well as an awareness of increased risk associated with oral contraceptive use, pregnancy, and hormone replacement therapy. Drawbacks may include medicolegal barriers to obtaining life insurance coverage, as well as over-anticoagulation exposure leading to unnecessary bleeding risk. Universal screening, even for women

considering hormonal therapy, oral contraceptives, or pregnancy, is not recommended, as it is not cost-effective and may deny women birth control options.
- **Consideration of a hypercoagulable workup** is usually recommended in patients with:
  - Recurrent VTE, especially unprovoked thrombosis, at a young age
  - Thrombosis at a young age (younger than 40 years of age)
  - Thrombosis at unusual sites (CVST, mesenteric vein, portal vein, hepatic vein)
  - Recurrent second or third trimester fetal loss, placental abruption, or severe preeclampsia (APS screening)
- The **optimal time for testing patients for hereditary defects** is not well defined. As discussed above, acute thrombosis can cause low levels of antithrombin, protein C, and protein S. Therapy with heparin reduces antithrombin levels, and warfarin reduces protein C and S levels. Therefore, it is usually recommended to test (if needed) at least 6 weeks after the thrombotic event. Anticoagulant therapy can affect thrombophilia testing results and should be avoided when possible.[24]

TREATMENT

There are few clinical trial data to provide evidence-based recommendations for the duration of anticoagulation in patients with hereditary thrombophilia.

- Many experts would recommend a **longer duration of anticoagulation in patients with:**
  - Active cancer
  - Multiple allelic abnormalities
  - Antithrombin deficiency
  - Protein C or S deficiency
  - More than one thrombotic event
  - APS
- Some experts recommend **lifelong anticoagulation for patients with:**
  - Two or more unprovoked VTEs
  - Unprovoked VTE with antithrombin deficiency
  - Multiple genetic abnormalities
  - One life-threatening VTE
- In all patients with a history of a thromboembolic event, regardless of the presence or absence of hereditary thrombophilias, prophylaxis should be considered (risk vs. benefit) with unfractionated heparin or LMWH during high-risk situations including surgery, trauma, and immobilization. Women should also be advised of the increased risk of recurrent thrombotic events with combination oral contraceptives, hormone replacement therapy, and pregnancy.

Arterial Thromboembolism

GENERAL PRINCIPLES

Definition

Arterial thromboses are those that lodge in the arterial side of the circulatory system. There are two types:

- In situ thrombosis due to a damaged artery (e.g., by trauma, vasculitis, or foreign body)
- Embolization from a proximal source (e.g., from the atria in atrial fibrillation, a ventricular or arterial aneurysm, a proximal clot formed in an area of damaged artery, or a venous clot that passes into the arterial circulation through a heart defect including atrial septal defect)

Etiology

Possible hypercoagulable states leading to arterial thrombosis include hyperhomocystein-emia, antiphospholipid syndrome, heparin-induced thrombocytopenia (HIT), myeloproliferative neoplasms, and paroxysmal nocturnal hemoglobinuria. Of note, these disorders may present with either venous or arterial thrombosis.

Risk Factors

- Smoking
- Hypertension
- Atherosclerosis
- Turbulent blood flow
- Diabetes
- Chronic inflammation
- Hyperlipidemia
- Hypercoagulable state

DIAGNOSIS

Clinical Presentation

Symptoms are typically related to end-organ damage from acute ischemia stemming from the location of the clot.

TREATMENT

The initial management of an arterial thrombus includes workup to establish the source, for embolic, or to determine the etiology of in situ clot. The presence of a hypercoagulable state as the etiology of the arterial thrombus may be considered if there are no readily identifiable risk factors.

Special Considerations

Hyperhomocysteinemia

GENERAL PRINCIPLES

Homocysteine is an intermediate amino acid formed in the metabolism of methionine. Elevated levels of homocysteine are associated with risk of arterial and venous thromboses. Hyperhomocysteinemia can be due to inheritance of enzyme defects involved in the homo-cysteine metabolic pathways or can be acquired. Severe hyperhomocysteinemia (plasma levels >100 µmol/L) is most commonly due to defects in cystathionine B-synthase, which results in homocystinuria, intellectual disability, and thromboses at a young age. The most common genetic defect in mild homocysteinemia (plasma levels, 15–40 µmol/L) results in reduced activity of the enzyme methylenetetrahydrofolate reductase (MTHFR). However, a large study found no association between mutations in MTHFR (MTHFR 677C → T) and risk of VTE.[25]

Acquired Causes

- Vitamin B_{12}, vitamin B_6, and folate deficiencies
- Chronic renal failure

- Hypothyroidism
- Cancer
- Increasing age
- Smoking
- Inflammatory bowel disease
- Psoriasis
- Rheumatoid arthritis
- Methotrexate, phenytoin, and theophylline

DIAGNOSIS

The **diagnosis** is made by measuring fasting homocysteine plasma levels.

TREATMENT

Patients deficient in folate, vitamin B_6, or vitamin B_{12} can be supplemented with these vitamins at sufficient doses to achieve normal levels. In the absence of specific deficiencies, plasma homocysteine levels can be reduced by up to 50% by administration of folate at doses of 1–2 mg/d. In patients with severe hyperhomocysteinemia due to cystathionine B-synthase deficiency, treatment with vitamin B supplements improves homocysteine levels. In several recent studies, patients with first-time events, either arterial (stroke, myocardial infarction [MI]) or VTE, treated with vitamin supplementation (e.g., folic acid, vitamin B_6, vitamin B_{12}) had reductions in homocysteine levels but no protection from recurrent MI, recurrent VTE, or progression of peripheral vascular disease. Therefore, the role of homocysteine in thrombosis is still debated.

Antiphospholipid Syndrome

GENERAL PRINCIPLES

Antiphospholipid syndrome is characterized by recurrent venous or arterial thrombosis and/or recurrent pregnancy morbidity/fetal loss and the presence of persistent antiphospholipid antibodies (anticardiolipin antibodies, lupus anticoagulants, anti–B_2-glycoprotein 1).[26] **Antiphospholipid antibodies** are autoantibodies that recognize phospholipids and/ or phospholipid-binding proteins. Lupus anticoagulants are IgG or IgM antibodies that react with negatively charged phospholipids. In vitro, they appear as anticoagulants and interfere with membrane surfaces in clotting assays, resulting in false prolongation of the aPTT and, rarely, the PT. The pathogenesis of antiphospholipid antibodies is thought to involve the binding and subsequent activation of endothelial cells, platelets, and complement to promote thrombosis and the inhibition of the fibrinolytic pathway. The syndrome is considered primary if there is no accompanying autoimmune disease and secondary if the patient has systemic lupus erythematosus (SLE).

DIAGNOSIS
Clinical Presentation

Although VTE is more common (DVT, PE, or both), patients may present with arterial occlusions, the most frequent involving the brain, followed by coronary occlusions. Any vessel or vascular bed may be involved and diverse presentations, such as intestinal, pancreatic, or splenic infarction, ARDS, retinitis, and acute renal failure may occur. Other features seen include thrombocytopenia, hemolytic anemia, cardiac valve vegetations or thickening, and livedo reticularis or vasculopathy. **Catastrophic antiphospholipid syndrome**, characterized by multiple simultaneous thromboses, occurs in <1% of patients and is associated with multiorgan failure and death.

Diagnostic Testing

Diagnosis relies on meeting at least one of the clinical and one of the laboratory criteria as below.

- **Clinical**
  - One or more episodes of venous, arterial, or small vessel thrombosis
  - Pregnancy morbidity—at least one unexplained death of a morphologically normal fetus beyond the 10th week of gestation; at least three unexplained spontaneous abortions before the 10th week of gestation; or one or more premature births secondary to eclampsia, preeclampsia, or placental insufficiency before the 34th week of gestation
- **Laboratory-positive testing must be present on two or more occasions at least 12 weeks apart with the first positive test no more than 5 years from the clinical event.**
  - **Lupus anticoagulant:** Testing should include two testing methods (e.g., dilute Russell viper venom assay or phospholipid neutralization assay). False positive results can occur in patients on an anticoagulant.
  - **Anticardiolipin antibody and Anti–B$_2$-glycoprotein** 1 of IgG or IgM isotype presents at medium or high titer (>40 GPL or MPL, or >99th percentile). The IgG isotypes have a higher association with clinical events versus the IgM isotypes. IgA isotypes are not considered part of the diagnostic criteria.

TREATMENT

The treatment of antiphospholipid syndrome is lifelong anticoagulation. Several trials have compared treatment with oral direct FXa inhibitors versus VKAs for the treatment of antiphospholipid syndrome. A systematic review and meta-analysis including these trials found that treatment with the direct oral FXa inhibitors versus VKAs was associated with a fivefold increased risk of subsequent arterial thromboembolic events, with stroke most predominant. This risk remained on subgroup analysis when analyzing patients with and without history of prior arterial events. There was not a significant difference in the odds of subsequent VTE between the two treatment groups. Finally, in subgroup comparison, the association of subsequent arterial events was more pronounced in "triple positive patients" (i.e., patients positive for each lupus anticoagulant, anticardiolipin antibodies, and anti–beta-2-glycoprotein antibodies) compared to those who were only single or double positive.[17] Given these findings, current practice supports the use of warfarin, INR goal 2–3, for patients with antiphospholipid syndrome. Future studies are needed to determine if subsets of patients could be considered for DOACs. Hydroxychloroquine and aspirin may be used as adjunct therapy in certain clinical circumstances. High-dose steroids, plasma exchange, and rituximab have been used to treat patients with catastrophic antiphospholipid syndrome, although these approaches are based on case studies and not on clinical trials.

REFERENCES

1. Cushman M. Epidemiology and risk factors for venous thrombosis. *Semin Hematol.* 2007;44:62–69.
2. Moser KM, Fedullo PF, LitteJohn JK, Crawford R. Frequent asymptomatic pulmonary embolism in patients with deep venous thrombosis. *JAMA.* 1994;271:223–225.
3. Meignan M, Rosso J, Gauthier H, et al. Systematic lung scans reveal a high frequency of silent pulmonary embolism in patients with proximal deep venous thrombosis. *Arch Intern Med.* 2000;160:159–164.
4. Weiner RS, Schwartz LM, Woloshin S. Time trends in pulmonary embolism in the United States. *Arch Intern Med.* 2011;171:831–837.

5. Francis CW. Clinical practice. Prophylaxis for thromboembolism in hospitalized medical patients. *N Engl J Med.* 2007;356:1438–1444.
6. Palareti G, Cosmi B, Legnani C. Diagnosis of deep vein thrombosis. *Semin Thromb Hemost.* 2006; 32:659–672.
7. Bounameaux H, Perrier A. Diagnosis of pulmonary embolism: in transition. *Curr Opin Hematol.* 2006;13:344–350.
8. Stein PD, Fowler SE, Goodman LR, et al; PIOPED II Investigators. Multidetector computed tomography for acute pulmonary embolism. *N Engl J Med.* 2006;354:2317–2327.
9. PIOPED investigators. Value of the ventilation/perfusion scan in acute pulmonary embolism—results of the prospective investigation of pulmonary embolism diagnosis (PIOPED). *JAMA.* 1990; 263:2753–2759.
10. Stein PD, Woodard PK, Weg JG, et al; PIOPED II investigators. Diagnostic pathways in acute pulmonary embolism: recommendations of the PIOPED II investigators. *Am J Med.* 2006;119:1048–1055.
11. van Belle A, Büller HR, Huisman MV, et al; Christopher Study Investigators. Effectiveness of managing suspected pulmonary embolism using an algorithm combining clinical probability, D-dimer testing, and computed tomography. *JAMA.* 2006;295(2):172–179.
12. Segal JB, Streiff MB, Hofmann LV, Thornton K, Bass EB. Management of venous thromboembolism: a systematic review for a practice guideline. *Ann Intern Med.* 2007;146:211–222.
13. Dolovich LR, Ginsberg JS, Douketis JD, Holbrook AM, Cheah G. A meta-analysis comparing low-molecular-weight heparins with unfractionated heparin in the treatment of venous thromboembolism: examining some unanswered questions regarding location of treatment, product type and dosing frequency. *Arch Intern Med.* 2000;160(2):181–188.
14. Ortel TL, Neumann I, Ageno W, et al. American Society of Hematology 2020 guidelines for management of venous thromboembolism: treatment of deep vein thrombosis and pulmonary embolism. *Blood Advances.* 2020;4:4693–4738.
15. Kahale LA, Hakoum MB, Tsolakian IG, et al. Anticoagulation for the long-term treatment of venous thromboembolism in people with cancer. *Cochrane Database Syst Rev.* 2018;6:CD006650.
16. Frere C, Farge D, Schrag D, Prata PH, Connors JM. Direct oral anticoagulant versus low molecular weight heparin for the treatment of cancer-associated venous thromboembolism: 2022 updated systematic review and meta-analysis of randomized controlled trials. *J Hematol Oncol.* 2022;15(1):69.
17. Khairani CD, Bejjani A, Piazza G, et al. Direct oral anticoagulants vs vitamin K antagonists in patients with antiphospholipid syndromes: meta-analysis of randomized trials. *J Am Coll Cardiol.* 2023;81(1):16–30.
18. Hann CL, Streiff MB. The role of vena caval filters in the management of venous thromboembolism. *Blood Rev.* 2005;19:179–202.
19. Stam J. Current concepts: thrombosis of the cerebral veins and sinuses. *N Engl J Med.* 2005;352: 1791–1798.
20. Pesavento R, Bernardi E, Concolato A, Valle FD, Pagnan A, Prandoni P. Postthrombotic syndrome. *Semin Thromb Hemost.* 2006;32:744–751.
21. Bauer K. The thrombophilias: well-defined risk factors with uncertain therapeutic implications. *Ann Intern Med.* 2001;135:367–373.
22. Seligsohn U, Lubetsky A. Genetic susceptibility to venous thrombosis. *N Engl J Med.* 2001;334: 1222–1231.
23. Heit JA, Sobell JL, Li H, Sommer SS. The incidence of venous thromboembolism among factor V Leiden carriers: a community-based cohort study. *J Thromb Haemost.* 2005;3:305–311.
24. Goodwin AJ, Adcock DM. Thrombophilia testing and venous thrombosis. *N Engl J Med.* 2017;377: 2297–2298.
25. Bezemer ID, Doggen CJM, Vos HL, Rosendaal FR. No association between the common MTHFR 677C→T polymorphism and venous thrombosis: results from the MEGA Study. *Arch Intern Med.* 2007;167(5):497–501.
26. Garcia D, Erkan D. Diagnosis and management of the antiphospholipid syndrome. *N Engl J Med.* 2018;378(21):2010–2021.

Coagulopathy

Joshua I. Siner

7

Coagulopathy refers to disorders with excessive bleeding because of alterations of proteins involved in the coagulation pathway. It can be divided into two main categories: hereditary and acquired.

- Hereditary
  - von Willebrand disease (vWD)
  - Hemophilia A
  - Hemophilia B
  - Rare factor deficiencies—factor XI, factor X, factor VII, factor XIII, combined factor V/VIII deficiency, dysfibrinogenemias
- Acquired
  - Liver disease
  - Vitamin K deficiency
  - Disseminated intravascular coagulation
  - Acquired inhibitors of coagulation
- The Bleeding Assessment Tool (BAT) is a standardized and validated clinical scoring system to screen patients for bleeding disorders and helps determine patients that require further testing and referral to a hematologist for evaluation (Table 7-1).[1]

Hereditary Coagulopathy

von Willebrand Disease

GENERAL PRINCIPLES

von Willebrand disease (vWD) is the most common inherited bleeding disorder, affecting between 1:100 and 1:400 individuals. It is caused by quantitative or qualitative abnormalities of von Willebrand factor (vWF), resulting in disorders of primary and secondary hemostasis. The usual inheritance pattern of vWD is autosomal dominant with incomplete penetrance due to complicated genetic/epigenetic regulators, most notably ABO blood groups. The symptoms of vWD can change over time as levels of vWF tend to increase with age, systemic alterations, and pregnancy. vWF has two primary functions. First, vWF mediates platelet activation and aggregation at high blood flow. Second, vWF complexes with factor VIII (FVIII) which prolongs the half-life of circulating FVIII by decreasing its clearance from plasma.

Classification

The subtypes of vWD are presented in Table 7-2.[2] Of note, the diagnosis of mild vWD type 1 can be difficult as vWF/FVIII are acute phase reactants that are elevated with systemic inflammation, pregnancy, and stress.

TABLE 7-1	BLEEDING ASSESSMENT TOOL				
			SCORE		
Symptoms (Up to the Time of Diagnosis	0	1	2	3	4
Epistaxis	No/trivial	>5/y or more than 10 min	Consultation only	Packing or cauterization of antifibrinolytic	Blood transfusion or replacement therapy (i.e., hemostatic blood components or FVIIa) or desmopressin
Cutaneous	No/trivial	For 5 or more bruises (>1 cm) in exposed areas	Consultation only	Extensive	Spontaneous hematoma requiring blood transfusion
Bleeding from minor wounds	No/trivial	>5/y or more than 10 min	Consultation only	Surgical hemostasis	Blood transfusion, replacement therapy or desmopressin
Oral cavity	No/trivial	Present	Consultation only	Surgical hemostasis or antifibrinolytic	Blood transfusion, replacement therapy, or desmopressin
GI bleeding	No/trivial	Present (not associated with ulcer, portal hypertension, hemorrhoids, or angiodysplasia)	Consultation only	Surgical hemostasis or antifibrinolytic therapy	Blood transfusion, replacement therapy, or desmopressin
Hematuria	No/trivial	Present (Macroscopic)	Consultation only	Surgical hemostasis or iron therapy	Blood transfusion, replacement therapy, or desmopressin

Tooth extraction	No/trivial or never done	Reported in <25% of all procedures, no intervention	Reported in >25% of all procedures, no intervention	Resuturing or packing	Blood transfusion, replacement therapy, or desmopressin
Surgery	No/trivial or never done	Reported in <25% of all procedures, no intervention	Reported in >25% of all procedures, no intervention	Surgical hemostasis or antifibrinolytic therapy	Blood transfusion, replacement therapy, or desmopressin
Menorrhagia	No/trivial	Consultation only, or: • Change pads more than every 2 h • Clot and flooding • PBAC score >100^a	Time off from work/school >2 times per year Or Requiring antifibrinolytics, hormonal or iron therapy	Requiring combined treatment with antifibrinolytics and hormonal therapy or present since menarche and >12 mo	Acute menorrhagia requiring hospital admission and emergency treatment; or blood transfusion, replacement therapy, or desmopressin; or requiring D&C or endometrial ablation/hysterectomy
Postpartum hemorrhage	Never	Consultation only Use of syntocinon Lochia >6 wk	Iron therapy or antifibrinolytics	Requiring blood transfusion, replacement therapy, or desmopressin; or requiring examination under anesthesia and/or inducing tamponade of the uterus	Any procedure requiring critical care or surgical intervention
Muscle hematomas	Never	Posttrauma, no therapy	Spontaneous, no therapy	Spontaneous or traumatic requiring desmopressin or replacement therapy	Spontaneous or traumatic requiring surgical intervention or blood transfusion

(continued)

TABLE 7-1 BLEEDING ASSESSMENT TOOL (*Continued*)

Symptoms (Up to the Time of Diagnosis	SCORE				
	0	1	2	3	4
Hemarthrosis	Never	Posttrauma, no therapy	Spontaneous, no therapy	Spontaneous or traumatic requiring desmopressin or replacement therapy	Spontaneous or traumatic requiring surgical intervention or blood transfusion
CNS bleeding	Never			Subdural, any intervention	Intracranial, any intervention
Other bleedings	No/trivial	Present	Consultation only	Surgical hemostasis or antifibrinolytics	Blood transfusion, replacement therapy, or desmopressin

Consultation: patient sought medical evaluation and was referred to specialist or had a detailed laboratory investigation.
Normal Range: <4 adult males, <6 adult females, <3 for children.
[a]PBAC, Pictorial Blood Assessment Chart.

TABLE 7-2 SUBTYPES OF vWD

Type	Description	Genetic Inheritance	DDAVP
1	Partial quantitative deficiency of vWF, ~70% of vWD cases	Autosomal dominant	Effective
1c	Increased clearance of mature vWF. Increased ratio of vWF propeptide : vWF:Ag		
2	Qualitative abnormalities of vWF	N/A	Not as effective, but a trial is reasonable, except for type 2B
2A	Abnormal assembly or reduced half-life of high–molecular-weight vWF multimers (HMWM)	Autosomal dominant	Not as effective, but a trial is reasonable
2B	Increased binding of vWF to platelet glycoprotein (GP) Ib, leading to deceased HMWM and platelets	Autosomal dominant	Contraindicated due to risk of potentiating thrombocytopenia
2M	Decreased binding of vWF to platelets, normal multimer distribution	Autosomal dominant	Not as effective, but a trial is reasonable
2N	Decreased binding of vWF to FVIII, low FVIII level	Autosomal recessive	Not as effective, but a trial is reasonable
3	Complete quantitative deficiency of vWF	Autosomal recessive or compound heterozygous	Ineffective
Platelet-type vWD	Abnormal platelet GP Ib-IX-V with increased affinity for large vWF multimers; phenotype indistinguishable from type 2B	N/A	N/A

vWD, von Willebrand disease.

Pathophysiology

vWF is a glycoprotein synthesized by endothelial cells and megakaryocytes. It is stored in the Weibel–Palade bodies of endothelial cells as well as platelet α granules. During primary hemostasis it mediates the adhesion of platelets at sites of vascular injury through activation by the GP 1b-IX-V receptor. vWF is synthesized as a 300-kD monomer and subsequently undergoes multiple posttranslational modifications (dimerization via disulfide bonds, N-linked glycosylation, and assembly into multimers of various sizes). Circulating vWF appears in a heterogeneous range of multimers and is negatively regulated by a disintegrin and metalloproteinase with thrombospondin motifs (ADAMTS)13. The largest multimers mediate platelet adhesion.

DIAGNOSIS

The majority of cases are quantitative defects with only mild symptoms.[3,4]

Clinical Presentation
- Recurrent mucocutaneous bleeding primarily identified at menarche with onset of menorrhagia.
- Easy bruising.
- Prolonged bleeding after trauma or surgery.
- Family history of a bleeding disorder is common.
- Use of antiplatelet medication (e.g., aspirin) can unmask the disease.
- Musculoskeletal bleeding is rare.
- Although the majority of affected patients have mild vWD and minor bleeding, patients with the most severe form may suffer life-threatening hemorrhage.

Differential Diagnosis
- Hemophilia A

Diagnostic Testing
Laboratories
(See Chapter 5 for details.) vWF levels vary with physiologic stress, estrogen levels (supplemental and pregnancy), and other medical comorbidities, and levels may need to be repeated for confirmation.

- Complete blood count (CBC)
- Prothrombin time (PT) (usually normal), Activated partial thromboplastin time (aPTT) (can be slightly prolonged)
- Quantitative vWF antigen (vWF:Ag)
- Qualitative vWF assay: Ristocetin cofactor assay (vWF:RCof), vWF collagen-binding assay (vWF:CBA), and/or vWF activity by immunoassay targeting vWF binding site to platelets
- Factor VIII level
- vWF multimer assay
- Ristocetin-induced platelet aggregation (RIPA) analysis
- Factor VIII–binding ELISA

TREATMENT

- **DDAVP (Desmopressin).** A Trial of DDAVP is indicated for type 1 and 2 only. It is contraindicated for type 2B as it can potentiate thrombocytopenia and bleeding risk.[5,6]
  - Mechanism of action: Analog of antidiuretic hormone (vasopressin) that lacks vasoactive properties. It acts by releasing endothelial stores of vWF transiently increasing plasma levels of FVIII and vWF by a factor of three to five, peaking 30–60 minutes post IV administration and 90–120 minutes post subcutaneous or intranasal injection.
  - Dosage: 0.3 µg/kg IV or SC or up to 300 µg intranasally (although as of 12/2023, the intranasal formulation is not currently available).
  - DDAVP should not be used in patients with unstable coronary artery disease, due to concern for ultralarge vWF multimer-mediated platelet aggregation in regions of high shear stress near atherosclerotic plaques.

- At the time of vWD diagnosis or before elective treatment, a test dose of DDAVP should be administered to establish the individual pattern of response. FVIII levels and vWF:RC should be measured at 1 and 4 hours after drug administration to determine peak factor levels and clearance rate.
- Typically limited to three successive doses owing to the development of tachyphylaxis as vWF stores from Weibel–Palade bodies are exhausted
- Attention should be kept on neurologic symptoms in the event patients develop hyponatremia.

- **FVIII/vWF replacement**
  - Used when DDAVP is inadequate or unsuitable for the vWD subtype.
  - The primary treatment for all vWD subtypes is when significant bleeding or major surgery is involved.
  - Virus-inactivated FVIII + vWF concentrates, such as *Humate-P,* have the greatest clinical experience. Vials are labeled by FVIII and vWD dose and the correct potency should be selected based on the desired factor being replaced.
  - Recombinant vWF, *Vonvendi,* was initially approved in 2015 for treatment of bleeding episodes and then expanded to prophylaxis. Notably, this product does not contain FVIII.
  - Initial dosing and maintenance regimens vary by severity of hemorrhage and subtype of vWD.
  - FVIII levels should be obtained every 12 hours on the day concentrates are administered and every 24 hours thereafter. Target FVIII levels are similar to those detailed for hemophilia A below.

- Cryoprecipitate, which contains 5–10 times more FVIII and vWF than fresh frozen plasma, can also be used, although techniques of virus inactivation are not routinely applied to this product.
- Platelet transfusion can be useful, especially when hemorrhage is not controlled despite adequate FVIII levels after FVIII and vWF concentrates.
- Antifibrinolytic amino acids (aminocaproic acid, tranexamic acid), in high doses, may be used for the treatment of patients with vWD and menorrhagia.
- Progestin-containing contraceptives are beneficial to support patients with menorrhagia and suppress endometrial cycling thereby limiting blood loss.
- Iron replacement may be indicated with menorrhagia and in patients presenting with excessive blood loss or symptoms of iron deficiency with or without anemia.

Hemophilia A

GENERAL PRINCIPLES

Hemophilia A is an inherited coagulation disorder caused by alterations of the gene encoding FVIII, leading to impaired intrinsic pathway function (see Figure 5-1 for intrinsic pathway).[7,8] The inheritance pattern is X-linked recessive; the gene that encodes FVIII is located on the long arm of the X chromosome (Xq28). Thirty percent of cases are the result of spontaneous mutations. The incidence is approximately 1 in 5,000 live male births worldwide.

DIAGNOSIS

Clinical Presentation

- Joint and muscle/soft tissue hemorrhages, easy bruising
- Prolonged bleeding after trauma or surgery with first challenge at time of circumcision

- Chronic disability can result from hemarthrosis-induced arthropathy and intramuscular bleeding

Diagnostic Criteria

- Laboratory evaluations include:
  - Platelet count—normal
  - PT—normal
  - PTT—prolonged
  - PTT mixing study—correct with normal plasma
  - FVIII level—decreased (confirmation of diagnosis)
  - Von Willebrand factor (vWF) level—normal
  - Genetic analysis is used for carrier detection, prenatal diagnosis and informs risk of inhibitor formation.
- Disease severity depends on FVIII level
  - Mild disease—level >5% of normal
  - Moderate disease—levels 1–5% of normal
  - Severe disease—≤1% of normal
- Inhibitors (development of neutralizing antibodies to replacement factor) are a driver of morbidity in patients with hemophilia
  - Measured in Bethesda units (1 B.U. is the amount of functional inhibition to neutralize 50% of factor function, 2 B.U. inhibits 75%, etc.)
  - Patients with greater than 5 B.U. are considered to have a high titer and cannot be treated with replacement factor

Differential Diagnosis

- Hemophilia B
- von Willebrand disease (vWD) type 2N
- Acquired hemophilia

TREATMENT

- **Factor VIII replacement**[7]
  - Used in severe hemophilia, for both major and minor bleeding, and is given either on demand for bleeding/procedures or as prophylaxis.
  - Options consist of recombinant FVIII including full-length, B-domain deleted, and extended half-life products (used for prophylaxis) or purified, virus-attenuated FVIII concentrates from pooled plasma.
  - Dosage for immediate replacement: Each unit/kg of FVIII replacement will raise the peak plasma FVIII level by 2%. Therefore, the bolus dose = (target FVIII level – baseline FVIII [as below]) × weight (kg) × 0.5.
  - Target FVIII level:
    - Minor bleeding: ≥30%
    - More severe bleeding (e.g., muscle and joint hemorrhages): ≥50%
    - Surgical procedures or life-threatening bleeding: ≥80%
  - The half-life of FVIII is 8–12 hours, therefore, following a loading dose, repeat doses are administered every 8–12 hours, adjusted to measured factor VIII levels.
  - Extended half-life formulations can tailor prophylaxis from one to three times weekly depending on patient needs.
  - FVIII replacement can also be provided by continuous infusion, such as during prolonged surgical procedures.
  - Intensive therapy (i.e., targeted replacement of >50%) should continue until hemostasis is achieved.

- Postoperative therapy is usually continued for 10–14 days. Measuring peak and trough FVIII levels after the first and selected subsequent doses permits dose adjustments to ensure cost-effective therapy.
- **Emicizumab**
  - Emicizumab[9] is a bispecific antibody that binds factor IX and factor X, designed to replace the colocalizing function of missing cofactor function and to restore hemostasis.
  - Due to its long half-life, a typical dosing schema involves a subcutaneous injection every 4–6 weeks. It is equally effective for patients with or without inhibitors.
  - Emicizumab interacts with standard coagulation and factor assays causing chromogenic and clotting-based activity assays to have falsely elevated levels. The only assay able to differentiate FVIII function/inhibitor levels in patients on emicizumab is a bovine-based chromogenic assay.
- **Gene therapies for hemophilia A**
  - The newest modality in the treatment of hemophilia is adenoviral-associated gene transfer vectors wherein a truncated FVIII gene is delivered to hepatocytes, ectopically expressed and secreted into circulation. The first product was FDA approved in June 2023 for patients over the age of 18 without an inhibitor.[10]
- **Recombinant factor VII**[11]
  - Recombinant factor VIIa promotes hemostasis by activating the extrinsic pathway.
  - It is currently approved for use in hemophilia A and B patients who have developed inhibitors to FVIII or factor IX (FIX) and are at risk of severe bleeding.
  - Dosage: 90 μg/kg every 2–3 hours until hemostasis is achieved.
- **Factor eight inhibitor bypassing agents (FEIBA)**
  - FEIBA or activated prothrombin complex concentrates (aPCC) is a mixture of FVIIa, prothrombin. Factor IX and Factor X in addition to small amounts of FVIII.
  - It is approved for patients with inhibitors to restore hemostasis prophylactically, for on-demand bleeding, and surgical hemostasis.
- **DDAVP (Desmopressin)**
  - Used in patients with mild disease (FVIII level >5%) and minor bleeding episodes occurring sporadically or in the setting of minor procedures.
  - Details as outlined above for vWD.

COMPLICATIONS

- Infection from factor concentrates—historically hepatitis C virus, hepatitis B virus, and HIV from contaminated blood products in the 1980s.
- Antibody formation, primarily in patients with severe factor deficiency[12]
- Thrombosis with overcorrection and bypassing agents (FEIBA, FVIIa)
- Hemophilic arthropathy
  - Recurrent hemorrhage into one or more joints leading to chronic effusion, joint space narrowing, limited range of motion, atrophy of adjacent musculature, and end-stage arthritis
  - Can be prevented by prophylactic factor infusions (three times a week for FVIII and twice a week for FIX), intra-articular steroid injection, synovectomy, and joint replacement.

Hemophilia B

GENERAL PRINCIPLES

Hemophilia B is the inherited loss of factor IX function. The clinical presentation, diagnostic criteria, disease severity, and morbidity are indiscernible from hemophilia A with the exception of loss of the factor IX function. Notably, inhibitors to factor IX are less frequent than in hemophilia A, but they have additional risks, including deposition of inhibitor complexes in renal tissue.

TREATMENT

- **Factor IX replacement**
  - Factor IX enzyme replacement therapy is available in multiple formulations. The standard plasma-derived and recombinant factor IX products have a longer half-life than FVIII. Administering 1 unit of factor will increase circulating activity by 1% (Table 7-3).
  - Extended half-life products using fusions of immunoglobulin Fc domains have been more successful in factor IX replacement than FVIII and allow for once-weekly dosing for prophylaxis.
- **Gene therapies for hemophilia B**
  - Gene therapy for hemophilia B was first approved in 2022.[13] It was first to market given its smaller gene size and the utilization of a hyperfunctional factor IX (factor IX-Padua) which lowers the required gene therapy dose and avoids the common adverse reactions, including immune responses to the capsid proteins.

TABLE 7-3	HEMOPHILIAS	
	Hemophilia A	**Hemophilia B**
Inherence pattern	X-linked recessive	X-linked recessive
Gene location	Xq28	Xq27
Incidence	1 in 5,000 live male births	1 in 30,000 live male births
Presentations	Recurrent hemarthrosis, soft tissue hematomas	Recurrent hemarthrosis, soft tissue hematomas
Diagnosis	Decreased FVIII level	Decreased FIX level
Treatment	• FVIII concentrates • Each unit/kg of FVIII replacement raises plasma FVIII level by 2% • Bolus dose = target FVIII level (as above) × weight (kg) × 0.5 • Dosing frequency every 8–12 h (except for long-acting formulations) • DDAVP can be used carefully in mild disease with minor bleeding • FVIIa or FEIBA for patients with inhibitors and bleeding	• FIX concentrates • Each unit/kg of FIX replacement raises plasma FIX level by 1% • Bolus dose = target FIX level (as above) × weight (kg) (multiply by 1.3 when recombinant is given) • Dosing frequency every 12–24 h • DDAVP is ineffective • FVIIa for patients with inhibitors and bleeding

Note: FIX is a small molecule with extensive extravascular distribution; therefore, multiplication by 1.3 is needed in dosage calculation. In addition, the corrective dosing for prophylaxis should be individualized for personal kinetics (recovery and half-life) and replacement product.

FUTURE OF ANTIHEMOPHILIC THERAPIES

There remain a number of unmet clinical needs in hemophilia, most notably how to treat patients with inhibitors—especially rare factor IX inhibitors. There are additional antibody and siRNA-based therapeutics in the clinical pipeline that attempt to "rebalance" hemostasis by reducing the activity of coagulation inhibitors (including tissue factor pathway inhibitor, protein C, and antithrombin). Further questions remain as to what the uptake among patients and the true duration of gene therapies will be. Finally, how will a newly aging cohort of patients with hemophilia encounter common diseases as their life expectancy approaches a population without bleeding disorders?

Acquired Coagulopathies

Acquired Hemophilia A

GENERAL PRINCIPLES

Acquired hemophilia is the result of a pathologic autologous inhibitory antibody that is capable of reducing factor function, most commonly FVIII. The most common risk factors are:

- Advanced age
- Lymphoproliferative malignancies
- Autoimmune disorders such as rheumatoid arthritis or lupus
- Drug reactions
- Postpartum

Presentation can occur with prolongation of PTT or PT, bruising, hematomas, or life-threatening bleeding. The diagnosis is made when a mixing study (1:1 patient-to-healthy control plasma) does not correct the clotting times. The inhibitor is then confirmed and quantified by Bethesda assay (as described above). Antiphospholipid antibodies such as lupus anticoagulant may also show a nonspecific inhibitor pattern (see Chapter 6 for more information on antiphospholipid syndrome). Mortality is high in acquired hemophilia primarily from infections related to immunosuppression and bleeding.

TREATMENT

There are two primary goals in the treatment of acquired hemophilia. The first is controlling bleeding which can be achieved in the acute setting with activated factor VII and then controlled with administration of recombinant porcine factor VIII (trade name Obizur) which evades most FVIII-directed inhibitors. The second is immunosuppression for inhibitor eradication which consists of high-dose steroids in the acute setting and then frequently transition to rituximab (anti-CD20 antibody) or cyclophosphamide to avoid the side effects of large steroid doses with prolonged taper.

Liver Disease

All coagulation factors, with the exception of vWF, are produced in the liver. Liver dysfunction leads to a number of coagulation abnormalities secondary to decreased factor synthesis (with the exception of FVIII), decreased clearance of activated factors, dysregulation of fibrinolytic pathways, and production of abnormal fibrinogen.[14] The coagulopathy of liver disease is usually stable unless the liver synthetic function is rapidly worsening, such as in fulminant hepatic failure. Patients with liver synthetic dysfunction frequently also have thrombocytopenia secondary to portal hypertension, splenic sequestration, and loss of thrombopoietin production in end-stage cirrhosis.

Vitamin K Deficiency

- Vitamin K is a fat-soluble vitamin involved in the posttranslational modification of pro-coagulant factors II, VII, IX, and X, and anticoagulant proteins C and S. These reactions take place in the liver, where vitamin K serves as a cofactor for the conversion of glutamic acid residues to gamma-carboxyglutamic acid, which facilitates binding of coagulation factors to phospholipid in the presence of calcium, an essential step in coagulation. Vitamin K must then be recycled by vitamin K epoxide reductase (VKOR) for further gamma-carboxylation to occur. It follows that vitamin K deficiency would render these so-called vitamin K–dependent coagulation factors ineffective.
- Disorders of vitamin K most commonly result from the use of warfarin, a VKOR inhibitor. Other causes of vitamin K deficiency are inadequate dietary intake, which may deplete vitamin K stores in as little as 7 days, malabsorption syndromes, or use of antibiotics, which can eliminate vitamin K–producing bowel flora.
- The presentation and initial diagnostic workup of vitamin K (bleeding, prolonged PTT, and PT/INR) can be indistinguishable, however, checking a factor V level can help differentiate as it relies on synthetic liver function and is not a vitamin K–dependent factor (factor V normal = vitamin K deficient; factor V low = liver dysfunction).
- Vitamin K deficiency results in prolonged PT that corrects during mixing studies. This is especially important for newborns, where vitamin K deficiency can lead to intracranial hemorrhage.
- Vitamin K repletion may be provided PO, SC, or IV. PO is the preferred route. IV vitamin K is effective but carries the risk of anaphylaxis. To minimize this risk, vitamin K may be diluted in a dextrose or saline solution and slowly administered via an infusion pump. If bleeding is significant or does not respond to vitamin K therapy, factor replacement in the form of fresh frozen plasma should be administered.

Disseminated Intravascular Coagulation

DIC is a hemostatic derangement of multiple etiologies characterized by small- and medium-vessel thrombosis with consumption of platelets and coagulation factors.[15] It leads to microangiopathic hemolytic anemia, thrombocytopenia, and coagulation abnormalities (see Chapter 4).

REFERENCES

1. Rodeghiero F, Tosetto A, Abshire T, et al. ISTH/SSC bleeding assessment tool: a standardized questionnaire and a proposal for a new bleeding score for inherited bleeding disorders. *J Thromb Haemost.* 2010;8:2063–2065.
2. Sadler JE, Budde U, Eikenboom JC, et al. Update on the pathophysiology and classification of von Willebrand disease: a report of the subcommittee on von Willebrand factor. *J Thromb Haemost.* 2006;4:2103–2114.
3. Budde U, Drewke E, Mainusch K, et al. Laboratory diagnosis of congenital von Willebrand disease. *Semin Thromb Hemost.* 2002;28:173–190.
4. Favaloro EJ. Laboratory assessment as a critical component of the appropriate diagnosis and sub-classification of von Willebrand's disease. *Blood Rev.* 1999;13:185–204.
5. Mannucci PM. Treatment of von Willebrand's disease. *N Engl J Med.* 2004;351:683–694.

6. Mannucci PM. Desmopressin (DDAVP) in the treatment of bleeding disorders: the first 20 years. *Blood.* 1997;90:2515–2521.

7. Hoyer LW. Hemophilia A. *N Engl J Med.* 1994;330:38–47.

8. Bolton-Maggs PH, Perry DJ, Chalmers EA, et al. The rare coagulation disorders—review with guidelines for management from the United Kingdom Haemophilia Centre Doctors' Organization. *Haemophilia.* 2004;10:593–628.

9. Blair HA. Emicizumab: a review in Haemophilia A. *Drugs.* 2019;79:1697–1707.

10. Ozelo MC, Mahlangu J, Pasi KJ, et al. Valoctocogene roxaparvovec gene therapy for hemophilia A. *N Engl J Med.* 2022;386:1013–1025.

11. Butenas S, Brummel KE, Branda RF, et al. Mechanism of factor VIIa-dependent coagulation in hemophilia blood. *Blood.* 2002;99:923–930.

12. Sahud MA. Laboratory diagnosis of inhibitors. *Semin Thromb Hemost.* 2000;26:195–203.

13. Pipe SW, Leebeek FWG, Recht M, et al. Gene therapy with etranacogene dezaparvovec for hemophilia B. *N Eng J Med.* 2023;388:706–718.

14. Lechner K, Niessner H, Thaler E. Coagulation abnormalities in liver disease. *Semin Thromb Hemost.* 1977;4:40–56.

15. Levi M, Ten Cate H. Disseminated intravascular coagulation. *N Engl J Med.* 1999;341:586–592.

Bone Marrow Failure

Constantine N. Logothetis and
Stefan P. Tarnawsky

GENERAL PRINCIPLES

- **Pancytopenia is the reduction in all three peripheral blood cell lineages:** Red blood cells (RBCs), white blood cells (WBCs), and platelets. Anemia can cause fatigue, shortness of breath, or lightheadedness. Thrombocytopenia can present with bleeding and bruising. Neutropenia is associated with recurrent infections and mucosal changes. The extent of the reduction is associated with the severity of symptoms.
- Pancytopenia may be due to defects in bone marrow production or from peripheral causes.
- Impaired bone marrow production may be caused by infiltrative processes including malignancies (e.g., carcinoma, leukemia), infections (e.g., tuberculosis), inflammatory conditions (e.g., sarcoidosis). Nutritional deficiencies can also prevent adequate bone marrow function, such as vitamin B_{12} deficiencies, folate deficiencies, and copper deficiencies.
- Causes of increased destruction of blood cells in the periphery include hypersplenism, autoimmune diseases, and overwhelming sepsis. Medications may also cause pancytopenia, with antipsychotics (clozapine), antibiotics (e.g., sulfamethoxazole), and chemotherapies being common culprits. Impaired production of blood cells is seen in bone marrow failure states, both inherited and acquired. **Bone marrow failure** is defined as the inability of the bone marrow to produce an adequate number of circulating blood cells. Inherited BM failure syndromes are described in Table 8-1.[1] Acquired bone marrow failure states include myelodysplastic neoplasms (MDS), acquired aplastic anemia (AA), and paroxysmal nocturnal hemoglobinuria (PNH). MDS will be discussed in more detail in the following chapter.
- In most cases, initial laboratory evaluation should include a complete blood count, serum chemistries, peripheral smear, and reticulocyte count. If clinically indicated, an evaluation of the patient's folate, B_{12}, and copper levels or an infectious workup (including HIV, hepatitis panel, and other viral or fungal serologies) should be undertaken. If an etiology is not apparent, a bone marrow biopsy and aspirate should be obtained. In cases where a hematologic malignancy is suspected, flow cytometry and cytogenetics performed on the aspirate may be useful.
- Treatment and further laboratory or imaging evaluations will depend on the etiology of the cytopenia(s). In cases where a medication is the underlying cause, discontinuation of the offending drug may be curative. Cytopenias resulting from bone marrow infiltration or suppression by other conditions may improve with treatment of the underlying condition. Cytopenias resulting from nutritional deficiencies can be treated by addressing the underlying nutritional deficiencies. In cases where bone marrow failure is the etiology of the cytopenias, treatment will depend on the diagnosis. Features and management of selected bone marrow failure syndromes are described in the following sections.

TABLE 8-1	FEATURES OF INHERITED BONE MARROW FAILURE SYNDROMES				
	Fanconi Anemia (FA)	**Dyskeratosis Congenital (DC)**	**Shwachman–Diamond Syndrome**	**Congenital Amegakaryocytic Thrombocytopenia**	**Diamond–Blackfan Anemia (DBA)**
Clinical effects	Microcephaly, thumb abnormalities, hypogonadism, skin changes	Triad of skin pigmentation, nail dystrophy, and mucosal leukoplakia	Exocrine pancreatic deficiency, skeletal abnormalities, skin changes	Cardiac and neurologic abnormalities	Craniofacial, thumb, growth abnormalities
Associated malignancies	Leukemia, SCC, GI adenocarcinoma liver, brain, Wilms tumor	Leukemia, lymphoma, SCC, GI adenocarcinomas, lung, skin, liver	Leukemia	Leukemia	Leukemia, osteosarcoma, soft tissue sarcoma
Inheritance	AR, rarely XLR	XLR, AD, AR	AR	AR	AD
Genetics	Multiple genes identified: FANCA, FANCC, FANCD1, FANCD2, FANCE, FANCF, FANCG, FANCI, FANCJ, FANCL, FANCM, FANCN, and FANCB. FA genes function coordinately to repair DNA damage. FA-B subtype is XLR	XLR form associated with mutations in dyskerin gene (DKC1); AD form associated with genes encoding RNA component of telomerase (TERC) and telomerase reverse transcriptase (TERT); AR form associated with NOP10/NOLA3 and NHP2/NOLA2	Up to 90% harbor biallelic mutations in the SBDS gene, which encodes a highly conserved protein thought to function in ribosome biogenesis	Mutations in c-MPL gene, which encodes the thrombopoietin receptor	Multiple genes identified: RPS19, RPS17, RPS24, RPL35A, and RPL11. DBA genes encode protein components of either the small 40S or large 60S ribosomal units
Additional tests	Chromosome breakage	Telomere length	Serum trypsinogen, pancreatic isoamylase, fecal elastase, pancreatic imaging		Erythrocyte adenosine deaminase

SCC, squamous cell carcinomas; GI, gastrointestinal; AR, autosomal recessive; XLR, X-linked recessive; AD, autosomal dominant.
Data from Shimamura A. Clinical approach to marrow failure. Hematology Am Soc Hematol Educ Program. 2009:329–337.

Schwachman–Diamond Syndrome

GENERAL PRINCIPLES

Schwachman–Diamond syndrome (SDS) is an inherited bone marrow failure disorder characterized by the triad of pancytopenia, skeletal malformations, and exocrine pancreas dysfunction. The diagnosis is made clinically but is supported by genetic analysis identifying biallelic mutations in ribosome biogenesis genes—most commonly SBDS. Patients struggle with GI upset, recurrent infections, and have a high risk of developing a hematologic malignancy, such as MDS or AML. Treatment of SDS is supportive, with allogeneic hematopoietic stem cell transplantation reserved for patients with life-threatening cytopenias or malignant transformation.

Epidemiology

SDS is a rare autosomal recessive condition with an estimated carrier frequency of 1/110.[2] The incidence of the disease in live births has been estimated between 1/75,000 and 1/200,000 with a male:female ratio of 1.7:1. There is no known geographic or ethnic variation in SDS incidence.

Classification

Over 90% of SDS patients have biallelic mutations in the SBDS gene. Patients with different causative ribosome gene mutations may have slightly different symptoms, resulting in a genotype-phenotype correlation. For instance, patients with SRP54 mutations, are at very high risk of neutropenia and recurrent infections with lower incidences of pancreatic insufficiency, whereas patients with DNAJC21 and EFL1 mutations have more skeletal abnormalities and cognitive symptoms.[3] Further, two distinct compensatory molecular pathways have been identified that mitigate the anemia in SDS patients.[4] EIF6 inactivation counteracts the ribosome defect in SDS patients and improves anemia without increasing leukemic potential. Other patients develop TP53 mutations that increase hematopoietic proliferation with a concomitant higher risk of developing leukemia.

Pathophysiology

Approximately 90% of patients have biallelic mutation in SBDS, which causes an absence of a key ribosome protein. The remaining patients may have mutations in other genes with important roles in ribosome assembly or protein synthesis, including DNAJC21, EFL1, and SRP54. Carriers for these mutations are usually asymptomatic. The precise mechanism whereby these mutations cause the triad of exocrine pancreatic dysfunction, skeletal abnormalities, and bone marrow failure is unknown.

DIAGNOSIS

Clinical Presentation

The median age of symptom onset is approximately 2 months, with cytopenias (96%), exocrine pancreatic dysfunction (83%), and skeletal deformities (57%) being the most common findings.[5] These features may cause recurrent infections, including otitis, sinusitis, cellulitis, and sepsis. Decreased stature, diarrhea, and failure to thrive are also common features. The median age of diagnosis is approximately 16 months; rarely patients may go undiagnosed into adolescence or early adulthood.

Diagnostic Testing

The diagnosis of SDS should be suspected in infants presenting with cytopenias with or without skeletal abnormalities and pancreatic insufficiency. Historically, this triad—in the context of an appropriate family history—was sufficient to make the diagnosis. Currently, genetic testing for the underlying genes (SBDS, DNAJC21, EFL1, and SRP54) should be performed. Ancillary testing should include a CBC, CMP, reticulocyte count, nutritional studies (iron, copper, folate, vitamins A, D, E, K, and B_{12}). If the mutation analysis is unrevealing, then a strong clinical suspicion for SDS should lead to consideration of whole genome sequencing to assess for as-yet unknown genetic causes of SDS. Patients with a confirmed diagnosis of SDS should be referred to genetic counselors, to discuss family planning and consideration of testing their siblings and parents.

TREATMENT

SDS is an inherited condition that affects multiple organ systems. As such, there is no cure for SDS. Management of patients with SDS focuses on nutritional support, symptom management, and risk reduction. Patients will benefit from exogenous pancreatic enzymes. Hematopoietic growth factors may be considered to reverse cytopenias. Care should be taken to minimize DNA damage through sun exposure and radiation, which will further increase the risk of malignancy. Severe bone marrow failure causing life-threatening cytopenias with recurrent infections may prompt consideration of an allogeneic hematopoietic stem cell transplant. The high morbidity associated with this treatment requires careful patient selection.

PROGNOSIS

The severity of SDS is variable making prognostic generalizations difficult. Estimates of overall survival vary between 24 and 38 years.[6] The cause of death in infancy is most commonly bone marrow failure, whereas in older children and adults the cause of death is more commonly MDS or AML. The presence of a concurrent TP53 mutation in hematopoietic cells in SDS patients is associated with a high risk of malignant transformation and is a poor prognostic factor.

Aplastic Anemia

GENERAL PRINCIPLES

AA is a deficiency of functional hematopoietic stem cells (HSCs) leading to cytopenias in one or more of the three peripheral blood lineages. The characteristic bone marrow finding is profound age-adjusted hypocelluarity, without evidence of infiltration or fibrosis. AA may be inherited as part of a bone marrow failure syndrome, or it may be acquired following an autoimmune condition, or exposure to toxins, medications, or infections. AA can coexist with other conditions such as PNH (discussed in the next section) and T-cell large granular lymphocytic leukemia (T-LGL). Approximately 40–50% of patients with acquired AA have expanded populations of PNH cells.[7]

Epidemiology

Acquired AA is a rare disease. The incidence is estimated to be about two cases per million per year in Western countries and about two- to threefold higher in Asia. Almost half of the cases occur during the first three decades of life.[7]

Classification

AA can be acquired or inherited. Table 8-1 outlines several forms of inherited AA. In the presence of an empty marrow, pancytopenia, and transfusion dependence, the severity of

TABLE 8-2　POTENTIAL CAUSES OF SEVERE APLASTIC ANEMIA

Infections
　　Hepatitis A, B, C—nonserologic
　　Epstein–Barr virus
　　Cytomegalovirus
　　Mycobacterial infections
　　Human immunodeficiency virus
　　Parvovirus B19

Drugs and chemicals
　　Gold salts
　　Chloramphenicol
　　Carbamazepine
　　Sulfonamides
　　Nonsteroidal anti-inflammatory drugs
　　Antiepileptic and psychotropic agents
　　Cardiovascular drugs
　　Penicillamine
　　Allopurinol
　　Benzene
　　Pesticides

PNH

Graft-versus-host disease (GVHD)

Pregnancy

Eosinophilic fasciitis

Modified from Valdez JM, Scheinberg P, Young NS, et al. Infections in patients with aplastic anemia. *Semin Hematol.* 2009;46:269–276.

the disease is based on the absolute neutrophil count (ANC). In nonsevere AA, the ANC is >0.5 × 10⁹/L. In severe AA, the ANC is between 0.2 and 0.5 × 10⁹/L. In very severe AA, the ANC is <0.2 × 10⁹/L.[8]

Etiology

The syndromes associated with inherited bone marrow failure are listed in Table 8-1. Acquired AA, is likely triggered by antigen exposure, leading to aberrant and dysregulated T-cell activation. Table 8-2 lists factors that have been implicated in causing acquired AA.[9]

Pathophysiology

The pathophysiology of acquired AA is an immune-mediated attack on the HSCs, in most cases caused by activated cytotoxic T-cells bearing the Th1 profile.[10] These activated T-cells produce cytokines such as interferon-gamma (IFN-γ) and tumor necrosis factor-alpha (TNF-α). These, in turn, increase Fas ligand expression, whose binding to Fas receptors on HSCs can trigger apoptosis. The precipitating cause of aberrant T-cell activation is often unknown, but common triggers are believed to be certain medications, toxins, and infections (see Table 8-2). HLA-DR2 is overexpressed in patients with AA. Recent data also implicate intrinsic defects in HSCs. Mutations in the genes for telomerase, TERC, and TERT have been described in patients without overt clinical stigmata of dyskeratosis congenita. Telomere shortening is observed in one-third to one-half of patients with AA. Accelerated telomere shortening may result in premature death of rapidly proliferating cells.

DIAGNOSIS

Clinical Presentation

Patients with AA present with symptoms related to pancytopenia. The presence of weight loss, pain, loss of appetite, or fever suggests another diagnosis. Physical examination usually reveals pallor, mucosal bleeding, petechiae, and ecchymoses. The presence of lymphadenopathy, hepatomegaly, or splenomegaly strongly suggests another diagnosis such as lymphoma, leukemia, or bone marrow infiltration.

Diagnostic Testing

The diagnosis is established by **bone marrow aspiration and biopsy**. The findings include a profoundly hypocellular marrow with morphologically normal residual hematopoietic cells. Severe AA is defined as a BM cellularity <25% with at least two of the following criteria: (i) ANC <500/ul, (ii) platelets <20,000/ul, absolute reticulocyte count <50,000/ul. There is no increased reticulin formation or infiltrative elements. Evaluation for other etiologies of pancytopenia includes viral serologies for hepatitis, CMV, EBV, parvovirus, HIV, and herpes. Serum B_{12} and folate levels should be determined. In young adults, chromosome fragility testing with diepoxybutane (DEB) should be considered to definitively rule out Fanconi anemia—an inherited cause of AA in infants and young children. Flow cytometry should be performed to evaluate for co-occurring PNH and/or T-LGL.

TREATMENT

Management of AA depends on the severity of symptoms and can include observation, immunosuppression, and allogeneic HSCT. Supportive care with transfusions and infection mitigation may be required as well.

- **Supportive care:** Patients with symptomatic anemia will need RBC transfusions. Patients with symptomatic thrombocytopenia or a platelet count of <10,000 should be given platelet transfusions. Expert consensus statements suggest irradiating all blood products for AA patients who are receiving ATG or other forms of immunosuppression to reduce the risk of alloimmunization and give a theoretical risk of transfusion-associated graft versus host disease.[11] Blood products from family members should be avoided to prevent alloimmunization. EPO and myeloid factors are not mainstays of treatment. No significant survival has been seen in patients receiving G-CSF as compared to those who did not receive G-CSF.
- **Immunosuppression:** First-line treatment of patients with acquired AA who are not candidates for allogeneic HSCT (see below) is immunosuppression with horse ATG and cyclosporine. A recent phase three trial showed that triplet therapy with the incorporation of the thrombopoietin mimetic eltrombopag improved hematologic CR from 10% to 22% at 3 months, and reduced the time to first response from 8.8 m to 3.0 m, compared to ATG, cyclosporine, and placebo.[12]
- **HSCT:** Patients with severe AA who are under 40 years of age with an HLA-matched sibling donor should be offered HSCT as first-line treatment. The 10-year survival of patients >40 years of age after matched sib transplant is 55% versus 86% for those aged 1–20 and 76% for those aged 21–40.[13] Acute GVHD occurs in about 20–30% of patients. Chronic GVHD is a major cause of morbidity and mortality in patients who survived more than 2 years post transplantation, and life-long immunosuppression may be needed. Chronic GVHD occurs in about 30–40% of patients. As a matched sibling donor is available in only about 20–30% of cases, alternative sources of HSCs have been

sought. HSCT from an unrelated donor carries higher morbidity and mortality than HSCT from a matched sibling donor and is reserved for patients who lack a matched sibling donor and who failed to respond to one or more rounds of immunosuppression. Bone marrow remains the preferred source of stem cells in severe AA given the higher rate of chronic GVHD observed with stem cell grafts from peripheral blood.[14]

PROGNOSIS

Spontaneous remissions have been seen in approximately 13% of AA patients, with the vast majority of these occurring within 8 weeks of diagnosis.[15] These spontaneous remissions occur most commonly in patients whose AA is temporally associated with a likely causative drug exposure or infection. For those without spontaneous remission, patients with severe AA will eventually succumb to infections or bleeding complications. Untreated severe AA has an estimated 2-year survival of 30%.[16] With treatment, the infections remain the leading cause of death, with some patients succumbing to clonal evolution of AA into a myeloid neoplasm.[17] For acquired AA, survival correlates with age of diagnosis, with 5-year survival >90% in patients 0–18 years of age versus 38% for patients >60 years of age.[18] Overall survival outcomes with allogenic transplants are noted above. The data for overall survival of patients treated with immunosuppression with eltrombopag remain immature, but at a follow-up of 4 years, the OS was 92.5%.

Paroxysmal Nocturnal Hemoglobinuria

GENERAL PRINCIPLES

PNH is an acquired disease characterized by nonmalignant clonal expansion of one or more HSCs that have undergone somatic mutation of the PIG-A gene. PNH can present with bone marrow failure, hemolytic anemia, smooth muscle dystonias, and thrombosis. PNH can arise de novo or in the setting of AA.[19]

Pathophysiology

The protein encoded by the PIG-A gene is essential for the synthesis of glycosylphosphatidylinositol (GPI), and therefore GPI-linked proteins are lacking in the PIG-A mutant clone. PNH RBCs lack two GPI-anchored complement regulatory proteins, CD55 and CD59. Hemolysis in PNH results from increased susceptibility of PNH RBCs to complement-mediated destruction. Intravascular hemolysis releases free hemoglobin into circulation. Free plasma hemoglobin scavenges nitric oxide (NO), and the depletion of NO at the tissue level is postulated to account for multiple PNH manifestations, including esophageal spasm, male erectile dysfunction, renal insufficiency, and thrombosis. Small PNH clones are present in a considerable proportion of the healthy general population. These clones are greatly expanded in patients with symptoms of PNH. It is postulated that PNH patients have some degree of marrow failure and the PNH clone is selectively protected from bone marrow injury as a result of the lack of GPI-linked proteins.[20]

DIAGNOSIS

Clinical Presentation

The clinical manifestations of PNH are **intravascular hemolytic anemia**, **marrow failure**, and **thrombosis**. The clinical course is unpredictable, and patients can have spontaneous remissions. Bone marrow failure can be transient, mild, or severe. Venous thromboembolism is the leading cause of morbidity and mortality in PNH and occurs in about 40% of PNH patients. Unusual sites of involvement characterize the thrombophilia in PNH and include hepatic vein thrombosis (Budd–Chiari syndrome), mesenteric vein thrombosis, and cerebral and dermal vein thromboses.[21,22] PNH can present with or without evidence of another disorder such as AA or MDS. PNH clones can be found in roughly 70% of adult patients with AA.[19] Subclinical PNH (without clinical or laboratory evidence of hemolysis) can occur in association with other bone marrow failure syndromes. PNH is not commonly associated with inherited bone marrow failure syndromes such as Fanconi anemia, dyskeratosis congenita, or Schwachman–Diamond syndrome.[19]

Diagnostic Testing

Flow cytometry is the most sensitive and specific test to identify the absence of GPI-anchored proteins on RBCs and neutrophils and thereby make the diagnosis of PNH. Fluorescein-labeled proaerolysin variant (FLAER) directly binds the GPI moiety on GPI-linked proteins and is increasingly replacing CD55 and CD59 monoclonal antibodies in the flow cytometric panels to diagnose PNH. The hemolysis is intravascular (high reticulocyte count, increased lactate dehydrogenase and unconjugated bilirubin, and decreased haptoglobulin) and is Coombs negative. Iron studies are needed to evaluate for iron-deficiency anemia, which can result from renal loss of hemoglobin. Bone marrow biopsy is helpful in assessing for marrow failure.

TREATMENT

The approach to therapy is dependent on the severity of symptoms and degree of hemolysis. For asymptomatic patients or those with mild symptoms, watchful waiting is reasonable. For patients with underlying AA, treatment is directed toward the underlying bone marrow failure. **Indications for treatment** in classic PNH include disabling fatigue, thromboses, transfusion dependence, frequent pain paroxysms, renal insufficiency, or other end-organ complications. Folic acid supplementation should be given to patients with ongoing hemolysis. Complement inhibition and HSCT are the only established effective therapies for PNH.

- **Complement inhibition: Eculizumab,** a humanized monoclonal antibody against complement C5, inhibits terminal complement activation.[23] It has been approved by the FDA for use in PNH. Eculizumab is effective in decreasing intravascular hemolysis, need for blood transfusions, and risk of thrombosis. Eculizumab is administered intravenously at a dose of 600 mg weekly for the first 4 weeks, then 900 mg biweekly starting on week 5. It is well tolerated but must be continued indefinitely as it does not treat the underlying cause. Its serious adverse effects include risk of infection by encapsulated organisms. Patients receiving eculizumab should be vaccinated against *Neisseria meningitides* prior to starting therapy.
- **Ravulizumab** is the most recent humanized monoclonal antibody approved by the FDA for the treatment of PNH. Similar to eculizumab, ravulizumab is effective at decreasing intravascular hemolysis, need for blood transfusions, and risk of thrombosis. In the trials that led to the approval of ravulizumab for the treatment of PNH, ravulizumab was compared to eculizumab and the results showed it was noninferior to eculizumab in both treatment naïve and previously treated PNH patients. In contrast to eculizumab, ravulizumab is administered every 8 weeks. The loading dose and maintenance dose of ravulizumab are dependent upon weight.[24,25]
- **HSCT:** Allogeneic HSCT remains the only curative therapy for PNH, but it is associated with significant morbidity and mortality. Currently, there is no definite indication for transplantation. Patients with life-threatening thrombosis and underlying severe BM failure should be considered for transplantation.

• **Treatment of thrombosis:** Thrombosis is a life-threatening complication of PNH and should be treated promptly with anticoagulation. However, anticoagulation is only partially effective in preventing clots, and treatment with eculizumab or ravulizumab should be strongly considered in patients with thrombosis. The duration of anticoagulation after initiation of eculizumab or ravulizumab is controversial in these patients. Likewise, the role of prophylactic anticoagulation in PNH is also controversial. Heparin and low–molecular-weight heparin products are preferred. Direct oral anticoagulants are thought to be safe and effective in PNH-induced thrombotic events; however, they have not been well studied.[19]

PROGNOSIS

The natural history of PNH is highly variable. Median survival was 10–15 years prior to the advent of C5 inhibitors. Currently, patients managed with complement inhibitors have a median survival similar to age-matched non-PNH controls. Thrombosis is the leading cause of death. Patients with PNH may also develop life-threatening bone marrow failure, MDS, or leukemia.[19] Patients with AA and a PNH clone typically do not exhibit signs or symptoms of PNH early in the natural history of their disease, but many will experience further expansion of the PIG-A mutant clone and progress to classic PNH.

REFERENCES

1. Shimamura A. Clinical approach to marrow failure. *Hematology Am Soc Hematol Educ Program.* 2009;329–337.
2. Burroughs L, Woolfrey A, Shimamura A. Shwachman-Diamond syndrome: a review of the clinical presentation, molecular pathogenesis, diagnosis, and treatment. *Hematol Oncol Clin North Am.* 2009; 23:233–248.
3. Kawashima N, Oyarbide U, Cipolli M, Bezzerri V, Corey SJ. Shwachman-Diamond syndromes: clinical, genetic, and biochemical insights from the rare variants. *Haematologica.* 2023;108(10):2594–2605.
4. Kennedy AL, Myers KC, Bowman J, et al. Distinct genetic pathways define pre-malignant versus compensatory clonal hematopoiesis in Shwachman-Diamond syndrome. *Nat Commun.* 2021;12:1334.
5. Han X, Lu S, Gu C, Bian Z, Xie X, Qiao X. Clinical features of Shwachman-Diamond syndrome: a systematic review. *BMC Pediatr.* 2023;23(1):503.
6. Furutani E, Liu S, Galvin A, et al. Hematologic complications with age in Shwachman-Diamond syndrome. *Blood Adv.* 2022;6:297–306.
7. Young NS, Scheinberg P, Calado RT. Aplastic anemia. *Curr Opin Hematol.* 2008;15:162–168.
8. Bacigalupo A. Aplastic anemia: pathogenesis and treatment. *Hematology Am Soc Hematol Educ Program.* 2007;23–28.
9. Valdez JM, Scheinberg P, Young NS, Walsh TJ. Infections in patients with aplastic anemia. *Semin Hematol.* 2009;46:269–276.
10. Patel BA, Giudice V, Young NS. Immunologic effects on the haematopoietic stem cell in marrow failure. *Best Pract Res Clin Haematol.* 2021;34:101276.
11. Marsh J, Socie G, Tichelli A, et al; European Group for Blood and Marrow Transplantation (EBMT) Severe Aplastic Anaemia Working Party. Should irradiated blood products be given routinely to all patients with aplastic anaemia undergoing immunosuppressive therapy with antithymocyte globulin (ATG)? A survey from the European Group for Blood and Marrow Transplantation Severe Aplastic Anaemia Working Party. *Br J Haematol.* 2010;150:377–379.
12. Peffault de Latour R, Kulasekararaj A, Iacobelli S, et al. Eltrombopag added to immunosuppression in severe aplastic anemia. *N Engl J Med.* 2022;386:11–23.
13. Bacigalupo A. How I treat acquired aplastic anemia. *Blood.* 2017;129:1428–1436.
14. Bacigalupo A, Socié G, Schrezenmeier H, et al; Aplastic Anemia Working Party of the European Group for Blood and Marrow Transplantation (WPSAA-EBMT). Bone marrow versus peripheral blood as the stem cell source for sibling transplants in acquired aplastic anemia: survival advantage for bone marrow in all age groups. *Haematologica.* 2012;97:1142–1148.
15. Lee JH, Lee JH, Shin YR, et al. Spontaneous remission of aplastic anemia: a retrospective analysis. *Haematologica.* 2001;86:928–933.

16. DeZern AE, Churpek JE. Approach to the diagnosis of aplastic anemia. *Blood Adv.* 2021;5:2660–2671.
17. Patel BA, Groarke EM, Lotter J, et al. Long-term outcomes in patients with severe aplastic anemia treated with immunosuppression and eltrombopag: a phase 2 study. *Blood.* 2022;139:34–43.
18. Vaht K, Göransson M, Carlson K, et al. Incidence and outcome of acquired aplastic anemia: real-world data from patients diagnosed in Sweden from 2000–2011. *Haematologica.* 2017;102:1683–1690.
19. Brodsky RA. How I treat paroxysmal nocturnal hemoglobinuria. *Blood.* 2021;137:1304–1309.
20. Bessler M, Hiken J. The pathophysiology of disease in patients with paroxysmal nocturnal hemoglobinuria. *Hematology.* 2008:104–110.
21. Hill A, Kelly RJ, Hillmen P. Thrombosis in paroxysmal nocturnal hemoglobinuria. *Blood.* 2013; 121:4985–4996.
22. Parker CJ. Paroxysmal nocturnal hemoglobinuria. *Curr Opin Hematol.* 2012;19:141–148.
23. Brodsky RA, Young NS, Antonioli E, et al. Multicenter phase 3 study of the complement inhibitor eculizumab for the treatment of patients with paroxysmal nocturnal hemoglobinuria. *Blood.* 2008; 111:1840–1847.
24. Kulasekararaj AG, Hill A, Rottinghaus ST, et al. Ravulizumab (ALXN1210) vs eculizumab in C5-inhibitor–experienced adult patients with PNH: the 302 study. *Blood.* 2019;133:540–549.
25. Lee JW, Sicre de Fontbrune F, Wong Lee Lee L, et al. Ravulizumab (ALXN1210) vs eculizumab in adult patients with PNH naive to complement inhibitors: the 301 study. *Blood.* 2019;133:530–539.

Myelodysplastic Neoplasms and Clonal Hematopoiesis

9

Constantine N. Logothetis and
Stefan P. Tarnawsky

Clonal Hematopoiesis

GENERAL PRINCIPLES

Clonal hematopoiesis (CH) occurs when genetic mutations in a hematopoietic stem cell (HSC) provide it with a growth advantage.[1] This causes the HSC to have a disproportionately large contribution to circulating blood cells. The genes implicated in CH are recurring, such that the 10 most commonly mutated genes in CH account for over 90% of cases.[2,3] Given that these CH genes provide a growth advantage, it is not surprising that many of them are also frequently found in blood cancers.[4,5] Although CH increases the risk of malignancy, most patients with CH do not develop blood cancers. Nevertheless, patients with CH may have a slightly higher mortality, primarily due to a higher risk of cardiovascular disease.[6] Poor prognostic features include cooccurring cytopenias and certain high-risk genetic features.

Classification

The key discriminators among CH patients are (i) the presence or absence of co-occurring cytopenias, and (ii) the identity of the underlying driver mutation(s). In a patient with normal blood counts, the condition is commonly referred to as clonal hematopoiesis of indeterminate potential (CHIP). As researchers continue to refine prediction models regarding which CH patients will progress to malignancy, the appropriateness of the "indeterminate potential" moniker has been questioned. Alternative names have been proposed such as age-related clonal hematopoiesis (ARCH). Herein, we will continue to use the term CHIP. In a patient with persistent cytopenias that cannot be explained through other causes, CH is termed clonal cytopenia of unknown significance (CCUS) and is discussed in the next section.

Epidemiology

CH is strongly associated with age.[2] The precise prevalence will vary depending on the threshold used to define clonality. For instance, CH becomes more common if the minimum clone size is reduced from >10% of peripheral blood cells to >0.1%.[7] Furthermore, not all genetic tests can identify all CH-associated mutations. For instance, the most prevalent CH gene alteration is loss of chromosome Y, which only occurs in males. This alternation can only be reliably detected with cytogenetic analysis, and is missed by targeted sequencing panels—which are the most frequently used test for CH. Nevertheless, the most common estimates of CH frequency are 1% at age 40, 5–15% at age 60, and 10–50% by age 80.[2,8] Certain exposures can also increase the incidence of CH, including smoking and chemotherapy.[9] In general, CH related to chemotherapy has distinct driver mutations—most commonly in DNA damage response genes such as TP53, PPM1D, and CHEK2—and has a higher risk of progression to malignancy.

Pathophysiology

The hallmark of CH is an HSC with a fitness advantage, meaning it has increased growth relative to other HSCs. Emerging evidence supports that the increased fitness in CH HSCs is caused by the underlying mutation(s) themselves. Understanding the precise cellular mechanism downstream of each individual CH mutation is an active area of research. However, the most common CH mutations converge on a handful of key growth pathways and hence can be classified into several signaling groups. For instance, DNMT3A, TET2, and ASXL1 are epigenetic modifiers that modulate global gene expression patterns by adding activating or repressive structures to specific areas of the genome. In contrast, U2AF1, SRSF2, and SF3B1 are components of the spliceosome, and mutations in these genes cause global alterations in mRNA splicing leading to preferential expression of alternative gene isoforms.[10] These isoforms can cause disease either by giving rise to a defective protein (hypomorph) or to a protein with atypical function (neomorph). Ongoing research aims to identify the precise downstream signals of each CH-associated mutation to determine how to promote fitness. This knowledge would lead to targeted therapies, which could slow the growth of a given CH clone.

DIAGNOSIS

The ability to detect CH relies on identifying the genetic feature(s) that distinguish a clonal HSC from nonaffected hematopoietic cells. These genetic features are highly variable and may include single nucleotide polymorphisms, chromosomal translocations, and aneuploidy, among others. In clinical practice, CH is usually identified by targeted sequencing of hotspot loci in the 40–60 genes that are most commonly implicated in CH. These tests can identify HSC clones with a corresponding variant allele frequency (VAF) as small as 0.1%, which means that a given mutation can be detected in as few as 1 in 1,000 sequencing reads for a given gene. Since each cell has two copies of almost all genes, a VAF of 0.1% generally corresponds to a clone size of one in 500 cells. The clinical significance of VAFs between 0.1% and 2% is uncertain, and most research studies use a VAF threshold of 2% to define CH. Whereas performing the genetic analysis on a bone marrow sample is preferred (since it allows morphologic analysis of this crucial hematopoietic compartment to look for evidence of malignancy or other pathologies), the VAFs obtained from peripheral blood correlate closely with those obtained from bone marrow.[11] Any patient being screened for CH must have a careful history, physical exam, and at a minimum a CBC and peripheral blood smear to assess for the presence of cytopenias or dysplastic cells.

PROGNOSIS

A patient with CHIP—who by definition has normal blood counts—has an estimated 0.5%/year chance of developing a hematologic malignancy (most commonly CLL).[2] Emerging data suggests this risk varies widely depending on the driver mutation.[1,12] CHIP patients with mutations in TP53 or spliceosome factors (notably U2AF1 and SRSF2) have much higher risk of progression to malignancy compared with unselected cohorts of CHIP patients, whereas those with a single DNMT3A mutation have a lower than average risk. CH that emerges following prior chemotherapy also has a worse prognosis.[9,13] Additional negative prognostic features include abnormal erythrocyte morphologies, namely high MCV and high RDW. Interestingly, CHIP has been implicated in nonhematopoietic disease processes, most notably a higher risk of cardiovascular disease, with an estimated hazard ratio of 1.9.[6] CH is rare among patients with Alzheimer dementia, and it has been hypothesized that CHIP may be protective against this disease.[14]

TREATMENT

Randomized trials have not addressed whether specific interventions can reduce the complications associated with CHIP. For example, it is unclear if CHIP alone—in the absence of other risk factors—should be an indication to start a statin to reduce cardiovascular events. Further, it is unknown whether interventions can reduce the risk of CHIP progressing to hematologic malignancy. The toxicities of current leukemia therapies preclude their use in CHIP. However, in the future, therapies targeting the specific underlying genetic changes may be able to reduce the risk of progression to hematologic malignancy. For now, observation with routine physical examination and laboratory assessment of CBC should be the preferred management.

Clonal Cytopenia of Unknown Significance

GENERAL PRINCIPLES

CCUS occurs when a patient with otherwise unexplained low blood counts is found to have an acquired mutation in blood cells.[15] The inference is that this mutation caused the cytopenia. The 10-year risk of progression to hematologic malignancy has been estimated at 50% to 95% in patients with CCUS, compared to 5% in patients with CHIP. Furthermore, the malignancies that develop following CCUS often affect the myeloid lineage (MDS or AML) and have a worse prognosis than CLL—the most common post-CHIP malignancy. As such, CCUS is emerging as a premalignant condition.[16] Ongoing studies are trying to identify which patients will progress to malignancy, when they will progress, and whether early intervention will mitigate this risk.

Epidemiology

CCUS—like CHIP—is a disorder of aging and becomes more prevalent in older populations. The precise prevalence has been difficult to estimate due to its recent conception and delayed implementation of consensus diagnostic criteria. In one well-cited study, 683 patients with unexplained cytopenias underwent a thorough examination.[15] Ultimately, 409 (60%) were diagnosed with a malignancy and 120 (17.5%) were found to have another clear cause of cytopenias. Among the 154 (22.5%) remaining patients with unexplained cytopenias, 56 (8.2%) had an acquired mutation in blood cells with a VAF >2% and thus met criteria for a diagnosis of CCUS.

DIAGNOSIS

To make the diagnosis of CCUS, a patient with thrombocytopenia, anemia, and/or neutropenia requires a thorough workup for potential causes of cytopenia. This includes a careful history to assess potential exposures or blood loss, lab tests looking for organ dysfunction (e.g., liver, kidneys), nutritional deficiencies (e.g., vitamin B_{12}, iron, copper), infections (e.g., HIV, ehrlichiosis), hemolysis, and a bone marrow biopsy to rule out malignancies and autoimmune conditions. If no cause of cytopenia is identified, then genetic testing should be performed on bone marrow cells with—at a minimum—karyotyping, targeted FISH, and sequencing panels looking for the 40–60 mutations most commonly implicated in CHIP, CCUS, and myeloid malignancies.[5] If such a mutation is found, then the patient is diagnosed with CCUS.

Classification

The mutation spectrum of CCUS differs from that of CHIP and MDS. In CCUS, TET2 is the most commonly mutated gene, followed by ASXL1 and DNMT3A.[15,16] SF3B1 is more commonly seen in MDS and is rare in CCUS patients. A recent study has proposed the Clonal Hematopoiesis Risk Score to classify the risk of CH and CCUS progressing to hematopoietic malignancy.[17] Patients were stratified as low-, medium-, and high-risk based on age, CBC parameters, and the number and type of acquired mutations. An online calculator helps with risk calculation, albeit it remains to be independently validated.[17]

PROGNOSIS

CCUS portends a much higher risk of progression to a hematologic malignancy than either CHIP or idiopathic cytopenia of uncertain significance (ICUS), the latter being patients with unexplained cytopenia and no known somatic mutations. The absolute 10-year risk of progression to a myeloid neoplasm in a cohort of 56 CCUS patients was 95%,[15] and another group noted a 4-year overall survival of approximately 80% among 78 CCUS patients.[16] Stratification of patients into low-risk and high-risk groups (the latter defined by the presence of mutation in splicing factors, TET2, ASXL1, or a DNMT3A mutation combined with one additional mutation), showed high-risk CCUS patients had a much higher rate of myeloid malignancy compared to the low-risk group (HR 4.12).[17] The more recent study that proposed the Clonal Hematopoiesis Risk Score had a much larger cohort of over 11,000 patients with CH or CCUS. Their 10-year risk of progressing to myeloid neoplasm in the low-, medium-, and high-risk groups were 0.67%, 7.8%, and 52.2%, respectively.

TREATMENT

No randomized clinical trials have determined whether early interventions can reduce the risk of CCUS progressing to malignancy. Given the new algorithms that can identify CCUS patients at high risk of evolution to malignancy, this is likely to be a very active area of research in the near future.

Myelodysplastic Neoplasms

GENERAL PRINCIPLES

Myelodysplastic neoplasms (MDS) are clonal stem cell disorders characterized by cytopenias and dysplastic bone marrow progenitors. Peripheral blood features include monocytosis, Pelger–Huet-like anomaly in neutrophils, circulating immature myeloid or erythroid cells, and macrocytosis. In MDS, the bone marrow is typically hypercellular, with "megaloblastoid changes," atypical megakaryocytes, erythroid hyperplasia, and defective maturation in the myeloid series. Increased blasts or ringed sideroblasts can also be seen. Despite increased cell proliferation, there is also increased apoptosis, leading to the discrepancy between the highly cellular bone marrow and peripheral cytopenias.

Epidemiology

The annual incidence rate of MDS is estimated to be 75/100,000 with 70 years being the median age at diagnosis.[18] Risk factors include exposure to chemotherapy (especially alkylating agents and topoisomerase II inhibitors), chloramphenicol, radiation, benzene, and other solvents, petroleum products, smoking, and immunosuppression. Inherited bone marrow failure syndromes are the primary risk factors for MDS in the pediatric age group.

TABLE 9-1	WHO 2022 CLASSIFICATION OF MYELODYSPLASTIC NEOPLASMS

Category	Blasts	Cytogenetics and Mutations
MDS with defining genetic abnormalities		
MDS with low blasts and isolated 5q deletion (MDS-5q)	<5% BM and <2% PB	Cytogenetics: 5q deletion alone, or with 1 other abnormality other than monosomy 7 or 7q deletion
MDS with low blasts and SF3B1 mutation (MDS-SF3B1)	<5% BM and <2% PB	Cytogenetics: Absence of 5q deletion, monosomy 7, or complex karyotype Mutations: SF3B1
MDS with biallelic TP53 inactivation (MDS-biTP53)	<20% BM and PB	Cytogenetics: Usually complex Mutations: Two or more TP53 mutations, or 1 mutation with evidence of TP53 copy number loss or copy neutral loss of heterozygosity
MDS, morphologically defined		
MDS with low blasts (MDS-LB)	<5% BM and <2% PB	
MDS, hypoplastic (MDS-h)	<5% BM and <2% PB	
MDS with increased blasts 1 (MDS-IB1)	5–9% BM or 2–4% PB	
MDS with increased blasts 2 (MDS-IB2)	10–19% BM or 5–19% PB or Auer rods	
MDS with fibrosis (MDS-f)	5–19% BM; 2–19% PB	

Adapted from Khoury JD, Solary E, Abla O, et al. The 5th edition of the World Health Organization Classification of haematolymphoid tumours: myeloid and histiocytic/dendritic neoplasms. *Leukemia.* 2022;36(7):1703–1719.

Classification

The World Health revised its classification of MDS in 2022. The revised classification is shown in Table 9-1.[19] **Therapy-related MDS** (tMDS) refers to MDS that arises after exposure to chemotherapy agents. tMDS differs from sporadic MDS in that it tends to be associated with distinct chromosomal abnormalities and carries a worse prognosis. tMDS after exposure to alkylating agents such as cyclophosphamide, melphalan, or nitrosoureas is associated with deletions or loss of chromosome 5 or 7 (sometimes as part of complex karyotypes), frequent somatic loss of TP53, and a longer latency of 3–10 years after therapy.[20] Topoisomerase II inhibitors such as doxorubicin, etoposide, and mitoxantrone cause tMDS/acute myeloid leukemia (AML) with translocations involving the MLL gene at chromosome 11q23, usually manifesting sooner, at about 1–3 years after treatment.[20]

Pathophysiology

MDS is a clonal stem cell disorder characterized by ineffective hematopoiesis leading to blood cytopenias. It carries a high risk of progression to AML. The pathophysiology of

MDS is complex and involves a multistep process of genetic changes. Somatic mutations have been detected in most MDS cases[5,21] and can involve genes encoding signaling molecules (*NRAS, KRAS, CBL, JAK2, FLT3*), epigenetic regulators (*TET2, EZH2, UTX, ASXL1, IDH1/2, DNMT3A, SETBP1*), transcription regulators (*RUNX1, NMP1, TP53*), and splicing factors (*SF3B1, SRSF2, ZRSF2, U2AF1*). Widespread gene hypermethylation is a major finding during progression of MDS to AML.[22]

DIAGNOSIS

Clinical Presentation

MDS is heterogeneous disorder due to its wide spectrum of severity (see Prognosis, below). Its main presenting clinical features (fatigue, bleeding, infections) are directly related to the severity of the cytopenias and the underlying bone marrow failure. Some patients with low-risk MDS may be asymptomatic and have only minor laboratory abnormalities on CBC. Lymph node involvement and hepatosplenomegaly are rare in MDS, and may suggest an alternate diagnosis, such as lymphoma, CMML, or an MDS/MPN overlap syndrome.

Diagnostic Testing

In the absence of other causes, marrow failure (as evidenced by cytopenias) with bone marrow findings of normal or increased cellularity with dysplastic myeloid cells is a cornerstone in establishing the diagnosis of MDS. The CBC often reveals cytopenias and an elevated mean corpuscular volume. Reticulocyte count is low. Peripheral blood smear may show oval macrocytic red cells, hypogranular neutrophils, and giant platelets. Distinct cytogenetic abnormalities can also help to confirm a diagnosis of MDS. Genetic analysis to identify the acquired mutations in MDS is now standard of care and provides prognostic information. As we refine our understanding of the genetics underlying MDS, it may be possible in the future to redefine MDS based solely on the complement of mutations. For now, however, pathologic identification of dysplasia remains a requirement for the diagnosis of MDS.

- **Bone marrow biopsy** is essential. The diagnosis of MDS requires the identification of dysplastic myeloid and/or erythroid progenitors, which distinguishes MDS from CCUS. Even among skilled hematopathologists, interobserver variability is high, which presents a major challenge to the diagnosis of MDS.[23] A molecular diagnosis of MDS—based solely on genetic abnormalities—would help eliminate this variability and will likely be proposed in the future. The marrow cellularity is usually increased; hypocellular MDS is rare and shares clinical and treatment similarities with aplastic anemia. The blast percentage is commonly normal (<5%), albeit MDS with excess blasts (5–9%) is associated with a worse prognosis. It is currently debated whether patients with 10–19% blasts should be classified as MDS or as AML, given the markedly poor prognosis in these patients.[19,24] Morphologic abnormalities include megaloblastic red cell precursors with multiple nuclei and asynchronous maturation of the nucleus or cytoplasm. Ringed sideroblasts (erythroid precursors with iron-laden mitochondria) are occasionally identified. There is often a predominance of immature myeloid cells, and granulocytic precursors may show asynchronous maturation of the nucleus and cytoplasm. Mature granulocytes are often hypogranular and hypolobulated. Megakaryocytes may be smaller and have fewer nuclear lobes.
- **Recurrent cytogenetic abnormalities** are present in 40–70% of de novo MDS and 95% of secondary MDS[5] (Table 9-2). The primary tools to assess for these are fluorescent in situ hybridization (**FISH**), and **metaphase karyotyping**. FISH can be performed on cells in interphase and can therefore be performed on terminally differentiated cells. However, FISH requires defined probes that look only for specific alterations. As such, FISH can only detect certain recurring chromosomal abnormalities, such as del(5), del(7), +(8),

TABLE 9-2	RECURRING CHROMOSOMAL ABNORMALITIES CONSIDERED AS PRESUMPTIVE EVIDENCE OF MDS IN THE SETTING OF PERSISTENT CYTOPENIA(S) OF UNDETERMINED ORIGIN

Unbalanced Abnormalities	WHO-Estimated Frequency in MDS (%)	Balanced Abnormalities	WHO-Estimated Frequency in MDS (%)
−7 or del(7q)	10; 50 in tMDS	t(11;16)(q23;p13.3)	3 in tMDS
−5 or del(5q)	10; 40 in tMDS	t(3;21)(q26.2;q22.1)	2 in tMDS
i(17q) or t(17p)	3–5	t(1;3)(p36.3;q21.1)	<1
−13 or del(13q)	3	t(2;11)(p21;q23)	<1
del(11q)	3	inv(3)(q21q26.2)	<1
del(12p) or t(12p)	3	t(6;9)(p23;q34)	<1
del(9q)	1–2		
idic(X)(q13)	1–2		

Reproduced with permission from Steensma DP. The changing classification of myelodysplastic syndromes: what's in a name? *Hematology Am Soc Hematol Educ Program.* 2009;2009(1):645–655.

among a handful of others. Metaphase karyotyping provides an unbiased global view of chromosomal abnormalities. However, usually, only 20 cells are assessed by karyotyping, whereas FISH will typically screen ~200 cells. FISH and metaphase cytogenetics remain complementary tools in the diagnosis and classification of MDS. Whole genome sequencing may be an alternative to FISH and metaphase cytogenetics.[25]

• **Targeted gene sequencing** is crucial for risk-stratifying MDS patients in the modern era. These next-generation sequencing (NGS) tests typically sequence mutation hotspots in the 40–60 genes that are most commonly mutated in MDS and AML. NGS can identify somatic mutations (Table 9-3) in the majority of MDS patients, including many with normal karyotypes.[26] Approximately 50% of MDS patients harbor a splicing factor mutation and a similar fraction carry more than one mutated epigenetic regulator.[5] Approximately 25% of patients have mutations of genes in both groups. In total, genetics tests can identify mutations in over 90% of MDS patients.[27]

TABLE 9-3	RECURRENT MUTATIONS IN MDS AND FREQUENCY

Splicing Factors (~50%)	Epigenetic Regulators (~45%)	Other Genes (~15%)
SF3B1 (18%)	TET2 (20%)	Transcription Factors
U2AF1 (12%)	ASXL1 (15%)	RUNX1, ETV6, PHF6,
SRSF2 (12%)	DNMT3A (12%)	GATA2
ZRSR2 (5%)	EZH2 (5%)	Kinase Signaling
Rarely co-occur with each other	IDH1/2 (5%)	NRAS, KRAS, JAK2, CBL
	Often co-occur except for TET2 and IDH	Cohesins
		STAG2, SMC3, RAD21

Data from Bejar R, Steensma DP. Recent developments in myelodysplastic syndromes. *Blood.* 2014;124(18):2793–2803.

TREATMENT

The Food and Drug Administration (FDA) has approved several drugs for the treatment of MDS patients including the hypomethylating agents 5-azacytidine (azaC), decitabine, and an oral preparation of decitabine-cedazuridine; the immunomodulator lenalidomide for patients with isolated del(5q) subtype; deferasirox, an iron chelator for treating chronic iron overload resulting from multiple transfusions; and luspatercept, an erythroid maturation agent. Supportive treatment with transfusions and growth factors is also part of MDS management. Allogeneic hematopoietic stem cell transplant (HSCT) is the primary curative treatment for patients with MDS. Features to consider for HSCT include patient's age, Revised International Prognostic Scoring System (IPSS-R) score, performance status, comorbidities, and availability of a suitable donor. Higher-risk patients should be considered for allogeneic stem cell transplant at diagnosis if a suitable donor is identified, whereas delaying transplantation for several years and prior to disease progression would be appropriate for lower-risk patients. In patients who require reduction of their disease burden prior to HSCT, hypomethylating agents, or participation in clinical trials can be used as bridges to transplant.

- **Lower-risk MDS**

  For patients with lower-risk MDS, treatment is aimed at reducing transfusions, restoring effective blood cell production, and maximizing quality of life. For lower-risk MDS patients with symptomatic anemia, treatment follows one of several pathways.

  ○ In patients with **isolated del(5q)** or **5q syndrome**, lenalidomide, a derivative of thalidomide, is the treatment of choice. In this population, approximately 70% of patients experience red blood cell (RBC) transfusion independence or a decline in transfusion needs when treated with lenalidomide, and 50–70% can achieve a cytogenetic response. Higher RBC transfusion independence and cytogenetic response are observed with a daily dose of 10 mg compared with 5 mg.[28] The median duration of response is approximately 2 years.[29] The major dose-limiting toxicity of lenalidomide is neutropenia and thrombocytopenia. Close monitoring of blood counts is required during treatment.[30] Additional side effects of lenalidomide include risk of venous thromboembolism, rash, and diarrhea.

  ○ In patients with **lower-risk MDS lacking del(5q)**, erythropoiesis-stimulating agents (ESAs), which include erythropoietin and darbepoetin, have historically been the first choice of treatment for anemia. Patients with low transfusion needs, defined as <2 units of packed red blood cells (PRBCs) monthly and a low baseline serum erythropoietin level (<500 IU) have a 74% chance of responding to ESAs. Most responses to ESA occur within 8–12 weeks of treatment and median duration of response is approximately 2 years.[30] The COMMANDS trial recently showed that luspatercept led to greater transfusion independence and improvements in hemoglobin compared to epoetin alfa in ESA-naïve, lower-risk MDS patients.[31]

  ○ For patients who experience ESA failure (primary resistance or relapse within 6 months), second-line treatments such as antithymocyte globulin (ATG), hypomethylating agents, and lenalidomide may be considered.[30] Of note, patients with higher transfusion needs (≥2 units of PRBCs) and high serum erythropoietin levels (≥500 IU) have only a 7% chance of responding to ESAs. Patients who are 60 years of age and younger with hypocellular marrows, HLA-DR15 histocompatibility type, or PNH clone positivity, have a good probability of responding to immunosuppressive therapy (IST) with ATG and cyclosporin A. Those who are deemed unlikely to respond to IST should be treated with hypomethylating agents or lenalidomide. In the recent MEDALIST trial, luspatercept was shown to reduce the severity of anemia in transfusion-dependent lower-risk MDS patients with ring sideroblasts who were refractory to or unlikely to respond to ESAs.[32]

- ○ Neutropenia (WBC <1.5 μL) is found in only 7% of lower-risk MDS and is rarely associated with life-threatening infection. Granulocyte colony–stimulating factor (G-CSF) can improve neutropenia in 60–75% of cases, but its prolonged use has not demonstrated an impact on survival, and there exists a theoretical risk of stimulating progression to higher-risk MDS or AML.[33] Thrombopoietin (TPO) receptor agonists such as romiplostim and eltrombopag have shown promising results in treating thrombocytopenia in MDS,[34] but are not approved for use in routine clinical practice.
  - ○ **Iron chelation therapy** may be used in patients who receive long-term RBC transfusions. Heavily RBC-transfused patients may develop significant iron overload which can lead to cardiac failure and liver cirrhosis. Iron chelation should be considered in patients with relatively favorable prognosis (low or INT-1 risk MDS) who have received at least 50–60 units of PRBCs, have a serum ferritin >2,500 U/L, or if cardiac MRI shows evidence of cardiac iron overload. Deferasirox, an oral iron chelator, offers a more convenient option than previous parenteral iron chelation. Deferasirox is commonly associated with gastrointestinal side effects and should not be used in patients with renal failure.[35]
- • **Higher-risk MDS**
  For patients with higher-risk MDS, the goals of treatment are similar to patients with AML, namely to prolong survival and maximize quality of life. For patients who are candidates for high-intensity therapy, allogeneic HSCT is recommended upfront if a suitable donor can be identified. Patients without a suitable donor or those who are not candidates for allogeneic HSCT should be treated with a hypomethylating agent or enrolled in a clinical trial. Decitabine/Cedazuridine (brand name Inqovi) was recently approved as an oral treatment option for patients with MDS.[36] The role of nonmyeloablative or reduced-intensity conditioning HSCT may be an option for older patients or those with comorbidities. Important questions such as optimal approaches to pretransplant therapy, donor selection, conditioning regimen, and posttransplant therapy to prevent relapse are areas of continued investigation.[37]

PROGNOSIS

Evolution to AML occurs in 10–50% of MDS cases and varies among MDS subtypes. The development of AML strongly correlates with survival. The International Prognostic Scoring System (IPSS) was developed in 1997 to stratify newly diagnosed and untreated patients into risk groups based on (i) percentage of BM blasts, (ii) the presence of cytopenias, and (iii) the presence of defined cytogenetic abnormalities (Table 9-4).[38] In 2012, the IPSS was revised (IPSS-R) to take into account age, the degree of cytopenias, and greater nuance in the BM blast percentage and cytogenetic categories (Table 9-5).[39] The estimated median overall survival for patients in the very low–, low-, intermediate-, high-, and very high–risk groups are 8.8 years, 5.3 years, 3 years, 1.6 years, and 0.8 years, respectively. As with the IPSS, those in the higher-risk categories (intermediate, high, very high) have a significantly higher risk of evolution to AML

A major limitation of the IPSS-R was that it did not consider the prognostic significance of specific gene mutations. This was overcome in 2022 with the publication of the IPSS-Molecular (IPSS-M).[27] An online tool permits calculation of a given patient's risk category as well as median AML-free survival and overall survival. Of note, given the lack of standardization among sequencing panels and cytogenetics techniques, the mutational status for all 31 relevant genes may not be known in some MDS patients. This is particularly notable for partial tandem duplications of MLL, whose presence harbors a particularly poor prognosis. As such, it is likely that the full adoption and routine implementation of IPSS-M will take several years.

TABLE 9-4	INTERNATIONAL PROGNOSTIC SCORING SYSTEM FOR MDS		
Points	Bone Marrow Blasts (%)	Karyotype[a]	Cytopenias[b]
0	<5	Good	0 or 1
0.5	5–10	Intermediate	2 or 3
1	—	Poor	
1.5	11–20		
2	21–30		

Percentage marrow blasts, karyotype, and cytopenias are each assigned point values, which are then added together to derive the patient's risk score. Scores for risk groups are as follows: Low 0; INT-1 0.5–1; INT-2 1.5–2; and High ≥2.5.
[a]Good prognosis karyotypes: normal, –Y only, del(5q) only, del(20q) only; intermediate, trisomy 8; Poor, complex defects, monosomy 7.
[b]Cytopenias defined as follows: hemoglobin <10 g/dL; absolute neutrophil count <1.5 × 10^9; platelet count <100 × 10^9/L.
Data from Greenberg P, Cox C, LeBeau MM, et al. International scoring system for evaluating prognosis in myelodysplastic syndromes. *Blood.* 1997;89:2079–2088.

TABLE 9-5	REVISED INTERNATIONAL PROGNOSTIC SCORING SYSTEM FOR MDS				
Points	Cytogenetics[a]	Bone Marrow Blast (%)	Hemoglobin (g/dL)	Platelets (Cells/μL)	Absolute Neutrophil Count (Cells/μL)
0	Very good	≤2	≥10	≥100	≥0.8
0.5				50–100	<0.8
1	Good	>2–<5	8–<10	<50	
1.5			<8		
2	Intermediate	5–10			
3	Poor	>10			
4	Very poor				

Scores for each risk group are as follows: Very low (≤1.5), Low (>1.5–3), Intermediate (>3–4.5), High (>4.5–6), and Very high (>6).
[a]Very good, –Y, del(11q); Good, Normal, del(5q), del(12p), del(20q), double including del(5q); intermediate, del(7q), +8, +19, i(17q), any other single or double independent clones; poor, –7, inv(3)/t(3q)/del(3q), double including –7/del(7q), complex/3 abnormalities; very poor, complex/>3 abnormalities.
From Greenberg PL, Tuechler H, Schanz J, et al. Revised international prognostic scoring system for myelodysplastic syndromes. *Blood.* 2012;120(12):2454–2465.

VEXAS Syndrome

GENERAL PRINCIPLES

Vacuoles, E1 enzyme, X-linked, Autoinflammatory, Somatic (VEXAS) syndrome is a novel disorder first described in 2020. VEXAS syndrome develops following a somatic mutation in the X-linked ubiquitin-activating enzyme gene, *UBA1*. The *UBA1* mutation is found in hematopoietic progenitor cells leading to a diverse array of hematologic manifestations, including macrocytic anemia, thrombocytopenia, thromboembolic disease, and progressive bone marrow failure which can evolve into hematologic malignancies. Roughly 24% of patients had myelodysplastic syndrome and about 20% of patients had either multiple myeloma or monoclonal gammopathy of undetermined significance.[40]

Clinical Presentation

Patients with VEXAS syndrome often present with severe autoinflammatory symptoms. Monocytes and neutrophils demonstrate highly activated inflammatory signatures illustrating severe myeloid inflammation, which can lead to constellation of symptoms including Sweet syndrome, relapsing polychondritis, polyarteritis nodosa, and giant cell arteritis in addition to the hematologic manifestations. The morbidity and mortality associated with VEXAS syndrome is considerably high.[40] Since the *UBA1* gene is located on the X chromosome, men are predominantly affected. Women can be affected due to lyonization of the X-chromosome.[41]

TREATMENT

There is no FDA-approved treatment for VEXAS syndrome and more management occurs via best clinical judgment. The literature contains many retrospective studies and case reports regarding the treatment of VEXAS syndrome. Currently, no benefit from disease-modifying antirheumatologic drugs has been observed. High-dose corticosteroids are frequently used with some clinical benefit. Unfortunately, steroids are associated with significant adverse events and patients are often refractory to tapers limiting their usefulness. Other treatments including azacitidine, tocilizumab, anakinra, and canakinumab have been explored retrospectively with mixed outcomes. Retrospective studies have suggested that janus kinase inhibitors (JAK-I), specifically JAK1/2 inhibitors, hold promising therapeutic benefits; clinical trials for these are ongoing.[41] Overall, the optimal treatment for VEXAS syndrome remains an active area of research.

REFERENCES

1. Fabre MA, de Almeida JG, Fiorillo E, et al. The longitudinal dynamics and natural history of clonal haematopoiesis. *Nature*. 2022;606(7913):335–342.
2. Jaiswal S, Fontanillas P, Flannick J, et al. Age-related clonal hematopoiesis associated with adverse outcomes. *N Engl J Med*. 2014;371(26):2488–2498.
3. Xie M, Lu C, Wang J, et al. Age-related mutations associated with clonal hematopoietic expansion and malignancies. *Nat Med*. 2014;20(12):1472–1478.
4. Cancer Genome Atlas Research Network; Ley TJ, Miller C, Ding L, et al. Genomic and epigenomic landscapes of adult de novo acute myeloid leukemia. *N Engl J Med*. 2013;368(22):2059–2074.
5. Ogawa S. Genetics of MDS. *Blood*. 2019;133(10):1049–1059.
6. Jaiswal S, Natarajan P, Silver AJ, et al. Clonal hematopoiesis and risk of atherosclerotic cardiovascular disease. *N Engl J Med*. 2017;377(2):111–121.
7. Young AL, Challen GA, Birmann BM, Druley TE. Clonal haematopoiesis harbouring AML-associated mutations is ubiquitous in healthy adults. *Nat Commun*. 2016;7(1):12484.

8. Watson CJ, Papula AL, Poon GYP, et al. The evolutionary dynamics and fitness landscape of clonal hematopoiesis. *Science*. 2020;367(6485):1449–1454.

9. Bolton KL, Ptashkin RN, Gao T, et al. Cancer therapy shapes the fitness landscape of clonal hematopoiesis. *Nat Genet*. 2020;52(11):1219–1226.

10. Yoshida K, Sanada M, Shiraishi Y, et al. Frequent pathway mutations of splicing machinery in myelodysplasia. *Nature*. 2011;478(7367):64–69.

11. Jansko-Gadermeir B, Leisch M, Gassner FJ, et al. Myeloid NGS analyses of paired samples from bone marrow and peripheral blood yield concordant results: a prospective cohort analysis of the AGMT study group. *Cancers (Basel)*. 2023;15(8):2305.

12. Abelson S, Collord G, Ng SWK, et al. Prediction of acute myeloid leukaemia risk in healthy individuals. *Nature*. 2018;559(7714):400–404.

13. Coombs CC, Zehir A, Devlin SM, et al. Therapy-related clonal hematopoiesis in patients with non-hematologic cancers is common and associated with adverse clinical outcomes. *Cell Stem Cell*. 2017;21(3):374–382.e4.

14. Bouzid H, Belk JA, Jan M, et al. Clonal hematopoiesis is associated with protection from Alzheimer's disease. *Nat Med*. 2023;29(7):1662–1670.

15. Malcovati L, Gallì A, Travaglino E, et al. Clinical significance of somatic mutation in unexplained blood cytopenia. *Blood*. 2017;129(25):3371–3378.

16. Choi EJ, Cho YU, Hur EH, et al. Clinical implications and genetic features of clonal cytopenia of undetermined significance compared to lower-risk myelodysplastic syndrome. *Br J Haematol*. 2022; 198(4):703–712.

17. Weeks LD, Niroula A, Neuberg D, et al. Prediction of risk for myeloid malignancy in clonal hematopoiesis. *NEJM Evid*. 2023;2(5):10.1056/evidoa2200310.

18. Cazzola M. Myelodysplastic syndromes. *N Engl J Med*. 2020;383(14):1358–1374.

19. Khoury JD, Solary E, Abla O, et al. The 5th edition of the World Health Organization classification of haematolymphoid tumours: myeloid and histiocytic/dendritic neoplasms. *Leukemia*. 2022; 36(7):1703–1719.

20. Churpek JE, Larson RA. The evolving challenge of therapy-related myeloid neoplasms. *Best Pract Res Clin Haematol*. 2013;26(4):309–317.

21. Bejar R, Stevenson K, Abdel-Wahab O, et al. Clinical effect of point mutations in myelodysplastic syndromes. *N Engl J Med*. 2011;364(26):2496–2506.

22. Shen L, Kantarjian H, Guo Y, et al. DNA methylation predicts survival and response to therapy in patients with myelodysplastic syndromes. *J Clin Oncol*. 2010;28(4):605–613.

23. Font P, Loscertales J, Soto C, et al. Interobserver variance in myelodysplastic syndromes with less than 5% bone marrow blasts: unilineage vs. multilineage dysplasia and reproducibility of the threshold of 2% blasts. *Ann Hematol*. 2015;94(4):565–573.

24. Arber DA, Orazi A, Hasserjian RP, et al. International consensus classification of myeloid neoplasms and acute leukemias: integrating morphologic, clinical, and genomic data. *Blood*. 2022;140(11):1200–1228.

25. Duncavage EJ, Schroeder MC, O'Laughlin M, et al. Genome sequencing as an alternative to cytogenetic analysis in myeloid cancers. *N Engl J Med*. 2021;384(10):924–935.

26. Bejar R, Steensma DP. Recent developments in myelodysplastic syndromes. *Blood*. 2014;124(18): 2793–2803.

27. Bernard E, Tuechler H, Greenberg PL, et al. Molecular international prognostic scoring system for myelodysplastic syndromes. *NEJM Evid*. 2022;1(7):EVIDoa2200008.

28. Fenaux P, Giagounidis A, Selleslag D, et al. A randomized phase 3 study of lenalidomide versus placebo in RBC transfusion-dependent patients with Low-/Intermediate-1-risk myelodysplastic syndromes with del5q. *Blood*. 2011;118(14):3765–3776.

29. Platzbecker U. Treatment of MDS. *Blood*. 2019;133(10):1096–1107.

30. Carraway HE, Saygin C. Therapy for lower-risk MDS. *Hematology*. 2020;2020(1):426–433.

31. Platzbecker U, Della Porta MG, Santini V, et al. Efficacy and safety of luspatercept versus epoetin alfa in erythropoiesis-stimulating agent-naive, transfusion-dependent, lower-risk myelodysplastic syndromes (COMMANDS): interim analysis of a phase 3, open-label, randomised controlled trial. *Lancet*. 2023;402(10399):373–385.

32. Fenaux P, Platzbecker U, Mufti GJ, et al. Luspatercept in patients with lower-risk myelodysplastic syndromes. *N Engl J Med*. 2020;382(2):140–151.

33. Fenaux P, Adès L. How we treat lower-risk myelodysplastic syndromes. *Blood*. 2013;121(21): 4280–4286.

34. Fenaux P, Muus P, Kantarjian H, et al. Romiplostim monotherapy in thrombocytopenic patients with myelodysplastic syndromes: long-term safety and efficacy. *Br J Haematol*. 2017;178(6):906–913.

35. Gattermann N, Finelli C, Porta MD, et al. Deferasirox in iron-overloaded patients with transfusion-dependent myelodysplastic syndromes: results from the large 1-year EPIC study. *Leuk Res.* 2010;34(9):1143–1150.

36. Garcia-Manero G, Griffiths EA, Steensma DP, et al. Oral cedazuridine/decitabine for MDS and CMML: a phase 2 pharmacokinetic/pharmacodynamic randomized crossover study. *Blood.* 2020; 136(6):674–683.

37. Sekeres MA, Cutler C. How we treat higher-risk myelodysplastic syndromes. *Blood.* 2014;123(6): 829–836.

38. Greenberg P, Cox C, LeBeau MM, et al. International scoring system for evaluating prognosis in myelodysplastic syndromes. *Blood.* 1997;89(6):2079–2088.

39. Greenberg PL, Tuechler H, Schanz J, et al. Revised international prognostic scoring system for myelodysplastic syndromes. *Blood.* 2012;120(12):2454–2465.

40. Beck DB, Ferrada MA, Sikora KA, et al. Somatic Mutations in UBA1 and severe adult-onset autoinflammatory disease. *N Engl J Med.* 2020;383(27):2628–2638.

41. Sujobert P, Heiblig M, Jamilloux Y. VEXAS: where do we stand 2 years later? *Curr Opin Hematol.* 2023;30(2):64–69.

Myeloproliferative Neoplasms 10

Imran Nizamuddin and Amy W. Zhou

GENERAL PRINCIPLES

Myeloproliferative neoplasms (MPNs) are a group of myeloid malignancies characterized by stem cell–derived clonal myeloproliferation. The diagnostic criteria for these diseases have evolved over the years. As of 2022, the predominant classification system is the International Consensus Classification (ICC) of Myeloid Neoplasms and Acute Leukemias.[1] An alternative classification proposed by the 5th edition of the World Health Organization (WHO) may be used.[2] Despite minor differences in diagnostic criteria, both systems recognize similar conditions under the category of MPNs. Major ICC categories are listed in Table 10-1. Philadelphia chromosome–positive chronic myeloid leukemia (CML) is discussed separately in the chapter on leukemias (see Chapter 32).

Collectively, these disorders are uncommon. They share the signs and symptoms of extramedullary disease, clonal marrow hyperplasia without dysplasia, and proliferation of one or more cell lines. The clinical course of these diseases is variable, and all carry a risk of leukemic transformation.

Polycythemia Vera

GENERAL PRINCIPLES

Definition

Polycythemia vera (PV) is a clonal stem cell disorder characterized by erythrocytosis and is defined by mutations in the JAK2 kinase.[3] *JAK2* (9p24) mutations were first identified in 2005 and found to be present in nearly all patients with PV. Over 95% of patients display somatic activating mutations in exon 14 (*JAK2* **V617F mutation**) and approximately 3% carry a mutation in exon 12.

Epidemiology

PV is the most common of the MPNs, with an incidence of approximately 2 in 100,000 people. The average age of PV patients is 60 years, but it occurs across all age groups, with a male predominance. Although familial clustering does exist, it is uncommon.

Etiology

Virtually all patients with PV have a *JAK2* mutation, the most common being *JAK2* V617F, which is located on exon 14 of chromosome 9. The JAK2 protein is an essential kinase in the erythropoietin (EPO) receptor signal transduction pathway. Constitutive JAK2 kinase activity results in EPO-independent proliferation of erythrocyte precursors. JAK2 is also involved in the JAK2-STAT5 pathways of the thrombopoietin (TPO) receptor and the granulocyte colony–stimulating factor receptor (GCSF-R), and patients with PV may have elevated platelets and leukocytes as well.[4]

TABLE 10-1	CLASSIFICATION OF MYELOPROLIFERATIVE DISORDERS	
BCR-ABL Positive	**BCR-ABL Negative**	**JAK2 V617F**
Chronic myeloid leukemia	Polycythemia vera	>95%
	Essential thrombocythemia	50–60%
	Primary myelofibrosis	35–55%
	Chronic neutrophilic leukemia	1–5%
	Chronic eosinophilic leukemia, not otherwise specified	
	Myeloproliferative neoplasm, unclassifiable	

Adapted from Arber DA, Orazi A, Hasserjian RP, et al. International Consensus Classification of myeloid neoplasms and acute leukemias: integrating morphologic, clinical, and genomic data. *Blood.* 2022;140:1200–1228.

Clinical Course

- PV is a chronic disorder and may be characterized as having distinct phases during its course. The **pre-erythrocytic phase** is generally asymptomatic, with an isolated increase in platelets or RBCs. This progresses to the **erythrocytic phase**, characterized by erythrocytosis requiring regular phlebotomy, as well as increased granulocytes and platelet counts. Splenomegaly, pruritus, thrombosis, and hemorrhage may be present. Eventually, this may progress to the **spent phase**, associated with fibrosis and characterized by a reduced need for phlebotomy.
- The Myeloproliferative Neoplasm Symptom Assessment Form (MPN-SAF) may be used to assess symptomatic burden in a standardized and reproducible manner.[5]
- Leukemic transformation rates at 20 years are estimated to be <10%, and the risk of transformation to secondary myelofibrosis (MF) is slightly higher.[6]
- Thrombotic risk is present throughout the course of PV, and patients can experience arterial or venous thrombosis. Thromboses can occur in unusual sites such as portal, splenic, mesenteric, or hepatic (Budd–Chiari syndrome) veins. For patients, especially young women (<45 years of age), who present with splanchnic vein thrombosis, a *JAK2* V617F mutation should be sent, as this can be the first clinical manifestation of MPN.[7]

DIAGNOSIS

Clinical Presentation

Patients are often asymptomatic at presentation; however, they may present with symptoms related to increased RBC mass and hyperviscosity. Symptoms may include headache, weakness, peptic ulcer disease, hyperhydrosis, vision changes, tinnitus, and vertigo. In addition, patients may experience pruritus, especially with exposure to hot water. **Erythromelalgia**, due to microarteriolar occlusion, is characterized by burning pain, increased skin warmth, and erythema of the hands and feet. Patients are also predisposed to thrombosis and, less often, hemorrhage. Many of these symptoms have been attributed to hyperviscosity, but dysfunction of leukocytes and platelets may also play an important role. Physical examination findings may include splenomegaly, hepatomegaly, and plethora, although splenomegaly generally is less common in PV and should prompt consideration for evaluation of MF if present.

TABLE 10-2 ICC 2022 DIAGNOSTIC CRITERIA FOR POLYCYTHEMIA VERA AND ESSENTIAL THROMBOCYTHEMIA

Polycythemia Vera

Diagnosis requires presence of all three major criteria OR the first two major criteria plus the minor criterion:

Major:
1. Increased hemoglobin level (>16.5 g/dL in men or >16.0 g/dL in women), hematocrit (>49% in men or >48% in women), or increased red blood cell mass (>25% above mean normal predicted value)
2. Presence of JAK2 V617F or JAK2 exon 12 mutation
3. Bone marrow biopsy showing hypercellularity for age with trilineage growth (panmyelosis) including prominent erythroid, granulocytic, and megakaryocytic proliferation with pleomorphic, mature megakaryocytes

Minor:
Subnormal serum EPO level

Essential Thrombocythemia

Diagnosis requires presence of all four major criteria OR the first three major criteria plus the minor criterion:

Major:
1. Platelet count ≥450 × 10⁹/L
2. Bone marrow biopsy showing megakaryocyte proliferation with large and mature morphology; no relevant bone marrow fibrosis
3. Not meeting diagnostic criteria for CML, PV, PMF, MDS, or other myeloid neoplasm
4. Demonstration of a *JAK2*, *CALR*, or *MPL* mutation

Minor:
Demonstration of another clonal marker or absence of secondary cause of thrombocytosis

EPO, serythropoietin; Hct, hematocrit; Hgb, hemoglobin; CML, chronic myelogenous leukemia.
Adapted from Arber DA, Orazi A, Hasserjian RP, et al. International Consensus Classification of myeloid neoplasms and acute leukemias: integrating morphologic, clinical, and genomic data. *Blood.* 2022;140:1200–1228.

Diagnostic Criteria

The 2022 ICC diagnostic criteria for PV is listed in Table 10-2.[1] Diagnosis of PV requires the presence of all three major criteria or the first two major criteria with the minor criterion. Overall, hallmarks of diagnosis include elevated hemoglobin (Hgb) level, presence of a *JAK2* gene mutation, and subnormal serum EPO level. Over 95% of patients with PV test positive for the *JAK2* V617F mutation, with a small minority testing positive for *JAK2* exon 12 mutations.[8,9]

Differential Diagnosis

Patients with secondary polycythemia typically have elevated EPO levels caused by chronic hypoxemia, heavy smoking, renal disease, or malignancies such as renal cell cancer, hepatocellular cancer, and hemangioblastoma. Rare conditions such as congenital polycythemia with augmented hypoxia-sensing and high-oxygen affinity (Hgb) mutants should be considered. Relative polycythemia, or pseudopolycythemia, is associated with a normal red cell mass and decreased plasma volume secondary to causes such as dehydration, diuretics, and burns. In cases of *JAK2*-negative polycythemia with low-normal EPO levels, a bone marrow (BM) biopsy should be considered.

Diagnostic Testing

- The diagnosis is suspected when blood counts reveal an elevated Hgb or hematocrit (Hct). The **EPO level is low** (<20 mU/mL) and often undetectable. The *JAK2* **V617F mutation** is seen in nearly all patients. Proliferation of other cell lines of myeloid lineage may be seen.
- Iron studies should be checked as virtually all patients are iron deficient at presentation or during the course of their disease.[10] Furthermore, iron deficiency may mask an otherwise increased Hgb or Hct.
- **Bone marrow (BM) biopsy** findings are not required for diagnosis of PV if other criteria are met; however, the detection of MF in the BM at the time of diagnosis has prognostic value.[11] Furthermore, it may be performed if a *JAK2* mutation is not detected in the peripheral blood and other etiologies need to be ruled out. In PV, the BM is characterized by trilineage myeloproliferation with pleomorphic megakaryocytes. Cytogenetic abnormalities are relatively uncommon in PV, with a recent large series showing about 12% with an abnormal karyotype, and they are associated with worse prognosis.[12]

TREATMENT

The goals of treatment are to reduce the blood volume to maintain Hct of <45% and to prevent thrombotic complications. Patients with an Hct target of less than 45% have a significantly lower rate of cardiovascular death and major thrombosis than those with higher targets.[13] **Thrombotic risk** has been associated with an age >60 years and prior thrombosis history. In addition, history of hypertension is associated with an increased risk of arterial thrombosis.[14]

- **Low-risk patients** are <60 years old and have no history of thrombosis. These patients are managed with phlebotomy to an Hct of <45% and low-dose aspirin. Iron deficiency via phlebotomy is a goal of treatment.
- **High-risk patients** are ≥60 years old or have a history of a thrombotic event. These patients typically require cytoreductive agents in addition to phlebotomy. Low-dose aspirin should be given to all patients with PV unless there is a specific contraindication.

Medications

Hydroxyurea is the most commonly used first-line cytoreductive agent. Additional second-line agents may include interferon alpha (IFN-α) or ruxolitinib.

- **Hydroxyurea** is added to phlebotomy in the treatment of high-risk PV patients. The usual starting dose is 500 mg daily. The dose of hydroxyurea is titrated to maintain the Hct <45 without the need for phlebotomy. Hydroxyurea is generally well tolerated but may cause rash, hyperpigmentation, and distal leg ulcers. Gastrointestinal symptoms of nausea, vomiting, constipation, and diarrhea are very common with doses >60 mg/kg. There is currently no controlled evidence to implicate hydroxyurea as being leukemogenic.
- **IFN-α** may be considered in patients who are intolerant or resistant to hydroxyurea. Pegylated preparations of IFN-α are preferred due to improved tolerability. Pegylated IFN-α is started at 45 μg once a week and titrated up to 180 μg once a week as tolerated. Ropeginterferon alfa-2b was recently approved by the Federal Drug Administration (FDA) based on high rates of complete hematologic response.[15] Compared to conventional interferons, this formulation has more favorable tolerability and convenience.
- **Ruxolitinib**, a JAK2 inhibitor previously approved for treatment of patients with MF, is FDA-approved for second-line treatment in PV patients who are either resistant or intolerant to hydroxyurea. Compared to best available therapy (which most commonly included hydroxyurea or IFN-α), ruxolitinib demonstrated greater reduction in

splenomegaly, fewer thromboembolic events, greater control of PV symptoms (fatigue, **pruritus**, and night sweats), and fewer patients requiring phlebotomy.[16] Ruxolitinib is well tolerated, with the most common side effect being myelosuppression; however, long-term safety data are not yet available.

- Additional agents can be useful in symptom management. **Hyperuricemia** may be treated with allopurinol. **Erythromelalgia** may be treated with aspirin or other nonsteroidal anti-inflammatory drugs.

SPECIAL CONSIDERATIONS

- **Surgery:** Patients with PV have a higher rate of hemorrhagic or thrombotic complications in the perioperative period; this risk should be considered when undergoing elective surgery.[17] Thromboembolic prophylaxis should be used as well. Aspirin is often held prior to surgery, and this period may increase risk for thrombotic events. Splenectomy is rarely recommended in PV patients because of the high risk of surgical complications and thrombosis.
- **PV and pregnancy:** There is an increased incidence of premature births, preeclampsia, and hemorrhage in PV patients.[18] Management should include phlebotomy and low-dose aspirin. Aspirin should be discontinued 5 days prior to delivery to limit hemorrhagic risk. If cytoreductive therapy is needed, IFN-α is the agent of choice as it has not been shown to be teratogenic or leukemogenic.

OUTCOME/PROGNOSIS

In general, life expectancy in PV is inferior to that of age- and sex-matched controls, but prognosis is still very good for the majority of patients. The overall median survival is approximately 14 years, and in patients <60 years, the median survival is approximately 24 years.[12] Risk factors for survival in PV include advanced age (>70 years), leukocytosis (WBC >13 $\times$ 10^9/L), thrombosis, and abnormal karyotype.[19] Morbidity and mortality are related to thrombotic events. Leukemic transformation rates at 20 years are estimated at <10% for PV; fibrotic transformation rates are slightly higher. Risk factors for leukemic transformation include advanced age, leukocytosis, and abnormal karyotype,[12] while risk factors for fibrotic transformation include *JAK2* V617F allele burden of more than 50%.[20]

Essential Thrombocythemia

GENERAL PRINCIPLES

Definition

Essential thrombocythemia (ET) is a stem cell disorder characterized by markedly elevated platelet count caused by excessive megakaryocyte proliferation. The activating *JAK2* V617F mutation is seen in nearly half of patients with ET. Mutations in myeloproliferative leukemia virus oncogene (*MPL*), located on chromosome 1p34, are found in 3–4% of ET patients.[21] Recently, mutations in calreticulin (*CALR*) have been described in a large percentage of ET patients that are *JAK2* and *MPL* mutation negative, with a frequency of approximately 20–25%.[22,23]

Epidemiology

ET occurs at an incidence of between 1.5 and 2.5 cases per 100,000. Most patients are >50 years of age, and there is a female predominance.[24]

Pathophysiology

Approximately 90% of cases have a somatically acquired driver mutation in *JAK2*, *CALR*, or *MPL*, resulting in constitutive activation of JAK-STAT pathway. However, the role of these specific mutations in pathogenesis and influence on disease phenotype is still being elucidated. *JAK2* and *MPL* mutations are believed to directly activate JAK-STAT and make myeloproliferation cytokine independent or hypersensitive. Mutant *CALR* is now known to interact directly with the TPO receptor (MPL) resulting in constitutive activation of MPL and downstream signaling molecules in the JAK/STAT pathway.[25]

DIAGNOSIS

Clinical Presentation

Symptoms generally are related to hemorrhage and vaso-occlusion, although most patients are asymptomatic at diagnosis. The risk of bleeding is increased when the platelet count is $>1,000 \times 10^9$/L secondary to acquired von Willebrand factor (vWF) deficiency. Vaso-occlusion may cause erythromelalgia, transient ischemic attacks, visual disturbances, headache, seizures, and dizziness. Large vessel involvement has also been reported with myocardial infarction and cerebrovascular accidents. A small percentage of patients may experience pruritus. Physical examination findings are generally limited to splenomegaly and easy bruising; however, splenomegaly is uncommon in ET and should prompt evaluation for MF if present.

Diagnostic Testing

- The 2022 ICC diagnostic criteria for ET are listed in Table 10-2.[1] **Other causes of reactive (secondary) thrombocytosis should be carefully investigated** and include splenectomy, trauma, cancer, acute and chronic inflammation, infection, and iron deficiency. C-reactive protein and erythrocyte sedimentation rate can be useful in this evaluation. If iron stores are absent, iron replacement is initiated, which may uncover PV in some patients.
- Clonal markers that should be tested include *JAK2* V617F (frequency 50%), *CALR* mutations (frequency 20–25%), and *MPL* mutations (frequency 3–4%).[26] The clinical presentation and course may somewhat differ based on the mutation present. If the above mutations are negative, but diagnosis is still suspected, clonality can be demonstrated by presence of other gene mutations (*ASXL1*, *EZH2*, *TET2*, *IDH1/2*, *SRSF2*, *SF3B1*). In addition, thrombocytosis might accompany CML, which should be ruled out with *BCR::ABL1* mutation screening.
- **BM findings** include hypercellularity with granulocyte hyperplasia and increased megakaryocytes. The megakaryocytes are large, often clustered, and may exhibit mild atypia.

TREATMENT

The goal of treatment in ET is to prevent thrombosis and alleviate symptoms. Risk factors for arterial thrombosis in ET include age >60 years, thrombosis history, cardiovascular risk factors, leukocytosis, and presence of *JAK2* V617F mutation. Interestingly, the major risk factor for venous thrombosis is male sex.[27] Patients with *CALR* mutations have a lower risk of thrombosis, despite having a higher platelet count.[28] The IPSET-thrombosis score can be utilized for risk stratification, which guides management.[29]

- **Very low–risk patients** are defined as <60 years old, no *JAK2* mutation, and no prior thrombotic history. **Low-risk patients** are defined as <60 years old and no prior thrombotic history, but with *JAK2* mutation detected. Both of these groups are managed with low-dose aspirin *or* observation alone depending on presence of *JAK2* V617F mutation, cardiovascular risk factors, and vasomotor symptoms.

- **Intermediate-risk patients** are defined as >60 years old, no *JAK2* mutation, and no prior thrombotic history. **High-risk patients** are defined as those with prior thrombotic history at any age or those >60 years old with *JAK2* V617F mutation. These patients require **cytoreductive agents** such as hydroxyurea or anagrelide in addition to low-dose aspirin.
- **Aspirin** is commonly used to prevent thrombosis but should be withheld once platelet counts are >1,500 × 10^9/L due to bleeding risk. Extreme thrombocytosis may promote the abnormal adsorption of large vWF multimers and result in a hemostatic defect.[30] Accordingly, such patients should be screened for the presence of acquired von Willebrand disease (vWD). Low-dose aspirin therapy (e.g., <100 mg/day) is acceptable if the ristocetin cofactor level is at least 30%; if <30%, all aspirin should be avoided. Aspirin therapy has also been shown to be effective in alleviating microvascular symptoms such as erythromelalgia and headaches. The optimal dose of aspirin is unknown, but generally, low-dose aspirin is utilized.
- **Hydroxyurea** is used first line in high-risk patients who need cytoreductive therapy. In a randomized controlled trial, hydroxyurea demonstrated a significant decrease in the incidence of thrombotic complications in high-risk ET patients, with an incidence of 3.6% compared to 24% in patients who received no hydroxyurea.[31]
- **Anagrelide** has been compared to hydroxyurea and found to be less effective in reducing the risk of arterial thrombosis, major bleeding, and fibrotic progression; however, it performed better in preventing venous thrombosis. Additionally, the adverse dropout rate was significantly higher in the anagrelide arm.[32] Therefore, anagrelide is generally considered second line for patients who are intolerant or resistant to hydroxyurea.
- **IFN-α** can be used to control platelet count and reduce thrombotic complications.[33] Nevertheless, no studies have compared it directly to hydroxyurea for ET. IFN-α is mainly used for those who desire to become pregnant or those who are intolerant or resistant to hydroxyurea. Pegylated forms are preferred due to ease of administration and more favorable toxicity profile.
- **Management of thrombosis** typically requires either lifelong aspirin, for arterial thrombosis, or anticoagulation with a direct oral anticoagulant or vitamin K antagonist for venous thrombosis. In addition, other risk factors should be aggressively managed, including platelet count, leukocyte count, and cardiovascular risk factors. Rarely, symptomatic, extreme thrombocytosis may be managed with plateletpheresis, although the results are short lived and must be combined with cytoreductive therapy for long-term control.

SPECIAL CONSIDERATIONS

- **Surgery:** Splenectomy poses a high risk for patients with ET and is associated with thrombotic complications.[17] In addition, splenectomy can lead to increased platelet counts and should be avoided.
- **Pregnancy:** Pregnant patients are at higher risk of early miscarriage complications and are often treated with aspirin.[18] As the pregnancy progresses, the platelet count usually decreases toward the normal range but may rebound quickly after delivery. Aspirin should be discontinued 5 days prior to delivery to limit hemorrhagic risk. Patients with intermediate or high-risk diseases are candidates for cytoreductive therapy. IFN-α is the only cytoreductive therapy considered safe in pregnancy.
- **Extreme thrombocytosis:** Patients with platelet counts of >1 million/μL may develop an acquired von Willebrand syndrome and have an increased risk of bleeding.[30] In some patients (e.g., ristocetin cofactor <30%), aspirin should be held due to risk of hemorrhage. Cytoreductive therapy should be considered for patients with extreme thrombocytosis and increased bleeding risk.

OUTCOME/PROGNOSIS

In the modern era, most patients have a normal life expectancy, although survival is affected by factors used for risk stratification.[34] Risk factors for survival in ET are similar to PV and include advanced age, leukocytosis, and thrombosis. Additionally, an Hgb concentration below normal value has also been associated with decreased survival. Morbidity and mortality are related to thrombotic and hemorrhagic events. Transformation to AML is relatively rare and occurs in approximately 5% of patients.

Primary Myelofibrosis

GENERAL PRINCIPLES

Definition

Primary myelofibrosis (PMF) is a clonal disorder characterized by ineffective erythropoiesis and extramedullary hematopoiesis leading to progressive BM failure, severe anemia, constitutional symptoms (e.g., night sweats, fevers, fatigue), marked hepatosplenomegaly, and thrombosis. MF can arise de novo as PMF or following a history of PV or ET.

Epidemiology

PMF is the least common of the MPNs, with an annual incidence of 0.2–1.5 cases per 100,000. The typical case is a male older than age 50 years. The median age at presentation is 67 years, and 70% of cases are diagnosed after age 60 years.[24,35] No common etiologic factor has been identified, although there are sporadic reports of an association with radiation and benzene exposure.

DIAGNOSIS

Clinical Presentation

Two-thirds of patients are symptomatic at diagnosis from the effects of hypercatabolism, cytopenias, or extramedullary hematopoiesis. The most common symptom is fatigue. Bone pain may also be a prominent feature. Splenomegaly is a common finding and can often lead to abdominal discomfort and early satiety.[36,37] A minority of patients will develop portal hypertension, with the associated signs and symptoms such as ascites and variceal bleeding. Progressive splenomegaly may lead to **splenic infarction**, which presents acutely with fever, nausea, and left upper quadrant pain. Patients may develop neutrophilic dermatoses, which appear as tender plaques. **Extramedullary hematopoiesis** may develop in many sites, including the spleen, liver, lymph nodes, serosal surfaces, paraspinal or epidural spaces, and urogenital system.

Diagnostic Criteria

The **2022 ICC diagnostic criteria** for PMF are listed below.[1] Diagnosis requires meeting all three major criteria and at least one minor criterion confirmed in two consecutive determinations:

- Major criteria:
  - BM biopsy showing megakaryocyte proliferation and atypia (small to large megakaryocytes with aberrant nuclear/cytoplasmic ratio and hyperchromatic and irregularly folded nuclei and dense clustering) accompanied by either reticulin and/or collagen fibrosis grades 2 or 3

- ○ Demonstration of *JAK2, CALR*, or *MPL* mutation or presence of other clonal marker or no evidence of reactive marrow fibrosis
  - ○ Not meeting WHO criteria for CML, PV, MDS, or other myeloid neoplasm
- Minor criteria
  - ○ Anemia
  - ○ Leukocytosis $\geq 11 \times 10^9$/L
  - ○ Palpable splenomegaly
  - ○ Increased serum LDH level
  - ○ Leukoerythroblastosis

Other causes of BM fibrosis should be excluded, including cancers metastatic to the marrow, CML, myelodysplasia with fibrosis, other MPNs, infection, autoimmune disorders, secondary hyperparathyroidism associated with vitamin D deficiency, and lymphoma. In addition, the marrow may not be fibrotic early in the course of the disease, further complicating the diagnosis. Thus, overt PMF must be differentiated from early/prefibrotic PMF. Careful morphologic examination of the BM, as well as cytogenetic studies, may help to differentiate among disorders. O**steosclerosis** is often seen on imaging and may be confused with metastatic carcinoma.

Diagnostic Testing

- The **complete blood count** is usually abnormal in PMF. Fifty percent to 70% of patients will be anemic at presentation, some severely, with 25% having an Hgb <8 g/dL. Other abnormalities are variably present: leukocytosis (50%), leukopenia (7%), thrombocytosis (28%), and thrombocytopenia (37%). The **peripheral smear** shows a leukoerythroblastic picture with teardrop poikilocytes, nucleated red cells, and anisocytosis. Patients with MF exhibit aberrant cytokine signaling which leads to chronic inflammation that is associated with constitutional symptoms and cytopenias characteristic of the disease.[38,39]
- A **BM biopsy** should be performed in all patients with PMF to assess for fibrosis and obtain cytogenetic studies which are important for prognosis. BM aspiration may result in a "dry tap" secondary to fibrosis. Findings on marrow examination include increased cellularity, granulocyte hyperplasia, and megakaryocyte dysplasia. Reticulin staining should be requested to evaluate for fibrosis.
- **Clonal markers** found in PV and ET are also present in PMF. The *JAK2* V617F mutation is found in approximately 50–60% of patients with PMF. *CALR* mutations are present in 20–25% and *MPL* mutations are present in <10%.[40,41] These mutations are mutually exclusive.

TREATMENT

Current drug therapies in PMF are not curative or disease-modifying. Relief of symptoms and improvement of quality of life are primarily goals of care. The only curative therapy remains hematopoietic stem cell transplantation (HSCT); however, transplant-related death or severe morbidity may occur in more than half of transplant recipients and necessitates risk justification.[42] Treatment recommendations are largely dependent on individual patient risk factors (see below under "Outcome/Prognosis"). Patients who are at low risk and asymptomatic may be managed with observation alone.

- **JAK2 inhibitors** have demonstrated efficacy in reducing spleen size and relieving constitutional symptoms (e.g., pruritus, fatigue). Efficacy is independent of *JAK2* mutation status.[43] Ruxolitinib, fedratinib, and pacritinib are all JAK2 inhibitors approved by the FDA for treatment of intermediate or high-risk MF. Ruxolitinib is associated with infections, myelosuppression, and carries the risk of withdrawal syndrome with sudden or rapid discontinuation and should be tapered.[44] Fedratinib has been associated with myelosuppression, GI side effects, and Wernicke-like encephalopathy and serum thiamine levels should be monitored. For patients with severe thrombocytopenia, pacritinib is less myelosuppressive and specifically approved for patients with a platelet count below 50×10^9/L. Momelotinib is a new JAK1/2 inhibitor that also inhibits ACVR1, a key regulator in iron homeostasis, and has demonstrated anemia benefits. It should be noted that none of the JAK2 inhibitors affect *JAK2* V617F allele burden, reverse marrow fibrosis, induce complete remissions, or decrease the risk of leukemic transformation.[45]

- **Hydroxyurea** can be used in patients who are not candidates for JAK2 inhibitors or HSCT. It typically does not improve symptoms or splenomegaly, but can be used for cytoreduction in patients with extreme leukocytosis or thrombocytosis.
- **IFN-α** can be considered in early/low-risk MF patients, although its use may be limited by side effects.[46] Some evidence suggests that recombinant IFN-α may slow progression of early PMF.[47]
- **Splenectomy** can be associated with serious perioperative complications, including bleeding, thrombosis, and infection. Therefore, it should be reserved for patients who have not responded to JAK inhibitors or other more conservative approaches.
- **Involved-field radiotherapy** (i.e., splenic irradiation) may offer temporary relief for drug-refractory organomegaly.[48]
- **Allogeneic stem cell transplantation** is the only curative therapy. HSCT is generally recommended only for high or intermediate-2 risk patients where the benefits of transplantation would outweigh the risks given the high rates of transplant-related morbidity and mortality. There are no randomized trials of HSCT versus symptom-based management in PMF. Most comparisons of transplantation versus other approaches in PMF are retrospective studies of younger, highly selected patient populations. In one such large retrospective study, transplantation resulted in long-term relapse-free survival in about one-third of patients.[42] Some studies suggest that survival with HSCT is not affected by adverse karyotype or high-risk mutations.[49] Despite earlier concerns that a fibrotic marrow would affect engraftment, studies do not currently suggest a difference in engraftment rates in patients with MF compared to those without.[42,50]
- Additional agents that have been used for MF-associated anemia include erythropoietin stimulating agents, luspatercept, androgens, prednisone, danazol, thalidomide with or without prednisone, or lenalidomide with or without prednisone. The expected response rates are variable, around 15–25%. Lenalidomide works best in the presence of del(5q31).[37]

OUTCOME/PROGNOSIS

- PMF carries the worst prognosis of all the MPNs. Its course is highly variable, and most of the morbidity and mortality is due to progressive marrow failure, thrombosis, hypersplenism, advanced age, and evolution into AML. The rate of progression to acute leukemia is about 20% over 10 years.[6]
- The International Working Group for Myelofibrosis Research and Treatment (IWG-MRT) initially devised a prognostic scoring system (**IPSS**) in 2009 to risk-stratify patients at the time of diagnosis.[51] The **DIPSS** scoring system was later developed in order to risk stratify patients at any time point during the disease course (Table 10-3).[52] Current comprehensive prognostic models in use for PMF include **GIPSS** and **MIPSS70+ v2.0**. GIPSS utilizes karyotype and molecular features to assign patients to one of four prognostic groups.[53] **MIPSS70+ v2.0** is a similar model but also incorporates clinical features (degree of anemia, presence of circulating blasts, constitutional

TABLE 10-3 IPSS AND DIPSS PROGNOSTIC SCORING SYSTEMS IN PMF

Risk Factors	Point value IPSS	Point value DIPSS	IPSS Risk Group	IPSS Risk Score	IPSS Median Survival	DIPSS Risk Group	DIPSS Risk Score	DIPSS Median Survival
Age >65 y	1	1	Low	0	11.3 y	Low	0	Not reached
Constitutional symptoms[a]	1	1	Intermediate-1	1	7 y	Intermediate-1	1–2	14.2 y
Hb <10 g/dL	1	2	Intermediate-2	2	4 y	Intermediate-2	3–4	4 y
WBC count >25 × 10^9/L	1	1	High	≥3	2.3 y	High	≥5	1.5 y
Blood blasts ≥1%	1	1						

[a]Constitutional symptoms defined as weight loss >10% of baseline value in the year preceding PMF diagnosis and/or unexplained fever or excessive sweats persisting for more than 1 month.

TABLE 10-4   NEWER PROGNOSTIC SCORING SYSTEM IN PMF

		GIPSS		
Risk Factors	Points	Risk Group	Risk Score	Median Survival
Karyotype[a]		Low risk	0	26.4 y
Favorable	0			
Unfavorable	1			
Very high risk (VHR)	2	Intermediate-1	1	10.3 y
Driver mutations		Intermediate-2	2	4.6 y
Absence of type 1–like CALR	1	High	≥3	2.6 y
High molecular risk (HMR)				
ASXL1 mutation	1			
SRSF2 mutation	1			
U2AF1 Q157 mutation	1			

		MIPSS70+ v2.0		
Risk Factors	Points	Risk Group	Risk Score	Median Survival
Clinical risk factors		Very low risk	0	Not reached
Severe anemia[b]	2	Low risk	1–2	10.3 y
Moderate anemia[c]	1	Intermediate risk	3–4	7 y
Circulating blasts ≥2%	1			
Constitutional symptoms	2	High risk	5–8	3.5 y
Karyotype[a]	3	Very high risk	≥9	1.8 y
Unfavorable				
Very high risk	4			
Mutations				
Absence of type 1-like CALR	2			
≥2 HMR mutations[d]	3			
One HMR mutation	2			

[a]Classification of karyotype—VHR: single or multiple abnormalities of -7, i(17q), inv(3)/3q21, 12p-/12p11.2, 11q-/11q23, or other autosomal trisomies not including +8/+9 (e.g., +21, +19); Favorable: Normal karyotype or sole abnormalities of +9, 13q-, 20q-, chromosome 1 translocation/duplication, or sex chromosome abnormality including -Y; Unfavorable: All other abnormalities.
[b]Severe anemia defined as Hb <9 g/dL in men and Hb <8 g/dL in women.
[c]Moderate anemia defined as Hb 9–10.9 g/dL in men and Hb 8–9.9 g/dL in women.
[d]HMR mutations include mutations in ASXL1, EZH2, SRSF2, IDH1/2, and U2AF1 genes.

symptoms).[54] MIPSS70+ 2.0 is often used to refine prognosis for patients assigned into the intermediate risk groups by GIPSS. Table 10-4 presents a comparison of these two scoring systems. Both GIPSS and MIPSS70+ v2.0 were shown to be superior to DIPSS. However, DIPSS may still be seen in clinical use in the absence of molecular data.

Hypereosinophilic Syndrome

GENERAL PRINCIPLES

Definition

Hypereosinophilia is defined as an absolute eosinophil count (AEC) of >1,500/μL and may be associated with tissue damage. Hypereosinophilic syndrome (HES) is defined as an AEC of >1,500/μL for more than 6 months with the presence of eosinophil-mediated organ damage.[55] Hypereosinophilia is considered a provisional diagnosis until a primary (clonal) or secondary cause of eosinophilia is identified. Historically, most of these primary disorders were considered MPNs. The 2022 ICC classification includes many of these conditions under a category entitled "Myeloid/lymphoid neoplasms with eosinophilia and tyrosine kinase gene fusions."[1] Nevertheless, entities with a similar presentation but without genetically defined features include chronic eosinophilic leukemia, not otherwise specified (CEL, NOS), idiopathic hypereosinophilic syndrome (iHES), lymphocyte-variant hypereosinophilia, and hypereosinophilia of unknown significance (HEus).

Epidemiology

The incidence and prevalence of HES are not well characterized, but SEER data suggest an incidence rate of approximately 0.036 per 100,000.[56] The incidence of eosinophilias with recurrent genetic abnormalities (*PDGFRA/B*, *FGFR1*) comprises a minority of patients with HES. *FIP1L1-PDGFRA* fusion occurs in approximately 10–20% of patients with idiopathic hypereosinophilia, and for reasons that are unknown, the overwhelming majority are seen in males.[56] Other eosinophilia subtypes exhibit no clear gender bias. CEL and idiopathic HES are usually diagnosed between the ages of 20 and 50 years, but may also arise at the extremes of age (i.e., infants and children or adults ages 65–74).[57]

Pathophysiology

Several mechanisms have been proposed to account for the dysregulated overproduction of eosinophils in patients with HES[58]:

- Clonal eosinophilic proliferation as a result of a primary molecular defect involving hematopoietic stem cells and/or defects in signal transduction from the receptors that mediate eosinophilopoiesis
- Overproduction of eosinophilopoietic cytokines, such as IL-5
- Functional abnormalities of the eosinophilopoietic cytokines, related to enhanced or prolonged biologic activity
- Defects in the normal suppressive regulation of eosinophilopoiesis or of eosinophil survival and activation

DIAGNOSIS

Clinical Presentation

Ninety percent of patients will have symptoms at diagnosis. Characteristically, patients will complain of various **nonspecific constitutional symptoms** such as fever, fatigue, cough, pruritus, diarrhea, rash, and muscle pains. Infiltrating eosinophils will produce end-organ damage in the majority of patients within 3 years of diagnosis. Cardiac disease is the major cause of death, but virtually every organ system may be involved (Table 10-5).[57,59]

Diagnostic Criteria

Diagnosis first relies on the exclusion of all possible causes of reactive or secondary eosinophilia. Secondary eosinophilia has numerous causes including infections such as tissue-invasive

TABLE 10-5	CLINICAL MANIFESTATION OF CHRONIC EOSINOPHILIC LEUKEMIA/HYPEREOSINOPHILIC SYNDROME (CEL/HES)

Cardiac	Skin
Constrictive pericarditis	Angioedema
Fibroblastic endocarditis	Urticaria
Myocarditis	Papulonodular lesions
Intramural thrombosis	Erythematous plaques
Central nervous system	Gastrointestinal
Mononeuritis multiplex	Ascites
Peripheral neuropathy	Diarrhea
Paraparesis	Gastritis
Cerebellar dysfunction	Colitis
Epilepsy	Pancreatitis
Dementia	Cholangitis
Cerebral vascular accident	Hepatitis
Eosinophilic meningitis	Musculoskeletal
Pulmonary	Arthritis
Infiltrates	Arthralgias
Fibrosis	Myalgias
Pleural effusions	Raynaud phenomenon
Pulmonary emboli	

parasites, allergy/atopy and hypersensitivity conditions, drug reactions, pulmonary eosinophilic diseases (i.e., idiopathic acute or chronic eosinophilic pneumonia, allergic bronchopulmonary aspergillosis), collagen vascular disease (i.e., eosinophilic granulomatosis with polyangiitis), allergic gastroenteritis (with associated peripheral eosinophilia), adrenal insufficiency, and nonmyeloid malignancies (i.e., T-cell lymphomas, Hodgkin disease, and acute lymphoblastic leukemia [ALL]). Eosinophilia associated with WHO-defined myeloid malignancy (i.e., acute myeloid leukemia [AML], MDS, systemic mastocytosis [SM], CML, and other MPNs and MDS/MPN disorders) must also be ruled out.

Diagnostic Testing

The diagnosis is usually suspected based on **peripheral hypereosinophilia** and some constellation of the symptoms reviewed in Table 10-5. Reactive or secondary causes as mentioned previously must be ruled out.

- If no secondary causes are identified, investigation for myeloproliferative variants should be pursued. Screening for *FIP1L1-PDGFRA* fusion by FISH or RT-PCR should be performed on the peripheral blood. A **BM aspirate and biopsy** should also be performed to evaluate for reciprocal translocations involving 4q12 (*PDGFRA*), 5q31–q33 (*PDGFRB*), 8p11–13 (*FGFR1*), and 9p24 (*JAK2*). It should be noted that these translocations may not be detected by routine karyotyping and may only be detected by FISH. An elevated serum tryptase level may be seen in HES patients with the *FIP1L1-PDGFRA* fusion.
- If no cytogenetic abnormalities are identified, **flow immunocytometry** and **T-cell clonality assessments** are performed to detect histopathologic or clonal evidence for an acute or chronic myeloid or lymphoproliferative disorder. If no other cytogenetic abnormalities are identified, the diagnosis of CEL may be entertained (Table 10-6). Presence of an abnormal T-cell population (demonstrated by peripheral blood lymphocyte immunophenotyping or T-cell receptor gene rearrangement studies), which may be associated with excessive eosinophilopoietic cytokine

TABLE 10-6	ICC 2022 DIAGNOSTIC CRITERIA FOR CHRONIC EOSINOPHILIC LEUKEMIA, NOS

Diagnosis requires all 6 criteria:

1. Peripheral blood hypereosinophilia (eosinophil count $\geq 1.5 \times 10^9$/L and eosinophils $\geq 10\%$ of white blood cells)
2. Blasts constitute <20% cells in peripheral blood and bone marrow
3. No tyrosine kinase gene fusions (e.g., BCR::ABL1, other ABL1, PDGFRA, PDGFRB, FGFR1, JAK2, or FLT3 fusions)
4. Not meeting criteria for other MPNs, chronic myelomonocytic leukemia, or systemic mastocytosis
5. Bone marrow shows increased cellularity with dysplastic megakaryocytes and often significant fibrosis, associated with an eosinophilic infiltrate or increased blasts $\geq 5\%$ in the bone marrow and/or $\geq 2\%$ in the peripheral blood
6. Demonstration of a clonal cytogenetic abnormality and/or somatic mutations

Reproduced with permission from Arber DA, Orazi A, Hasserjian RP, et al. International Consensus Classification of myeloid neoplasms and acute leukemias: integrating morphologic, clinical, and genomic data. *Blood*. 2022;140(11):1200–1228.

production in vitro (i.e., IL-5), is consistent with a diagnosis of lymphocyte-variant hypereosinophilia.

TREATMENT

- Treatment is dependent on the subtype of eosinophilic disorder. **Imatinib should be used first line in patients with *PDGFRA/B* rearrangement**, given the exquisite sensitivity of these disorders to imatinib therapy. Lower doses of imatinib 100 mg daily may be sufficient to produce complete molecular remission in some patients.[60] Imatinib may be considered in CEL, NOS, or HES; however, hematologic responses in these groups are often partial and short lived. Rare complete responses have been observed in patients with diagnostically occult *PDGFRA* or *PDGFRB* mutations or other unknown pathogenetic targets.[61] Imatinib is not generally effective for patients with lymphocyte-variant hypereosinophilia.
- **Corticosteroids** reduce peripheral eosinophil numbers and the toxicity of the eosinophilic granules. Steroids are used as **first-line therapy in idiopathic HES and lymphocyte-variant hypereosinophilia**. For those who are unable to tolerate or are refractory to steroid therapy, second-line agents include steroid-sparing immunosuppressive agents (cyclophosphamide) or IFN-α.[62]
- **Hydroxyurea** is an effective first-line agent for HES in conjunction with corticosteroids or as second line in steroid nonresponders. It is also used first line in CEL, NOS. A typical starting dose is 500–1,000 mg daily. Hydroxyurea is typically not effective for lymphocyte-variant hypereosinophilia.[62]
- **IFN-α** can produce hematologic and cytogenetic remissions in HES and CEL, NOS patients refractory to other therapies including prednisone and/or hydroxyurea. It can also be used in conjunction with corticosteroids or a steroid-sparing immunosuppressive agent.[62]
- **Pemigatinib**, a selective inhibitor of FGFR1-3, is approved by the FDA for treatment of relapsed/refractory myeloid and lymphoid neoplasms with eosinophilia that *FGFR1* rearrangements in adults based on durable clinical and cytogenetic responses.[63]
- **HSCT** has been utilized in rare cases to successfully treat HES or CEL, NOS.[64]

OUTCOMES/PROGNOSIS

The clinical course is variable and differs based on the subtype of eosinophilic disorder. For patients with rearranged *PDGFRA/B*, prognosis may be very good, given the sensitivity to imatinib and achievement of complete molecular remissions.[60]

For patients with HES, reports of survival have been variable, ranging from a 3-year survival of 12% to a 5-year survival rate of 80%, decreasing to 42% at 15 years. Factors predictive of a worse outcome included corticosteroid-refractory hypereosinophilia, cardiac disease, and male sex.[65] These data are less relevant currently in the era of molecularly defined eosinophilias and improved medical and surgical interventions for cardiovascular sequelae.

The prognosis of CEL, NOS is poor, with a median survival of 22.2 months. Up to half of the patients transformed to AML at 20 months from diagnosis.[66]

Lymphocyte-variant hypereosinophilia has a relatively indolent course; however, rarely, some patients may develop either T-cell lymphoma or Sézary syndrome.[67]

Mast Cell Disorders

GENERAL PRINCIPLES

Definition

Mast cell activation disorders can be primary, secondary, or idiopathic. Primary mast cell disorders are characterized by clonal proliferation of mast cells with abnormal genetic or surface makers. Mastocytosis is the most common primary mast cell disorder, referring to the pathologic accumulation of mast cells in tissues.[1] Patients may be diagnosed either with cutaneous mastocytosis (CM) or SM. CM is classified into urticaria pigmentosa/maculopapular cutaneous mastocytosis (UP/MPCM), diffuse CM, and mastocytoma of the skin.[68] SM has numerous subtypes, including indolent SM, smoldering SM, aggressive SM, SM with associated myeloid neoplasm (SM-AHN), and mast cell leukemia.[1] Aggressive SM, SM-AHN, and mast cell leukemia are often grouped as advanced SM.

Epidemiology

Mastocytosis is rare, with an estimated prevalence of 1 per 10,000 persons; however, underdiagnosis is assumed.[69] The vast majority of adults with mastocytosis tend to have systemic forms. In contrast, children with mastocytosis almost uniformly have isolated cutaneous disease. CM in pediatric patients frequently resolves spontaneously.

Pathophysiology

Mast cells are granulocytes that are present in mucosal tissues and vascularized connective tissues. They have numerous functions; while they are best known for mediating allergic response, they are also involved in wound healing, angiogenesis, and defense against pathogens, among other roles. Activation of mast cells can be driven by a number of processes, including allergens binding to surface IgE receptors, physical injury, pathogens binding to pathogen-associated molecular patterns, and complement activation. When activated, mast cells degranulate to release vasoactive mediators, including histamine, tryptase, and heparin; they also generate cytokines that recruit other inflammatory cells. These mediators are responsible for many of the signs and symptoms of allergic reaction. For example, histamine leads to increased blood vessel permeability and endothelial activation, resulting in localized edema, warmth, and redness.[70]

Molecular pathogenesis of mast cell disorders is not completely understood. Mast cells express KIT (CD117) on their surface, a receptor for stem cell factor (also known as kit ligand), a growth factor stimulating development and expansion of mast cells from precursors. Gain-of-function mutations in *KIT* are associated with both CM and SM.[71] The most common mutation is D816V, and allele burden predicts survival.[72] *KIT* mutations are somatic in the vast majority of cases.

DIAGNOSIS

Clinical Presentation

Patients present with signs or symptoms caused either by the activation of mast cells or the infiltration of mast cells into organs leading to impaired function.

- The most common cutaneous finding is the development of maculopapular CM/urticaria pigmentosa. This is characterized by the **presence of multiple monomorphic macules**.
- Mast cell mediators may lead to symptoms such as **flushing, fatigue, or gastrointestinal symptoms**. In rare cases, recurrent anaphylactic episodes can be seen.
- Patients with SM may have **cutaneous findings as well as cytopenias** related to BM infiltration or hepatosplenomegaly related to organ infiltration.
- Episodes of idiopathic anaphylaxis or anaphylaxis to stings from *Hymenoptera* insects are more likely to develop in patients with SM compared to the general population.[73]

Diagnostic Criteria

Diagnostic criteria for SM are listed in Table 10-7.[1] Diagnosis requires tissue biopsy, either from the BM or other extracutaneous organs. For CM, diagnosis requires characteristic skin lesions. A skin biopsy is not entirely necessary for diagnosis but is typically pursued.

Diagnostic Testing

- A **complete blood count with differential** should be obtained on all patients to evaluate for cytopenias, proliferation of other cell lines, and presence of circulating mast cells.
- **BM biopsy and aspirate** are obtained in almost all cases. Morphologically abnormal spindle-shaped mast cells are identified. The classic immunophenotype of mast cells in SM is KIT, tryptase, CD2, and CD25 positivity.[74] While tryptase and KIT immunostaining cannot differentiate between normal and neoplastic mast cells, CD25 is a reliable marker for discrimination of neoplastic cells.[75] BM biopsy also allows for diagnosis of SM-AHN.
- **Elevated serum tryptase levels** are seen in the vast majority of patients with SM, regardless of subgroup.[76] Nevertheless, this is not specific as elevations can be seen in other myeloid neoplasms. Of note, tryptase should only be tested when a patient is at a baseline state.
- **Molecular studies** including mutational analysis for *KIT* D816V should be completed.

  This is often done with a high-sensitivity PCR assay on a peripheral blood sample; nevertheless, a negative result in the peripheral blood does not exclude the possibility of a *KIT* mutation present in the BM.[77]

TREATMENT

Treatment is individualized based on the patient and the type of disease (CM vs. SM, subgroup of SM). Given the rarity of SM, clinical trials are encouraged.

- General measures include **avoidance of triggers**, such as heat, cold, stress, exercise, dehydration, alcohol, and others. Certain medications, such as anesthetic agents, opioid analgesics, vancomycin, and NSAIDs, as well as contrast dye, may also precipitate episodes.[73]

TABLE 10-7	ICC 2022 DIAGNOSTIC CRITERIA FOR MAST CELL DISORDERS

Systemic Mastocytosis

Diagnosis requires major criterion or at least three minor criteria:

Major:
1. Multifocal dense infiltrates of tryptase- and/or CD117 positive mast cells (≥15 mast cells in aggregates) detected in sections of bone marrow and/or other extracutaneous organ(s)

Minor:
1. In bone marrow biopsy or in section of other extracutaneous organs, >25% of mast cells are spindle shaped or have an atypical immature morphology
2. Mast cells in bone marrow, peripheral blood, or other extracutaneous organs express CD25, CD2, and/or CD30, in addition to mast cell markers
3. *KIT* D816V mutation or other activating *KIT* mutation detected in bone marrow, peripheral blood, or other extracutaneous organs
4. Elevated serum tryptase level, persistently >20 ng/mL. In cases of SM-AMN an elevated tryptase does not count as an SM minor criterion.[a]

Systemic Mastocytosis with an Associated Myeloid Neoplasm

Diagnosis requires all of the following criteria:
1. Meets the diagnostic criteria for SM
2. Meets the criteria for an associated myeloid neoplasm (e.g., CMML or other MDS/MPN, MDS, MPN, AML, or other myeloid neoplasm)
3. The associated myeloid neoplasm should be fully classified according to established criteria

[a]In cases of SM-AMN, an elevated tryptase does not count as an SM minor criterion.
Adapted with permission from Arber DA, Orazi A, Hasserjian RP, et al. International Consensus Classification of myeloid neoplasms and acute leukemias: integrating morphologic, clinical, and genomic data. *Blood*. 2022;140:1200–1228.

- **Symptom-directed treatment** is utilized to alleviate mast cell degranulation symptoms in all patients with mastocytosis. Treatment options include epinephrine, corticosteroids, histamine receptor blockers, cromolyn sodium, and leukotriene modifying agents. Aspirin may be used in refractory cases.[78]
- **Observation** is recommended for indolent SM and smoldering SM. However, cytoreductive therapy may be used for patients with refractory symptoms. **Avapritinib**, an oral inhibitor of D816V-mutated *KIT*, was recently approved by the FDA for the treatment of indolent SM based on improvement in symptoms and mast cell burden.[79] Midostaurin (off-label), cladribine, or IFN-α are other available options.[78]
- **Advanced SM is typically treated with targeted therapies.** Avapritinib is FDA-approved and associated with rapid and durable reduction in SM-associated symptoms, improved quality of life, reduced spleen size, and ≥50% improvement in BM mast cells and serum tryptase in approximately 90% of patients.[80] It should be avoided in patients with platelet count <50 K/μL due to increased risk of intracranial hemorrhage. **Midostaurin**, a multikinase inhibitor, achieves responses in up to two-thirds of patients; however, it is less commonly used than avapritinib given its greater toxicity and worse tolerability.[81] Imatinib **should not be used** for patients with the *KIT* D816V mutation, but may be used in rare cases without this mutation (e.g., transmembrane KIT mutations).[82]

- **HSCT** has the potential to cure advanced SM, but it is generally reserved for patients with relapsed/refractory disease.[83]

SPECIAL CONSIDERATIONS

- In patients with SM-AHN, the SM and AHN components are typically treated at separate times due to concerns for overlapping toxicities. HSCT may be used in settings in which SM responds to treatment, but AHN does not.[83]
- Pregnancy may lead to worsening mastocytosis symptoms. Mastocytosis has not been linked to decreased fertility, pregnancy complications, or effects on infant health.[84]

OUTCOMES/PROGNOSIS

Adult SM patients have a shorter life expectancy as a group compared to age-matched controls. Prognosis is thought to be associated with disease subtype, although some of these studies were done prior to current classification systems.[76] Patients with indolent SM have similar survival compared to the general population with overall low rates of transformation to acute leukemia or aggressive SM.[76,85] Those with smoldering SM may have worse survival compared to those with indolent disease, although this may be related to older age at diagnosis.[86] Advanced SM patients typically have worse prognosis compared to indolent and smoldering forms. In one study, patients with aggressive SM had a median overall survival of 41 months, compared to 24 months and 2 months for those with SM-AHN and mast cell leukemia, respectively.[76] Category of AHN (i.e., MPN, chronic myelomonocytic leukemia, myelodysplastic syndrome, etc.) influences survival as well.[87]

Certain clinical features, such as advanced age, weight loss, anemia, thrombocytopenia, hypoalbuminemia, and excess BM blasts are reported as independent adverse prognostic factors for survival.[76] A commonly used prognostic model incorporating some of these variables (age, WHO-defined subgroup, platelet count, Hgb level, serum alkaline phosphatase) is the Mayo alliance prognostic system, with a greater number of adverse clinical features associated with worse survival.[88] Molecular and cytogenetic features are also associated with outcomes in patients with advanced SM. Worse outcomes are seen in patients with abnormalities besides *KIT* D816V, such as poor-risk karyotype and mutations in *SRSF2*, *ASXL1*, or *RUNX1*.[89]

REFERENCES

1. Arber DA, Orazi A, Hasserjian RP, et al. International Consensus Classification of Myeloid Neoplasms and Acute Leukemias: integrating morphologic, clinical, and genomic data. *Blood.* 2022; 140(11):1200–1228.
2. Khoury JD, Solary E, Abla O. The 5th edition of the World Health Organization Classification of Haematolymphoid Tumours: myeloid and histiocytic/dendritic neoplasms. *Leukemia.* 2022;36(7): 1703–1719.
3. Tefferi A, Barbui T. Polycythemia vera and essential thrombocythemia: 2021 update and diagnosis, risk-stratification, and management. *Am J of Hematol.* 2020;95(12):1599–1613.
4. Spivak JL. Narrative review: thrombocytosis, polycythemia vera, and JAK2 mutations: the phenotypic mimicry of chronic myeloproliferation. *Ann Intern Med.* 2010;152(5):300–306.
5. Scherber R, Dueck AC, Johansson P, et al. The Myeloproliferative Neoplasm Symptom Assessment Form (MPN-SAF): international prospective validation and reliability trial in 402 patients. *Blood.* 2011;118(2):401–408.
6. Tefferi A, Guglielmelli P, Larson DR, et al. Long-term survival and blast transformation in molecularly annotated essential thrombocythemia, polycythemia vera, and myelofibrosis. *Blood.* 2014;124(16): 2507–2513.
7. Smalberg JH, Arends LR, Valla DC, et al. Myeloproliferative neoplasms in Budd-Chiari syndrome and portal vein thrombosis: a meta-analysis. *Blood.* 2012;120(25):4921–4928.

8. Scott LM, Tong W, Levine RL, et al. JAK2 exon 12 mutations in polycythemia vera and idiopathic erythrocytosis. *N Engl J Med.* 2007;356(5):459–468.

9. Pardanani A, Lasho TL, Finke C, Hanson CA, Tefferi A. Prevalence and clinicopathologic correlates of JAK2 exon 12 mutations in JAK2V617F-negative polycythemia vera. *Leukemia.* 2007;21(9): 1960–1963.

10. Ginzburg YZ, Feola M, Zimran E, Varkonyi J, Ganz T, Hoffman R. Dysregulated iron metabolism in polycythemia vera: etiology and consequences. *Leukemia.* 2018;32(10):2105–2116.

11. Barraco D, Cerquozzi S, Hanson CA, et al. Prognostic impact of bone marrow fibrosis in polycythemia vera: validation of the IWG-MRT study and additional observations. *Blood Cancer J.* 2017;7(3):e538.

12. Tefferi A, Rumi E, Finazzi G, et al. Survival and prognosis among 1545 patients with contemporary polycythemia vera. *Leukemia.* 2013;27:1874–1881.

13. Marchioli R, Finazzi G, Specchia G, Masciulli A, Mennitto MR, Barbui T. The CYTO-PV: a large-scale trial testing the intensity of CYTOreductive therapy to prevent cardiovascular events in patients with polycythemia vera. *Thrombosis.* 2011;2011:794240.

14. Barbui T, Carobbio A, Rumi E, et al. In contemporary patients with polycythemia vera, rates of thrombosis and risk factors delineate a new clinical epidemiology. *Blood.* 2014;124(19):3021–3023.

15. Gisslinger H, Klade C, Georgiev P, et al. Ropeginterferon alfa-2b versus standard therapy for polycythemia vera (PROUD-PV and CONTINUATION-PV): a randomised, non-inferiority, phase 3 trial and its extension study. *Lancet Haematol.* 2020;7(3):e196–e208.

16. Vannucchi AM, Kiladjian JJ, Griesshammer M, et al. Ruxolitinib versus standard therapy for the treatment of polycythemia vera. *N Engl J Med.* 2015;372(5):426–435.

17. Ruggeri M, Rodeghiero F, Tosetto A. Postsurgery outcomes in patients with polycythemia vera and essential thrombocythemia: a retrospective survey. *Blood.* 2008;111(2):666–671.

18. Gangat N, Tefferi A. Myeloproliferative neoplasms and pregnancy: overview and practice recommendations. *Am J Hematol.* 2021;96(3):354–366.

19. Bonicelli G, Abdulkarim K, Mounier M, et al. Leucocytosis and thrombosis at diagnosis are associated with poor survival in polycythaemia vera: a population-based study of 327 patients. *Br J Haematol.* 2013;160(2):251–254.

20. Passamonti F, Rumi E, Pietra D, et al. A prospective study of 338 patients with polycythemia vera: the impact of JAK2 (V617F) allele burden and leukocytosis on fibrotic or leukemic disease transformation and vascular complications. *Leukemia.* 2010;24(9):1574–1579.

21. Pardanani AD, Levine RL, Lasho T, et al. MPL515 mutations in myeloproliferative and other myeloid disorders: a study of 1182 patients. *Blood.* 2006;108(10):3472–3476.

22. Nangalia J, Massie CE, Baxter EJ, et al. Somatic CALR mutations in myeloproliferative neoplasms with nonmutated JAK2. *N Engl J Med.* 2013;369(25):2391–2405.

23. Klampfl T, Gisslinger H, Harutyunyan AS, et al. Somatic mutations of calreticulin in myeloproliferative neoplasms. *N Engl J Med.* 2013;369(25):2379–2390.

24. Srour SA, Devesa SS, Morton LM. Incidence and patient survival of myeloproliferative neoplasms and myelodysplastic/myeloproliferative neoplasms in the United States, 2001–12. *Br J Haematol.* 2016; 174(3):382–396.

25. Chachoua I, Pecquet C, El-Khoury M, et al. Thrombopoietin receptor activation by myeloproliferative neoplasm associated calreticulin mutants. *Blood.* 127(1):1325–1335.

26. Rumi E, Cazzola M. Diagnosis, risk stratification, and response evaluation in classical myeloproliferative neoplasms. *Blood.* 2017;129(6):680–692.

27. Carobbio A, Thiele J, Passamonti F. Risk factors for arterial and venous thrombosis in WHO-defined essential thrombocythemia: an international study of 891 patients. *Blood.* 2011;117(22):5857–5859.

28. Pérez Encinas MM, Sobas M, Gómez-Casares MT, et al. The risk of thrombosis in essential thrombocythemia is associated with the type of CALR mutation: a multicentre collaborative study. *Eur J Haematol.* 2021;106(3):371–379.

29. Barbui T, Vannucchi AM, Buxhofer-Ausch V, et al. Practice-relevant revision of IPSET-thrombosis based on 1019 patients with WHO-defined essential thrombocythemia. *Blood Cancer J.* 2015; 5(11):e369.

30. Budde U, Schaefer G, Mueller N. Acquired von Willebrand's disease in the myeloproliferative syndrome. *Blood.* 1984;64(5):981–985.

31. Cortelazzo S, Finazzi G, Ruggeri M, et al. Hydroxyurea for patients with essential thrombocythemia and a high risk of thrombosis. *N Engl J Med.* 1995;332(17):1132–1136.

32. Gisslinger H, Gotic M, Holowiecki J, et al; ANAHYDRET Study Group. Anagrelide compared to hydroxyurea in WHO-classified essential thrombocythemia: the ANAHYDRET study, a randomized controlled trial. *Blood.* 2013;121(10):1720–1728.

33. Saba R, Jabbour E, Giles F, et al. Interferon alpha therapy for patients with essential thrombocythemia: final results of a phase II study initiated in 1986. *Cancer.* 2005;103(12):2551–2557.

34. Passamonti F, Rumi E, Pungolino E, et al. Life expectancy and prognostic factors for survival in patients with polycythemia vera and essential thrombocythemia. *Am J Med.* 2004;117(10):755–761.

35. Mesa RA, Silverstein MN, Jacobsen SJ, Wollan PC, Tefferi A. Population-based incidence and survival figures in essential thrombocythemia and agnogenic myeloid metaplasia: an Olmsted County Study, 1976-1995. *Am J Hematol.* 1999;61(1):10–15.

36. Tefferi A. Myelofibrosis with myeloid metaplasia. *N Engl J Med.* 2000;342(17):1255–1265.

37. Tefferi A. Primary myelofibrosis: 2023 update on diagnosis, risk-stratification, and management. *Am J Hematol.* 2023;98(5):801–821.

38. Mascarenhas J, Gleitz HFE, Chifotides HT, et al. Biological drivers of clinical phenotype in myelofibrosis. *Leukemia.* 2023;37(2):255–264.

39. Fisher DAC, Fowles JS, Zhou A, Oh ST. Inflammatory pathophysiology as a contributor to myeloproliferative neoplasms. *Front Immunol.* 2021;12:683401.

40. Tefferi A, Lasho TL, Finke CM. CALR vs JAK2 vs MPL-mutated or triple-negative myelofibrosis: clinical, cytogenetic and molecular comparisons. *Leukemia.* 2014;28(7):1472–1477.

41. Cazzola M, Kralovics R. From Janus kinase 2 to calreticulin: the clinically relevant genomic landscape of myeloproliferative neoplasms. *Blood.* 2014;123(24):3714–3719.

42. Ballen KK, Shrestha S, Sobocinski KA, et al. Outcome of transplantation for myelofibrosis. *Biol Blood Marrow Transplant.* 2010;16(3):358–367.

43. Guglielmelli P, Biamonte F, Rotunno G, et al; COMFORT-II Investigators; Associazione Italiana per la Ricerca sul Cancro Gruppo Italiano Malattie Mieloproliferative (AGIMM) Investigators. Impact of mutational status on outcomes in myelofibrosis patients treated with ruxolitinib in the COMFORT-II study. *Blood.* 2014;123(14):2157–2160.

44. Tefferi A, Pardanani A. Serious adverse events during ruxolitinib treatment discontinuation in patients with myelofibrosis. *Mayo Clin Proc.* 2011;86(12):1188–1191.

45. Tefferi A. JAK inhibitors for myeloproliferative neoplasms: clarifying facts from myths. *Blood.* 2012;119(12):2721–2730.

46. Bewersdorf JP, Giri S, Wang R, et al. Interferon therapy in myelofibrosis: systematic review and meta-analysis. *Clin Lymphoma Myeloma Leuk.* 2020;20(10):e712–e723.

47. Silver RT, Vandris K, Goldman JJ. Recombinant interferon-α may retard progression of early primary myelofibrosis: a preliminary report. *Blood.* 2011;117(24):6669–6672.

48. Elliott MA, Chen MG, Silverstein MN, Tefferi A. Splenic irradiation for symptomatic splenomegaly associated with myelofibrosis with myeloid metaplasia. *Br J Haematol.* 1998;103(2):505–511.

49. Tefferi A, Partain DK, Palmer JM, et al. Allogeneic hematopoietic stem cell transplant overcomes the adverse survival effect of very high risk and unfavorable karyotype in myelofibrosis. *Am J Hematol.* 2018;93(5):649–654.

50. Soll E, Massumoto C, Clift RA, et al. Relevance of marrow fibrosis in bone marrow transplantation: a retrospective analysis of engraftment. *Blood.* 1995;86(12):4667–4673.

51. Cervantes F, Dupriez B, Pereira A, et al. New prognostic scoring system for primary myelofibrosis based on a study of the International Working Group for Myelofibrosis Research and Treatment. *Blood.* 2009;113(13):2895–2901.

52. Passamonti F, Cervantes F, Vannucchi AM, et al. Dynamic international prognostic scoring system (DIPSS) predicts progression to acute myeloid leukemia in primary myelofibrosis. *Blood.* 2010;116(15):2857–2858.

53. Tefferi A, Guglielmelli P, Nicolosi M, et al. GIPSS: genetically inspired prognostic scoring system for primary myelofibrosis. *Leukemia.* 2018;32(7):1631–1642.

54. Tefferi A, Guglielmelli P, Lasho TL, et al. MIPSS70+ Version 2.0: mutation and karyotype-enhanced international prognostic scoring system for primary myelofibrosis. *J Clin Oncol.* 2018; 36(17):1769–1770.

55. Valent P, Klion AD, Horny HP, et al. Contemporary consensus proposal on criteria and classification of eosinophilic disorders and related syndromes. *J Allergy Clin Immunol.* 2012;130(3):607–612.

56. Crane MM, Chang CM, Kobayashi MG, et al. Incidence of myeloproliferative hypereosinophilic syndrome in the United States and an estimate of all hypereosinophilic syndrome incidence. *J Allergy Clin Immunol.* 2010;126(1):179–181.

57. Shmali W, Gotlib J. World Health Organization-defined eosinophilic disorders: 2022 update on diagnosis, risk stratification, and management. *Am J Hematol.* 2012;97(1):129–148.

58. Ackerman SJ, Bochner BS. Mechanisms of eosinophilia in the pathogenesis of hypereosinophilic disorders. *Immunol Allergy Clin North Am.* 2007;27(3):357–375.

59. Podjasek JC, Butterfield JH. Mortality in hypereosinophilic syndrome: 19 years of experience at Mayo Clinic with a review of the literature. *Leuk Res.* 2013;37(4):392–395.

60. Baccarani M, Cilloni D, Rondoni M, et al. The efficacy of imatinib mesylate in patients with FIP1L1-PDGFRalpha-positive hypereosinophilic syndrome. Results of a multicenter prospective study. *Haematologica.* 2007;92(9):1173–1179.

61. Jain N, Cortes J, Quintás-Cardama A, et al. Imatinib has limited therapeutic activity for hyper-eosinophilic syndrome patients with unknown or negative PDGFRα mutation status. *Leuk Res.* 2009;33(6):837–839.

62. Ogbogu PU, Bochner BS, Butterfield JH, et al. Hypereosinophilic syndrome: a multicenter, ret-rospective analysis of clinical characteristics and response to therapy. *J Allergy Clin Immunol.* 2009; 124(6):1319–1325.

63. Verstovsek S, Gotlib J, Vannucchi AM, et al. FIGHT-203, an ongoing phase 2 study of pemigati-nib in patients with myeloid/lymphoid neoplasms (MLNs) with fibroblast growth factor receptor 1 (FGFR1) rearrangement (MLNFGFR1): a focus on centrally reviewed clinical and cytogenetic responses in previously treated patients. *Blood.* 2022;140(Supplement 1):3980–3982.

64. McLornan DP, Gras L, Martin I, et al. Outcome of allogeneic haematopoietic cell transplantation in eosinophilic disorders: a retrospective study by the chronic malignancies working party of the EBMT. *Br J Haematol.* 2022;198(1):209–213.

65. Lefebvre C, Bletry O, Degoulet P. Prognostic factors of hypereosinophilic syndrome. Study of 40 cases. *Ann Med Interne (Paris).* 1989;140(4):253–257.

66. Helbig G, Soja A, Barkowska-Chrobok A, Kyrcz-Krzemień S. Chronic eosinophilic leukemia-not otherwise specified has a poor prognosis with unresponsiveness to conventional treatment and high risk of acute transformation. *Am J Hematol.* 2012;87(6):643–645.

67. Lefèvre G, Copin MC, Staumont-Sallé D; French Eosinophil Network. The lymphoid variant of hypereosinophilic syndrome: study of 21 patients with CD3-CD4+ aberrant T-cell phenotype. *Medicine (Baltimore).* 2014;93(17):255–266.

68. Castells M, Metcalfe DD, Escribano L. Diagnosis and treatment of cutaneous mastocytosis in chil-dren: practical recommendations. *Am J Clin Dermatol.* 2011;12(4):259–270.

69. Brockow K. Epidemiology, prognosis, and risk factors in mastocytosis. *Immunol Allergy Clin North Am.* 2014;34(2):283–295.

70. Da Silva EZ, Jamur MC, Oliver C. Mast cell function: a new vision of an old cell. *J Histochem Cyto-chem.* 2014;62(10):698–738.

71. Lanternier F, Cohen-Akenine A, Palmerini F, et al. Phenotypic and genotypic characteristics of masto-cytosis according to the age of onset. *PLoS One.* 2008;3(4):e1906.

72. Hoermann G, Gleixner KV, Dinu GE, et al. The KIT D816V allele burden predicts survival in patients with mastocytosis and correlates with the WHO type of the disease. *Allergy.* 2014;69(6):810–813.

73. Brockow K, Jofer C, Behrendt H, et al. Anaphylaxis in patients with mastocytosis: a study on history, clinical features and risk factors in 120 patients. *Allergy.* 2008;63(2):226–232.

74. Parker RI. Hematologic aspects of mastocytosis: I: Bone marrow pathology in adult and pediatric systemic mast cell disease. *J Invest Dermatol.* 1991;96(3):47S–50S.

75. Sotlar K, Horny HP, Simonitsch I, et al. CD25 indicates the neoplastic phenotype of mast cells: a novel immunohistochemical marker for the diagnosis of systemic mastocytosis (SM) in routinely processed bone marrow biopsy specimens. *Am J Surg Pathol.* 2004;28(10):1319–1325.

76. Lim KH, Tefferi A, Lasho TL, et al. Systemic mastocytosis in 342 consecutive adults: survival studies and prognostic factors. *Blood.* 2009;113(23):5727–5736.

77. Kristensen T, Vestergaard H, Bindslev-Jensen C, et al. Prospective evaluation of the diagnostic value of sensitive KIT D816V mutation analysis of blood in adults with suspected systemic mastocytosis. *Allergy.* 2017;72(11):1737–1743.

78. Pardanani A. Systemic mastocytosis in adults: 2021 Update on diagnosis, risk stratification and man-agement. *Am J Hematol.* 2021;96(4):508–525.

79. Gotlib J, Castells M, Elberink HO, et al. Avapritinib versus placebo in indolent systemic mastocytosis. *NEJM Evid.* 2023;2(6):1–15.

80. Gotlib J, Reiter A, Radia DH, et al. Efficacy and safety of avapritinib in advanced systemic mastocy-tosis: interim analysis of the phase 2 PATHFINDER trial. *Nat Med.* 2021;27(12):2192–2199.

81. Gotlib J, Kluin-Nelemans HC, George TI, et al. Efficacy and safety of midostaurin in advanced sys-temic mastocytosis. *N Engl J Med.* 2016;374(26):2530–2541.

82. Akin C, Fumo G, Yavuz AS, et al. A novel form of mastocytosis associated with a transmembrane c-kit mutation and response to imatinib. *Blood.* 2004;103(8):3222–3225.

83. Ustun C, Gotlib J, Popat U, et al. Consensus opinion on allogeneic hematopoietic cell transplantation in advanced systemic mastocytosis. *Biol Blood Marrow Transplant.* 2016;22(8):1348–1356.

84. Ferrari J, Benvenuti P, Bono E, et al. Mastocytosis: fertility and pregnancy management in a rare disease. *Front Oncol.* 2022;12:874178.

85. Escribano L, Alvarez-Twose I, Sánchez-Muñoz L, et al. Prognosis in adult indolent systemic mastocytosis: a long-term study of the Spanish Network on Mastocytosis in a series of 145 patients. *J Allergy Clin Immunol.* 2009;124(3):514–521.

86. Tefferi A, Shah S, Reichard KK, Hanson CA, Pardanani A. Smoldering mastocytosis: survival comparisons with indolent and aggressive mastocytosis. *Am J Hematol.* 2019;94(1):E1–E2.

87. Pardanani A, Lim KH, Lasho TL, et al. Prognostically relevant breakdown of 123 patients with systemic mastocytosis associated with other myeloid malignancies. *Blood.* 2009;114(18):3769–3772.

88. Pardanani A, Shah S, Mannelli F, et al. Mayo alliance prognostic system for mastocytosis: clinical and hybrid clinical-molecular models. *Blood Adv.* 2018;2(21):2964–2972.

89. Schwaab J, Schnittger S, Sotlar K, et al. Comprehensive mutational profiling in advanced systemic mastocytosis. *Blood.* 2013;122(14):2460–2466.

Transfusion Medicine

11

Nathan B. McLamb and
Suzanne R. Thibodeaux

INTRODUCTION

Blood Banking and Transfusion Medicine is a medical subspecialty that encompasses blood banks, apheresis services, and cellular therapy laboratories. Blood banks allow for transfusion of donated blood products to treat many disorders, including anemia and impaired hemostasis. Apheresis can be used therapeutically to treat many disorders involving blood that can be removed and/or replaced as well as for donation of blood components and cellular therapy products. In cellular therapy laboratories, cellular therapy products can be processed and stored for recipients. Transfusion medicine services provide consultation on blood banking (including appropriate use, testing, storage, and delivery of blood products), apheresis (including discussions on indications and procedure parameters), and cellular therapy laboratories (including processing, handling, and storage of cellular therapy products) to optimize patient safety.

BLOOD BANKING

Blood banking is an integral component of transfusion medicine and encompasses the processes by which donated blood is processed, tested, and selected in ways that maximize safety to the blood donor and recipient.

Donor Screening

Blood donors undergo extensive screening and testing to optimize safety of both the donors and the eventual recipients. At the time of donation, donors must meet requirements for age, weight, vital signs, hematologic indices, and time from last donation. A donor history questionnaire is administered to assess risk of transfusion-transmitted diseases and other conditions that may compromise transfusion safety. The questionnaire reflects current guidance from the Food and Drug Administration (FDA) and the Association for the Advancement of Blood and Biotherapies (AABB) *Standards for Blood Banking and Transfusion Services*.[1,2] Donated blood products are tested for infectious diseases prior to transfusion. Every blood product is screened for hepatitis B virus, hepatitis C virus, human immunodeficiency virus (HIV), human T-lymphotropic virus (HTLV), West Nile virus, and syphilis (Treponema *pallidum*). Every blood donor is tested at least once for Chagas disease (*T. cruzi*). In certain geographic areas, blood may also be tested for *Babesia*. The risk of transfusion-transmitted infection is extremely low due to effective screening; however, laboratory screening may not identify new infections acquired during the initial "window period," where infectious microorganisms are present in blood but undetectable by current testing methods. Although the risk cannot be completely eliminated, donor screening and testing as well as new technologies in both testing and blood product modifications offer ways for the transfusion medicine community to optimize blood supply safety.

Pretransfusion Testing

Characterizing the blood of intended transfusion recipients is essential to guiding the selection of the safest blood for transfusion. As part of standard pretransfusion workups, routine laboratory testing is performed on samples from potential transfusion recipients to prevent hemolytic transfusion reactions due to anti-ABO antibodies and other clinically relevant antibodies against red blood cell (RBC) antigens. Antibodies to RBC antigens are typically IgM or IgG isotypes and can be alloantibodies or autoantibodies. RBC alloantibodies are directed against foreign (nonself) RBC antigens and typically form from exposure from previous pregnancies or transfusions. RBC autoantibodies are directed against RBCs regardless of self or nonself. IgM antibodies are pentamers that are characterized by the ability to bind complement and potentially cause intravascular hemolysis. IgG antibodies are monomers that can potentially cause extravascular hemolysis and in some cases hemolytic disease of the fetus and newborn.

Most blood bank testing is performed by serologic methods based on agglutination, formation of visibly clumped RBCs caused by interactions between antigens on RBCs and antibodies in plasma (Table 11-1). Potential for antibodies in plasma to cause RBC agglutination can be visualized by mixing RBCs with known antigen expression with patient plasma and centrifugation. If IgM antibodies are present agglutination may be easily visualized. The addition of antihuman globulin (AHG, also known as Coomb reagent) augments the agglutination process by bridging IgG antibodies bound to RBC antigens to create larger and more visible clumps. Generally, the magnitude of agglutination indicates the strength of the reaction.

ABO/Rh(D) typing always consists of two steps, the forward and reverse types. The forward type is performed on the patient's RBCs with reagent anti-A, anti-B, and anti-Rh(D) antibodies and indicates the patient's ABO/Rh(D) type. The forward type indicates which ABO antigens (A, B, A and B, or neither A nor B) and if the Rh(D) antigen is present (indicating Rh(D) positivity) are present on the patient's RBCs. The reverse type is performed with the patient's plasma and reagent type A or B RBCs and indicates the naturally occurring antibodies to the A and/or B antigen that the patient does not have on their own RBCs. Of note, the Rh type is only performed as a forward type due to the lack of naturally forming anti-Rh(D) antibodies. The forward and reverse types must be consistent with each other. If an ABO discrepancy is detected between the forward and reverse types, no type can be determined. A commonly encountered scenario in hematology/oncology is an ABO discrepancy during the engraftment process of a nonidentical ABO allogeneic hematopoietic stem cell transplant.

RBC antibody screening and identification are intended to detect unexpected antibodies against common, clinically significant RBC antigens including but not limited to those in the Rh system (e.g., D, C, c, E, e), Kell (e.g., K), Kidd (e.g., Jk^a), Duffy (e.g., Fy^a), MNS (e.g., M), Lewis (e.g., Le^a), and Lutheran (e.g., Lu^a). Testing involves mixing patient plasma with RBCs with known antigen expression profiles and evaluating for agglutination. The RBC antibody screen consists of two to three reagent RBCs expressing the most clinically significant RBC antigens, and a positive screen indicates that RBC antibodies may be present but further testing is required for characterization. RBC antibody identification (known as the indirect antiglobulin test or IAT, may be referred to as indirect Coomb test) consists of a panel of 10–20 reagent RBCs of known antigen expression, the goal of which is to have enough variability in RBC antigen profiles that an antibody can be identified from the pattern of reactivity seen across one to several panels. The antibody panel also has an "autocontrol," in which the patient's plasma is tested with their own RBCs to detect potential antibodies binding RBCs in the patient.

In cases of positive autocontrols, a direct antiglobulin test (DAT, may also be called direct Coomb test) may be performed to detect antibodies bound to RBCs in the patient's circulation. Washed patient RBCs are mixed with anti-IgG and/or anti-C3. If either IgG or C3 (a surrogate for IgM attachment) is present on the surface of the patient's RBCs, agglutination will be observed and measured. If IgG is bound to RBCs, an elution can be performed to remove bound antibodies from RBCs. The resulting eluate can then undergo RBC antibody screening and identification to characterize the antibody.

TABLE 11-1 COMMON BLOOD BANK TESTS

Test	Purpose	Indication	Technique
Pretransfusion testing			
ABO/Rh type	To identify ABO and Rh(D) antigens on a patient's RBCs	All recipients, within 3 d of transfusion	Immediate spin on recipient's RBCs
Antibody screen	To detect clinically relevant non-ABO antibodies in a patient's plasma	All recipients, within 3 d of transfusion	Indirect antiglobulin test on 2–3 donor RBC lines with known antigen expression profiles
Antibody identification	To identify the specificity of antibodies detected by a screen	Recipients with positive antibody screens	Indirect antiglobulin test on ≥10 donor RBC lines with known antigen expression profiles
Direct antiglobulin test	To detect antibodies coating recipients' RBCs in vivo	Suspected autoimmune or alloimmune hemolysis	Direct antiglobulin test on recipient's RBCs
Compatibility testing			
Full crossmatch	To confirm that a potential recipient lacks antibodies against a product's RBC antigens	When the recipient's antibody screen is positive, or the recipient has a history of previous antibodies	Indirect antiglobulin test on product (donor's) RBCs using patient's plasma
Immediate spin crossmatch	To confirm that a potential recipient lacks anti-ABO antibodies against a product's RBC ABO antigens	When the recipient has no history of antibodies and has a negative antibody screen	Immediate spin on product (donor's) RBCs using patient's plasma
Electronic/computer crossmatch	To confirm that a potential recipient lacks anti-ABO antibodies against a product's RBC ABO antigens	When the recipient has no history of antibodies and has a negative antibody screen	Computer comparison of records of recipient and product (donor's) ABO type

Adsorption can be performed to remove autoantibodies present in plasma and allow for identification of any RBC alloantibodies. Autoadsorption is a process by which the patient's own RBCs are used to "sponge" off autoantibodies from the patient's plasma, allowing for any alloantibodies to remain in the patient's plasma and be identified through antibody panels. Alloadsorption is a process by which reagent RBCs known antigen expression profiles are used to selectively sponge off antibodies potentially present in the patient's plasma.

If a patient has a finding other than a straightforward ABO/Rh(D) type and a negative antibody screen, additional time is needed to identify the cause of positivity. For additional tests that might be required, such as DATs and subsequent elutions or adsorptions, additional samples might be needed. In cases of rare or multiple antibodies, the RBC antibody identification process could span several hours to days.

Compatibility Testing

Once a blood product is selected for transfusion, testing for compatibility between the donated blood product and the intended recipient is critical to optimize safety for that specific transfusion event. Compatibility testing is performed by crossmatching, either by serologic or electronic methods (Table 11-1). Serologic crossmatch involves incubating donor RBCs with plasma from the intended recipient. Alternatively, RBCs from either the donor or recipient may be incubated with a commercially prepared reagent known to contain specific antibodies of interest. Immediate spin (IS) crossmatch is primarily used to rapidly identify clinically significant pentameric IgM antibodies (such as anti-A or anti-B antibodies) that can cause acute intravascular hemolysis. If IgM antibodies (such as anti-ABO antibodies) are present against an antigen on the RBCs, antibody binding will cause visible agglutination and clot formation in the test tube after centrifugation. Electronic crossmatch involves blood product selection based on ABO/Rh type using an FDA-approved computer system validated for use on site at the blood bank distributing the blood. Electronic or IS crossmatch can only be utilized if the intended recipient has no history of RBC antibodies and has a negative antibody screen.

In certain critical, life-threatening situations, the immediate need for blood products supersedes the requirement for thorough and potentially time-consuming compatibility testing. In these situations, it may be appropriate for clinicians to request emergency release of blood products before compatibility testing has been completed. In these cases, to avoid an acute hemolytic transfusion reaction due to anti-ABO antibodies, type O RBCs (which lack ABO antigens) and type AB plasma (or type A plasma if AB plasma is not available) are transfused until testing is complete. Obtaining a sample before transfusion if possible is important so blood bank testing can be performed in parallel and blood products can be tailored to the patient as soon as new information regarding ABO/Rh type and RBC antibodies becomes available.

Blood Products

Blood products can be collected from whole blood and subsequently separated into components by centrifugation and manual separation, or specific blood components can be collected by automated apheresis.[3] Most units of packed RBCs, plasma and cryoprecipitate in the US are derived from whole-blood collections, while the majority of platelet units and granulocytes are collected by apheresis. Each blood product is intended to replace or restore the component lost or dysfunctional. The most common blood products, descriptions, indications, and doses are described in Table 11-2.

Blood Product Modifications

Blood products can undergo modifications either in all situations or in certain circumstances to optimize transfusion safety for recipients (Table 11-3).[3] Blood product undergoes leukoreduction by filtration before storage (prestorage leukoreduced) to remove residual white blood cells that could contain immunogenic antigens on them (i.e., human leukocyte

TABLE 11-2   BLOOD PRODUCTS

Blood Product	Description	Indication	Dosing
Packed RBCs (pRBCs)	~200 mL of RBCs suspended in plasma and additives to a final volume of ~300 mL	To augment O_2 delivery to tissues	1 unit is expected to increase Hgb by ~1 g/dL or Hct by 3%
Platelets	Pooled platelets: concentrates separated from multiple units of whole blood Single-donor platelets: obtained from a single donor by apheresis Shelf life: 5 d Stored agitated at room temperature to prevent activation	To reduce the risk of spontaneous hemorrhage in individuals with thrombocytopenia To facilitate hemostasis in patients with acute bleeding	1 unit is expected to increase platelet count by ~30,000–50,000/μL Transfusion thresholds: Intracranial bleeding: <100,000/μL Other bleeding or preprocedure: <50,000/μL All others: <10,000/μL
Fresh-frozen plasma (FFP)	Fluid portion of blood that is separated and stored at <−18°C 1 mL undiluted plasma contains ~1 IU of each coagulation factor	To provide coagulation factors for patients with coagulopathy who are actively bleeding	Recommendations vary, usually starting with 2–4 units, depending on severity of bleeding and coagulopathy
Cryoprecipitate	Produced by thawing FFP at 1–6°C and recovering the cold-insoluble precipitate A rich source of factor VIII, fibrinogen, von Willebrand factor, and factor XIII usually pooled in 5 or 10 units	Bleeding associated with fibrinogen deficiency and factor XIII deficiency	1 unit increases fibrinogen by ~7–8 mg/dL in a 70-kg patient 10 units are usually given at one time Goal fibrinogen concentration is >100 mg/dL

Granulocytes	Collected by apheresis in stimulated donors Irradiated to prevent transfusion-associated graft-vs.-host disease Shelf life: 24 hours	Patients with severe neutropenia (ANC <500/µL) and infection who do not respond to growth factors and antibiotic treatment Patients with a reasonable chance of recovery	Must be infused within 24 hours of collection, preferably within 8 hours of collection due to rapid loss of function One product per day until ANC >500/µL or clinical improvement
Whole blood	Collected by whole-blood donation Type O, low titer anti-A Variable availability and inventory	Massive trauma with acute blood loss	1 unit replaces 1 unit of whole-blood loss Dosing may be dependent upon available inventory and local policies

ANC, absolute neutrophil count.

143

TABLE 11-3 · BLOOD PRODUCT MODIFICATIONS AND SPECIFICATIONS

	Purpose	Indication	Products	Process
Modification				
Leukoreduction	To prevent transfusion complications due to presence of residual donor WBCs[a]	All patients (recommended)	pRBCs, platelets	Leukoreduction filter before storage (majority) or at time of transfusion
Irradiation	To prevent transfusion-associated graft-vs.-host disease (TA-GVHD) due to donor WBCs	Certain neonatal and immunosuppressed patients[b]	pRBCs, platelets, granulocytes	Gamma or x-ray irradiation of product (25–50 Gy)
Washing/saline-replacement	To reduce transfusion of potentially allergenic plasma proteins	Patients with history of repeated, severe allergic/anaphylactic reactions	pRBCs	Centrifugation, removal of plasma, and replacement with saline
Volume reduction	To decrease potassium, reduce overall volume, or remove plasma proteins	Neonates, pediatric patients, patients with history of severe allergic reactions	pRBCs, platelets	Centrifugation, removal of supernatant
Pathogen reduction	To reduce risk of certain transfusion-transmitted infections[c] and an alternative to irradiation	Recommended for most patients with some neonatal and hypersensitivity contraindications[d]	Apheresis platelets and whole-blood–derived plasma or apheresis plasma	Products are treated with a chemical photosensitizer that crosslinks nucleic acids when exposed to UVA light
Specification				
HLA matching	To prevent platelet refractoriness due to HLA antibodies	Patients with platelet refractoriness and positive HLA antibody screen	Platelets	Platelet crossmatching or matching of donor HLA antigens against recipient antibodies
IgA deficient	To prevent anaphylaxis in IgA-deficient recipients with anti-IgA	IgA-deficient patients	All plasma-containing products	Collection of products from IgA-deficient donors

CMV seronegative	To prevent transmission of CMV[e]	CMV-negative patients receiving CMV-negative transplants, neonates, and pregnant women	pRBCs, platelets, granulocytes	Donor testing (CMV serology) at time of donation
Sickledex negative	To prevent transfusion of Hgb S to recipients with sickle cell disease	Patients with sickle cell disease	pRBCs	Hb S solubility (Sickledex) testing of product

[a]Leukoreduction is used to reduce the risk of viral infections (e.g., CMV), HLA alloimmunization, febrile transfusion reactions, and other forms of transfusion-related immunomodulation.
[b]Generally accepted indications for irradiation include intrauterine transfusions, premature neonates, patients with hematologic malignancies and solid tumors, and bone marrow transplant recipients.
[c]Examples of resistant pathogens include hepatitis A, hepatitis E, human parvovirus B19, poliovirus, and *Bacillus cereus* spores.
[d]Contraindicated in neonatal patients being treated with phototherapy or patients with hypersensitivity to amotosalen or other psoralens.
[e]It is generally accepted that leukoreduction and CMV seronegativity are equally efficacious at preventing CMV transmission.

TABLE 11-4   CAUSES OF PLATELET REFRACTORINESS

Immunologic	Nonimmunologic
ABO antibodies	Acute bleeding
Anti-HLA antibodies	DIC
Antiplatelet antibodies	Infection
Drug-induced antibodies	Medications
Plasma protein antibodies	Fever
	Splenomegaly (sequestration)
	Bone marrow transplant
	GVHD

DIC, disseminated intravascular coagulation; GVHD, graft-vs.-host disease.

antigen, or HLA) or cytomegalovirus. Most platelet products are processed with pathogen reduction technology, which inactivates many potential microbial organisms, including bacteria and viruses, as well as lymphocytes. Irradiation, volume reduction, and washing are other modifications that can be considered in certain clinical scenarios (Table 11-3).

Blood Product Specifications

Blood products can also be requested with certain specifications depending on clinical scenario (Table 11-3). IgA-deficient products can be requested for patients with demonstrated history of allergic reaction to transfusion, documented IgA deficiency, and evidence of anti-IgA in their plasma.

A major consideration for many hematology/oncology patients is platelet refractoriness, where response to platelet transfusion is less than expected. If platelet counts do not increase by ~20,000/μL within 10–60 minutes following transfusion on at least two separate occasions, platelet refractoriness may be considered. Platelet refractoriness is often multifactorial, and the most common causes are nonimmune mediated (Table 11-4). Platelets express HLAs on their surfaces, and exposure to HLA antigens by previous transfusions or pregnancies can lead to development of HLA antibodies. Patient with suspected HLA-mediated platelet refractoriness may benefit from screening for HLA antibodies, and if present, selection of HLA-matched platelets. Since ABO antigens can also adsorb and therefore be present on platelets, platelet-refractory patients may also respond better to ABO-matched platelet transfusions.

Transfusion Complications

Every blood product transfusion carries with it the risk of complications, some of which may be severe and life-threatening. Recognizing signs and symptoms of a transfusion complication, treating it appropriately, and evaluation of the blood product by the blood bank is important to ensure transfusion safety (Table 11-5). Additional information can be found in the CDC's National Healthcare Safety Network Biovigilance Component Hemovigilance Module Surveillance Protocol.[4] In all cases, if a suspected transfusion reaction occurs at any point during transfusion, the transfusion should be stopped immediately and appropriate measures are taken, including sending the blood product and a sample of the patient's plasma to the blood bank for evaluation.

APHERESIS

Apheresis is the process by which individual components (RBCs, platelets, white blood cells, and plasma) of a patient's blood are removed via centrifugation. High-flow bidirectional

TABLE 11-5 TRANSFUSION COMPLICATIONS

Reaction[a]	Mechanism	Signs/Symptoms	Diagnosis	Treatment/Prevention
Acute hemolytic transfusion reaction	Preformed (usually ABO) antibody against incompatible product	Fever Hypotension Flank or chest pain Shock Renal failure	Clerical check Direct antiglobulin test (+) Hemoglobinuria Hemoglobinemia Repeat ABO type	Hydration Pressors
Delayed hemolytic transfusion reaction	Delayed (~2–28 d following transfusion) RBC antibody response	Usually asymptomatic	Unexplained decrease in hemoglobin Increased indirect bilirubin Direct antiglobulin test (usually +) New detection of an antibody to an RBC antigen	Monitor hemoglobin, renal status Identify antibody Provide antigen-negative blood in future
Febrile nonhemolytic transfusion reaction	Cytokines or antibodies against donor WBCs	Fever Chills	Exclude hemolytic reaction or bacterial contamination	Antipyretics (e.g., acetaminophen) Transfuse leukoreduced products
Bacterial contamination	Transmission of bacteria during donation	Fever Shock DIC	Culture of product Culture of patient	Broad-spectrum antibiotics
Allergic reaction	Allergy to donor plasma proteins	Urticaria Pruritus Hypotension	Exclude acute hemolytic reaction	Antihistamines (e.g., diphenhydramine) Corticosteroids if severe

(continued)

TABLE 11-5	TRANSFUSION COMPLICATIONS (*Continued*)			
Reaction[a]	Mechanism	Signs/Symptoms	Diagnosis	Treatment/Prevention
Anaphylactic reaction	Allergy to donor plasma proteins or antibody to IgA in IgA-deficient recipients	Wheezing Hypotension Shock	Exclude acute hemolytic reaction Evaluate for IgA deficiency	Hydration Pressors Oxygen Intubation if necessary
Transfusion-associated circulatory overload (TACO)	Volume overload, especially in patients with a history of congestive heart failure	Hypertension Dyspnea Hypoxia	Pulmonary edema	Diuretics Transfuse slowly
Transfusion-related acute lung injury (TRALI)	Presumed to be due to donor anti-HLA or other antibodies directed against recipient neutrophils, causing lung damage	Acute respiratory distress within 6 h of transfusion With or without fever	Pulmonary edema Exclude TACO HLA antibody screen on donor	Supportive care Usually self-limited
Transfusion-associated graft-vs.-host disease (TA-GVHD)	Donor lymphocytes cause GVHD in immunosuppressed recipients ~2 wk following transfusion	Fever Rash Diarrhea Pancytopenia	Usually clinical diagnosis	Supportive care Mortality ~100% Prevent with irradiation
Hypotensive transfusion reaction	Mechanism unclear, but may involve vasoactive mediators	Unexplained hypotension	Exclude acute hemolytic transfusion reaction, anaphylaxis	Volume support Pressors if needed

[a]If a transfusion reaction is suspected, the transfusion should be stopped immediately.

vascular access is required for the procedure, which can be achieved with large-bore peripheral intravenous lines, central venous lines able to support apheresis flow rates, or a capable surgically embedded intravenous access device.

Apheresis can be used for donations as discussed previously to collect plasma, platelets, RBCs, and granulocytes. Apheresis is the major modality by which hematopoietic progenitor cells are collected for autologous or allogeneic hematopoietic cell transplant as well as lymphocytes for chimeric antigen receptor T-cell manufacturing.

Apheresis is utilized for a multitude of diseases to quickly remove or reduce the pathogenic component in blood.[5] Therapeutic plasma exchange (TPE) involves removal of plasma and replacement with albumin and/or fresh-frozen plasma for many different disease states, especially conditions caused by pathologic antibodies. When albumin is the only replacement fluid, coagulation factors and highly protein-bound drugs will be decreased during each procedure and should be taken into consideration when coordinating care. ACE inhibitor administration is avoided due to the apheresis instrument potential to activate bradykinin, which can lead to profound hypotension with concurrent ACE inhibitor administration. Transient hypocalcemia is the most common and easily managed side effect from apheresis due acid citrate dextrose-solution A (ACD-A) as the anticoagulant (primary or in conjunction with heparin) for the procedure. Transfusion reactions are also of concern when blood products are used as replacement fluids.

Other therapeutic apheresis procedures are used for certain clinical conditions. RBC exchange involves removal and replacement of RBCs and is primarily indicated for acute and chronic conditions in patients with sickle cell disease. Erythrocytapheresis may be used in patients with very high hematocrits where phlebotomy may not be possible. Platelets are removed during thrombocytapheresis procedure in patients with symptomatic thrombocytosis. White blood cells are removed therapeutically during a leukocytapheresis procedure for symptomatic leukocytosis.

CELLULAR THERAPY LABORATORY

The cellular therapy laboratory plays an important part in storage and processing of cellular therapies for recipients of those therapies.[6] After cells are collected, many times by apheresis, the cellular therapy product is transported to the cellular therapy laboratory for characterization. Depending on the disposition, cell therapy products may undergo RBC reduction, plasma reduction, or both. Many cellular therapy products are cryopreserved and stored in liquid nitrogen for future use. Since every cellular therapy product is specific to the patient who receives it, most cellular therapy processes, including dose calculations and reformulations, are manual and individualized. As cellular therapies grow in volume and variety, cellular therapy laboratories grow in tandem to support clinical care.

CONCLUSION

Blood banking maximizes safety of donated blood and blood products through donor screening, blood product testing, recipient pretransfusion testing, compatibility testing, blood product modifications and specifications, and transfusion reaction evaluations. Apheresis offers ways by which blood products and cellular therapy products can be donated and offers an automated way to quickly reduce or replace pathogenic blood components. The cellular therapy laboratory processes and stores cell therapy products for use in hematopoietic stem cell transplants or other cell therapies. In summary, transfusion medicine is a vital service to patients, including those receiving hematology/oncology clinical care.

REFERENCES

1. Recommendations for Evaluating Donor Eligibility Using Individual Risk-Based Questions to Reduce the Risk of Human Immunodeficiency Virus Transmission by Blood and Blood Products: Guidance for Industry. Center for Biologics Evaluation and Research, Food and Drug Administration, U.S. Department of Health and Human Services, May 2023. www.fda.gov/media/164829/download. Accessed August 15, 2023.
2. Association for the Advancement of Blood and Biotherapies Standards for Blood Banks and Transfusion Services. https://www.aabb.org/standards-accreditation/standards/blood-banks-and-transfusion-services
3. Association for the Advancement of Blood and Biotherapies Circular of Information for the Use of Human Blood and Blood Components. https://www.aabb.org/news-resources/resources/circular-of-information
4. National Healthcare Safety Network, Biovigilance Component, Hemovigilance Module Surveillance Protocol. https://www.cdc.gov/nhsn/pdfs/biovigilance/bv-hv-protocol-current.pdf
5. Connelly-Smith L, Alquist CR, Aqui NA, et al. Guidelines on the use of therapeutic apheresis in clinical practice—evidence-based approach from the writing Committee of the American Society for Apheresis: the ninth special issue. *J Clin Apher*. 2023;38:77–278.
6. Association for the Advancement of Blood and Biotherapies Circular of Information for the Use of Cellular Therapy Products. https://www.aabb.org/news-resources/resources/circular-of-information

Sickle Cell Disease

Oladipo Cole

12

Sickle Cell Disease

GENERAL PRINCIPLES

Sickle cell disease (SCD) is a term for a group of autosomal recessive inherited red blood cell disorders characterized by the presence of at least one sickle gene and the predominance of hemoglobin (Hgb) S. This is manifested by chronic hemolytic anemia and vaso-occlusive events resulting in ischemic tissue injury. Common examples of SCD include sickle cell anemia (homozygous Hgb SS), sickle β-thalassemia syndromes (Hgb S-β^+ or S-β^0), and Hgb SC disease.[1] There is tremendous variability in clinical severity among disease groups and among individual patients with the same Hgb abnormalities.

Epidemiology

In the United States, these disorders are most commonly observed in African American and Hispanic people from the Caribbean, Central America, and parts of South America and less commonly in Mediterranean, Indian, and Middle Eastern populations. Approximately 300,000 infants are born annually worldwide with SCD and about 100,000 persons are affected by SCD in the United States.[2] Sickle cell trait is present in 8–10% of African Americans. The incidence of Hgb SS and Hgb SC disease is 1 of every 500 live births and 1 of every 835 live births, respectively. In Hispanic Americans, the incidence of SCD is much less, at 1 of every 36,000 live births.

Pathophysiology

- The normal Hgb is a tetramer consisting of two α- (chromosome 16) and two β-chains (chromosome 11). **Hgb S** results from a single nucleotide substitution (A to T) on the sixth codon of the β-globin gene, altering amino acid expression. This substitution results in the expression of a hydrophobic valine in place of the normal hydrophilic glutamic acid. The change in the molecular structure of Hgb S results in the polymerization and aggregation of the Hgb tetramers. This leads to RBC deformity ("sickling") and increased whole-blood viscosity. The poor deformability of the RBC containing Hgb S results in occlusion of the microvasculature and ischemic tissue injury.
- **Factors that contribute to Hgb S polymerization** include decreased O_2 tension, low pH, RBC dehydration, and cold temperatures.
- The rate of hemolysis is dependent on the relative percentage of other Hgb, Hgb S concentration, and oxygen saturation.
- Proinflammatory interactions among the sickled cells, vascular endothelium, and circulating leukocytes contribute to vaso-occlusion. Sickled RBCs adhere to and activate vascular endothelium. This results in upregulation of endothelial adhesion molecules. WBCs are recruited, activated, and adhere to the vasculature. These adherent WBCs aggregate with sickled RBCs in the microvasculature, leading to obstructed blood flow and continued hypoxia. Abnormal vasomotor tone favoring vasoconstriction also contributes to vaso-occlusion. Organs prone to venous stasis such as spleen and bone marrow are susceptible to frequent vaso-occlusion and infarction.

DIAGNOSIS

Clinical Presentation

The hallmarks of SCD are **anemia** due to decreased RBC lifespan and chronic hemolysis, and **vaso-occlusion**, leading to acute and chronic complications secondary to end-organ dysfunction.[3] The major causes of morbidity are acute vaso-occlusive pain crises, symptomatic anemia, cerebrovascular accidents, and infections. The clinical manifestations of SCD vary tremendously both within and among the major genotypes. Even within genotypes regarded as being the most severe, some patients are entirely asymptomatic, whereas others are disabled by recurrent pain and chronic complications. SCD is associated with a shortened life expectancy due to multisystem failure from acute and chronic vaso-occlusion. One autopsy series[4] reported **causes of death in sickle cell patients**, in decreasing order of frequency, as infection, stroke, therapy complications, splenic sequestration, pulmonary emboli/thrombi, renal failure, pulmonary hypertension, hepatic failure, red cell aplasia, and left ventricular dysfunction. Of note, death was sudden in 40% of the cases. In 1973, the mean survival was only 14.3 years. Currently, the life expectancy has been extended into mid-50s. **Risk factors for mortality in SCD** are frequent pain crises, acute chest syndrome (ACS), renal disease, pulmonary disease and other comorbid conditions.[5]

- **Sickle cell trait**
  - Sickle cell trait is a benign carrier condition with no hematologic manifestations. Red cell morphology, red cell indices, and the reticulocyte count are normal. In individuals who appear to have sickle cell trait but are symptomatic, the laboratory diagnosis must be verified. Hgb other than Hgb S that polymerize may account for reports of "sickle cell trait" associated with clinical problems, and these patients should be further evaluated. Patients with sickle cell trait have a normal life expectancy. Clinical complications of sickle cell trait include splenic infarction, hematuria, increased frequency of urinary tract infection, especially in pregnancy, and a mild defect in ability to concentrate urine. Sickle cell trait has been described as a risk factor for sudden death in African Americans. It is associated with a 30-fold increased incidence of sudden death during basic training of African American military recruits. This is thought to be related to exercise-induced vaso-occlusion and rhabdomyolysis during exertion under extreme conditions. The risk of sudden death can be reduced with measures to prevent exertional heat illness. Sickle cell trait is not a contraindication to competitive sports, and mandatory screening prior to participation is not supported by the American Society of Hematology.
- **Hemoglobin SC disease**
  - Hgb SC disease is approximately one-fourth as frequent among African Americans as Hgb SS and is typically less severe than homozygous Hgb SS disease. Although deoxygenated Hgb C forms crystals, Hgb C does not participate in polymerization with deoxy-Hgb S. The lifespans of Hgb SC and Hgb SS red cells are 27 and 17 days, respectively. The predominant red cell abnormality on the peripheral smear is an abundance of target cells and crystal-containing cells. The degree of anemia and leukocytosis is frequently mild. Splenomegaly may be the only physical finding, and clinical complications may be less frequent than in sickle cell anemia. The frequency of acute painful episodes is approximately one-half that of sickle cell anemia, and the life expectancy is two decades longer. However, there is a higher incidence of peripheral retinopathy in Hgb SC disease than Hgb SS disease. These patients may present with splenic sequestration and infarction in adulthood.
- **Hemoglobin S-β thalassemia**
  - Hgb S-β thalassemia represents approximately 10% of SCD patients. Hgb Sβ^0 patients have no normal β-globin production while Hgb Sβ$^+$ patients produce some normal β-globin. Hgb Sβ$^+$ is distinguished from Hgb Sβ^0 by electrophoresis (Table 12-1). Hgb S-β thalassemia can be distinguished from Hgb S homozygous patients by the presence

TABLE 12-1 CLINICAL AND HEMATOLOGIC FINDINGS IN THE COMMON VARIANTS OF SICKLE CELL DISEASE

Morphology	Clinical Severity	Hgb Electrophoresis (%)				Hematologic Value[a]		
		S	F	A_2	A	Hgb (g/dL)	MCV (fL)	RBC
SS	Usually marked	>90	<10	<3.5	0	6–11	>80	Sickle cells, target cells
SC	Mild to moderate	50	<5	—[b]	0	10–15	75–95	Sickle cells, target cells
AS	None	40–50	<5	<3.5	50–60	12–15	>80	Normal
S-β^0	Marked to moderate	>80	<20	>3.5	0	6–10	<80	Sickle cells, target cells
S-β^+	Mild to moderate	>60	<20	>3.5	10–30	9–12	<80	No sickle cells, target cells

Hgb, hemoglobin; MCV, mean corpuscular volume.
[a]Hematologic values are approximate.
[b]Fifty percent Hgb C.

of HbA2 (typically >3.5 g/dL). HbA levels correlate with clinical severity of Hgb S-β thalassemia, with higher levels associated with fewer hematologic abnormalities and less severe disease.

Diagnostic Testing

- SCD is identified through laboratory testing alone. There are no findings on physical examination that suggest the presence or absence of SCD.
- **Neonatal screening** resulting in timely definitive diagnosis and appropriate comprehensive care has been shown to reduce the morbidity and mortality of SCD in early childhood. All states provide universal screening for newborns. When a screening test indicates SCD, a definitive diagnosis is established through further blood testing.
- The **peripheral smear** is normal in sickle cell trait (Hgb AS), but sickle cells are seen in each of the major SCD syndromes. **Solubility testing** is abnormal in all syndromes having at least one sickle cell gene and thus detects all carriers of the Hgb S gene as well as those with the SS phenotype.
- **Hgb electrophoresis** is able to provide the clinician with the exact phenotype of SCD. Typical electrophoretic profiles are listed in Table 12-1.

TREATMENT

Chronic Management

- Many patients can live for long periods without experiencing acute or severe exacerbations of SCD. Increased awareness of the disease and its long-term complications is contributing to the prolonged survival seen in sickle cell patients today.[6]
- All patients with SCD should have routine office appointments to establish baseline physical findings, laboratory data, and develop a patient–physician relationship. Patients with Hgb SS should have regular medical evaluations every 3–6 months, depending on the symptoms or manifestations of the disease.
- Preventive care is essential. A vaccination history should be maintained. Adults should have seasonal influenza vaccines. The pneumococcal vaccination should be offered and given at intervals based on the recommendations of the Advisory Committee on Immunization Practices (ACIP). Patients with SCD have an increased risk of SARS-CoV-2, also known as COVID-19, related hospitalization and death. The ACIP recommends that SCD patients older than age 16 be vaccinated.[7] Retinopathy screening should be performed by an ophthalmologist beginning at age 10. Subsequent retina examinations should occur every 1–2 years if normal, and referral should be made to a retina specialist for abnormal findings. Screening for renal disease with a urinalysis examining for proteinuria should begin at age 10 and continue annually. All patients should be screened for hypertension. It is recommended to keep patients' blood pressure at a goal of ≤130/80 mm Hg to minimize risk of stroke and other renal/cardiovascular complications.[8] Patients should be counseled during routine clinic visits about red flags for which they should seek further medical attention (Table 12-2).
- Daily **folic acid** (1 mg PO daily) should be administered for the prevention of folate deficiency in the chronic hemolytic state.
- **Hydroxyurea** is a cytotoxic medication that has been shown to decrease the frequency of acute pain crisis, ACS, hospital admissions, and erythrocyte transfusions, and to decrease mortality in adults with Hgb SS. The mechanism by which hydroxyurea influences sickle cells and vaso-occlusion is likely multifactorial, including increases in Hgb F synthesis, improved red cell deformability, modulation of sickle cell adherence properties, increased nitric oxide production, and effects on WBCs. Indications for hydroxyurea therapy include three or more severe pain crises per year, daily life affected by pain, symptomatic anemia, and recurrent ACS. Hematologic effects of hydroxyurea include decreased

TABLE 12-2	CONDITIONS THAT REQUIRE MEDICAL ATTENTION FOR PATIENTS WITH SICKLE CELL DISEASE

Fever >101°F
Lethargy
Dehydration
Worsening pallor
Severe abdominal pain
Acute pulmonary symptoms
Neurologic symptoms
Pain associated with extremity weakness or loss of function
Acute joint swelling
Recurrent vomiting
Pain not relieved by conservative measures or home medications
Priapism lasting >3 h

reticulocyte, platelet, and WBC counts. It will also result in an elevated MCV and HbF concentration, both of which are useful to monitor medication compliance, but a lack of response should not be used as a sole reason to stop therapy. Hydroxyurea is typically started at low doses (15 mg/kg/d) and is titrated to achieve clinical effect and target mild myelosuppresion (demonstrated by an ANC between 2,000 and 4,000/µL with minimal toxicity). Not all patients respond to this therapy. Hydroxyurea has been shown to be teratogenic in mice and should be avoided in pregnancy. Hydroxyurea may have a carcinogenic risk to humans (leukemia has been reported).

- **Novel Disease Modifying Agents** have been developed to improve quality of health and decrease healthcare costs. L-Glutamine, crizanlizumab, and voxelotor have recent FDA-approval in treatment of SCD with or without hydroxyurea use. Crizanlizumab is a humanized monoclonal antibody that binds to P-selectin and blocks its interaction with P-selectin glycoprotein ligand 1 (PSGL-1). In a phase III multicenter study, Crizanlizumab significantly lowered the rate of sickle cell–related pain crises versus placebo.[9] A Hgb oxygen-affinity modulator, Voxelotor, is an oral drug that increases Hgb affinity for oxygen and inhibits Hgb S polymerization. Voxelotor was shown to significantly increase Hgb levels and reduce markers of hemolysis in SCD patients.[10] Lastly, L-glutamine, which is an essential amino acid required for synthesizing NAD (nicotinamide adenine dinucleotide) in RBC, was shown to reduce the median number of pain crises over 48 weeks.[11] Updates in societal guidelines are pending real-word data and continued prospective studies.

- **Hematopoietic Stem Cell Transplantation (HSCT)** is the only curative therapy option available to patient with SCD. HSCT restores normal hematopoiesis halting, or in some cases, reversing end-organ damage caused by SCD. It is important to screen patients for matched sibling donors early, rather than later in their life. It is suggested that, when available, HLA-matched sibling transplant should be considered for patients who have frequent pain crisis, recurrent ACS, or have experienced overt stroke/abnormal transcranial Doppler ultrasound. Other HSCT donor sources and gene therapy can be considered under appropriate clinical trials with high-volume center experience.[12]

SPECIAL CONSIDERATIONS

Surgery and Anesthesia

Surgery and anesthesia are stress states that can provoke a sickle pain crisis. Currently, it is recommended that patients with SCD undergo simple transfusion to an Hgb of 10 mg/dL before elective surgery. Studies comparing aggressive transfusion (Hgb S levels <30%) versus conservative transfusion (to Hgb 10 mg/dL) showed no benefit of the more aggressive regimen.[13] More recent studies have compared transfusion to Hgb 10 mg/dL versus no preoperative transfusion in patient undergoing surgery.[14] The transfusion arm was associated with markedly less serious adverse events and episodes of ACS. In patients undergoing high-risk surgery, patients will likely benefit from more aggressive transfusion (either simple or exchange) to achieve Hgb S concentration <30% and Hgb >10 mg/dL. Intraoperative overexpansion of blood volume should be avoided, particularly in patients with decreased cardiac function. Hypothermia must also be avoided intraoperatively to prevent sickling. After surgery, IV fluid management must ensure adequate hydration, with the avoidance of volume overload and pulmonary complications. Also, adequate O_2 saturation should be maintained at all times with particular attention being paid to the immediate postoperative sedation period. Incentive spirometry (IS) should also be employed in all patients.

Dental Procedures

Procedures requiring local anesthesia can be performed in the dentist's office. However, any dental procedure requiring general anesthesia warrants hospital admission.

Transfusion Therapy

- Transfusion of RBCs has been used for almost every complication of SCD, although clinical trials have not been performed supporting efficacy for each complication.[15] Indications for transfusion include the need to improve O_2-carrying capacity (as in aplastic crisis or ACS), increase blood volume (as in splenic sequestration), or improve blood rheology (to prevent stroke recurrence, prior to surgery). **Simple transfusion** can be sufficient to improve O_2-carrying capacity and blood volume and is generally indicated in aplastic crisis, acute splenic and hepatic sequestration, milder cases of ACS, and prior to surgery. RBC transfusion is not routinely recommended for asymptomatic anemia, uncomplicated acute pain crisis, avascular necrosis, priapism, leg ulcers, or acute kidney injury (in absence of multiorgan failure). **Partial exchange transfusion** has the advantage of decreasing the percentage of Hgb S without increasing the blood volume or causing hyperviscosity. It is generally recommended for acute indications such as ACS, acute ischemic stroke, retinal artery occlusion, and multiorgan failure. It may be recommended for chronic transfusion programs, in which avoiding hyperviscosity and iron overload is important.
- **Indications for chronic transfusion**, which may be either simple or exchange, are primary stroke prevention for at-risk children and secondary stroke prevention in children. Many clinicians apply the same principles to adults with stroke. The use of chronic transfusion, with a goal Hgb S level of 30%, in combination with iron chelators has been shown to reduce risk of stroke in comparison to hydroxyurea and phlebotomy. Patients with pulmonary hypertension and recurrent ACS may also benefit from chronic transfusion. The goal of transfusion is to raise the Hgb to a level of approximately 10 g/dL. Levels >10 g/dL can lead to hyperviscosity and increased vaso-occlusion.
- **Transfusion complications** in sickle cell patients are common and include the following:
  - **Alloimmunization** in transfused sickle cell patients is due in part to minor blood-group incompatibilities (Rh, Kell, Duffy, and Kidd antigens) resulting from antigenic discrepancy in the donor (mostly Caucasian) and recipient (mostly African American) pool. Five percent to 50% of SCD patients who have received multiple transfusions develop alloimmunization, which is a risk for delayed hemolytic reactions and can make obtaining compatible blood difficult. Some centers utilize RBC phenotyping or directed donor programs to minimize risk of alloimmunization.
  - **Hyperviscosity syndrome** is characterized by a posttransfusion elevation in blood pressure and congestive heart failure, mental status change, or stroke. Treatment is exchange transfusion.

- ○ **Iron overload** and its complications become a problem in those patients who are chronically transfused. If transfusion is given without chelation, portal fibrosis can develop as early as 2 years after transfusion. Traditionally, liver iron concentration (LIC) was measured by ultrasound-guided transcutaneous needle biopsy. Biopsy has the advantage of providing both histologic assessment of liver damage and iron quantification. However, life-threatening hemorrhages may occur. A noninvasive and clinically accepted approach is to quantify the LIC using a specific MRI protocol to measure liver R2, such as FerriScan. Chelation is recommended when the total-body iron level is elevated.[16] Chelation therapy with deferoxamine (Desferal), which requires subcutaneous overnight infusion, is a time-consuming and inconvenient therapy. Oral iron chelators, such as deferasirox (Exjade, Jadenu), are effective treatments, although not all patients can afford or tolerate this medication. Patients with iron overload on chelation therapy are at increased risk for infection with *Yersinia enterocolitica*. Serial assessments (i.e., liver MRI), with timing and modality based on patients' individual clinical characteristics, should be performed in patients receiving chronic transfusions.

COMPLICATIONS

Hematologic Complications

Acute exacerbations of anemia in patients with SCD are a significant cause of morbidity and mortality. The most common causes of these exacerbations are splenic sequestration and aplastic crises.

- **Acute splenic sequestration** of blood is characterized by an exacerbation of anemia, increased reticulocytosis, and a tender, enlarging spleen. Acute sequestration can progress to hypovolemic shock and death. It is associated with a 15% mortality rate, accounted for 6.6% of deaths in one autopsy series, and is more common in children. Patients susceptible to splenic sequestration are those whose spleens have not undergone fibrosis (i.e., young patients with sickle cell anemia and adults with Hgb SC disease or S-β+ thalassemia). Treatment is **simple transfusion to restore blood volume and red cell mass**. Transfusion should be used judiciously as this can lead to release of sequestered cells with resultant hyperviscosity. Splenic sequestration recurs in 50% of cases and consideration should be given to prophylactic splenectomy after the resolution of the acute event.
- **Aplastic crises** are transient arrests of erythropoiesis characterized by abrupt falls in Hgb levels and decreased reticulocytosis. Given the decreased lifespan of RBC in SCD, aplastic crises place patients at risk for severe anemia that is frequently symptomatic. **Parvovirus B19** accounts for the majority of aplastic crises in children with SCD, but the high incidence of protective antibodies in adults makes parvovirus a less frequent cause of aplasia. Intravenous immune globulin (IVIG) can be used to treat parvovirus infection. Other infections have been reported to cause transient aplasia. Aplastic crisis can also be the result of bone marrow necrosis, which is characterized by fever, bone pain, reticulocytopenia, and a leukoerythroblastic response. The mainstay of treating aplastic crises is simple **transfusion to correct severe anemia**. SCD patients in the peri-infection period are at increased risk for complications, including pain crisis, ACS, and stroke. In parvovirus B19 infection, reticulocytopenia lasts 7–10 days, and as reticulocyte count recovers, the need for supportive transfusion should fade. A patient having an exacerbation of chronic anemia with an elevated absolute reticulocyte count is less likely to require urgent transfusion than one with a normal or low absolute reticulocyte count.
- **Hyperhemolytic crisis** is the sudden exacerbation of anemia with increased reticulocytosis and elevated bilirubin level. The mechanism for this is largely unknown but is thought to be related to hemolysis of transfused and endogenous RBCs. The diagnosis of a delayed hemolytic transfusion reaction should be considered in any patient receiving a recent blood transfusion. Treatments include supportive care, IVIG, and corticosteroids.

Simple transfusion should also be utilized with caution for severe symptomatic anemia. Most of these patients recover within 14 days.

- **Subacute anemia:** The gradual onset of worsening anemia may be due to the developing renal insufficiency or folic acid deficiency. Chronic hemolysis results in increased use of folic acid stores and can lead to megaloblastic crises if nutritional supplementation is not used.

Acute Painful Crisis

- Acute pain is the first symptom of disease in more than 25% of patients. The acute painful episode is the most frequent reason that patients with SCD seek medical attention. There is tremendous variability of painful episodes within genotypes and within the same patient over time. Some patients will rarely have painful episodes and can be managed solely in the outpatient setting, while others are hospitalized more than six times per year. Early recognition of a pain crisis, combined with careful management and titration of narcotics as an outpatient, can reduce the number of hospitalizations. More frequent pain crises are associated with higher mortality rates.
- Pain episodes may be precipitated by temperature extremes, dehydration, infection, hypoxia, acidosis, psychosocial stress, menses, and alcohol consumption. In addition, patients may report that anxiety, depression, or physical exhaustion cause pain crises. In many instances, no precipitating factors can be identified. The painful episodes can occur in any area of the body, most commonly the back, chest, extremities, and abdomen. In approximately 50% of painful episodes, patients will present with objective clinical signs such as fever, joint swelling, tenderness, tachypnea, hypertension, nausea, and vomiting. There is no clinical or laboratory finding that is pathognomonic for painful crises.
- In general, the management of acute painful crises includes the **identification and treatment of possible precipitating factors**, **IV fluid hydration**, and **analgesics**. All patients should have a CXR, urinalysis, complete blood count (CBC), and comprehensive metabolic panel (CMP) performed. Other laboratory testing (i.e., pregnancy test for females) and microbiology studies should be performed, as guided by the patient's symptoms. The possibility that the pain is precipitated by a concurrent medical condition such as an infection should be considered, and the physician should search for a precipitating illness in every instance. When a patient presents complaining of pain, the physician is charged with ruling out etiologies other than vaso-occlusion. Acute painful episodes generally last 4–6 days but may vary in intensity and duration.
- Providing aggressive relief of pain often requires the use of parenteral narcotics. Patients will often be aware of the medications and dosages that have provided adequate relief in the past. Of note, **patients with SCD do not respond to conventional doses of analgesia**, and patients are often underdosed by providers who do not routinely care for SCD patients. They typically are on chronic oral narcotics and may have developed a tolerance to conventional doses of narcotics. **Patient-controlled anesthesia (PCA) pumps** are effective in the treatment of an acute painful crisis. Appropriate conversion between chronic PO medications and IV doses of narcotics must be used to ensure adequate and prompt pain relief. The cases in which there is no nausea or vomiting, patients are continued on the PO regimen prescribed for continuous relief at home, and PCA-demand-only doses can be added. Home doses of long-acting narcotics should be typically continued in the absence of contraindications. If chronic pain was poorly controlled, consideration should be given to uptitrating long-acting narcotics for basal pain control. Patients should be monitored frequently, and objective pain scores should be followed closely for titration of effective analgesia.
- Painful events are not commonly associated with changes in the patient's Hgb levels, and transfusions are not indicated for simple acute painful crises. **Hydroxyurea reduces the frequency of painful crises.**

Infections

Infections are a leading cause of morbidity and mortality in SCD patients. Outcomes for children improved with the use of prophylactic penicillin to prevent *Streptococcal pneumoniae* sepsis. Prophylactic antibiotics are not routinely used in adults. Adults with Hgb SS disease are functionally asplenic, and fever should be worked up aggressively with the appropriate cultures, imaging studies, and consideration of prompt antibiotic coverage. Patients with other genotypes are also at risk for infection, although they are not always functionally asplenic. Sources of fever include sepsis, meningitis, ACS, osteomyelitis, and urinary tract infection. In meningitis, empiric coverage should include *Streptococcus pneumoniae* and *Haemophilus influenzae*. The coverage for ACS and osteomyelitis is discussed below.

Neurologic Complications

- Neurologic complications are common in patients with SCD, including transient ischemic attacks, cerebral infarction, silent strokes, cerebral hemorrhage, seizures, spinal cord infarction or compression, CNS infections, vestibular dysfunction, and sensory hearing loss.[17] Stroke, silent cerebral infarcts (silent strokes), and cognitive morbidity are the most common permanent sequelae of SCD in children and adults. The risk of stroke by age 20 is 11% and increases to 24% by the age of 45.[18,19] Ischemic strokes are more common in children and those >30 years old, whereas hemorrhagic stroke is more common between 20 and 30 years of age.
- **Risk factors** for strokes include severe anemia, low reticulocyte counts, low Hgb F levels, high WBC counts, the Hgb SS genotype, ACS within the previous 2 weeks, and systolic hypertension. Strokes are fatal in approximately 20% of initial cases, and 67% of patients will have a recurrence within 3 years. Patients with symptoms and signs of an acute stroke should be evaluated immediately.
- In those with a hemorrhagic stroke, initial management depends on the site and amount of bleeding. Possible presenting symptoms include severe headache, nausea, vomiting, neck stiffness, and alterations in consciousness. Angiography should be employed to determine the locations of the bleed. Outcomes are typically poor with mortality being 25–50%.
- Acute management of ischemic stroke includes urgent transfusion (to reduce Hgb S <30%), preferably via partial exchange transfusion. Simple transfusion (to Hgb not greater than 10–11 g/dL) should be administered if exchange transfusion is delayed or unavailable. Other etiologies should also be investigated, and a lipid panel, Hgb A1C, transthoracic echocardiogram, electrocardiogram, and urine drug screen should also be obtained. Antiplatelet and IV tissue plasminogen activator (tPA) agents may be considered with shared-decision making however the risk of hemorrhagic conversion is slightly higher in SCD patients.
- **Chronic exchange transfusion therapy** to maintain Hgb S levels below 30% and Hgb concentration >9 g/dL has been shown to prevent recurrent thrombosis in children and adults. At this time, it is unclear how long chronic transfusion should be maintained and there is a paucity of data as to if this should be continued as an adult. Prophylactic transfusions to reduce Hgb S to <30% in children with abnormal transcranial Doppler velocity measurements in cerebral blood vessels have been shown to reduce the risk of first clinical stroke. Guidelines recommend chronic blood transfusion goals for secondary stroke prevention of Hgb >9 g/dL at all times and maintaining the HbS level at <30% of total Hgb until the time of the next transfusion.[19]

Pulmonary Complications

ACS is one of the most feared acute pulmonary complications.[15,17,20,21] ACS is defined as a new radiographic infiltrate on CXR and one or more of the following: fever (T ≥38.5°C), cough, chest pain, dyspnea, tachypnea, and hypoxemia. Of note, the initial CXR may be negative, and there should be a low threshold for repeat imaging as clinically indicated. The definitive etiology of ACS is not known, but infection, vaso-occlusion and infarct, fat embolism from necrotic marrow, or a combination of these factors have been implicated. It has been reported to occur in 29% of patients with SCD and can progress to respiratory failure and death. ACS is the second most frequent cause of hospitalization and the most frequent complication of surgery in SCD. It should be noted, however, that nearly 50% of cases occur during hospitalization for other causes. The use of IS is one of the MOST IMPORTANT intervention in preventing ACS and reducing in-patients morbidity and mortality in hospitalized SCD patients. Risk factors include prior episodes of ACS, Hgb SS, leukocytosis, hospitalization for acute pain crisis, and high-baseline Hgb concentrations.

- Atypical and typical bacterial pathogens and viruses, especially respiratory syncytial virus (RSV), have been found in patients with ACS. **Antibiotics** are indicated as initial therapy, preferably a cephalosporin and a macrolide or fluoroquinolone. Hypoxemia should be corrected by **supplemental oxygen**.
- **Analgesics** and IS to correct splinting from chest pain should be initiated. Either **simple or exchange transfusion** should be considered promptly if there is a change in oxygen status from baseline. Simple transfusion can be used if there is a need for increased O_2-carrying capacity such as mild hypoxemia or worsened anemia. Severe hypoxemia, clinical deterioration, or impending respiratory failure should lead to urgent consideration of exchange transfusion.
- Care in an intensive care unit and ventilator support may be required. ACS has a mortality rate of approximately 30%. Chronic therapy with hydroxyurea can reduce the frequency of episodes and should be administered in patients with multiple episodes of ACS. Chronic transfusions have not been evaluated in a prospective fashion. They could be considered in a patient who has failed hydroxyurea therapy and has had multiple episodes of very severe ACS.

Chronic pulmonary disease is an important cause of morbidity and mortality in patients with SCD. SCD patients may have restrictive and obstructive lung diseases, pulmonary fibrosis, and pulmonary hypertension. Pulmonary disease is more common in those with a history of ACS and it correlates with intensity of chronic hemolysis.

- Pulmonary hypertension occurs in up to 30% of SCD patients, with up to 10% of these patients having moderate to severe range pressures. The etiology of pulmonary hypertension in SCD is unknown, although chronic intravascular hemolysis, which impairs normal vasodilation through its effects on the nitric oxide pathway, may contribute. Patients presenting with dyspnea on exertion and findings of right heart failure should be evaluated promptly. Pulmonary pressure rises during acute vaso-occlusive crises. Diagnosis is made with cardiac catheterization or transthoracic echocardiogram Doppler studies. Brain natriuretic peptide (BNP) correlates with pulmonary pressures, and elevated levels are associated with increased risk of death. The American Society of Hematology suggests obtaining a right heart catheterization for patients with peak tricuspid regurgitation jet velocity (TRJV) ≥2.5 m/s and also a 6-minute walk desaturation and/or elevated NT-BNP. There are few data on the efficacy of different treatment modalities, maximizing supportive care, treating comorbid conditions, and employing medications used in other patient populations with pulmonary hypertension may be of benefit. These patients may be considered for hydroxyurea, pulmonary vasodilators, anticoagulation, and home O_2 therapy. Prompt referral to a pulmonologist experienced in the management of pulmonary hypertension is beneficial.[8]

Hepatobiliary Complications

- The prevalence of pigmented **gallstones** in SCD is directly related to the rate of hemolysis. In sickle cell anemia, gallstones occur in children as young as 3–4 years and are eventually found in approximately 70% of patients. Patients presenting with fever, nausea, vomiting, and right upper quadrant (RUQ) pain should be evaluated for acute cholecystitis. Cholecystectomy should be considered even for asymptomatic gallstones.

- **Hepatomegaly and liver dysfunction** in SCD can be caused by multiple etiologies, including intrahepatic blood sequestration, transfusion-acquired hepatitis, transfusion-related iron overload, and, very rarely, autoimmune liver disease.
- **Hepatic sequestration:** Acute sequestration can also occur in the liver. Sickled RBC causes vaso-occlusion in the liver sinusoids resulting in infarction and sinusoidal obstruction. This results in RBC sequestration. Patient will present with severe RUQ pain, hepatomegaly, elevated liver enzymes, hyperbilirubinemia, and worsened anemia. Diagnosis is difficult, as CT and ultrasound show only a diffusely enlarged liver, liver function tests may be normal to moderately elevated, and the liver is variably tender. Treatment is supportive care and simple transfusion. Exchange transfusions should be considered in severe cases. Very rarely this results in severe hepatic dysfunction requiring liver transplantation.
- **Benign cholestasis of SCD** results in severe, asymptomatic hyperbilirubinemia without fever, pain, leukocytosis, or hepatic failure. Progressive cholestasis with RUQ pain, marked elevations in bilirubin and alkaline phosphatase, and progression to liver failure have been reported. These patients are treated with exchange transfusion and supportive care. Another serious complication is the **hepatic crisis**, in which hepatic ischemia results in fever, RUQ pain, leukocytosis, severe hyperbilirubinemia, and abnormal liver function tests. It may progress to fulminant liver failure, which has a dismal prognosis. Because of the nearly uniform mortality of this type of hepatic crisis, exchange transfusion, plasmapheresis, and liver transplantation have been used as therapy, but no controlled data are available to support this approach.

Obstetric and Gynecologic Complications

- Delayed menarche, dysmenorrhea, ovarian cysts, pelvic infection, and fibrocystic disease of the breast are more common in women with SCD.[22] However, the major reproductive concern in these patients is pregnancy. The improvement in fetal and maternal outcomes is largely due to improved prenatal and high-risk obstetric care. The incidence of spontaneous abortion, intrauterine growth retardation, preeclampsia, placental abruption, low birth weight, and intrauterine fetal death is higher in women with SCD.
- **Maternal complications during pregnancy** include increased rates of acute painful episodes, severe anemia, infections, and even death. The course of pregnancy is more benign in Hgb SC disease.
- All SCD patients should undergo reproductive counseling. Progestin-only methods, levonorgestrel IUDs, and barrier methods have no restrictions. Long-acting reversible contraception methods have low failure rates and are preferred contraception methods. Combined hormonal agents are generally considered safe in SCD.
- Management of pain crises during pregnancy should be identical to those in nonpregnant women, with IV hydration, attention to complications, and adequate pain control. Opiates can affect fetal movement and heart rate but are not teratogenic. Transfusions are generally reserved for patients with worsening anemia (Hgb <6 g/dL) and in anticipation of surgery. Hydroxyurea has been shown to be teratogenic in animals and should be stopped in pregnancy. Newer disease-modifying agents have either limited data or insufficient studies to warrant use during pregnancy and should also be avoided until more evidence is provided to suggest use during pregnancy.
- There is a very high incidence of acute painful episodes associated with therapeutic abortions. Inpatient IV hydration immediately before the procedure and for the 24 hours after the procedure is recommended.

Renal Complications

- The kidney is particularly vulnerable to complications of SCD, with manifestations that result from medullary, distal and proximal tubular and glomerular abnormalities leading to the **inability to concentrate the urine**. Papillary infarction with hematuria, renal tubular acidosis, and abnormal potassium metabolism occur more commonly in patients with SCD or sickle cell trait. Patients with hematuria should be evaluated with ultrasound.
- Patients with SCD cannot excrete acid and potassium normally but usually do not develop systemic acidosis or hyperkalemia without an additional acid load, such as in the setting of renal insufficiency. **Chronic renal insufficiency** may be predicted by albuminuria and should be suspected in the setting of hypertension and worsening anemia. In children and adults with SCD and worsening anemia associated with chronic kidney disease, using a combination therapy with hydroxyurea and erythropoiesis-stimulating agents may be utilized to treat worsening anemia. An Hgb goal threshold of 10 g/dL (hematocrit of 30%) is recommended to reduce the risk of vaso-occlusion–related complications, stroke, and VTE.[8]
- Risk factors for the development of chronic renal failure include hypertension and the use of anti-inflammatory drugs. The average age at onset of chronic renal failure is 23 years in sickle cell anemia and 50 years in Hgb SC disease.
- The use of ACE inhibitors was found to diminish proteinuria and pathologic glomerular changes; it is unclear whether their use slows the progression of sickle nephropathy. There is no general consensus on the value of protein:creatinine ratio, but it is recommended to refer patients to a renal specialist for evaluation when values are consistently elevated. Renal transplantation is recommended for patients with end-stage renal failure.[8]

Priapism

- Priapism affects 29–42% of males with SCD. It peaks in frequency at 1–5 years of age and at 13–21 years of age.[23] Priapism is most likely to develop in patients with lower Hgb F levels and reticulocyte counts, increased platelet counts, and the Hgb SS genotype.
- First-line therapy is conservative, including increasing PO fluid intake and analgesia. If the episode persists for 3 hours, the patient should seek medical care. IV fluids, parenteral narcotics, and a Foley catheter to promote bladder emptying are the initial treatments for acute priapism. If the episode lasts 4–6 hours, penile aspiration and irrigation as well as intracavernous injection of an α-adrenergic agonist by a urologist should be performed. Partial exchange transfusion can be considered, although efficacy has not been proved in randomized controlled trials, and it can be associated with complications in this setting.
- ASPEN syndrome (*a*ssociation of *S*CD, *p*riapism, *e*xchange transfusion, and *n*eurologic events), which involves headache, mental status change, neurologic deficits, and stroke, has been described in SCD patients with priapism undergoing exchange transfusion. It is important that initiation of transfusion does not delay more definitive treatment.
- If detumescence does not occur with nonsurgical management, a spongiosum–cavernosum or cavernosaphenous vein shunt may be recommended.
- Despite interventions, impotence remains a frequent complication of priapism. There is a paucity of clinical trials for the secondary prevention of priapism, although chronic transfusion, hydroxyurea, ketoconazole, and vasoactive agents such as pseudoephedrine are used at some centers.

Ocular Complications

- Anterior chamber ischemia, retinal artery occlusion, and proliferative retinopathy with the risk of subsequent hemorrhage and retinal detachment can lead to vision loss in SCD.

Sickle retinopathy is most frequently found between 15 and 30 years of age. Although found in all SCD subtypes, it is most frequent in Hgb SC.
- All patients who sustain eye trauma must be evaluated by an ophthalmologist urgently because they are at increased risk of visual loss. Patients should undergo a yearly retinal examination performed by an ophthalmologist. Sickle cell retinopathy may require vision-improving therapy with laser photocoagulation.

Bone Complications

- Bone and joint problems are a common cause of both acute and chronic pain in SCD. Erythroid hyperplasia secondary to chronic hemolytic anemia leads to widening of the medullary space and thinning of the trabeculae and cortices. This results in bony distortion, especially in the skull, vertebrae, and long bones. Vaso-occlusion and subsequent bone and marrow infarcts are common, especially in the spine, ribs, and long bones.
- **Dactylitis**, painful swelling of the hands and feet, is caused by microinfarcts of the phalanges and metatarsals and usually occurs in early childhood.
- **Osteonecrosis** occurs in all SCD phenotypes but most frequently in sickle cell anemia with coexistent α-thalassemia. Osteonecrosis occurs in both the femoral and humeral heads, as well as in the vertebral bodies. The femoral heads more commonly undergo progressive destruction as a result of chronic weight bearing. MRI is the most accurate imaging study to diagnose avascular necrosis of the femoral head. Core decompression procedures to relieve increased intraosseous pressure can be used in early-stage osteonecrosis. A patient with more advanced disease is a candidate for total hip arthroplasty. This decision must take into account the likelihood that a second hip revision may be required and that there are more complications and a relatively high failure rate in patients with SCD compared to other patient populations. Vertebral infarction also occurs and leads to chronic back pain.
- **Osteomyelitis** must be differentiated from the more common bone infarction, because the two syndromes present with similar clinical and imaging findings but are treated very differently. *Staphylococcus* and *Salmonella* are common pathogens for osteomyelitis in sickle cell patients. Increasing antibiotic resistance to *Salmonella* is a major problem in SCD. Septic arthritis must also be distinguished from the more common joint effusion associated with acute painful episodes. Bone biopsy and culture are the most reliable tests to establish the diagnosis before starting long-term antibiotics.

Dermatologic Complications

Skin ulcers are a major cause of morbidity in SCD. Ulcers occur commonly near the medial or lateral malleolus and are frequently bilateral. About 2.5% of patients age 10 and older develop leg ulcers. Ulcers may begin spontaneously or as a result of trauma. They are commonly infected with *Staphylococcus aureus, Pseudomonas, Streptococci,* or *Bacteroides* species. Males have a threefold greater risk of developing leg ulcers. Therapy with gentle debridement, wet-to-dry dressings, and compression bandages is typically effective. Compression stockings may be used to prevent recurrence. Antibiotics should be reserved for patients with culture-proven wound infection.

Cardiac Complications

An important cardiac consideration in the management of patients with SCD is the high cardiac output related to chronic anemia. Chronic high cardiac output can result in four-chamber enlargement and cardiomegaly. Age-dependent loss of cardiac reserve can lead to a greater risk of heart failure in adult patients during fluid overload, transfusion, or other reduced O_2-carrying capacity states. Acute myocardial infarction with epicardial coronary disease has been reported but is rare. Patients with chronic iron overload syndromes are at risk for restrictive cardiomyopathy.

REFERENCES

1. Natarajan K, Townes TM, Kutlar A. Disorders of hemoglobin structure: sickle cell anemia and related abnormalities. In: Lichtman MA, Kipps TJ, Seligsohn U, et al., eds. *Williams Hematology.* 8th ed. McGraw-Hill; 2010.
2. Kavanagh PL, Fasipe TA, Wun T. Sickle cell disease: a review. *JAMA.* 2022;328(1):57–68.
3. Stuart MJ, Nagel RL. Sickle cell disease. *Lancet.* 2004;364:1343–1360.
4. Manci EA, Culberson DE, Yang YM, et al. Causes of death in sickle cell disease: an autopsy study. *Br J Haematol.* 2003;123(2):359–365.
5. Elmariah H, Garrett ME, De Castro LM, et al. Factors associated with survival in a contemporary adult sickle cell disease cohort. *Am J Hematol.* 2014;89(5):530–535.
6. Yawn BP, Buchanan GR, Afenyi-Annan AN, et al. Management of sickle cell disease: summary of the 2014 evidence-based report by expert panel members. *JAMA.* 2014;312(10):1033–1048.
7. COVID-19 ACIP vaccine recommendations Atlanta, GA: US Department of Health and Human Services, CDC; 2021. https://www.cdc.gov/vaccines/hcp/acip-recs/vacc-specific/covid-19.html
8. Liem RI, Lanzkron S, D Coates T, et al. American Society of Hematology 2019 guidelines for sickle cell disease: cardiopulmonary and kidney disease. *Blood Adv.* 2019;3(23):3867–3897.
9. Ataga KI, Kutlar A, Kanter J, et al. Crizanlizumab for the prevention of pain crises in sickle cell disease. *N Engl Med.* 2017;376:429–439.
10. Vichinsky E, Hoppe CC, Ataga KI, et al. A phase 3 randomized trial in sickle cell disease. *N Engl Med.* 2019;381:509–519.
11. Niihara Y, Miller ST, Kanter J, et al; Investigators of the Phase 3 Trial of l-Glutamine in Sickle Cell Disease. A phase 3 trial of L-glutamine in sickle cell disease. *N Engl J Med.* 2018;379:226–235.
12. Kanter J, Liem RI, Bernaudin F, et al. American Society of Hematology 2021 guidelines for sickle cell disease: stem cell transplantation. *Blood Adv.* 2021;5(18):3668–3689.
13. Vichinsky EP, Haberkern CM, Neumayr L, et al. A comparison of conservative and aggressive transfusion regimens in the perioperative management of sickle cell disease. The preoperative transfusion in sickle cell disease study group. *N Engl J Med.* 1995;333:206–213.
14. Howard J, Malfroy M, Llewelyn C, et al. The Transfusion Alternatives Preoperatively in Sickle Cell Disease (TAPS) study: a randomised, controlled, multicentre clinical trial. *Lancet.* 2013;381(9870): 930–938.
15. Chou ST. Transfusion therapy for sickle cell disease: a balancing act. *Hematology Am Soc Hematol Educ Program.* 2013;2013:439–446.
16. Porter J, Garbowski M. Consequences and management of iron overload in sickle cell disease. *Hematology Am Soc Hematol Educ Program.* 2013;2013(1):447–456.
17. Verduzco LA, Nathan DG. Sickle cell disease and stroke. *Blood.* 2009;114(25):5117–5125.
18. Ohene-Frempong K, Weiner SJ, Sleeper LA, et al. Cerebrovascular accidents in sickle cell disease: rates and risk factors. *Blood.* 1998;91(1):288–294.
19. DeBaun MR, Jordan LC, King AA, et al. American Society of Hematology 2020 guidelines for sickle cell disease: prevention, diagnosis, and treatment of cerebrovascular disease in children and adults. *Blood Adv.* 2020;4(8):1554–1588.
20. Gladwin MT, Vichinsky E. Pulmonary complications of sickle cell disease. *N Engl J Med.* 2008; 359(21):2254–2265.
21. Gladwin MT, Sachdev V, Jison ML, et al. Pulmonary hypertension as a risk factor for death in patients with sickle cell disease. *N Engl J Med.* 2004;350:886–895.
22. Smith-Whitely K. Reproductive issues in sickle cell disease. *Blood.* 2014;124(24):3538–3543.
23. Rogers Z. Priapism in sickle cell disease. *Hematol Oncol Clin North Am.* 2005;19(5):917–928.

Drugs That Affect Hemostasis: Anticoagulants, Thrombolytics, and Antifibrinolytics

13

Sasha Haarberg

GENERAL PRINCIPLES

Hemostasis is a regulatory process with two functions: (1) maintain clot-free blood flow and (2) aggressively respond to localized vascular injury with formation of a hemostatic plug. Aberrancies in this system can cause either thrombus formation or uncontrolled bleeding. When hemostasis is inappropriately or over exuberantly activated, **anticoagulants** or **thrombolytics** are used to moderate this process. **Procoagulants** are used to stop bleeding, reverse the effects of anticoagulation medications, or replenish factors required for clot formation and stabilization.

Normal Hemostasis

Endothelial cells line the inner surface of blood vessels. These cells produce vasodilators that prevent platelet aggregation and block thrombus formation and fibrin deposition. Damage to the endothelial layer exposes the subendothelial extracellular matrix (ECM), which promotes platelet adherence and activation and exposes tissue factor (TF), a membrane-bound procoagulant factor. TF, in conjunction with secreted platelet factors, induces platelet aggregation and activates the coagulation cascade, ultimately leading to conversion of prothrombin to thrombin (factor IIa), forming the initial hemostatic plug. Thrombin then converts fibrinogen to insoluble fibrin, forming a permanent plug.

The **coagulation cascade** (Fig. 13-1) is a series of enzymatic reactions with feedback promotion and inhibition that regulate and restrict the process of hemostasis to the site of vascular injury. A deficiency of procoagulant factors or cofactors can cause bleeding; whereas low levels or decreased function of factors involved in limiting coagulation can trigger thrombosis.

The **adhesion of platelets** (Fig. 13-2) to exposed collagen is mediated by von Willebrand factor (vWF), which links collagen fibrils to the surface of platelets. Activated platelets release factors such as thromboxane A_2 (TXA_2) and adenosine diphosphate (ADP), which bind to their respective receptors. This initiates a series of enzymatic reactions that decrease cyclic adenosine monophosphate (cAMP) levels and promote the release of the same factors to recruit additional platelets. Recruited platelets are connected by fibrin cross-linking of glycoprotein (GP) IIb/IIIa receptors.

Anticoagulants: Agents That Prevent Thrombosis

ANTIPLATELET DRUGS

Aspirin

Mechanism of Action

Aspirin (acetylsalicylic acid) irreversibly inhibits cyclo-oxygenase-1 (COX-1), blocking the conversion of arachidonic acid to TXA_2, which is involved in the recruitment and aggregation of platelets.[1] A minimum dose of 160 mg of aspirin is required to maximally inhibit platelet function within 30 minutes. The effect of aspirin remains for the life span of the

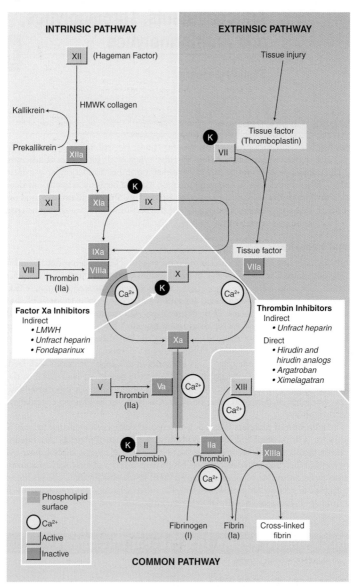

FIGURE 13-1. The coagulation cascade. The coagulation cascade is divided into two pathways: extrinsic and intrinsic, which converge at factor X, the start of the common pathway leading to thrombin formation and fibrin cross-linking. The extrinsic pathway is activated by tissue factor. Contact with subendothelial surfaces or a negatively charged surface activates factor XII (Hageman factor) and starts the intrinsic coagulation cascade. (Diagram modified from Kumar V. *Robbins & Cotran Pathologic Basis of Disease*. W. B. Saunders; 2004, Fig. 4-9.)

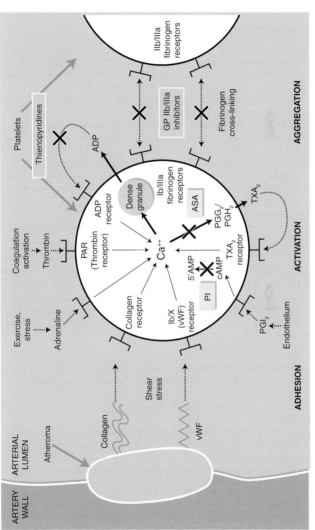

FIGURE 13-2. Mechanisms implicated in platelet adhesion, activation, and aggregation. Aspirin irreversibly inhibits thromboxane A_2 (TXA_2) synthesis, dipyridamole increases cAMP levels, clopidogrel irreversibly modifies the ADP receptor, and abciximab antagonizes the glycoprotein IIb/IIIa receptor. (Hankey GJ, Eikelboom JW. Antiplatelet drugs. *Med J Aust.* 2003;178:568–574. © Copyright 2003 The Medical Journal of Australia, reproduced with permission.)

platelet (8–10 days). Normal hemostasis is regained when 20% of platelets have normal COX-1 activity.

Preparation and Dosage

Aspirin is absorbed in the gastrointestinal tract, achieving peak levels between 30 and 60 minutes, depending on dosage, formulation, and physiologic factors. Aspirin is hydrolyzed in the plasma, conjugated in the liver, and then primarily cleared by the kidneys. In the United States, aspirin is available as 81- or 325-mg doses.

Clinical Indications

- **Ischemic stroke and transient ischemic attack (TIA).**[2,3] In patients with a history of stroke or ischemia due to fibrin platelet emboli, aspirin therapy (50–325 mg daily) reduces the combined end point of TIA, stroke, and death by 13–18%.
- **Suspected acute myocardial infarction (MI).** Aspirin treatment in patients with acute coronary syndrome reduces vascular mortality by 23%. Patients are asked to chew the aspirin tablet(s) (160–325 mg) to enhance absorption due to formulation variability.
- **Prevention of recurrent MI and unstable angina.** Aspirin therapy (75–325 mg daily) in patients with a history of MI is associated with a 20% reduction in death and reinfarction. A 5–10% decrease in event rate is observed in patients with unstable angina.
- **Chronic stable angina.** Aspirin reduces the risk of nonfatal MI, fatal MI, and sudden death by 34%. The secondary end point for vascular events (first occurrence of MI, stroke, or vascular death) is decreased by 32%.
- **Revascularization procedure.** Lifelong aspirin is recommended for patients who undergo cardiac or peripheral revascularization, if there is a pre-existing condition for which aspirin is already indicated.

Adverse Effects

Common side effects of aspirin include stomach pain, nausea, vomiting, dyspepsia, and risk of gastrointestinal bleeding. Some of these effects can be moderated by enteric coating, which protects the gastric mucosa. Aspirin may cause urticaria, angioedema, and bronchospasm. It is contraindicated in patients with a known allergy to nonsteroidal anti-inflammatory drugs and in patients with the syndrome of asthma, rhinitis, and nasal polyps. Aspirin should not be used in children with viral illness because of the risk of Reye syndrome.

Overdose

The earliest sign of salicylate toxicity is tinnitus (ringing in the ears). Respiratory alkalosis occurs early but is quickly followed by metabolic acidosis. Treatment is supportive.

Dipyridamole

Mechanism of Action

Dipyridamole (Aggrenox, Persantine) reversibly inhibits the uptake of adenosine into platelets and endothelial cells, increasing cAMP levels and, therefore, inhibiting platelet response to recruitment factors. Dipyridamole also inhibits tissue phosphodiesterase, augments the antiplatelet adhesion effects of nitric oxide, and stimulates prostacyclin release, thereby inhibiting TXA_2 formation.

Preparation and Dosage

Peak levels of dipyridamole are generally achieved 2 hours after ingestion, with a range of 1–6 hours. Metabolism occurs by liver conjugation and excretion through the gastrointestinal tract. Aggrenox is available as a capsule containing 25 mg of aspirin and 200 mg of extended-release dipyridamole. Persantine is available as 25-, 50-, and 75-mg tablets.

Clinical Indications

In patients with a history of ischemic stroke or TIA, Aggrenox reduces the risk of subsequent stroke compared to therapy with aspirin alone.[4]

Adverse Effects

Aggrenox and Persantine have a gastrointestinal side-effect profile similar to that of aspirin, with twice the rate of headache and dizziness. Serious side effects include thrombocytopenia.

P2Y$_{12}$ Antagonist

Mechanism of Action

Clopidogrel, cangrelor, prasugrel, and ticagrelor modify the ADP receptor on platelets, inhibiting the binding of ADP to its receptor involved in platelet aggregation.

Preparation and Dosage

- Clopidogrel is available in 75-mg tablets. No dose adjustment for renal or hepatic impairment.
- Cangrelor is available as a solution for intravenous administration. No dose adjustment for renal or hepatic impairment. Critical properties include quick onset (~2 minutes) and quick return to normal platelet function after discontinuation (~1 hour).
- Prasugrel is available in 5- and 10-mg tablets. No dose adjustment for renal or mild to moderate hepatic impairment. Use with caution in severe renal or hepatic impairment.

Ticagrelor is available in 60- and 90-mg tablets. No dose adjustments for renal or mild hepatic impairment; however, due to hepatic metabolism use with caution in moderate to severe impairment.

Clinical Indications

- **Clopidogrel. Recent MI, recent stroke, or established peripheral vascular disease.** The CAPRIE study compared a daily dose of 325-mg aspirin to 75-mg clopidogrel and demonstrated a relative risk reduction of 7% for fatal and nonfatal MI, stroke, and over-all event rate in the clopidogrel-treated group. **Acute coronary syndrome.** The CURE study demonstrated that patients presenting with a non—ST-elevation MI within 24 hours of the onset of symptoms had a 20% relative risk reduction in cardiovascular death, MI, or stroke when treated with an oral load of clopidogrel in addition to standard therapies (aspirin and heparin, no GPIIb/IIIa-receptor blocker 3 days prior to random-ization) compared to patients receiving only standard therapies.
- **Cangrelor. Percutaneous coronary intervention (PCI).** In the CHAMPION PHOE-NIX trial, cangrelor significantly reduced rate of ischemic events during PCI as compared to clopidogrel with no significant increase in severe bleeding.
- **Prasugrel. Acute coronary syndrome with PCI.** In the TRITON TIMI-38 trial, pra-sugrel showed reduced risk of cardiovascular events compared to clopidogrel in patients with ACS managed with PCI; however, higher rates of serious bleeding were seen in comparison to clopidogrel.
- **Ticagrelor. Recent MI, recent stroke, or coronary artery disease with high risk of stroke.** In the PLATO trial, ticagrelor significantly reduced cardiovascular death when compared to clopidogrel. In the THALES trial, ticagrelor was shown to have a relative risk reduction of 17% in subsequent stroke or death compared to aspirin alone.

Adverse Effects

Clopidogrel and ticagrelor carry a risk of thrombotic thrombocytopenic purpura. Clopido-grel and prasugrel have a risk of hypersensitivity reactions. Ticagrelor carries risk of brad-yarrhythmias and respiratory effects. All drugs carry a risk of bleeding at varying rates.

Glycoprotein IIb/IIIa Antagonists

Mechanism of Action

Abciximab (ReoPro), **tirofiban** (Aggrastat), and **eptifibatide** (Integrilin) are GPIIb/IIIa antagonists. Abciximab is the Fab fragment of the chimeric human–murine monoclonal antibody, which binds to and causes a conformational change in the GPIIb/IIIa receptor, preventing the binding of platelet "glue"—fibrinogen or vWF. Abciximab also blocks other procoagulant properties of platelets and leukocytes. Tirofiban (a nonpeptide) and eptifibatide (a cyclic heptapeptide) are reversible antagonists of the GPIIb/IIIa receptor. GPIIb/IIIa inhibitors are intended for use with aspirin and heparin.

Preparation and Dosage
Following IV bolus administration, plasma levels of abciximab decrease rapidly, with a half-life of <10 minutes. The second half-life is about 30 minutes, likely related to dose-dependent reversible binding of the GPIIb/IIIa receptor. Platelet function recovers over 48 hours, although abciximab remains in the circulation for 15 days. Within 30 minutes of tirofiban infusion, >90% platelet inhibition is obtained. The half-life is about 2 hours, with clearance largely influenced by renal function; however, tirofiban can be dialyzed out of circulation, if needed. The pharmacokinetics of eptifibatide is essentially the same as that of tirofiban.

Clinical Indications
- **Abciximab.** Following PCI or atherectomy, an IV abciximab bolus (0.25 mg/kg) followed by an infusion (0.125 μg/kg/min × 12 hours) decreases the composite of death, MI, and urgent intervention for recurrent ischemia in the first 48 hours postprocedure, a benefit that extended to 3 years. The CAPTURE trial demonstrated a lower preintervention and 30-day postintervention MI rate with IV abciximab.[3] However, there was no mortality benefit at 1 or 6 months and no difference in event rate between the abciximab-treated and the placebo groups.
- **Tirofiban.** In a study of patients undergoing PCI or arthrectomy, tirofiban (with heparin therapy) decreased the composite end point (death, new MI, refractory ischemia, and repeat cardiac procedure) by 32%.
- **Eptifibatide.** Eptifibatide infusion prior to PCI decreased the composite end point of death, MI, and urgent intervention by 1% at 30 days, and this benefit extended to 1 year.

Adverse Effects
GPIIb/IIIa receptor blockers are associated with thrombocytopenia, which can be severe.

ANTICOAGULATION DRUGS

Anticoagulants interfere with the coagulation cascade, reducing the generation of thrombin and the buttressing effects of fibrin.

Warfarin
Mechanism of Action
Warfarin (Coumadin) is an anticoagulant that acts by inhibiting the synthesis of vitamin K–dependent coagulation factors (II, VII, IX, and X, proteins C and S). Since the half-lives of proteins C and S are about one-third the half-life of the other vitamin K–dependent procoagulation factors, patients are briefly hypercoagulable before anticoagulation effects take place. For this reason, patients are often bridged with heparin as they become therapeutic on warfarin.

Preparation and Dosage
The anticoagulation effects of warfarin occur within 24 hours of ingestion, peaking at 72–96 hours and lasting 2–5 days. Cytochrome P-450 is involved in the metabolism of warfarin. Drugs that affect P-450 expression will alter the metabolism of warfarin and affect International Normalized Ratio (INR) levels. Warfarin is available in multiple-dose tablets, and therapy requires periodic INR monitoring. For more detailed suggestions on dosage initiation for warfarin, visit www.WarfarinDosing.org

Clinical Indications
- **Deep venous thrombosis (DVT) and pulmonary embolism (PE).** Current recommendation for anticoagulation in patients with an initial event and reversible risk factor for DVT or PE is 6–12 months. Recurrent thromboembolic disease warrants a hypercoagulable workup, and studies suggest a benefit of lifelong anticoagulation therapy (goal INR, 2–3).
- **Atrial fibrillation.** Prospective trials of patients with atrial fibrillation show a risk reduction of 60–86% in systemic thromboembolism and less bleeding in the low INR range (1.4–3) compared to the high INR range (2–4.5).
- **MI.** Warfarin can be used postinfarction to reduce the risk of recurrent MI and stroke. Some cardiologists would consider discontinuing anticoagulation 2–3 months postinfarction if wall motion abnormalities on echocardiography have resolved.
- **Mechanical and bioprosthetic valves.** Anticoagulation with warfarin is generally not required in the management of bioprosthetic valves. A goal INR of 2.5–3.5 is generally recommended for mechanical aortic and mitral valve replacements, with the exception that aortic St. Jude and other bileaflet aortic valves can be maintained with an INR of 2–3. If the INR is subtherapeutic or anticoagulation needs to be changed quickly, patients are usually managed with IV heparin.

Adverse Effects
Warfarin is associated with a significant risk of hemorrhage, which is associated with higher INR levels. The anticoagulation effects of warfarin can be reversed within 1–3 days with oral or IV vitamin K (Table 13-1). Immediate reversal of anticoagulation can be achieved with administration of fresh-frozen plasma (FFP). Warfarin is contraindicated in pregnancy due to teratogenic effects and the risk of fetal hemorrhage. **Warfarin-induced skin necrosis** (microthrombi due to earlier deficiency of proteins C and S compared to other vitamin K factors) is a rare complication of therapy; it occurs in areas of high-percentage adipose tissue and may become life threatening.

Unfractionated Heparin
Mechanism of Action
Unfractionated heparin is a polysaccharide that binds to antithrombin III (ATIII) and increases the rate of ATIII inactivation of thrombin (II) and factor Xa.

Preparation and Dosage
Heparin is administered IV or SC, based on patient lean body weight and clinical context (Table 13-2). IV heparin is monitored by measuring the partial thromboplastin time (PTT). Discontinuation of IV heparin results in normalization of anticoagulation within 2–3 hours.

TABLE 13-1	REVERSAL OF WARFARIN
No bleeding	
INR >5	Hold warfarin
5 < INR < 9	Vitamin K, 1–2.5 mg PO redose if INR high at 48 h
INR ≥9	Vitamin K, 2–10 mg PO or IV
	Follow INR q8h
Minor bleeding	Vitamin K, 1–5 mg PO or IV
Major bleeding	Vitamin K, 10 mg IV, and FFP or factor VII concentrate

FFP, fresh-frozen plasma.

TABLE 13-2 HEPARIN NOMOGRAM

PTT (s)	Bolus (U)	Infusion Rate
<40	3,000	↑ 3 U/kg/h
40–50	2,000	↑ 2 U/kg/h
51–59	None	↑ 1 U/kg/h
60–94	None	No change
95–104	None	↓ 1 U/kg/h
105–114	Hold 30 min	↓ 2 U/kg/h
≥114	Hold 1 h	↓ 3 U/kg/h

Typical heparin bolus, 60 U/kg (80 U/kg for pulmonary embolus/deep venous thrombosis); maximum, 5,000 U. Typical infusion, 14 U/kg/h. Monitor PTT q6h until two consecutive PTTs are therapeutic (60–96) and at least once daily thereafter. Monitor CBC, q48h.
PTT, partial thromboplastin time.

Clinical Indications
- **Anticoagulation bridge therapy.** Heparin is used as bridge therapy to initiate and discontinue anticoagulation in patients with prosthetic heart valves (to prevent valve thrombosis) and thrombotic disease.
- **Prophylaxis.** Hospitalized patients at significant risk for developing DVT and associated sequelae are given SC heparin (5,000 U bid or tid) to decrease the incidence of thrombotic disease.
- **Acute coronary syndrome and vascular surgery.** The advantage of heparin is immediate anticoagulation.
- **Invasive lines and catheters.** Invasive pressure catheters and lines are flushed with heparin to prevent catheter clotting.

Adverse Effects
Heparin is associated with a risk of bleeding. Rapid reversal of heparin can be achieved by infusion of protamine sulfate (1-mg protamine reverses 100 units of circulating heparin). Heparin-induced thrombocytopenia (HIT) is a complication that results in a rapid fall in platelet number (see Chapter 4). Suspicion of HIT should prompt discontinuation of heparin; platelet counts generally recover within 1–2 weeks. Warfarin should be avoided in acute HIT, unless combined with another anticoagulant while the INR is subtherapeutic.

Low–Molecular-Weight Heparin
Mechanism of Action
Enoxaparin (Lovenox) is a low–molecular-weight heparin that inhibits thrombin (factor IIa) and factor Xa.

Preparation and Dosage
Enoxaparin is administered SC. Maximum activity occurs 3–5 hours after SC injection, and it is administered every 12 hours, except in patients with renal impairment, in whom once-daily dosing is sufficient for anticoagulation.

Clinical Indications
- **Prophylaxis of DVT.** Enoxaparin is used to prevent thrombosis complications in patients with orthopedic, general surgical, or medical problems requiring prolonged immobilization (walking ≤10 m for ≤3 days). The prophylactic dose is 40 mg SC every 24 hours or 30 mg SC every 12 hours.

- **Prophylaxis of ischemic complications of unstable angina.** Dose is 1 mg/kg lean body weight SC every 12 hours.
- **Treatment of DVT and PE.** 1 mg/kg lean body weight SC every 12 hours.

Adverse Effects
Bleeding is a complication of enoxaparin, and no therapy to reverse anticoagulation is available. Thrombocytopenia occurs in about 1% of patients. A drop in platelet count to <100,000/μL should prompt discontinuation of this medication. Patients with HIT from heparin therapy are at risk for enoxaparin-induced thrombocytopenia; thus, other anticoagulation drugs are preferred in these situations. The use of enoxaparin for thromboprophylaxis in pregnant women and in patients with mechanical valves has not been thoroughly studied.

Fondaparinux
Mechanism of Action
Fondaparinux (Arixtra) binds to ATIII and selectively inhibits factor Xa.

Preparation and Dosage
A therapeutic level of fondaparinux is achieved within 2 hours of SC injection and is eliminated by renal excretion. Multiple prefilled syringe doses are available. Dosing is based on body weight: 5 mg (<50 kg), 7.5 mg (50–100 kg), and 10 mg (>100 kg) SC daily.

Clinical Indications
- **Prophylaxis.** Fondaparinux is indicated for DVT prophylaxis in patients undergoing orthopedic and general surgery procedures.
- **DVT and PE.** Fondaparinux is approved as bridge therapy for anticoagulation with warfarin.

Adverse Effects
Fondaparinux carries a slightly higher risk of hemorrhage compared to enoxaparin (4% vs. 3%, respectively) and similar rates of thrombocytopenia. There is no antidote for fondaparinux.

Direct Thrombin Inhibitors
Mechanism of Action
Argatroban and **bivalirudin** directly inhibit thrombin by reversibly binding to the thrombin active site.

Preparation and Dosage
Argatroban comes in premixed and concentrated solutions. The concentrated vial must be diluted to 1 mg/mL prior to administration. No dosage adjustment is necessary in renal dysfunction; however, the dosage should be adjusted in hepatic impairment (0.5 μg/kg/min).

Bivalirudin comes in vials for reconstitution or premixed frozen solution. There are dosage adjustments for continuous infusions in the setting of renal dysfunction and dialysis which vary based on indication. No dose adjustments are needed in hepatic impairment.

Clinical Indications
- **Argatroban**. For prophylaxis or treatment of thrombosis in patients with HIT (0.5–2 μg/kg/min until PTT is 1.5–3 × baseline) or as an anticoagulant in patients with HIT undergoing PCI.[5]
- **Bivalirudin**. In patients with HIT, dosing is 0.08–0.1 mg/kg/h for CrCl ≥30 mL/min or 0.04–0.06 mg/kg/h for CrCl <30 mL/min, to target PTT of 45–70 seconds. Bivalirudin can also be used in patients undergoing PCI (0.75 mg/kg bolus prior to intervention, then 1.75 mg/kg/h for the duration of the procedure, and up to 4 hours postprocedure);

in acute coronary syndrome (0.1 mg/kg bolus, then 0.25 mg/kg/h); and as an anticoagulant with streptokinase thrombolysis in ST-elevation MI and known HIT (0.25 mg/kg bolus 3 minutes before streptokinase, followed by 0.5 mg/kg/h × 12 hours, then 0.25 mg/kg/h × 36 hours).

Adverse Effects
These agents prolong the INR. Fever and diarrhea are frequent side effects of argatroban. Hypotension can occur with infusion.

Dabigatran
Mechanism of Action
Dabigatran is an oral direct thrombin inhibitor.

Preparation and Dosage
The approved dose is 150 mg PO bid. Dose reduction to 75 mg bid is indicated in patients with renal insufficiency (creatinine clearance 15–30 mL/min).

Clinical Indications
Atrial Fibrillation. Dabigatran is indicated to reduce the risk of stroke in patients with atrial fibrillation, reducing the risk of stroke by 34% compared to warfarin, with no difference in major bleeding events.[6]

    DVT and PE. In a randomized trial, dabigatran was as effective as warfarin in the treatment of acute DVT.[7]

Adverse Effects
The primary risk is bleeding. Dabigatran should be discontinued 1–2 days before an invasive procedure or surgery (3–5 days in patients with renal insufficiency). No INR monitoring is required.

Rivaroxaban
Mechanism of Action
Rivaroxaban is an oral direct factor Xa inhibitor.

Preparation and Dosage
The approved dose is 15 mg PO bid for 21 days followed by 20 mg PO daily for treatment of venous thromboembolism (VTE). Treatment in atrial fibrillation is 20 mg PO daily. The VTE prophylaxis dose following knee or hip replacement surgery is 10 mg PO daily for 14–35 days. Use is contraindicated in patients with severe renal insufficiency (creatinine clearance <30 mL/min).

Clinical Indications
Atrial Fibrillation. Rivaroxaban is noninferior to warfarin for the reduction of ischemic stroke in patients with nonvalvular atrial fibrillation.[8]

    DVT and PE. In a randomized trial, rivaroxaban was noninferior to oral vitamin K antagonist for the treatment of acute VTE.[9]

Adverse Effects
The primary risk is bleeding. Rivaroxaban should be discontinued at least 24 hours before an invasive procedure or surgery (longer in patients with renal insufficiency). No INR monitoring is required.

Apixaban
Mechanism of Action
Apixaban is an oral direct factor Xa inhibitor.

Preparation and Dosage
The approved dose is 10 mg PO bid for 7 days followed by 5 mg PO bid for treatment of VTE. Treatment in atrial fibrillation is 5 mg PO bid except in patients at least 80 years of age, with a creatinine of ≥1.5 mg/dL, or weight ≤60 kg, for which dosing should be 2.5 mg PO bid. VTE prophylaxis following knee or hip replacement surgery is treated with 2.5 mg PO bid for 12 or 35 days, respectively.

Clinical Indications
Atrial Fibrillation. Apixaban is indicated to reduce the risk of stroke in patients with atrial fibrillation, reducing the risk of stroke by 21% compared to warfarin, with a statistically significant difference in major bleeding events.[10]

DVT and PE. Apixaban is noninferior to warfarin for acute treatment of VTE and reduced the risk of major bleeding in a phase III trial.[11]

Adverse Effects
The primary risk is bleeding. Apixaban should be discontinued at least 24–48 hours prior to invasive procedure or surgery. No INR monitoring is required.

Edoxaban
Mechanism of Action
Edoxaban is an oral direct factor Xa inhibitor.

Preparation and Dosage
The approved dose is 60 mg PO daily following 5- to 10-day treatment with a parental anticoagulation for VTE. Treatment in atrial fibrillation is 60 mg PO daily. Patients with VTE weighing ≤60 kg should receive 30 mg PO daily.

Clinical Indications
Atrial Fibrillation. Edoxaban is indicated to reduce the risk of stroke in patients with atrial fibrillation.[12] There is a Boxed Warning of reduced efficacy in nonvalvular atrial fibrillation in patients with a creatinine clearance >95 mL/min.

DVT and PE. Edoxaban is noninferior to standard therapy for acute treatment of VTE and reduced the risk of bleeding in a phase III trial.[13]

Adverse Effects
The primary risk is bleeding. Edoxaban should be discontinued at least 24 hours prior to invasive procedure or surgery. No INR monitoring is required. There is a Boxed Warning for spinal/epidural hematoma in patients undergoing neuraxial anesthesia or spinal puncture.

Thrombolytics and Fibrinolytics: Agents That Disintegrate Clot

Thrombolytics and fibrinolytics convert plasminogen to the active enzyme plasmin, which digests fibrin clots (Table 13-3). Allergic reactions to these agents have been reported, particularly streptokinase and urokinase. The most commonly reported reactions to streptokinase are fever and shivering (1–4%). Anaphylactic shock is much rarer, occurring in <0.1% of patients. To anticipate allergic reaction to streptokinase, an intradermal test dose of 100 IU has been suggested. Hypersensitivity reactions should be treated with adrenergic, corticosteroid, and/or antihistamine agents as needed.

The major risk of thrombolytics and fibrinolytics is bleeding. Relative **contraindications** to their use include the following:

• Recent surgery (within 10 days)
• Gastrointestinal bleeding

TABLE 13-3	THROMBOLYTICS AND FIBRINOLYTICS		
Drug	Mechanism of Action	Indication	Dose[a]
Streptokinase	Binds plasminogen, increases conversion to plasmin	Acute MI[3]	1,500,000 IU
		PE	250,000 IU, then 100,000 IU/h × 24 h
		DVT	250,000 IU, then 100,000 IU/h × 72 h
Urokinase	Same as streptokinase	PE	4,400 IU/kg, then 4,400 IU/kg/h × 12 h
Alteplase	Tissue plasminogen activator (tPA)	Acute MI[3]	15 mg; then 0.75 mg/kg over 30 min; then 0.5 mg/kg over 1 h
		PE	100 mg over 2 h
		Acute stroke	0.9 mg/kg over 60 min
		PAD	Given intra-arterially for limb-threatening ischemia
Reteplase	Recombinant tPA that binds fibrin with less affinity than alteplase, allowing it to penetrate clots better	Acute MI[3]	10 U × 2 doses, 30 min apart
Tenecteplase	Recombinant tPA with decreased plasma clearance and increased binding to fibrin	Acute MI[3]	One-time, weight-based dose

[a]All doses are IV.
MI, myocardial infarction; PE, pulmonary embolus; DVT, deep vein thrombosis; PAD, peripheral arterial disease.

- Trauma, including intracranial or intraspinal trauma, or surgery within the previous 3 months
- Known intracranial neoplasm, arteriovenous malformation, or aneurysm
- Known bleeding diathesis or INR >1.7
- Platelet count <100,000/ μL
- Systolic blood pressure >180 mm Hg or diastolic pressure >110 mm Hg
- Subacute bacterial endocarditis
- Pregnancy
- Cerebrovascular disease

In these situations, the bleeding risk must be weighed against the benefits of thrombolysis.

Coagulants: Agents that Treat Bleeding

DESMOPRESSIN

Mechanism of Action

Desmopressin (DDAVP) is a synthetic version of the naturally occurring pituitary hormone vasopressin (ADH). In patients with some types of von Willebrand disease (VWD) and mild hemophilia A, desmopressin transiently increases plasma levels of vWF and factor VIII.

Preparation and Dosage

The dose and route of administration depend on the clinical context. The half-life of desmopressin given IV is 3 hours, and the drug is metabolized primarily by the kidney.

Clinical Indications

- **Hemophilia A.** Desmopressin is used in patients with hemophilia A prior to surgery or patients who have spontaneous bleeding.
- **VWD (type 1 and some type 2).** In general, type 1 VWD patients are more likely to respond than type 2 VWD patients. Desmopressin should be avoided in patients with type 2B VWD because of the risk of thrombocytopenia. Type 3 VWD patients lack endogenous vWF and do not respond (see Chapter 7).

Adverse Effects

Desmopressin has been associated with headaches, tachycardia, and facial flushing. Other side effects include rhinitis, stomach cramps, vulvar pain, and vomiting. In patients receiving repeated doses of the medication, tachyphylaxis can occur. Patients taking desmopressin should be educated to limit fluid intake to satisfaction of thirst only, as hyponatremia may occur via the ADH effect of the drug. Consequently, children taking this medication should have their body weight routinely monitored. Rarely, water intoxication and coma can occur.

VITAMIN K

Mechanism of Action

Phytonadione (vitamin K) is a fat-soluble vitamin required by the liver for synthesis of clotting factors II, VII, IX, and X. Vitamin K is derived from green, leafy vegetables and is also produced by bacteria in the digestive tract. It is given to reverse the effects of warfarin.

Preparation and Dosage

Vitamin K can be taken orally from 2.5 mg to a maximum dose of 25 mg. Alternatively, the drug can be given SC, IM, or IV at doses ranging from 1 to 10 mg. Vitamin K is metabolized in the liver and excreted in the bile.

Clinical Indications

Vitamin K can be administered to reverse the effects of warfarin. See section on warfarin (above) for more details.

Adverse Effects

Reactions to vitamin K include taste changes, flushing, dizziness, and hypotension. Severe anaphylaxis reactions and death have been reported following parenteral administration of the drug. Hyperbilirubinemia can be seen in infants, following administration of the drug.

AMINOCAPROIC ACID

Mechanism of Action

Aminocaproic acid (Amicar) inhibits fibrinolysis by inhibiting plasminogen activators. It is often used to treat excessive postoperative bleeding, as well as gingival bleeding in hemophiliacs undergoing dental work.

Preparation and Dosage

Aminocaproic acid can be administered orally or IV. The drug comes in 500- or 1,000-mg tablets and 250-mg syrup or injectable vials. Aminocaproic acid is metabolized in the liver and is primarily excreted in urine. For treatment of acute bleeding, dosing is 5 g IV or PO over 1 hour, followed by 1 g/h IV or PO for 8 hours or until bleeding is controlled.

Clinical Indications

Aminocaproic acid can improve hemostasis when hemorrhage is due in part or whole to fibrinolysis, including the following situations: after cardiac surgery, thrombocytopenic hematologic disorders, severe abruption placentae, hepatic cirrhosis, and various malignancies. Studies have shown aminocaproic acid to be safe and efficacious as an adjunctive therapy for hemophiliacs undergoing dental procedures.

Adverse Effects

Side effects include abdominal pain, diarrhea, pruritus, headache, malaise, allergic reactions, thrombocytopenia, hypotension, convulsions, dyspnea, rash, and tinnitus. Rarely, rhabdomyolysis and acute renal failure can occur with this medication. **Creatinine phosphokinase (CPK) monitoring** should occur regularly in patients undergoing long-term therapy, and the drug should be discontinued if elevations of the enzyme are noted.

PROTAMINE

Mechanism of Action

Protamine sulfate is a parenterally administered medication used to treat heparin overdose. It binds heparin and forms a stable complex, which negates the anticoagulation effects of heparin. When given alone, protamine has a mild anticoagulant effect.

Preparation and Dosage

Protamine has a rapid onset of action, and the reversal of heparin occurs within 5 minutes after administering the drug. One milligram of protamine neutralizes approximately 100 units of heparin. It is given at a rate of 5 mg/min IV over 10 minutes, and the dose should not exceed 50 mg at one time.

Clinical Indications

Protamine is used to treat heparin overdose. It can also be used to treat bleeding complications in patients undergoing PCI.

Adverse Effects

Following administration of protamine, patients may experience hypotension and bradycardia. Other effects include nausea, vomiting, dyspnea, flushing, and fatigue. Severe reactions to protamine include anaphylaxis and anaphylactoid reactions. Some penicillins and cephalosporins have been shown to be incompatible with protamine. Protamine overdoses may cause bleeding.

HUMATE-P

Mechanism of Action

Humate-P (antihemophilic factor/vWF complex) is a product pooled from human plasma, which contains factor VIII and vWF. Administration of Humate-P promotes coagulation. It is approved for the treatment of (1) bleeding in hemophilia A patients, (2) bleeding in patients with severe vWD, and (3) patients with mild to moderate vWD in whom desmopressin is ineffective.

Preparation and Dosage

Dosage of Humate-P depends on patient weight, severity of bleeding, and vWF:RCo (ristocetin cofactor) activity. Dosage is calculated as (patient's weight [kg] × desired% increase in vFW activity)/1.5. The dose can be adjusted for the extent of bleeding.

Clinical Indications

Humate-P has >95% efficacy when used to control bleeding in patients with vWD (types 1, 2A, 2B, and 3).

Adverse Effects

As Humate-P is derived from human plasma, it carries a risk of transmission of infectious agents. Common side effects include flushing, chills, fever, dizziness, and headache. Although allergic reactions have been reported, severe anaphylaxis is rare.

RECOMBINANT COAGULATION FACTOR VIIA

Mechanism of Action

Coagulation factor VIIa (NovoSeven) is a recombinant human coagulation factor approved for bleeding in patients with hemophilia A or B with inhibitors or in patients with congenital factor VII deficiency. NovoSeven works by activating the extrinsic pathway of coagulation.

Preparation and Dosage

NovoSeven is administered IV, and the dosage depends on the clinical context. For hemophiliacs with bleeding episodes, 90 μg/kg is given every 2 hours until bleeding stops. In patients with congenital factor VII deficiency, NovoSeven is given at 15–30 μg/kg every 4–6 hours until cessation of bleeding.

Clinical Indications

NovoSeven has been shown to be at least partially effective in 85% of serious bleeding episodes.

Adverse Effects

As with any recombinant product, anaphylaxis is a potential side effect. NovoSeven is contraindicated in patients who have a known allergic reaction to mouse, hamster, or cow products. Common side effects include bleeding, fever, and hypertension. There is a slightly increased risk of thrombosis after administration of the medication.

REFERENCES

1. Patrano C, Baigent C, Hirsh J, Roth G. Antiplatelet drugs: American College of Chest Physicians evidence-based clinical practice guidelines (8th Edition). *Chest.* 2008;133(6 Suppl):199S–233S.

2. US Preventive Services Task Force. Aspirin for the prevention of cardiovascular disease: U.S. Preventive Services Task Force recommendation statement. *Ann Intern Med.* 2009;150:396–404.
3. Goodman SG, Menon V, Cannon CP, Steg G, Ohman EM, Harrington RA. Acute ST-segment elevation myocardial infarction: American College of Chest Physicians evidence-based clinical practice guidelines (8th Edition). *Chest.* 2008;133(6 Suppl):199S–233S.
4. ESPRIT Study Group; Halkes PH, van Gijn J, Kappelle LJ, Koudstaal PJ, Algra A. Aspirin plus dipyridamole versus aspirin alone after cerebral ischemia of arterial origin (ESPRIT): randomized controlled trial. *Lancet.* 2006;367:1665–1673.
5. Warkentin TE, Greinacher A, Koster A, Lincoff AM. Treatment and prevention of heparin-induced thrombocytopenia: American College of Chest Physicians evidence-based clinical practice guidelines (8th Edition). *Chest.* 2008;133(6 Suppl):340S–380S.
6. Connolly S, Ezekowitz M, Yusuf S, et al; RE-LY Steering Committee and Investigators. Dabigatran versus warfarin in treatment of patients with atrial fibrillation. *N Eng J Med.* 2009;361(12):1139–1151.
7. Schulman S, Kearon C, Kakkar AK, et al; RE-COVER Study Group. Dabigatran versus warfarin in the treatment of acute venous thromboembolism. *N Engl J Med.* 2009;361(24):2342–2352.
8. Patel M, Mahaffey KW, Gard J, et al; ROCKET AF Investigators. Rivaroxaban versus warfarin in nonvalvular atrial fibrillation. *N Engl J Med.* 2011;365(10):883–891.
9. EINSTEIN investigators. Oral rivaroxaban for symptomatic venous thromboembolism. *N Engl J Med.* 2010;363:2499–2510.
10. Granger CB, Alexander JH, McMurray JJ, et al; ARISTOTLE Committees and Investigators. Apixaban versus warfarin in patients with atrial fibrillation. *N Engl J Med.* 2011;365(11):981–992.
11. Agnelli G, Buller H, Cohen A, et al; AMPLIFY Investigators. Oral apixaban for the treatment of acute venous thromboembolism. *N Engl J Med.* 2013;369(9):799–808.
12. Giugliano RP, Ruff CT, Braunwald E, et al; ENGAGE AF-TIMI 48 Investigators. Edoxaban versus warfarin in patients with atrial fibrillation. *N Engl J Med.* 2013;369(22):2093–2104.
13. The Hokusai-VTE Investigators; Büller HR, Décousus H, Grosso MA, et al. Edoxaban versus warfarin for the treatment of symptomatic venous thromboembolism. *N Engl J Med.* 2013;369(15):1406–1415.

Plasma Cell Disorders

14

Michael J. Slade

Plasma cell disorders encompass a group of hematologic malignancies characterized by neoplastic clonal proliferation of plasma cells producing a monoclonal protein (M-protein). The range and severity of diseases are broad and include multiple myeloma (MM), monoclonal gammopathy of undetermined significance (MGUS), lymphoplasmacytic lymphoma (LPL), and amyloid light chain (AL) amyloidosis. The M-protein varies by disease entity; MM generally produces IgG, IgA, or isolated light chains (LC) whereas Waldenström macroglobulinemia (WM) is associated with monoclonal IgM.

Monoclonal Gammopathy of Undetermined Significance

GENERAL PRINCIPLES

MGUS is a clinically asymptomatic, premalignant condition characterized by the presence of a neoplastic clonal population of plasma cells in the bone marrow. The pathophysiology of the clonal population is the same as in MM; however, the diagnosis of MGUS requires the absence of myeloma-defining clinical characteristics. MGUS is common in the general population and increases with age; based on data from the iSTOP screening study in Iceland, the prevalence of MGUS in patients age >40 is 4.5% and increases to 10%–15% in patients aged ≥80 years.

DIAGNOSIS

Clinical Presentation

Patients with MGUS are clinically asymptomatic. It is typically diagnosed during routine workup of elevated total serum protein or proteinuria.

Diagnostic Criteria

The International Myeloma Working Group (IMWG) updated diagnostic criteria for MGUS in 2014.[1] **The following criteria must be met:**

- Presence of a serum M-protein IgA, IgG, or IgM <3 mg/dL **or** abnormal serum free light chain (sFLC) (κ or γ) **with** appropriately abnormal sFLC κ/γ ratio (i.e., ↑ for κ, ↓ for γ)
- Presence of fewer than 10% clonal bone marrow plasma cells
- Absence of myeloma-defining events
- Urinary M-protein <500 mg/24 hours (light chain only)
- Absence of signs or symptoms consistent with LPL (IgM only)

Diagnostic Testing

Approach to Testing

The workup for patients with MGUS should be guided by the risk of discovering occult MM on invasive/extensive investigation. In general, asymptomatic patients with IgG

MGUS, M-protein <1.5 g/dL, and normal sFLC or LC MGUS and sFLC ratio <8 can defer imaging and bone marrow biopsy at diagnosis.[2] However, unexplained symptoms or patient concerns are an indication for complete workup.

Laboratories

All patients should undergo testing to rule out MM and define risk of progression. Initial laboratory workup should include a complete blood count (CBC), serum electrolytes, blood urea nitrogen (BUN), serum creatinine, and serum calcium. An SPEP and a 24-hour urine collection with UPEP and immunofixation, quantitative immunoglobulins, and measurement of serum-FLCs should be performed.

Imaging

The IMWG updated the imaging recommendations for suspected MGUS in 2018 and skeletal surveys are no longer recommended due to their poor sensitivity for subtle skeletal lesions.[3] Cross-sectional imaging with a **low-dose full-body CT** is preferred, but if this is unavailable either a **PET scan** or **full-body MRI** are reasonable alternatives. If these modalities are not approved or available, **skeletal surveys** can still be used.

Diagnostic Procedures

In patients meeting the above criteria, a **bone marrow aspirate and biopsy** should be done with immunophenotyping and cytogenetics with fluorescence in situ hybridization (FISH) performed on CD138+-sorted cells.

TREATMENT

There is currently **no treatment indicated for MGUS**. The vast majority of patients with MGUS die from other causes without ever progressing to MM or requiring treatment. Guidelines on follow-up vary, but it is accepted practice to follow these patients annually with evaluation including SPEP, UPEP, CBC, and creatinine. If patients develop symptoms concerning progression to myeloma or rapidly rising M-protein, they should undergo more extensive evaluation.

PROGNOSIS

In general, the rate of progression for patients diagnosed with MGUS ranges from <1% to 10% per year and decreases over time. Multiple models are available to stratify patients using routine laboratory values, including CBC, BMP, M-protein, sFLCs, and immunoglobulins.

Multiple Myeloma

GENERAL PRINCIPLES

MM results when there is neoplastic clonal proliferation of plasma cells resulting in production of a monoclonal immunoglobulin (Ig), also known as the M-protein, which is present in the blood and/or urine. The effects of myeloma stem from direct impact of the M-protein and associated light chains, as well as clonal proliferation of plasma cells.

Epidemiology

In the United States, the annual incidence of MM is approximately 6–7 per 100,000 people. In 2023, an estimated 35,730 new cases will be diagnosed, and 12,590 deaths will occur. The median age at diagnosis is approximately 70.[4]

DIAGNOSIS

Clinical Presentation

Presentation of MM can be nonspecific, including complaints of fatigue, bone pain, weight loss, paraesthesia/neuropathy, and recurrent bacterial infections. The hallmark of the disease is bone destruction, and 85% of patients have **lytic lesions** or **diffuse osteopenia** at diagnosis. Approximately 60% of patients develop **pathologic fractures** and 66% have symptomatic **bone pain**. MM can be associated with **plasmacytomas** that invade vertebrae, which may result in vertebral fracture or neurologic emergencies such as cord compression. Often the diagnosis is made on evaluation of anemia or renal failure when workup reveals the presence of an M-protein.

Diagnostic Criteria

Historically defined by the presence of an M-protein and one of the CRAB criteria (hypercalcemia, renal failure, anemia, or bone lesions), the definition of MM has been recently updated. The IMWG **diagnostic criteria** for MM were refined in 2014 to include biochemical, imaging, and further pathologic criteria.[1] **Current criteria include:**

- Clonal bone marrow plasma cells ≥10% OR extramedullary plasmacytoma AND one of the following:
  - ○ Hypercalcemia (>11 mg/dL or >1 mg/dL above the ULN)
  - ○ Renal insufficiency (creatinine >2 mg/dL or <40 mL/min)
  - ○ Anemia (hemoglobin <10 mg/dL >2 g/dL below the LLN)
  - ○ Bone lesions: one or more osteolytic lesions on skeletal radiography, CT, or PET-CT
  - ○ One or more of the following biomarkers of malignancy:
    - ▪ Clonal bone marrow plasma cell percentage ≥60%
    - ▪ Serum-free light chain (FLC) ratio ≥100
    - ▪ ≥2 focal bone or bone marrow lesions on MRI studies

A diagnosis of **smoldering MM** (SMM), sometimes called asymptomatic MM, is made by meeting both of the following criteria[1]:

- Serum M-protein ≥3 g/dL or urinary M-protein ≥500 mg per 24 hours or clonal bone marrow plasma cells 10–60%
- Absence of myeloma defining events or amyloidosis

SMM progresses to MM at a rate of approximately 10% per year and varies based on a number of risk factors, including M-protein >2 mg/dL, >20% BMPCs, and FLCr >20 at diagnosis.[5]

Diagnostic Testing

Laboratories

All patients suspected of having MM should undergo an extensive workup. Initial laboratories should include CBC, electrolytes, BUN, creatinine, and calcium. Examination of the peripheral blood smear may reveal presence of Rouleaux formation. A serum protein electrophoresis (SPEP) with immunofixation, quantitative immunoglobulins, and measurement of serum-FLCs should be performed. Once the diagnosis of a plasma cell disorder is established, 24-hour urine with urine protein electrophoresis (UPEP), and immunofixation are needed. LDH, serum β_2-microglobulin, and albumin serve as important prognostic markers. The vast majority (>95%) of patients with newly diagnosed MM will have a detectable M-protein, with IgG 50%, 20% IgA, and 20% LC only.

Imaging

The IMWG updated the imaging recommendations for suspected sMM and/or MM in 2019 and skeletal surveys are no longer recommended due to their poor sensitivity for subtle skeletal lesions.[3] Cross-sectional imaging with a **low-dose full-body CT** or **FDG PET/CT** is preferred, followed by a **full-body or axial MRI** if initial imaging is negative to rule out disease meeting SLiM criteria. If these modalities are not approved or available, **skeletal surveys** can still be used.

Diagnostic Procedures

A **bone marrow aspirate and biopsy** should be done with immunophenotyping, cytogenetics, and FISH, as certain translocations have prognostic significance.

TREATMENT

The initial decision in treatment of MM is stratified based on patient fitness and eligibility for autologous hematopoietic cell transplantation (AHCT). While some studies have suggested that early treatment may be beneficial for patients with SMM, observation remains the standard of care.[3,4]

- **Initial therapy.** Patients should undergo treatment at presentation as median survival without therapy is 6 months. The goals of induction therapy include decreasing tumor burden, alleviating symptoms, preventing end-organ damage, and prolonging survival. Initial therapy varies depending on whether patients are transplant eligible or ineligible.
  - **Fit/AHCT eligible.** High-dose chemotherapy with AHCT is considered standard of care for transplant-eligible patients. The main deciding factors for eligibility to undergo AHCT include age, performance status, and presence of comorbidities. Initial induction therapy for patients suitable for transplant includes therapy with 4–6 months of multiagent chemotherapy. The current standard of care in the United States is a three-drug regimen with bortezomib, lenalidomide, and dexamethasone (VRd), plus or minus the anti-CD38 monoclonal antibody daratumumab. However, this backbone should be readily customized to account for patient comorbidities and preferences (e.g., preexisting peripheral neuropathy or financial toxicity).
  - **Autologous hematopoietic cell transplant.** AHCT has been shown in multiple randomized trials to extend progression-free survival in patients with newly diagnosed MM when compared with non-AHCT approaches, though the impact of AHCT on overall survival is unclear in the modern era. Currently, most patients deemed suitable for AHCT proceed to the harvesting of stem cells after two to four cycles of induction therapy. Patients should achieve at least a 50% reduction in M-protein (i.e., partial response) prior to proceeding to cell collection and/or AHCT. Response rates to SCT approach 90%, with one-third of patients experiencing a complete response. Indefinite maintenance therapy with lenalidomide has a proven progression-free and overall survival benefit, though only 50% of patients remain on maintenance therapy 2 years after transplant.[6] In patients with high-risk cytogenetics, two-drug maintenance with bortezomib is often used.[7] Allogeneic transplants are no longer commonly used given other treatment options.
  - **Unfit/AHCT ineligible.** Many newly diagnosed patients are ineligible for transplant. The goals of therapy in this setting are to protect organ function and improve symptoms while minimizing side effects and treatment burden. In elderly patients, comorbid medical conditions are common, and therapy should be carefully selected based on geriatric assessment and detailed discussion of patient preferences. In general, our approach is to combine lenalidomide and dexamethasone (Rd) with bortezomib reduced dose intensity (VRD-lite) or daratumumab (DRd) per the MAIA trial.[8,9] DRd is often preferred due to daratumumab's favorable side-effect profile and monthly dosing after the step-up period, which may significantly reduce treatment burden versus weekly bortezomib in VRD-lite.

- **Relapsed and refractory disease**. While treatment is improving, MM remains incurable, and relapse is inevitable (in absence of competing risk). There is no standard of care for relapsed disease and clinical trials are encouraged. For patients undergoing standard-of-care salvage therapy, the choice of agents should be made after careful consideration of previous treatments and functional status.
- **Supportive care**. Appropriate adjunctive treatment is vital to preserving patient's quality of life following the diagnosis of MM. Pain related to skeletal involvement is common and should be treated aggressively with opioid and nonopioid pain medications. Bisphosphonates and other antiresorptive agents play a vital role in decreasing skeletal events (i.e., fractures, lytic lesions, and osteoporosis) and in decreasing bone pain due to lytic lesions. Patients with MM are at increased risk for venous thromboembolism (VTE) and patients receiving immunomodulatory agents (thalidomide, lenalidomide, or pomalidomide) should be on VTE prophylaxis (aspirin or anticoagulants). VZV reactivation occurs in a high proportion of patients receiving proteasome inhibitor or anti-CD38 antibody treatment in the absence of prophylaxis and the use of acyclovir or valacyclovir is recommended. Radiation therapy is effective in decreasing bony pain from discrete lesions and can be used during complications such as spinal cord compression.

FOLLOW-UP

Follow-up of MM should be done by serial measurement of the M-protein level and other markers of disease progression including serum-FLCs, CBC, and serum creatinine. PET-CT scans are useful for measuring disease activity, especially in the setting of new skeletal pain with or without a history of trauma.

PROGNOSIS

- **International Staging System (ISS).** The ISS was developed in 2005 and is based on a database of more than 10,000 patients. The staging system also serves as an important prognostic tool. Median survivals are 62, 44, and 29 months for stages I, II, and III, respectively.[10]
  - Stage I: β_2-Microglobulin <3.5 mg/L and serum albumin ≥3.5 g/dL
  - Stage II: Neither stage I nor stage III
  - Stage III: β_2-Microglobulin ≥5.5 mg/L
- **Revised International Staging System (R-ISS).** In 2015, an updated version of the ISS was proposed integrating high-risk cytogenetic features and LDH.[11] High-risk cytogenetics were defined as the presence by FISH of t(4;14), t(14;16), or del(17p). The 5-year OS rate was 82%, 62%, and 40% for R-ISS groups I, II, and III, respectively.
  - Stage I: ISS stage I **and** normal LDH **and** no high-risk cytogenetic features
  - Stage II: Neither R-ISS stage I nor stage III
  - Stage III: ISS stage III **and** either elevated LDH **or** high-risk cytogenetics

Solitary Plasmacytoma

GENERAL PRINCIPLES

Solitary plasmacytoma is a collection of monoclonal plasma cells localized in tissue without evidence of MM. There are two types of solitary plasmacytoma: solitary plasmacytoma of bone (SBP) and solitary extramedullary plasmacytoma (SEP). Plasmacytomas in the bone are more common than in extramedullary sites, with both types combined constituting <10% of all plasma cell dyscrasias.

Epidemiology

The incidence of solitary plasmacytoma occurs at an annual rate of approximately 0.45 per 100,000 persons in the United States. The average age of diagnosis is 55 years, with incidence higher in males versus females and non-Hispanic Black versus non-Hispanic White individuals.[12]

DIAGNOSIS

Clinical Presentation

Solitary plasmacytomas of bone often present with bony pain, pathologic fracture, or spinal cord compression. Bones undergoing increased hematopoiesis are more commonly involved in SBP, with the three most commonly involved sites including vertebrae, pelvis, and upper extremities. While SEP has a predilection for the aerodigestive tract, the most common location tends to be in the head and neck area.

Diagnostic Criteria

Diagnostic criteria for solitary plasmacytoma were updated by the IMWG in 2014 and include the following:

- Presence of biopsy-proven plasmacytoma showing a population of clonal plasma cells
- Clonal plasma cells either absent from marrow or involving <10% of marrow
- Absence of end-organ damage that can be attributed to an underlying plasma cell disorder such as hypercalcemia, renal insufficiency, or anemia
- Absence of other lytic lesions on skeletal survey and MRI of the spine/pelvis

Diagnostic Testing

Laboratories

Diagnostic workup for solitary plasmacytoma is focused on evaluation of organ compromise and to rule out the concomitant diagnosis of MM. It should include a CBC and BMP to evaluate for CRAB criteria. SPEP and UPEP with immunofixation should be performed since approximately three-quarters of cases have detectable M-protein. sFLC and immunoglobulin levels may provide additional prognostic information.

Imaging

Per the updated imaging recommendation from the IMWG, the choice of staging imaging modality is guided by solitary plasmacytoma presentation: **FDG PET/CT scan** is the preferred imaging modality for SEP, while **full-body MRI** is preferred for SBP.[3] Follow-up imaging should be performed using the same technique as initial staging.

Diagnostic Procedures

Biopsy of the suspected solitary lesion should be performed at the onset of workup to establish the working diagnosis. A bone marrow biopsy and aspiration should be performed to delineate disease risk and rule out underlying MM.

TREATMENT

The mainstay of therapy for solitary plasmacytoma is **localized radiation therapy** at a dose of 40–50 Gy over 20–25 treatments from which response exceeds 90%.[13] Approximately 50% of patients remain alive and disease free 5 years after completing radiation therapy.[14] Surgery is an alternative if immediate tumor debulking is needed for complications such as fracture or spinal cord compression, with adjuvant radiation therapy considered. At present, there is no established role for systemic therapy in solitary plasmacytoma.

PROGNOSIS

More than 50% of patients with SBP will progress to MM, compared to fewer than 30% with SEP, with median time to progression of 2–4 years. Recently, two prognostic indicators have been identified to predict who will develop MM. A study at Mayo Clinic identified that patients with SBP who have an abnormal serum-FLC ratio or presence of a urinary M-protein at diagnosis have higher risk of progression at 5 years (44% vs. 25%).[15] Patients whose serum M-protein is still elevated 1 year after treatment also have an increased risk of progression. Overall survival is higher in SEP than in SBP (10-year survival 70% vs. 50%).

Waldenström Macroglobulinemia

GENERAL PRINCIPLES

WM is a rare malignant lymphoproliferative disorder characterized by the production of an IgM paraprotein by lymphocytic population with plasmacytoid features. It is currently classified as the subset of LPL patients with a detectable IgM M-protein in the serum, though this nomenclature has changed over time. It is biologically distinct from IgM MM, which is associated with excess plasma cells in the bone marrow.

Epidemiology

There are approximately 1,400 new cases of WM annually in the United States. The median age at diagnosis is 70 years. The rate is higher in men than in women and higher in those of European versus African ancestry.

DIAGNOSIS

Clinical Presentation

The presenting symptoms of WM are nonspecific and can be attributed to infiltration of lymphocytes or plasmacytoid cells into tissue and organs, blood viscosity changes due to the monoclonal IgM-protein, or paraneoplastic neuropathy. Infiltration into organs can lead to hepatosplenomegaly, lymphadenopathy, or dermatologic findings. At high quantities, the IgM-protein can lead to hyperviscosity of the blood, causing signs of stasis including stroke, transient ischemic attacks, respiratory failure, and VTE. There is a correlation between hepatitis C infection and increased incidence of WM, and 10% of patients with WM will have cryoglobulinemia.

Diagnostic Criteria

Two diagnostic criteria must be fulfilled to establish a diagnosis of WM:

- IgM M-protein of any value in the serum
- ≥10% lymphocytes with plasmacytoid differentiation in the bone marrow with a typical immunophenotype

Diagnostic Testing

Laboratories

Diagnostic testing should include **SPEP/UPEP with immunofixation, sFLC measurement, and bone marrow biopsy with aspiration** to establish the diagnosis. Testing for MYD88 may help clarify diagnosis and guide therapy. Ancillary testing should focus on evaluating for end-organ damage, risk stratification and diagnosis of related conditions, and includes CMP, CBC, LDH, β_2-microglobulin, viral serologies, and serum viscosity.

Imaging
A CT chest/abdomen and pelvis should be performed in all patients to define lymph node and organ involvement.

TREATMENT

As subset of patients with WM have an indolent course and, like MM, WM has a recognized asymptomatic stage (i.e., "smoldering" WM). Treatment of WM should **only be initiated when symptoms develop or there is evidence of significant end-organ damage**.[16] If a patient presents with symptoms of hyperviscosity, they should be evaluated for urgent plasmapheresis to lower IgM levels before initiating therapy due to risk of IgM flair phenomena. Current guidelines recommend treatment with fixed duration chemoimmunotherapy (i.e., bendamustine and rituximab or similar) or indefinite Bruton tyrosine kinase inhibitor (ibrutinib or zanubrutinib) plus or minus rituximab.[16] Choice of initial therapy is based on patient preference, medical comorbidities, and provider experience. Therapy for refractory or relapsed disease is based on prior treatment and response with high-dose chemotherapy followed by autologous HCT utilized in a subset of fit patients. No treatment has been shown to cure WM, though the median survival from time of diagnosis has been improving with the introduction of new agents and likely now approaches 10 years.

Immunoglobulin Light Chain Amyloidosis

GENERAL PRINCIPLES

Amyloidosis is characterized by the tissue deposition of amyloid fibrils in a β-pleated sheet configuration which is resistant to proteolysis. Notably, the term amyloidosis represents a broad **clinicopathologic diagnosis** (similar to other broad diagnostic categories such as "chronic kidney disease" or "diabetes mellitus") and does not differentiate the underlying cause of abnormal protein deposition. If amyloidosis is suspected, early referral to a center with multidisciplinary expertise in the workup and treatment of amyloidosis is essential.

Epidemiology

Amyloidosis is a rare disorder, though the incidence is increasing over time due to better diagnostics and increased awareness.[17] Over 35 subtypes of amyloidosis have been identified, including heritable and acquired variants. Of these, immunoglobulin light chain (AL) amyloidosis accounts for 55% of cases. The estimated incidence of AL amyloidosis is approximately three to five cases per million people.[18]

DIAGNOSIS
Clinical Presentation

Clinical presentation of amyloid is heterogeneous and nonspecific, leading to significant diagnostic delays in most patients. The majority of symptoms are defined by the predominant organ affected and can include nephrotic syndrome, cardiomyopathy, peripheral or autonomic neuropathy, hepatic dysfunction, and bleeding diatheses. Specific physical examination findings may include hepatomegaly, periorbital ecchymoses, macroglossia, and edema.

Diagnostic Criteria

Diagnostic criteria for AL amyloidosis were updated in 2014 and include[1]:

- Presence of amyloid-related systemic syndrome (i.e., renal, cardiac, hepatic, neurologic, gastrointestinal symptoms).
- Positive amyloid staining by Congo red in any tissue (regardless of organ presentation).
- Evidence that amyloid deposits are secondary to light chain–related, established by direct examination using mass spectrometry-based proteomic analysis or immunoelectron microscopy.
- Evidence of a monoclonal plasma cell disorder per above. Notably, AL amyloidosis can coexist with a range of plasma cell disorders, ranging from MGUS to MM.

Diagnostic Testing

General Principles

Diagnostic testing for amyloidosis should proceed in two stages: (1) establish amyloid deposition and (2) define subtype and organ involvement. Pathologic examination of the affected tissue is preferred, but may not be safe or feasible (especially in case of renal or cardiac disease). Biopsy of bone marrow and abdominal fat pad have a combined sensitivity of >90% in some series and may be a reasonable alternative. Once the presence of amyloid has been confirmed, **amyloid typing** via mass spectrometry or similar technology is **absolutely essential**, as amyloid subtype determines treatment options and varies significantly for AL (combination chemotherapy) versus other subtypes of amyloidosis.

Laboratories

Laboratory testing should establish the presence and define the features of a monoclonal gammopathy. Consequently, it should include an SPEP, IFIX, sFLC, and a 24-hour urine with UPEP and total protein measurement. A bone marrow biopsy with aspiration should be performed in all patients with suspected AL amyloidosis and cytogenetics with FISH should be obtained on CD138+ sorted plasma cells, as some genetic changes impact prognosis. The workup should also rule out the presence of other CRAB features. Other laboratory workup, including cardiac biomarkers, should be guided by the suspected scope of organ involvement.

Imaging

Imaging should be guided by the identity of the suspected comorbid monoclonal gammopathy as outlined in prior sections.

TREATMENT

The current standard of care of AL amyloidosis is combination chemotherapy with daratumumab, cyclophosphamide, bortezomib, and dexamethasone (dara-CyBorD) for 6 months, followed by an additional 18 months of daratumumab maintenance per the ANDROMEDA trial.[19] In fit patients without significant cardiac involvement, AHCT may have additional benefit and can be considered on a case-by-case basis.

REFERENCES

1. Rajkumar SV, Dimopoulos MA, Palumbo A, et al. International Myeloma Working Group updated criteria for the diagnosis of multiple myeloma. *Lancet Oncol.* 2014;15:e538–e548.
2. Go RS, Vincent Rajkumar S. How I manage monoclonal gammopathy of undetermined significance. *Blood.* 2018;1312):163–173.
3. Hillengass J, Usmani S, Rajkumar SV, et al. International myeloma working group consensus recommendations on imaging in monoclonal plasma cell disorders. *Lancet Oncol* 2019;20(6):e302–e312.

4. Munshi PN, Vesole D, Jurczyszyn A, et al. Age no bar: a CIBMTR analysis of elderly patients undergoing autologous hematopoietic cell transplantation for multiple myeloma. *Cancer.* 2020;126:5077–5087.

5. Lakshman A, Vincent Rajkumar S, Buadi FK, et al. Risk stratification of smoldering multiple myeloma incorporating revised IMWG diagnostic criteria. *Blood Cancer J.* 2018;8.

6. McCarthy PL, Holstein SA, Petrucci MT, et al. Lenalidomide maintenance after autologous stem-cell transplantation in newly diagnosed multiple myeloma: a meta-analysis. *J Clin Oncol.* 2017; 35(29):3279–3289.

7. Nooka AK, Kaufman JL, Muppidi S, et al. Consolidation and maintenance therapy with lenalidomide, bortezomib and dexamethasone (RVD) in high-risk myeloma patients. *Leukemia.* 2014;28:690–693.

8. Facon T, Kumar S, Plesner T, et al. MAIA Trial: daratumumab plus lenalidomide and dexamethasone for untreated Myeloma. *N Engl J Med.* 2019;380(22):2104–2115.

9. O'Donnell EK, Laubach JP, Yee AJ, et al. A phase 2 study of modified lenalidomide, bortezomib and dexamethasone in transplant-ineligible multiple myeloma. *Br J Haematol.* 2018;182:222–230.

10. Greipp PR, Miguel JS, Durie BGM, et al. International staging system for multiple myeloma. *J Clin Oncol.* 2005;23:3412–3420.

11. Palumbo A, Avet-Loiseau H, Oliva S, et al. Revised international staging system for multiple myeloma: a report from international myeloma working group. *J Clin Oncol* 2015;33:2863–2869.

12. Ellington TD, Henley SJ, Wilson RJ, Wu M, Richardson LC. Trends in solitary plasmacytoma, extra-medullary plasmacytoma, and plasma cell myeloma incidence and myeloma mortality by racial-ethnic group, United States 2003–2016. *Cancer Med.* 2021;10:386–395.

13. Soutar R, Lucraft H, Jackson G, et al. Guidelines on the diagnosis and management of solitary plasmacytoma of bone and solitary extramedullary plasmacytoma. *Br J Haematol.* 2004;124:717–726.

14. Katodritou E, Terpos E, Symeonidis AS, et al. Clinical features, outcome, and prognostic factors for survival and evolution to multiple myeloma of solitary plasmacytomas: a report of the Greek myeloma study group in 97 patients. *Am J Hematol.* 2014;89:803–808.

15. Dingli D, Kyle RA, Rajkumar SV, et al. Immunoglobulin free light chains and solitary plasmacytoma of bone. *Blood.* 2006;108:1979–1983.

16. Dimopoulos MA, Kastritis E. How I treat Waldenström macroglobulinemia. *Blood.* 2019;134: 2022–2035.

17. Ravichandran S, Lachmann HJ, Wechalekar AD. Epidemiologic and survival trends in amyloidosis, 1987–2019. *N Engl J Med.* 2020;382(16):1567–1568.

18. Wechalekar AD, Gillmore JD, Hawkins PN. Systemic amyloidosis. *Lancet.* 2016;387:2641–2654.

19. Kastritis E, Palladini G, Minnema MC, et al. ANDROMEDA: daratumumab-based treatment for immunoglobulin light-chain amyloidosis. *N Engl J Med.* 2021;385:46–58.

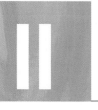

Oncology

Introduction and Approach to Oncology

15

Mia C. Weiss

Approach to a Cancer Patient

GENERAL PRINCIPLES

There have been enormous advances in our understanding of cancer biology and genomics over the past few decades. The novel treatment approaches, including newer targeted agents, immunotherapies, and advancement in supportive care strategies have given rise to increasing optimism. Yet a new diagnosis of cancer raises emotional and spiritual issues in a manner that few other diagnoses do, giving the medical oncologist a unique role in caring for the patient. While caring for a cancer patient, it is important to individualize management to the patient's needs and disease state. Listening and taking the time to explain terminology, prognosis, and treatment options are key components in the relationship between the oncologist and the patient. The oncologist's knowledge and experience with the behavior of advanced malignancies, combined with the use of complex medical regimens, often leads the oncologist serving as the primary care physician during treatment. Oncologists are central in providing palliative care for symptom relief as well as facilitating end-of-life discussions. A trusting relationship thus builds between the patient and the treating physician. This chapter provides an overview of this widely expanding field and provides a platform to understanding basic oncology terminologies and approaches. The chapters following this will provide further details on the management of specific cancers and associated clinical conditions.

Definition

Cancer or malignant tumors are defined as uncontrolled growths of cells with potential for local invasion and distant metastases.

Classification

- The classification of tumors in medical oncology is primarily based on the site of origin of the malignancy. Tumors are further classified based on the histopathologic characteristics of the tissue of origin. A pathologic diagnosis is one of the most important steps in management of the cancer, along with the identification of the primary site. Improvements in immunohistochemical (IHC) staining techniques and genomic techniques have aided in uniform identification and classification of tumors in general. It is important to remember that the individual characteristics and biology of the tumor, their ability to invade and metastasize, and their response to various therapies vary widely across tumor types.
- Two important terminologies used to refer to tumor characteristics are **stage** and **grade**.
  - **Stage** describes the extent of the disease in an individual patient. Unlike hematologic malignancies, staging is used for most solid tumors. Staging is essential for the oncologist to plan optimal treatment strategies and prognosis discussions. Stage is also the most important predictor of survival. The most commonly used staging system is the **TNM classification system** developed by the **American Joint Committee**

on **Cancer (AJCC)**. "T" represents the primary tumor characteristics including size. "N" represents the presence and extent of nodal sites of the disease. "M" represents metastasis or distant sites of spread. It is recommended that the reader consults an up-to-date staging manual when evaluating a patient because of frequent revisions for each individual malignancy. **Clinical staging** primarily uses radiographic data to describe the extent of gross disease. **Pathologic staging**, on the other hand, provides additional information gained by the pathologist through microscopic examination of the tumor.

- The **grade** of a tumor is a pathologic description of the cellular characteristics of a given malignancy. It is a measure of the degree of anaplasia or deviation of the growth and differentiation characteristics of a cancer from the parental cell type. Thus, a **low-grade tumor** retains many of the characteristics of the originating cell type and tends to be associated with a less aggressive behavior and more favorable prognosis. A **high-grade tumor** is characterized by loss of the characteristics of the originating cell type, as evidenced by a higher mitotic activity. High-grade tumors are often associated with a poorer prognosis, given the more aggressive behavior of the cells.

Epidemiology

Cancer is the second leading cause of death in the United States after heart disease. The lifetime risk of developing cancer in US is one in two for men and one in three for women. In the United States, the Surveillance, Epidemiology, and End Results (SEER) Program has been collecting population-based data, including cancer-related data, since 1975 and provides an important source of cancer trends in the population.

Terminologies Used in Cancer Epidemiology and Statistics

It is important to make a distinction between cancer incidence and cancer prevalence.

- The **cancer incidence rate** is the number of newly diagnosed cancers in a set population in a finite amount of time. It is usually expressed as number of new cancer diagnoses per 100,000 people in 1 year.
- **Cancer prevalence** is the number or percentage of people alive with a cancer diagnosis on any given date. This includes new cases and existing cases and is therefore a function of incidence and survival. Cancer prevalence cannot differentiate persons with cured cancer from those with active cancer.
- **Cancer mortality rate**, as expected, is the number of cancer-related deaths in a specified population over a defined period of time.
- **Survival is described in four broad terms: relative 5 year survival, median survival, overall survival, and progression free survival.** These statistics are based on observational studies.
  - **Relative 5-year survival rates** compare the survival among cancer patients with survival among the general population matched in age, gender, and race, adjusted for comorbidities. This statistic method is used for monitoring the progress of cancer detection and treatment in the population.
  - The **median survival** is more indicative of prognosis and is the statistic that is most commonly quoted to cancer patients. According to the National Cancer Institute, median survival is the time from diagnosis or treatment at which half of the patients with a given disease are found to be alive. In a clinical trial, the median survival time is one way to measure the effectiveness of a given treatment.
  - **Overall survival** is the percentage of people in a study or treatment group who are alive for a specific period of time, usually 5 years, after being diagnosed with or treated for a cancer. This is also referred to as the **cancer survival rate**.
  - **Progression-free survival** is another term that is often used in clinical studies which refers to the duration of time during and after treatment when the cancer has not worsened in a patient.

Epidemiologic Factors

The risk of developing cancer is affected by important demographic and geographic factors, in addition to other specific risk factors associated with individual cancers.

- **Age is both an important epidemiologic factor and a risk factor.** The highest incidence of certain cancers varies with age. For example, acute lymphoblastic lymphoma and neuroblastomas have their highest incidence in young children, while testicular cancers and Hodgkin lymphoma have their peak incidence in young adulthood. On the other hand, the risk of common adult cancers increases with age, likely from a combination of accumulating effects of environmental carcinogens and internal factors such as genetic mutations, hormonal influences, and immune system impairments.
- Cancer affects both **sexes**, with some cancers being gender specific. While overall incidence of cancer is higher in men than women, the gender distribution of individual cancers varies.
- **Race and ethnicity** are other important epidemiologic factors that influence both cancer incidence and death rates. Although it is not understood completely at this time, this factor is possibly related to interaction of the genetic and biologic characteristics of the individual patient with environmental factors such as exposure to certain dietary products or infectious agents.
- **Socioeconomic factors**, such as lack of education and unemployment, also play a very intricate role in the above factor. Societies with lower socioeconomic status are at a higher risk, which is attributable to inadequate use of screening tests, high-risk behavior such as alcohol use and smoking, and delays in seeking medical attention.
- **Geographic location** influences certain cancers, primarily from the environmental exposure to certain carcinogens, and indirectly by the socioeconomic status and racial and ethnic background of its population composition.

Cancer Statistics

According to the American Cancer Society, a total of 1,958,370 new cancer cases and 609,820 deaths from cancer are projected to occur in the United States in 2023.[1] Overall cancer incidence rates have changed based on trends in medical practice including the use of cancer screening tests. Cancer incidence in men spiked in the 1990s due to an increase in detection of prostate-specific antigen (PSA) in asymptomatic previously unscreened men. Following this, cancer incidence decreased in men until around 2013 and then stabilized through 2019. In women, the cancer incidence rate was stable until the mid-1980s but has since increased by <0.5% per year. Although differences vary widely by age, the gap between genders and cancer incidence is slowly narrowing from 1.59 in 1992 to 1.14 in 2019 (95% confidence interval [CI] 1.57–1.61 vs. 95% CI 1.14–1.5).[1] See Table 15-1.

TABLE 15-1	**INCIDENCE AND MORTALITY RATES OF CANCER IN 2020[13]**	
	Men	**Women**
Incidence rates	• Lung (14.3%) • Prostate (14.1%) • Colon and rectum (10.6%) • Stomach (7%)	• Breast (24%) • Colon and rectum (9.4%) • Lung (8.4%) • Cervix/Uteri (6.5%)
Mortality rates	• Lung (22%) • Liver (11%) • Colon and rectum (9%)	• Breast (16%) • Lung and bronchus (14%) • Colon and rectum (10%)

The cancer death rate has continued to decline from 2019 to 2020 by 1.5%, which translates to a 33% overall reduction since 1991 and an estimated 3.8 million deaths averted reflecting significant advances in treatment. There remain large racial disparities in mortality among certain cancer types including breast, prostate, and uterine cancers reflecting the disparities among equitable healthcare access and prevention programs.

Pathophysiology

Few concepts in medicine are as complex as the pathophysiology of cancer. Chapters 16 and 17 discuss the molecular and genomic basis of carcinogenesis.

Risk Factors

Certain risk factors have been associated with specific cancers, such as tobacco use with lung and head and neck cancers, cytotoxic therapy with secondary hematologic malignancies, HPV infection with cervical dysplasia, and head and neck cancers. There are, however, still several unknown risk factors that contribute to the natural history of cancer. The individual risk factors for specific cancers are elucidated in the following chapters.

DIAGNOSIS

Common Clinical Presentation

Lymphadenopathy

Lymphadenopathy may cause a patient to seek medical attention, may be found incidentally on physical examination, or may be found by imaging. The differential diagnosis is broad, including infectious etiologies, autoimmune diseases, sarcoidosis, drug hypersensitivity, benign or clonal lymphoproliferative disorders, and malignancy. Malignant causes of lymphadenopathy include lymphoma and metastatic solid tumors. Features that suggest a malignant etiology of lymphadenopathy include lymph nodes >2 cm in size, lymph nodes that are hard or fixed to adjacent structures, and supraclavicular or epitrochlear lymphadenopathy. Lymphadenopathy may be localized or generalized, and the differential diagnosis varies depending on the location and distribution of the enlarged lymph nodes. When biopsy is indicated, an excisional biopsy is preferred over a core biopsy or aspiration, especially if the suspicion for lymphoma is high, as it allows for evaluation of the lymph node architecture, which is often necessary for classification of lymphoma.[2]

Brain Mass

- The differential diagnosis for a brain mass includes metastatic disease, primary brain tumors, CNS lymphoma, hamartoma, AV malformation, demyelination, cerebral infarction, bleeding, and infection.
- Brain **metastases** are the most common intracranial tumors in adults, accounting for 50% of all brain tumors. The presence of blood–brain barrier prevents penetration of chemotherapeutic agents into the CNS, thus providing a sanctuary site for metastatic tumor cells. The incidence of brain metastases is increasing, perhaps due to the increasing sensitivity of MRI. Lung, kidney, and breast carcinomas and melanoma frequently metastasize to the brain. Cancer of the prostate, esophagus, oropharynx, sarcomas, and nonmelanoma skin cancers rarely metastasize to the brain.
- Signs and symptoms of a brain mass include headache, focal neurologic deficits, altered mental status, seizures, and stroke.
- The imaging study of choice is a contrast-enhanced MRI, which will delineate the location, presence of other lesions, margins of the lesion, and presence of vasogenic edema. Brain metastases are usually located in the gray and white matter junction and have a large amount of vasogenic edema.[3]
- A brain biopsy should be performed whenever the diagnosis is in doubt. This is particularly important in patients who have a single lesion or have a cancer that rarely

metastasizes to the brain. Often, a brain lesion is the primary presentation of a malignancy. Evaluation for a source of a metastatic focus, particularly in lung and breast cancer, should precede biopsy.

- Basic initial workup includes staging CT of the chest, abdomen, and pelvis, colonoscopy, comprehensive skin examination, and mammogram.

Liver Metastases

- The differential diagnosis of a focal liver lesion includes primary malignant liver tumors (such as hepatocellular carcinoma, cholangiocarcinoma, lymphoma, and sarcoma), metastatic liver lesions, benign hepatic cysts, cavernous hemangioma, hepatic adenoma, and abscesses.
- Before proceeding to diagnostic testing, it is important to assess the clinical scenario. For example, is this an incidental finding? Does the patient have any risk factors such as hepatitis C, cirrhosis, oral contraceptive use, travel history, history of malignancy, or constitutional symptoms?
- Diagnostic modalities include liver ultrasound, triphasic CT of the liver, and MRI of the liver. If there is a likelihood of malignancy, a fine-needle biopsy can be done. It is important to note that if a patient has a remote history of cancer, one cannot assume that a new liver lesion is due to metastases. A new liver lesion has to be definitively diagnosed, as a second unrelated malignancy cannot be ruled out.

Bone Lesions

- Bone lesions can be the initial presentation of metastatic cancer or can present later in advanced malignancy. Bone metastases are commonly due to multiple myeloma, breast cancer, or prostate cancer, but almost any solid malignancy can metastasize to the bone. They are classified as osteolytic or osteoblastic lesions. Osteolytic lesions refer to the destruction of normal bone, whereas osteoblastic lesions are the result of deposition of new bone. Multiple myeloma lesions are purely osteolytic. Metastases from prostate cancer are usually osteoblastic. Breast cancer metastases are usually a combination of both. Bone is a preferential site for metastasis because tumor cells express and produce various chemokines and adhesive molecules that bind corresponding molecules on the stromal cells of the bone. For example, expression of RANKL (receptor activator of nuclear factor kappa B ligand) in bone facilitates development of metastasis by binding RANK (receptor activator of nuclear factor kappa B) on the surface of tumor cells. Also, tumor cells can become more adhesive by expressing bone sialoprotein and binding to collagen type I in the extracellular matrix of the bone.[4]
- Signs and symptoms of bone involvement include focal pain, pathologic fractures, hypercalcemia, and cord compression.
- Diagnosis is usually made by radiologic testing, including plain films, which diagnose osteolytic lesions, and bone scans, which detect osteoblastic lesions only.
- Treatment includes systemic therapy for the underlying malignancy. Local radiation can be used to palliate symptoms and prevent pathologic fractures. Bisphosphonates and the RANKL inhibitor denosumab are used to treat hypercalcemia, treat bone pain, prevent fractures, and prevent further destruction of the normal bone. Jaw osteonecrosis is a rare but severe side effect of these agents.[5]

History

The importance of a thorough history taking cannot be stressed enough. The duration of symptoms can provide some insight into the aggressiveness of the malignancy. The associated symptom complex can provide information on the extent of the disease, especially organ-specific symptoms, which can point toward metastatic involvement by the disease. For example, new-onset neurologic symptoms in a lung cancer patient should prompt imaging of the head. In a patient with metastatic disease, it may be important to first address the most bothersome symptom(s), for the purpose of pallia-tion, before starting definitive treatment for the cancer. Assessment of nutritional status and weight changes is an integral part of cancer management. Performance scales, as mentioned below, are used to assess the functional status of the patient either before starting treatment or during ongoing treatment. While evaluating a patient on active treatment, it is important for the treating physician to first familiarize with the most common side effects of that treatment in order to dose adjust or change treatment if necessary.

Evaluation of Performance Status
Performance status describes the functional abilities of the oncology patient. It is frequently used to provide a standardized assessment of patients considered for inclusion in protocols or to characterize patients at diagnosis or during treatment or follow-up. The initial per-formance status score predicts survival. The Karnofsky Performance Status and the Eastern Cooperative Oncology Group (ECOG) Performance Status Scales (Table 15-2) are two of the most frequently used scales.[6,7]

Physical Examination

A complete physical examination is performed on any newly diagnosed cancer patient with particular attention to the organ involved. In metastatic cancers where the **primary site** is not yet identified, a physical examination may provide the first clue as to the diagnosis. This should include a breast and pelvic examination in women, a genital examination in men, and rectal examination in both men and women. In other instances, a physical exam-ination may provide clues as to the **extent** of the primary malignancy. They may also point toward **metastatic spread** of tumors, for example, enlargement of the liver in a patient with colon cancer or bone tenderness in a breast cancer patient. A physical examination can also aid in **following response** to treatment, such as the decreasing size of the breast mass or lymph nodes.

TABLE 15-2	**KARNOFSKY AND EASTERN COOPERATIVE ONCOLOGY GROUP (ECOG) PERFORMANCE STATUS SCALES**

The **Karnofsky scale** runs in increments of 10 from 0 (death) to 100 (no impairment) and can be divided into three broad ranges.

80–100:	Normal activity without the need for special assistance and no or minimal symptoms of disease
50–70:	Unable to work but able to live at home and capable of self-care, although varying levels of assistance may be required
10–40:	Incapable of self-care, requiring acute or chronic care in a hospital or institutional setting, with rapidly progressive disease process
0:	Death

The **ECOG scale** runs in increments of 1 from 0 (no impairment) to 5 (death).
0: Full activity, without symptoms
1: Ambulatory, able to carry out light activity, minimal symptoms
2: Unable to work, ambulatory for >50% of daytime activity
3: In bed or chair for >50% of daytime activity, limited self-care
4: Completely disabled, confined to bed or chair, unable to do any self-care
5: Death

Diagnostic Testing

Pathology Diagnosis

The treatment of a malignancy requires a **diagnosis based on tissue pathology**. Only in rare emergent situations is treatment started without a diagnosis. Consultation from the surgical, medical, and radiation oncology team members is essential. It is crucial to include these oncology professionals in such cases where prompt therapy should be delivered to the patient to reduce the risk of morbidity or mortality in certain oncologic emergencies.

- **Light microscopy** is central to diagnosis. It delineates the microscopic structure of the malignancy, such as nuclear-to-cytoplasm ratio in leukemia, invasion into the micro-vasculature, or extent of glandular crowding in adenocarcinoma. Additional studies, including IHC staining, flow cytometry, cytogenetic, and molecular studies for gene rear-rangements can corroborate a suspected diagnosis and assist in further subclassification.
- **IHC staining** identifies specific proteins in the tissue based on the principle of antigen–antibody complex. The development of fluorescent and nonfluorescent chromogens along with various amplification techniques has increased the sensitivity and specificity of this procedure. This technique is widely used in surgical pathology for typing tumors based on the principle of differential expression of proteins in different biologic tissues. They help provide such fundamental information as: Is this a tumor? Is it benign or malignant? What type of tumor is it? They also provide information on the tissue of origin of the tumor. For example, cytokeratin stains are used to identify carcinomas from sarcomas, CD20 for B-cell lymphoma, etc. Others provide prognostic information such as Ki67, which is a marker of proliferation.
- **Flow cytometry** characterizes and sorts individual cells suspended in liquid as they flow in a narrow stream that passes through a beam of laser light. It is most frequently applied in hematologic malignancies where certain antigen profiles are diagnostic (e.g., CD5/CD23 coexpression in chronic lymphocytic leukemia). In **cytogenetic testing**, chromosomes from blood, bone marrow, or solid tissue can be isolated to identify deletions, translocations, trisomies, or insertions into the genome. In this process, chromosomes of 20 cells are counted in metaphase. The bands within the chromosomes are studied to identify any of the aforementioned abnormalities. Cytogenetic testing has been taken one step further with the advent of **FISH** (fluorescence in situ hybridization). The cellular DNA from the biopsy specimen is prepared on glass and mixed with known DNA probes that are fluorescently labeled, such as t9;22 rearrangement for chronic myeloid leukemia. If the DNA contains that translocation, the probes lit up under fluorescent microscopy will align differently than if the translocation is not present. The advantage of this test is that it can identify subtle changes in the chromosome. However, it can only identify one abnormality at a time (unlike cytogenetic testing) so the investigator must know which abnormality to look for. **Polymerase chain reaction (PCR)** is a sensitive test to detect specific DNA sequences, such as epidermal growth factors receptor (*EGFR*) mutation. **Reverse transcriptase PCR (RT-PCR)** can pick up minute amounts of RNA and is fre-quently used in chronic myelogenous leukemia to monitor treatment response.

Laboratory Testing

Routine evaluation with complete blood counts (CBCs) and a comprehensive metabolic panel is important for baseline information about organ function. Any abnormal laboratory data may provide additional information on organ infiltration by the tumor. For example, an elevated alkaline phosphatase may provide indication of bony metastasis, transaminitis may be indicative of liver involvement, and low blood counts may point toward bone mar-row infiltration. **Tumor markers** may provide additional information in some cases. Tumor markers are useful in **diagnostic workup** of certain germ cell tumors, such as testicular and neuroendocrine tumors. The majority of tumor markers, however, **lack** sensitivity and spec-ificity for cancer diagnosis. Some tests may provide **prognostic information** as they reflect tumor burden, such as an Lactate dehydrogenase (LDH) in lymphoma, and LDH, human chorionic gonadotropin (hCG), and alpha fetoprotein (AFP) in testicular germ cell tumors. Most tumor markers are used in clinical practice for the purpose of **monitoring treatment** response and progression of cancer. The only tumor marker that was part of **screening** in the United States is prostate-specific antigen (PSA) for prostate cancer, which is now controversial.

Imaging Modalities

- **CT** allows cross-sectional imaging of the patient.[8] Additional applications of CT include three-dimensional reconstructions and CT angiography. Intravenous radiocontrast medium is frequently utilized to enhance the sensitivity of the imaging. Risks of radiocontrast media include allergic reaction and nephrotoxicity.
- **MRI** is widely used in imaging the brain for either primary CNS tumors or metastases. MRI also has an emerging role in evaluation of breast cancer with breast MRI.[9] MRI of the liver has a role in hepatocellular carcinoma as well as evaluation of solitary liver metastases in colon and other cancer types. Absolute contraindications to MRI scanning include pacemakers, aneurysm clips, certain metallic cardiac prosthetic valves, and intraocular metal fragments.
- **PET** (positron emission tomography) is a functional imaging modality that images the distribution of intravenously administered radiolabeled tracers. 18-Fluorodeoxyglucose (FDG) is the most widely utilized metabolic tracer. PET is most sensitive in aggressive and metabolically active tumors such as melanoma, head and neck, breast, lung, esophageal, cervical, and colorectal cancer, as well as aggressive subtypes of lymphoma. FDG-PET has a lower sensitivity in slower-growing tumors such as low-grade lymphomas, neuroendocrine tumors, and bronchioalveolar cell lung carcinoma. PET scans can be performed with concurrent CT (PET-CT) to merge both functional and anatomic imaging.
- **Radionuclide bone scans** are frequently used to detect bone metastases. They are less sensitive to pure osteolytic lesions, such as in multiple myeloma.
- **Skeletal survey** includes plain x-rays of the skull, spine, pelvis, and extremities. It is utilized in multiple myeloma to survey for osteolytic bone lesions.

Utilization of other forms of medical imaging including volumetric (3D) anatomical imaging, dynamic contrast imaging, and functional (molecular) imaging is in the process of being tested and validated in clinical trials. If successful, the use of medical imaging may serve as surrogate endpoint in clinical trials and aid clinicians in making earlier treatment decisions.

Diagnostic Procedures

An array of diagnostic procedures is available to establish a cancer diagnosis in a given patient. This may range from simple blood tests or bone marrow biopsies obtained by the treating physician in hematologic malignancies to a multispecialty approach. Tissue for pathologic evaluation can be obtained by surgical approaches, such as lymph node biopsy or surgical resection specimen. Image-guided—such as CT—or ultrasound-guided biopsy of a target lesion is an attractive option when feasible, as these are less invasive. Evaluations of luminal tumors are aided by the use of various endoscopic procedures. Some clinical situations may pose special clinical challenges requiring more than one attempt and involvement of more than one specialty. Other diagnostic procedures such as lumbar puncture, pleural fluid thoracentesis, or ascitic fluid paracentesis are done as part of diagnostic workup or for palliation of symptoms.

TREATMENT

Approach to Oncology Treatment

The majority of adult solid malignancies are best managed through a multidisciplinary approach involving surgical oncologists, radiation oncologists, and medical oncologists.

There are often multiple different treatment options, and patients should be an active part of the decision-making process. An important element in the treatment of cancer patients is to define the goals of treatment, addressing the possibility of cure, prolongation of survival, or improvement in quality of life in individual cases. Treatment recommendations should be carefully tailored to the individual patient, taking into account comorbid conditions, performance status, and other psychosocial issues.

Principles of Surgical Approach in Cancer

Surgery still remains the most effective modality for curing cancer confined to a local site. In many instances, the surgical removal of the primary cancer also involves the removal of a regional lymph node area. Appropriate patients can be identified for **definitive or curative surgery**. The goal is for the surgeon to remove all neoplastic cells, including the resection of a complete margin of normal tissue around the primary tumor. Depending on the primary tumor, patients with a solitary or limited number of metastases to sites such as the brain, liver, and lung can be cured by the surgical resection of the metastatic disease. **Cytoreductive surgery or tumor debulking** can facilitate subsequent radiation and/or chemotherapy in some malignancies such as ovarian cancer. Surgery may also be necessary in the **palliative setting** to relieve symptoms, such as intestinal obstruction from colon cancer.

Principles of Radiation Therapy

Radiation therapy is the treatment of choice for some cancers. The use of this treatment modality is based on the responsiveness of the cancer to ionizing radiation. Some cancers are extremely sensitive, including lymphomas and seminomas, whereas others are relatively resistant. Radiation therapy can be the sole **curative local modality** in malignancies such as cervical cancer and prostate cancer. It is also useful in the **adjuvant setting** to increase the likelihood of local or regional control after surgery. Radiation therapy also plays a key role in the **palliation of symptoms** from primary or metastatic tumor masses, including spinal cord compression and bone metastases. Further details of the principles and uses of radiation therapy are elucidated in Chapter 19. See Table 15-3 for list of radiosensitive tumors.

Principles of Systemic Therapy

In contrast to surgery or radiation therapy, which has only local effects on the tumor, the role of systemic therapy is to treat both the local tumor and potential or actual areas of metastatic disease throughout the body. Systemic therapy for treatment of cancers refers to traditional cytotoxic chemotherapy, immunotherapy, and targeted therapy. The use of different systemic therapies in various cancers and the side effects are discussed in subsequent chapters. **Clinical trials** are important tools in medical oncology to test novel treatment approaches in the management of cancer. Important clinical trials in the past

TABLE 15-3	SENSITIVITY OF MALIGNANT TUMORS TO RADIATION	
Very Responsive	**Moderately Responsive**	**Poorly Responsive**
Hodgkin lymphoma	Head and neck cancer	Melanoma
Non-Hodgkin lymphoma	Breast cancer	Glioblastoma
Seminoma, dysgerminoma	Prostate cancer	Renal cancer
Neuroblastoma	Cervical cancer	Pancreatic cancer
Small-cell cancers	Esophageal cancer	Sarcoma
Retinoblastoma	Rectal cancer	Hepatoma
	Lung cancer	

decade have paved the way for more effective and less toxic regimens. Trials have also uncovered important biologic information which has helped individualize treatment approaches. It is important to screen patients for eligibility for the clinical trials available at your institution.

Chemotherapy

Before the initiation of chemotherapy, the **goal of treatment** must be clearly defined and discussed with the patient. Not all patients are candidates for chemotherapy. Potential risks and benefits must be considered when deciding to treat a patient with cytotoxic agents. The performance status and overall nutritional state of the cancer patient are extremely important when making the decision to use chemotherapy. Patients with performance status scores of 3–4 on the ECOG scale are usually not candidates for systemic therapy unless they have previously untreated tumors known to be especially responsive to chemotherapy. See Table 15-4 for a list of chemosensitive tumors.

Immunotherapy

Immunotherapy exploits the intricate interplay between cancer cells and the immune system, aiming to stimulate the body's own immune response to recognize and eliminate cancer cells. Immunotherapy approaches vary widely and can include use of immune checkpoint inhibitors, adoptive cell transfer, and cancer vaccines among others. In certain neoplastic subtypes such as melanoma, immunotherapy has revolutionized the management of this aggressive malignancy leading to durable responses and improved survival rates. Enhancing efficacy of immunotherapy in other tumor types, identifying predictive biomarkers, and overcoming resistance to these therapies remain some of the most important aspects of oncologic research to date.

Targeted Therapies

These therapies interfere with specific pathways needed for the growth and survival of cancer cells. These therapies may include monoclonal antibodies or small molecule inhibitors, which target specific receptors or kinases such as the EGFR, the vascular endothelial growth factor receptor (VEGFR), the anaplastic lymphoma kinase (ALK), and the Bcr-Abl tyrosine kinase. The past decade has seen the approval of several targeted agents in the treatment of various cancers either as single agent or in combination with chemotherapy. Endocrine therapies used in the treatment of prostate and breast cancer are among the oldest forms of targeted agents. They are very effective treatment strategies in these hormone-sensitive cancers and are used widely in multiple clinical settings.

TABLE 15-4	CANCERS CURABLE OR OCCASIONALLY CURABLE WITH CHEMOTHERAPY ALONE

Curable with chemotherapy alone
- Gestational choriocarcinoma
- Hodgkin lymphoma
- Germ cell cancer of the testis
- Acute lymphoid leukemia
- Non-Hodgkin lymphoma (some subtypes)
- Hairy cell leukemia

Occasionally curable with chemotherapy alone
- Acute myeloid leukemia
- Ovarian cancer
- Small-cell lung cancer

Chemotherapy

Systemic chemotherapy has been used in various clinical settings.

- **Adjuvant therapy** refers to the use of systemic therapy following complete surgical resection to improve both disease-free and overall survival. The goal is to **eliminate undetected local and micrometastatic foci of tumor**. There is no way to measure or follow response to therapy, and thus duration of treatment is determined empirically by clinical trials. Cancers for which adjuvant chemotherapy has proven to benefit survival include colorectal, breast, lung, ovarian cancers, rhabdomyosarcoma, Ewing sarcoma, and osteosarcoma. Similarly, adjuvant hormonal therapy is effective in improving survival in breast cancer patients whose tumors are estrogen receptor positive.

- **Neoadjuvant therapy** refers to systemic therapy that is administered before surgery. The goal of neoadjuvant therapy is to decrease the tumor burden for the definitive surgical procedure, thus minimizing complications and making **organ preservation** more feasible. In addition, the clinician can monitor the **tumor responsiveness** to the systemic agent and can deliver systemic treatment immediately to eliminate micrometastatic disease. Neoadjuvant chemotherapy is used in breast, esophageal, gastric, rectal, and bladder cancers, as well as some sarcomas.

- **Combined modality therapy** refers to the combination of chemotherapy and radiotherapy used to treat bulky disease, especially when curative resection is not possible or less effective or when **organ preservation** is considered. For example, combination therapy can be curative and organ preserving in certain tumors such as laryngeal and anal cancers. Combined modality therapy improves survival for some patients with locally advanced lung, esophageal, head and neck, pancreatic, and cervical cancers. The combined modality therapy can also be used to decrease the size of the tumor for either a curative or a salvage surgical procedure later.

- **Palliative chemotherapy** is typically administered in metastatic setting or advanced stage of malignancy. This treatment modality is not intended for cure, but for **slowing progression of disease and to prolong life**. The chemotherapy agents are either administered as a combination or single agents sequentially in this setting.

- **Induction chemotherapy** is used as the initial treatment of a malignancy to achieve complete remission or significant cytoreduction. It is commonly used in the treatment of acute leukemia and lymphoma. **Consolidation chemotherapy** is given after a patient is in remission to prolong the duration of remission and overall survival. **Maintenance chemotherapy** is the use of prolonged, low-dose chemotherapy to prolong the duration of remission and achieve a cure in those patients; it is currently only utilized in certain leukemias. **Salvage chemotherapy** is given with the intent to control disease or palliate symptoms after the failure of initial treatments.

- **High-dose chemotherapy** is typically used in the treatment of hematologic malignancies. High doses of chemotherapy are used to ablate the bone marrow requiring rescue with **allogeneic** or **autologous** bone marrow or stem cell replacement to repopulate the marrow. Allogeneic transplants have been curative in selected patients with chronic myelogenous leukemia and acute leukemias. Autologous stem cell transplants have been most successful for aggressive lymphomas and multiple myeloma. The use of bone marrow transplant in solid organ malignancies remains controversial.

MONITORING/FOLLOW-UP

Response to Therapy

In general, responses to therapy are measured by objective changes in tumor size and increases in disease-free and overall survival. RECIST 1.1 (response criteria in solid tumors) is a widely utilized tool for describing changes in solid tumor size in response to therapy. RECIST is a voluntary, international standard that is not an NCI standard. They are based on a simplification of former methods (WHO, ECOG) and based on measurable disease.[10,11] Alternative response criteria are utilized in hematologic malignancies. The single most important indicator of the effectiveness of chemotherapy is the complete response rate. No patient with advanced cancer can be cured without attaining complete remission. There are frequent changes in the definitions of response criteria assessment. The reader is advised to look for updated guidelines in this regard. The present information is currently available and defined on the NCI website.[12]

- **Complete response** is defined as the disappearance of all target lesions on imaging studies.
- **Partial response** is defined by at least a 30% reduction in the sum of the longest diameter of a target lesion when compared to the baseline study.
- **Progressive disease** is defined by at least a 20% increase in the sum of the longest diameter of target lesions, appearance of new lesions, or the death of the patient as a result of the tumor. Chemotherapy is discontinued in the setting of progression, and the patient is reevaluated.
- The term **stable disease** is used when the measurable disease does not meet the criteria for complete response, partial response, or progression. Stable disease represents a difficult challenge to oncologists. If therapy is tolerated with no significant side effects, it is often continued, provided it is recognized that progressive disease will eventually occur.

OUTCOME/PROGNOSIS

Goals of Care

When a patient is diagnosed with cancer, one of the first questions an oncologist will be asked is: "How long do I have?" It is not the oncologist's place to assign a life expectancy to any one patient. Each clinical scenario is different; to speculate on life expectancy can have serious emotional ramifications. An individual's prognosis is based on staging, comorbidities, performance status, and response to treatment. Although it is possible to predict curability or median survival, long-term follow-up is essential to get a more accurate sense of prognosis for any given patient. Even when the overall prognosis is poor, an honest and compassionate discussion with the patient and family members is essential. The role of the medical oncologist is to provide up-front and honest answers to even the most difficult questions and to allow the patient and family to set realistic goals that will help guide future healthcare decisions.

Palliative Care

Palliative care of cancer patients entails the management of all of the symptoms related to the cancer itself and the toxicities of treatment. It also includes the multidisciplinary care of psychosocial issues, with the primary goal of optimizing the quality of life and minimizing the morbidity and symptoms related to cancer and its treatments. Prolongation of survival is a secondary goal, which may or may not be achieved, but cure is not the primary intent in palliative care. Chemotherapy, hormonal therapy, radiation, and surgery are still useful in palliation. Patient selection for interventions is crucial. For patients with advanced cancer and poor performance status, aggressive treatment may be detrimental rather than beneficial.

Hospice

Hospice is a philosophy of care based on a coordinated program of support services for terminally ill patients and their families. Palliative care is provided with the aim to improve quality of life and allow a comfortable death. Any patient with a limited life expectancy (≤6 months) may be eligible for hospice care. The interdisciplinary hospice team consists of nurses trained in pain and symptom management, physicians, home health aides, social workers, chaplains, and volunteers. Care is generally given in the home but may be imparted in nursing homes or hospitals if necessary. Medicare hospice benefits also include complete coverage for all medications pertaining to the hospice diagnosis, durable medical equipment, and oxygen. Most hospice agencies provide 24-hour on-call service, brief respite care, and bereavement counseling for up to 1 year after the patient dies.

REFERENCES

1. Siegel RL, Miller KD, Wagle NS, et al. Cancer statistics, 2023. *CA Cancer J Clin*. 2023;73(1):17–48.
2. Brown JR, Skarin AT. Clinical mimics of lymphoma. *Oncologist*. 2004;9(4):406–416.
3. Barajas RF Jr, Cha S. Metastasis in adult brain tumors. *Neuroimaging Clin N Am*. 2016;26(4):601–620.
4. Keller F, Bruch R, Clauder F, et al. Extracellular matrix components regulate bone sialoprotein expression in MDA-MB-231 breast cancer cells. *Cells*. 2021;10(6):1304.
5. Castellano D, Sepulveda JM, García-Escobar I, et al. The role of RANK-ligand inhibition in cancer: the story of denosumab. *Oncologist*. 2011;16(2):136–145.
6. Karnofsky DA, Burchenal JH. The clinical evaluation of chemotherapeutic agents in cancer. In: MacLeod CM, ed. *Evaluation of Chemotherapeutic Agents*. Columbia University Press; 1949.
7. Oken MM, Creech RH, Tormey DC, et al. Toxicity and response criteria of the Eastern Cooperative Oncology Group. *Am J Clin Oncol*. 1982;5(6):649–656.
8. Torigian DA, Huang SS, Houseni M, et al. Functional imaging of cancer with emphasis on molecular techniques. *CA Cancer J Clin*. 2007;57(4):206–224.
9. Ray KM, Hayward JH, Joe BN. Role of MR imaging for the locoregional staging of breast cancer. *Magn Reson Imaging Clin N Am*. 2018;26(2):191–205.
10. Schwartz LH, Seymour L, Litière S, et al. RECIST 1.1 – Standardisation and disease-specific adaptations: perspectives from the RECIST working group. *Eur J Cancer*. 2016;62:138–145.
11. Eisenhauer EA, Therasse P, Bogaerts J, et al. New response evaluation criteria in solid tumours: revised RECIST guideline (version 1.1). *Eur J Cancer*. 2009;45(2):228–247.
12. Imaging Response Criteria. 2023. Accessed July 4, 2023. https://imaging.cancer.gov/clinical_trials/imaging_response_criteria.htm
13. Sung H, Ferlay J, Siegel RL, et al. Global Cancer Statistics 2020: GLOBOCAN estimates of incidence and mortality worldwide for 36 cancers in 185 countries. *CA Cancer J Clin*. 2021;71(3):209–249.

Cancer Biology

16

Jared Cohen

S ince the initial discovery of oncogenes in the 1970s, our understanding of cancer biology has expanded exponentially. Cancer is a disease that is characterized by the accumulation of genetic and epigenetic changes culminating in malignant transformation through alterations of cellular programs responsible for growth, survival, invasion, and metastasis.[1] Ongoing research aims to better understand the molecular basis of this reprogramming and develop novel therapeutics. The objective of this chapter is to briefly outline some of the characteristic biologic features of cancers.

HALLMARKS OF CANCER

Cellular proliferation is tightly regulated by signaling mechanisms that are intrinsic to the cell and its extrinsic microenvironment. Uncoupling of these regulatory mechanisms is critical to oncogenic transformation. Cancer cells acquire certain "hallmark" capabilities owing to genomic alterations accrued over time, liberating them from homeostatic control and endowing them with the ability to employ the local microenvironment in supporting ongoing proliferation.[2-4]

- **Self-sufficiency in growth signals:** Tumor cells can constitutively activate growth signaling pathways by generation of their own growth factors, which stimulate the release of additional growth factors bound to the extracellular matrix. This leads to increased sensitivity to growth signals by overexpressed receptors or by constitutively activated signaling pathways.
- **Evading growth inhibitors:** Aberrant cell proliferation is normally constrained by growth inhibitors such as transforming growth factor beta (TGFβ) that are secreted by cells in the microenvironment. These factors help maintain cells in a quiescent phase (G0) and inhibit uncontrolled progression from the G1 to S phase. Tumor cells can evade TGFβ inhibition by downregulating TGFβ receptors, displaying mutant receptors, or inactivating downstream signaling proteins.
- **Avoiding apoptosis:** Signals evoked by activation of oncogenes, DNA damage, detachment from the basement membrane, or hypoxia often trigger apoptosis, a form of programmed cell death. Apoptotic pathways often involve tumor suppressors such as TP53, RB1, and the BCL2 family proteins. Such control mechanisms are usually impaired in cancer cells by loss of TP53 or overexpression of antiapoptotic proteins such as BCL2.
- **Limitless replication potential:** Telomeres are structures composed of highly repetitive DNA sequences and specialized proteins at the ends of chromosomes that protect them from degradation. Each cycle of DNA replication results in gradual and progressive attrition of the telomere length. When the length of the telomere reaches a critically low threshold, cells undergo senescence or apoptosis. Cancer cells, however, prevent telomere attrition by either increasing the activity of *telomerase*—an enzyme that lengthens telomeres by adding DNA repeats—or by mechanisms such as alternative lengthening of telomeres (ALT) which allow cancer cells to replicate indefinitely.
- **Angiogenesis:** Tumors cannot grow larger than 0.2 mm in diameter, the diffusion limit of oxygen, without access to blood vessels. Tumor cells are capable of inducing formation of new blood vessels, termed angiogenesis, to support their growth. Angiogenesis is often

induced by hypoxia and requires upregulation of proangiogenic factors, such as vascular endothelial growth factor (*VEGF*) or fibroblast growth factors (*FGF1* and *FGF2*), with simultaneous inhibition of antiangiogenic factors such as angiopoietin-1 and thrombospondin-1. Inhibiting angiogenesis using anti-VEGF agents, such as bevacizumab, is a common strategy in cancer treatment.[5]

- **Tissue invasion and metastasis:** A defining feature of the malignant phenotype is the ability of cancer cells to invade their surrounding tissues and metastasize. A study of the clonal architecture of cancers suggests that metastatic clones evolve through the progressive accumulation of genetic alterations by the parent clone. Cancer cells acquire the ability to invade by undergoing epithelial–mesenchymal transition (EMT) and disrupt basement membranes by upregulating matrix metalloproteases (MMPs). Others acquire the ability to intravasate, survive in the bloodstream/lymphatic system, evade immune destruction, and extravasate into distal organs.

- **Evasion of the immune system:** To survive, cancer cells must escape immune surveillance, by either preventing immune recognition or inducing immune tolerance. Escape from immune recognition is mediated by downregulating mechanisms necessary for antigen presentation. Examples include downregulation of major histocompatibility complex (MHC) molecules or inhibition of costimulatory molecules on tumor cells. Generation of immune tolerance involves altering the complex cellular and cytokine network of antigen presentation. Examples include production of inhibitory cytokines, or suppression of stimulatory cytokines, and contributions from myeloid-derived suppressor and T-regulatory cells.

- **Reprogramming of metabolism:** Unlike normal cells that generate ATP through oxidative phosphorylation in the mitochondria, cancer cells are often reprogrammed to derive their energy from glycolysis in the cytoplasm (Warburg phenomena). Such transformation not only helps cancer cells adapt to their hypoxic microenvironment, but also provides them with essential substrates required for the synthesis of macromolecules such as amino acids and nucleosides, to sustain rapid proliferation.[6] Such reprogramming is usually driven by oncogenes such as *AKT1, NRF2, mTOR*, and *MYC*. The high dependence of cancer cells on glucose metabolism serves as the basis for [^{18}F] fluorodeoxyglucose positron emission tomography (FDG-PET) imaging.

- **Unlocking phenotypic plasticity:** Cancer cells can undergo reprogramming of their state of differentiation to enhance replicative potential. For example, cancer cells originating from normal cells approaching a terminally differentiated state can dedifferentiate back toward a progenitor state. Alternatively, cancer cells derived from a progenitor cell programmed for terminal differentiation may subvert this process to remain in a partially differentiated progenitor state. Some cancer cells undergo developmental reprogramming allowing for the acquisition of traits not predetermined by their cell of origin in a process termed transdifferentiation. This phenotypic plasticity provides survival advantage and promotes tumorogenesis.[7]

- **Senescent cells:** Cellular senescence, characterized by irreversible proliferative arrest and induced by a variety of conditions, including DNA damage, has long been thought to be protective against neoplasia. However, a growing body of evidence suggests that senescent cells may aid in tumorigenesis through paracrine signaling using cytokines, chemokines, and proteases to neighboring viable cancer cells and stromal cells within the tumor microenvironment.[8] In addition, cancer cells may enter a transitory and reversible senescent state to provide protection against chemotherapies targeting actively proliferating cells.

GENETIC AND EPIGENETIC ALTERATIONS

An abnormal gain or loss of gene function can occur as a result of alterations in genetic sequence (mutation, translocation, amplification, etc.) or through the impairment of the regulatory processes that control gene expression (epigenetic alterations).[9]

Acquisition of Genetic Changes

- **Inherited defects:** Germline alterations are inheritable alterations and are present both in the cancer cells and other normal tissues of an individual. Germline mutations in certain crucial genes can predispose to developing cancer and are the cause of most familial cancer syndromes. (See Table 16-1.)
- **Exogenous damage:** Exposure to chemicals such as aromatic hydrocarbons that are present in cigarette smoke, heavy metals, substances such as asbestos fibers, chemotherapy agents, or radiation in the form of ultraviolet (UV) rays and radiation treatments damage DNA. UV-A produces reactive oxygen species (ROS), while UV-B produces cyclobutane pyrimidine dimers and pyrimidine pyrimidone photoproducts. Platinum and alkylating chemotherapies cause DNA crosslinks.

TABLE 16-1	GENE LOSS AND FAMILIAL CANCER SYNDROMES[15]	
Syndrome	**Gene Altered**	**Associated Cancers**
Ataxia-telangiectasia	*ATM*	Non-Hodgkin lymphoma, ALL, CLL
Basal cell nevus syndrome (Gorlin syndrome)	*PTCH*	Basal cell carcinoma
Bloom syndrome	*BLM*	Lymphoid malignancies, Wilms tumor, head and neck, lung, esophagus, colon, cervix
Carney syndrome	*PRKAR1A*	Testicular tumors (Sertoli and Leydig cell tumors) Benign tumors: nevi, atrial myxoma
Cowden syndrome	*PTEN*	Breast, thyroid
Hereditary breast/ovarian cancer	*BRCA1 and BRCA2*	Breast, ovarian, fallopian tube, pancreatic
Hereditary nonpolyposis colon cancer (Lynch syndrome)	*MLH1, MSH2, MSH6, and PMS2*	Colorectal, endometrial, gastric
Familial adenomatous polyposis (FAP)	*APC*	Colorectal
Li–Fraumeni syndrome	*TP53*	Skin, soft tissue sarcoma, breast, GBM, leukemias, lymphomas, adrenocortical carcinoma
Neurofibromatosis type 1	*NF1*	Malignant peripheral nerve sheath tumor, astrocytoma, carcinoids
Neurofibromatosis type 2	*NF2*	Glioma, ependymoma
Peutz–Jeghers syndrome	*STK11*	Gastrointestinal, pancreatic, lung
Retinoblastoma	*RB1*	Retinoblastoma, osteosarcoma
Tuberous sclerosis complex	*TSC1/TSC2*	Subependymal giant cell astrocytomas, renal cell cancer
von Hippel–Lindau syndrome	*VHL*	Renal cell carcinoma

- **Oncogenic viruses:** Cells infected with certain DNA viruses and retroviruses can ultimately become cancerous. Infection with human oncogenic viruses can result in certain hallmark changes such as uncontrolled growth and evasion of apoptosis that are necessary for malignant transformation. Prominent examples include HPV in cervical and head and neck cancers, EBV in lymphomas and nasopharyngeal cancers, HBV and HCV in hepatocellular carcinoma, HTLV-1 in T-cell leukemia, and KSHV (HHV8) in Kaposi sarcoma.

- **Genomic instability:** DNA replication is error prone. Replication errors such as point mutations, chromosomal translocations, or copy number changes can occur spontaneously and are normally kept in check through DNA repair mechanisms. DNA damage response (DDR) pathways are triggered in response to such damage, which arrest cell cycle progression or program cells to undergo apoptosis if DNA damage is beyond repair. As expected, cells with germline or acquired defects in DNA maintenance pathways (such as *ATM, ATR, TP53, RB1*, etc.) are much more likely to accumulate and propagate replication errors. Chromothripsis refers to a rare, single catastrophic event that results in the shattering of a chromosome or chromosomal segment, followed by imperfect reassembly that results in massive genomic rearrangement.

Epigenetic Changes

Gene expression is regulated by epigenetic mechanisms such as gene promoter/enhancer methylation, histone modifications, or through microRNAs at the posttranscriptional level.[10]

- **Histone modification:** Acetylation/deacetylation of lysine residues on histone by histone acetyltransferases (HATs) and histone deacetylases (HDACs), can alter gene expression. Deacetylation causes histones to wrap more tightly around DNA, which blocks access of transcription factors to DNA. Tumor suppressor genes silenced by histone deacetylation can theoretically be reactivated by HDAC inhibitors. Currently, HDAC inhibitors such as Vorinostat and Romidepsin are approved for treatment of cutaneous T-cell lymphoma.

- **DNA methylation:** Methylation of cytosines in CpG dinucleotides by DNA methyltransferases generally leads to transcriptional silencing. Repetitive CpG dinucleotides are often found within the upstream promoter regions of most genes. When methylated, these regions become inaccessible to transcription factors and can also attract histone-modifying proteins that lead to formation of compact, inactive chromatin. DNA methylation is essential in normal developmental processes such as genomic imprinting and cellular differentiation. However, when the promoter of a tumor suppressor gene is hypermethylated, gene transcription is shut down and cells are propelled toward malignant transformation. For example, hypermethylation of the promoter for *MLH1*, a gene involved in DNA mismatch repair, has been implicated in the pathogenesis of hereditary nonpolyposis colorectal cancer (HNPCC). Two DNA methyltransferase inhibitors, 5-azacytidine, and decitabine (2′-deoxy-5-azacytidine), are approved therapies for the treatment of myelodysplastic syndrome and acute myeloid leukemia.

- **Posttranscriptional regulation through microRNAs:** MicroRNAs, are a species of short, single-stranded, non-(protein) coding RNAs that can bind to the complementary sequences within target mRNAs and generally lead to their degradation. More than half of human genes are now believed to be regulated by microRNAs at the posttranscriptional level. Aberrant expression of microRNAs is found in many human cancers.[11] For example, miR-15a and miR-16–1, which negatively regulate *BCL2*, an antiapoptotic gene, are often deleted or downregulated in B-cell chronic lymphocytic leukemia (CLL). On the other hand, miR-9, which is overexpressed in breast cancer, promotes metastasis by downregulating E-cadherin. Therapies targeting microRNAs are still under investigation.

Alterations in Oncogenes and Tumor Suppressor Genes

The two major classes of genes that are subject to alteration in the process of malignant transformation are oncogenes and tumor suppressors. In principle, tumorigenic changes involve gain of oncogene function and loss of tumor suppressor function.

- **Oncogenes** are altered versions of normal genes (termed proto-oncogenes) that have acquired "gain-of-function" point mutations, gene copy amplifications, translocations, or hypomethylation, resulting in cellular proliferation, growth, survival, invasion, and angiogenesis. Several categories of oncogenes have been described:
  ○ Growth factors: PDGF (platelet-derived growth factors), etc.
  ○ Growth-factor receptors: *EGFR, HER2, KIT, PDGFR, VEGFR*, etc.
  ○ Tyrosine kinases: *BCR-ABL1, SRC, SYK, BTK*, etc.
  ○ Serine-threonine kinases: *BRAF, AKT, MAPK*, cyclin-dependent (CDKs) and Aurora kinases, etc.
  ○ GTPases: *KRAS, HRAS, NRAS, CDC42, RAC1, RALA*, etc.
  ○ Cytoplasmic proteins: *BCL2*, Survivin (*BIRC5*), etc.
  ○ Transcription factors: *MYC, JUN, SOX2, FOS, NFKB1*, etc.
- **Tumor suppressor genes** or gate-keeper genes function to restrain cellular proliferation and maintain cellular homeostasis. Classic examples include *PTEN, NF1, NF2*, and *APC*, which are negative regulators of proliferation, *CDKN2A*, which controls cell cycle, *BRCA1* and *BRCA2*, which are key players in DDR, *VHJ*, which negatively regulates angiogenesis, and *TP53*, which plays a central role in many of these pathways and controls cell apoptosis. In cancer cells, expression of tumor suppressor genes is usually lost by biallelic gene deletion or loss-of-function mutations or is transcriptionally silenced by epigenetic mechanisms. While loss of tumor suppressor genes alone is not sufficient for malignant transformation, it does predispose cells to accumulate further genetic changes and cooperates with oncogenes to complete neoplastic transformation.

TP53 Mutations

The tumor suppressor *TP53* is the most frequently mutated gene in human cancer. *TP53* encodes a transcription factor that primarily activates genes responsible for cell cycle arrest and apoptosis; it is activated in response to stresses such as DNA damage, hypoxia, or oncogene activation. Inactivating mutations in *TP53* are found in more than 50% of all cancers. Hypermethylation of the promoter for *TP53* and upregulation of its inhibitors, such as MDM2, are also found in human cancers. Patients with **Li–Fraumeni** syndrome have germline mutations in the *TP53* gene and are at high risk for developing cancers including breast, bone, soft tissue, head and neck, and brain and, less commonly, lung, stomach, colon, and blood (leukemia). In sporadic cancers, the timing of *TP53* loss can differ. *TP53* alteration is usually an early event in lung, esophageal, head and neck, breast, cervical, bladder, and stomach cancers, but a late event in brain, thyroid, prostate, and ovarian cancers.

TUMOR METASTASIS

Tumor metastasis accounts for more than 90% of cancer deaths. In most cancers, metastatic traits are acquired late in the multistep oncogenic process. Metastasis is a consummation of multiple distinct properties acquired during clonal evolution from a genetically heterogeneous parent population.[12] These properties include:

- **Detachment from the primary tumor:** Adherence of tumor cells to adjacent cells and the extracellular matrix is almost always altered. Intercellular adhesion is greatly diminished by downregulation of normal adhesion proteins such as E-cadherin. These changes facilitate detachment of tumor cells from their native site.

- **Invasion, migration, and intravasation:** Expression of integrins such as α6β4 can greatly augment the invasion of cancer cells through the stroma. Disruption of the basement membrane is usually achieved via activation of metalloproteases. By undergoing epithelial-to-mesenchymal transition, cancer cells of epithelial origin acquire a mesenchymal cell phenotype that allows for motility and invasion.[12] Migration is further directed by various growth factors such as EGF, FGF, HGF, and IGF. Subsequently, cancer cells can penetrate vascular endothelial lining (intravasation) and enter the bloodstream or lymphatic system.
- **Survival in the vasculature or lymphatic system:** Once in the circulation or lymphatic system, cancer cells must evade immune recognition. By abrogating their major apoptotic machinery, cancer cells can avoid anoikis, a type of apoptosis triggered by loss of contact with extracellular matrix. Most cancer cells succumb to high-velocity shear stress within the circulation, and only a small number survive to reach target organs.
- **Arrest at the metastatic site and extravasation:** The orientation of blood and lymphatic vasculature and expression of specific chemokines help direct cancer cells to their site of metastasis. For example, breast cancer cells show high expression of the chemokine receptor CXCR4, while its ligand, CXCL12, is highly expressed in organs to which it most commonly metastasizes such as the lung, liver, bone, and regional lymph nodes. Once at the target organ site, cells must arrest the vasculature and extravasate in a process involving alterations in cell adhesion molecules and proteases.
- **Survival in the metastatic microenvironment:** After arriving at a distant site, tumor cells (seeds) must successfully interact with their microenvironment (soil) to initiate colonization. In addition, an angiogenic "switch" must be triggered by secretion of various angiogenic factors to sustain metastatic growth.

FUTURE DIRECTIONS

Advancements in next-generation genome-sequencing technologies have made it possible to study cancer genomes at high resolution leading to new classification of cancers based on their molecular profile in addition to cell-of-origin. Single-cell and multiplex spatial technologies continue to uncover the contributions of nonmalignant inflammatory and stromal cells in the tumor microenvironment to the acquisition of hallmark capabilities. In addition, research into the tumor microbiome has highlighted important associations between resident tissue microbes in both primary and metastatic sites and proliferative signaling and growth suppression modulation in certain cancers.[13,14]

Since the discovery that aberrant signaling pathways support malignant transformation, targeted inhibitors such as imatinib, trastuzumab, erlotinib, sorafenib, etc., have been developed which have transformed outcomes in patients with several different cancers. Likewise, agents targeting apoptosis (BH3 mimetics), the DDR (PARP inhibitors), unrestricted cell-cycling (CKD inhibitors), and replicative potential (telomerase inhibitors) are in various stages of development and have demonstrated efficacy in numerous cancers. However, most cancers consist of highly heterogeneous subpopulations of transformed cells resulting in the development of escape mechanisms and consequent treatment refractoriness.

Immunotherapies have also transformed the treatment landscape, abrogating a hallmark capability of immune evasion. Checkpoint inhibitors, cellular therapies, and T-cell redirectors are in widespread use for a variety of cancers however, durable responses remain limited. Efforts to identify predictive biomarkers of response and mechanisms of resistance are ongoing.

REFERENCES

1. Fearon ER, Vogelstein B. A genetic model for colorectal tumorigenesis. *Cell.* 1990;61:759–767.
2. Hanahan D, Weinberg RA. The hallmarks of cancer. *Cell.* 2000;100:57–70.
3. Hanahan D, Weinberg RA. Hallmarks of cancer: the next generation. *Cell.* 2011;144:646–674.

4. Hanagan, D. Hallmarks of cancer: new dimensions. *Cancer Discov.* 2022;12:31–46.

5. Folkman J. Angiogenesis: an organizing principle for drug discovery? *Nat Rev Drug Discov.* 2007; 6(4):273–286.

6. Cairns RA, Harris IS, Mak TW. Regulation of cancer cell metabolism. *Nat Rev Cancer.* 2011;11(2): 85–95.

7. Harris TJR, McCormick F. The molecular pathology of cancer. *Nat Rev Clin Oncol.* 2010;7(5): 251–265.

8. Wang B, Kohli J, Demaria M. Senescent cells in cancer therapy: friends or foes? *Trends Cancer.* 2020;6(10):838–857.

9. Jones PA, Baylin SB. The epigenomics of cancer. *Cell.* 2007;128(4):683–692.

10. Inui M, Martello G, Piccolo S. MicroRNA control of signal transduction. *Nat Rev Mol Cell Biol.* 2010;11(4):252–263.

11. Chiang AC, Massagué J. Molecular basis of metastasis. *N Engl J Med.* 2008;359(26):2814–2823.

12. Polyak K, Weinberg RA. Transitions between epithelial and mesenchymal states: acquisition of malignant and stem cell traits. *Nat Rev Cancer.* 2009;9(4):265–273.

13. Dzutsev A, Badger JH, Perez-Chanona E, et al. Microbes and cancer. *Annu Rev Immunol.* 2017; 35:199–228.

14. Zhang Q, Ma C, Duan Y, et al. Gut microbiome directs hepatocytes to recruit MDSCs and promote cholangiocarcinoma. *Cancer Discov* 2021;11:1248–1267.

15. Nagy R, Sweet K, Eng C. Highly penetrant hereditary cancer syndromes. *Oncogene.* 2004;23(38): 6445–6470.

Introduction to Cancer Genomics

17

Giordano F. Cittolin Santos and Daniel Morgensztern

T he human genome contains approximately 3.2 billion nucleotide base pairs, within which are contained approximately 20,000 protein-coding genes. Genomic sequence refers to the exact sequence in which these base pairs are arranged. Cancer is essentially a disease of the genome. Therefore, a systematic study of the genomic alterations in cancer is crucial for understanding the mechanisms that underlie malignant transformation for the development of new targeted therapies. With the advent of advanced computing and sequencing technologies, it is now possible to study the genomes of cancer cells at an unprecedented level of detail.[1-4] The objective of this chapter is to discuss some of the fundamentals of cancer genomics, how sequencing works, the different methods for sequencing, and its application and in clinical practice.

TYPES OF GENOMIC ALTERATIONS[5,6]

- Point mutations are single-nucleotide substitutions in the genome sequence. Depending on how they impact mRNA transcription and protein translation, point mutations are classified as either silent or synonymous if they are predicted to encode for the same amino acid, missense if they lead to the substitution of a different amino acid, nonsense if they result in premature termination of protein synthesis, frameshift if they affect the reading frame, or splice-site if they alter mRNA splicing sites.
- Diploid cells are traditionally expected to harbor two copies of every gene. Copy number alterations (CNAs) refer to a deviation in this number. Deletions refer to a decrease in the number of copies, which can be heterozygous due to the loss of one copy or homozygous if both copies are deleted, while gains refer to an increase in this number. High-level gains are called amplifications. Translocations refer to the abnormal transfer of chromosomal material from one chromosomal location to a different site on that or another chromosome.
- Focal DNA amplifications are observable in linear intrachromosomal or circular extrachromosomal form. Cytogenetically, those are classified as homogeneous staining regions (HSR) or double minutes, respectively. Extrachromosomal DNA (ecDNA) refers to a type of a structure of circular DNA that contains full-length genes or regulatory elements. Genes amplified in the ecDNA form exhibit distinct characteristics from intrachromosomal amplifications. They exhibit heightened mRNA transcript levels due to enhanced chromatin accessibility and can increase intratumor heterogeneity by randomly distributing to daughter cells, which is attributed to their absence of centromeres.
- Germline alterations are inherited from parents and present in all cells of the organism. Somatic alterations are noninherited postfertilization sequence changes that are acquired by the cancer cell during the process of malignant transformation. Comparison of the genomic sequence of a tumor to a noncancer-derived sample, such as white blood cells, obtained from the same individual is critical to differentiate these alterations since germline alterations would be present in both samples, while somatic alterations would be restricted to the tumor. While certain germline alterations are associated with familial cancer syndromes, targetable somatic alterations form the cornerstone of targeted therapies.
- Epigenetic regulation refers to the control of gene expression without altering its sequence. One example is the promoter regions of genes are rich in CpG (C occurring

next to G) sequences that are silenced by methylation, while demethylation promote gene expression. Furthermore, DNA is coiled around histone proteins, and chemical modification of histones through methylation or acetylation can result in the uncoiling or coiling of DNA, making genes more or less accessible for transcription, respectively.

SEQUENCING TECHNOLOGIES

First Generation

- Sanger sequencing, also referred to as a chain-termination method, forms the basis for first-generation sequencing technologies that were used in the human genome project.
- The workflow of first-generation sequencing starts with DNA fragmentation with restriction endonucleases. These fragments are then amplified in a bacterial host and incubated with deoxynucleotide triphosphates (dATP, dGTP, dCTP, dTTP), fluorescent or radio-active tagged di-deoxynucleotide triphosphates (ddATP, ddGTP, ddCTP, ddTTP), and DNA polymerase, to facilitate synthesis of a complementary DNA strand. However, the deoxynucleotides and di-deoxynucleotides compete for incorporation into the nascent strand, and incorporation of a di-deoxynucleotide interrupts chain elongation. Since this incorporation is a random process, complementary strands of varying lengths are synthesized that are later ordered by size through electrophoresis. Finally, the identity of terminal di-deoxynucleotide in each strand is determined by analyzing the unique radioactive or fluorescent tag attached to these molecules. The sequence of the DNA strand is finally assembled using computerized algorithms.
- It is possible to establish the sequence of a given nucleotide strand de novo (since no prior knowledge of the sequence is required for sequence assembly) through Sanger sequencing.
- The high operational costs, greater sequencing time, and the inability to process multiple samples simultaneously are some of the limitations of first-generation technologies.

Next-Generation Sequencing

- Next-generation sequencing (NGS) technologies are cheaper, faster, and capable of a higher throughput compared to first-generation sequencing, making them suitable for application in research and clinical practice.
- The workflow for NGS starts with DNA fragmentation. Oligonucleotide "adapter" sequences are ligated to the ends of DNA fragments, which are complementary to oligonucleotide sequences that are embedded on a surface such as a bead or chip. Base pairing between these sequences results in the immobilization of the DNA fragment, which is then amplified, resulting in the formation of "polonies" (resembling colonies). Then, synthesis of a strand complementary to the immobilized DNA strand with fluorescent-tagged nucleotides is initiated using the embedded oligonucleotide sequence as a primer. Each of the four nucleotides used in this reaction is tagged with unique fluorescent labels, and the process of chain elongation is periodically uncoupled to detect the fluorescent signal from the last bound nucleotide. Data gathered are mapped onto a reference genome, to assemble the sequence.[2]

Types of Sequencing

- Depending on the extent to which the nucleic acid repertoire of a cell is sequenced and the type of nucleic acid sequenced, sequencing can be described as whole-genome sequencing (WGS), whole-exome sequencing (WES), or transcriptome sequencing.
- WGS refers to the sequencing of the entire genome of a cell and aids in the detection of structural variations (SVs) and single-nucleotide variations (SNVs), and CNAs. It is also possible to study splice-site variations using WGS since intergenic regions are also sequenced.

- Sequence information from the exonic portion of the genome, referred to as the "exome," which constitutes nearly 20,000 genes and makes up 1% of the entire genome, is captured through WES.
- Transcriptome sequencing refers to the sequencing of mRNA and noncoding RNA transcripts. Transcriptome sequencing can be particularly useful in evaluating gene expression, gene fusion, and splice variants.

CANCER GENOME SEQUENCING[1,3,5,7]

- Cells accumulate randomly distributed mutations as a result of cell division. However, some of these mutations provide a growth advantage to cancer cells and are positively selected during cancer evolution. Since these mutations are predicted to play a crucial role in the initiation and maintenance of the malignant phenotype, they are referred to as driver mutations. *Passenger* mutations, in contrast, are referred to as bystander mutations that are co-inherited by cancer cells along with driver mutations. Among the oncogenic driver mutations, a subset of those are a predictive biomarker for drug response and are called clinically actionable mutations.
- With the help of complex statistical approaches that take into account background mutation rates and a variety of other parameters such as recurrence of mutations and gene expression, it is possible to identify those mutations that are enriched in cancer cells.
- Furthermore, it is possible to use transcriptome data to identify gene expression patterns to classify tumors using clustering statistical methods.

APPLICATIONS

The success of novel therapies would depend on the ability to effectively target driver alterations. Complex computational biology-based approaches aid in assigning genes to cell-signaling pathways that can facilitate the identification of novel driver alterations and therapeutic vulnerabilities in cancer cells. This information is also of great value in designing appropriate functional studies to validate the biologic role of new genes and pathways in cancer pathogenesis. NGS is starting to emerge as an important clinical tool. Some of the applications of NGS in the clinic include variant detection, screening for the presence of multiple genomic alterations simultaneously, evaluation of tumor heterogeneity, and characterization of mechanisms of acquired resistance to therapy.

- **Variant detection:** It is possible to capture oncogenic alterations in potentially targetable genes using NGS. Apart from the possibility of being able to determine the sequence of a gene in an unbiased manner, NGS is also extremely sensitive and can identify alterations, which can be missed by other diagnostic modalities.
- **Facilitating clinical trial enrollment:** The ability to sequence tumors to screen for the presence of multiple genetic alterations simultaneously, in a timely and cost-efficient fashion, is crucial for designing and implementing biomarker-driven clinical trials.
- **Intratumoral heterogeneity:** Cancers are best viewed as a collection of neoplastic subclones. Subclones can harbor unique alterations that provide them the ability to metastasize or resist cytotoxic therapy. It is possible to construct the clonal architecture of a tumor using NGS technologies.[8–10] This information can prove useful from a prognostic standpoint, and in designing better therapies. The association of an increased number of subclones and tumor-distant metastasis, recurrence, drug resistance, and outcomes varies depending on the tumor type.[11]
- **Rebiopsy and surveillance:** While the advent of targeted therapies has significantly altered the landscape of oncology, most patients who receive targeted therapies eventually develop tumor resistance, mostly through a second mutation in the target gene or activation of bypass signaling pathways. The ability to rebiopsy samples at recurrence and

resequence them to characterize mechanisms of drug resistance can aid in the selection of appropriate therapies. Furthermore, since it is possible to identify DNA from tumor cells in the circulation, periodic "liquid" biopsies can be obtained to track tumor response to therapy and emergence of resistant clones.[12]

CLINICAL IMPACT OF NEXT-GENERATION SEQUENCING[13,14]

Genomic sequencing is an integral component of clinical oncology and is included in guidelines for multiple malignancies where this information help decide the treatment, especially in non–small cell lung cancer, advanced colon, and melanoma.

CHALLENGES

Despite its advantages, NGS is associated with its own share of challenges.

- **Privacy:** It is possible to establish a person's identity using genome-sequencing data. This is especially a concern with data that are available on the public domain for research purposes.
- **Detection of deleterious germline alterations:** It is possible that deleterious genetic alterations are incidentally discovered during NGS such as *BRCA* or *TP53* mutations. If these alterations were likely to pose a significant health risk to biologic relatives, disclosing such information would be of critical importance. Such situations can pose ethical and confidentiality-related challenges, especially if the patient is not interested in finding or disclosing such information.
- **Detection of potentially deleterious alterations:** NGS results in the generation of massive amounts of data. Often, variants speculated to be deleterious or of questionable clinical importance are discovered during this process. Discussing each of these variants with patients is not feasible, as it can result in a great amount of stress and unnecessary testing. At the same time, withholding such information can carry legal implications.

REFERENCES

1. Meyerson M, Gabriel S, Getz G. Advances in understanding cancer genomes through second-generation sequencing. *Nat Rev Genet.* 2010;11(10):685–696.
2. Lander ES, Linton LM, Birren B, et al. Initial sequencing and analysis of the human genome. *Nature.* 2001;409(6822):860–921.
3. Stratton MR, Campbell PJ, Futreal PA. The cancer genome. *Nature.* 2009;458(7239):719–724.
4. Deshpande V, Luebeck J, Nguyen N-PD, et al. Exploring the landscape of focal amplifications in cancer using AmpliconArchitect. *Nat Commun.* 2019;10:392.
5. Garraway LA, Lander ES. Lessons from the cancer genome. *Cell.* 2013;153:17–37.
6. Noer JB, Hørsdal OK, Xiang X, Luo Y, Regenberg B. Extrachromosomal circular DNA in cancer: history, current knowledge, and methods. *Trends Genet.* 2022;38(7):766–781.
7. Chakravarty D, Solit DB. Clinical cancer genomic profiling. *Nat Rev Genet.* 2021;22(8):483–501.
8. Greaves M, Maley CC. Clonal evolution in cancer. *Nature.* 2012;481(7381):306–313.
9. Yates LR, Campbell PJ. Evolution of the cancer genome. *Nat Rev Genet.* 2012;13:795–806.
10. Swanton C. Intratumor heterogeneity: evolution through space and time. *Cancer Res.* 2012;72(19):4875–4882.
11. Yu T, Gao X, Zheng Z, et al. Intratumor heterogeneity as a prognostic factor in solid tumors: a systematic review and meta-analysis. *Front Oncol.* 2021;11:744064.
12. Krebs MG, Malapelle U, Andre F, et al. Practical considerations for the use of circulating NDA in the treatment of patients with cancer: a narrative review. *JAMA Oncol.* 2022;8:1830–1839.
13. Colomer R, Miranda J, Romero-Laorden N, et al. Usefulness and real-world outcomes of next generation sequencing testing in patients with cancer: an observational study on the impact of selection based on clinical judgement. *EClinicalMedicine.* 2023;60:102029.
14. Gibbs SN, Peneva D, Carter GC, et al. Comprehensive review on the clinical impact of next-generation sequencing tests for the management of advanced cancer. *JCO Precis Oncol.* 2023;7:e220071.

Cancer Therapeutics

18

Sasha Haarberg

GENERAL PRINCIPLES

- The management of malignancy with systemic therapy is the specific specialty of hematologists and medical oncologists. The appropriate and safe use of anticancer agents requires an understanding of various factors including, but not limited to, principles of the cell cycle and tumor growth kinetics, response assessment, and pharmacology of these agents, including mechanisms of action, pharmacokinetic/pharmacodynamic properties, adverse effects, and mechanisms of drug resistance. Therefore, the prescription and administration of these agents should only be done by specifically trained and experienced health care professionals. The intent of this chapter is to provide a brief overview of some of the general principles of anticancer therapy, their respective mechanisms of action, and selected adverse effects.[1-3] For the purposes of this text, we will divide anticancer agents into four classifications: chemotherapy, targeted therapy, immunotherapy, and hormonal therapy. See Table 18-1 for anticancer agent classification, mechanism(s) of action, selected toxicities, and other pertinent information relating to these agents.

- Chemotherapy agents are toxic to rapidly proliferating cells of the human body. These agents interfere with normal cell processes, typically DNA synthesis or repair either at a specific phase of the cell cycle or during multiple phases (cell-cycle nonspecific agents). The justification for using substances that are toxic to normal cells is that malignant cells are preferentially sensitive to the effects of chemotherapy. A balance must be struck between toxicity to malignant cells and harm to the normal tissues that are intended to be spared. This concept is described as the therapeutic index, which is the ratio of toxicity to tumor cells to that of normal cells. The therapeutic index is quite narrow for many antineoplastic agents.

- Target agents (small molecule inhibitors and monoclonal antibodies) are targeted to specific receptors in or on the cancer cell, often in signal transduction pathways that regulate tumor cell growth, proliferation, migration, angiogenesis, and apoptosis. Recent advances in cancer have led to the identification of several specific molecular targets for drug therapy and continue to evolve.

- Immunotherapy stimulates the host's immune system to directly attack cancer cells in a multitude of mechanisms.

- Endocrine-related tumors are often affected by hormone therapy (e.g., antiestrogens in breast cancer, thyroid hormone to suppress thyroid cancer, and antiandrogens to inhibit prostate cancer).

TABLE 18-1 PHARMACOLOGIC AGENTS IN ONCOLOGY

Drug Classification/ Subclassification/Agents	Mechanism of Action	Selected Toxicities	Other Pertinent Information
Antimetabolites	Interfere with normal synthesis pathways of tumor cells; often inhibit DNA or RNA synthesis; S-phase specific		
Hypomethylating agents	Hypomethylation of DNA, restoring normal gene differentiation and proliferation	Myelosuppression, N/V, diarrhea, fever, elevated LFT, fatigue, constipation, diarrhea, headache	
5-Azacitidine		Renal tubular acidosis	IV, SC, or Oral
Decitabine		Edema, cough	Oral
Decitabine/Cedazuridine			
Pyrimidine antagonists	Inhibits thymidylate synthase	Myelosuppression, N/V, stomatitis, mucositis, diarrhea	
Capecitabine		Palmar-plantar erythrodysesthesia, cardiotoxicity	Oral. Dosed in mg/m² rounded to nearest tablet size. Take within 30 min of a meal
Cytarabine		Cerebral and cerebellar toxicity, conjunctivitis	IV or intrathecally. High-dose regimens are toxic to the cerebellum and need to be monitored closely. Conjunctivitis associated with high-dose cytarabine may be prevented with prophylactic corticosteroid eye drops

Drug	Mechanism	Toxicity	Notes
Floxuridine		Cardiotoxicity	May be administered via a hepatic artery infusion pump
5-Fluorouracil		Palmar-plantar erythrodysesthesia, cardiotoxicity, neurologic toxicity	
Gemcitabine		Hepatotoxicity, flu-like syndrome, rash, hemolytic uremic syndrome, pulmonary toxicity, peripheral edema	Flu-like symptoms may last up to 48 h
Trifluridine/Tipiracil			Oral. Dosed in mg/m^2 rounded to nearest tablet size
Purine antagonists			
Cladribine	Inhibits ribonucleotide reductase and DNA synthesis; cell-cycle nonspecific	Myelosuppression, opportunistic infections, fever, fatigue, neurotoxicity, rash, nausea	IV or SC
Clofarabine	Inhibits ribonucleotide reductase and DNA polymerase	Myelosuppression, opportunistic infections, N/V, diarrhea, constipation, headache, fatigue, cardiotoxicity, dyspnea, renal tubular acidosis, elevated LFT, rash	Corticosteroids may be useful to treat capillary leak syndrome associated with therapy
Fludarabine	Inhibits ribonucleotide reductase, DNA polymerase, primase, and ligase I	Myelosuppression, opportunistic infections, neurotoxicity	
6-Mercaptopurine	Inhibits purine synthesis	Myelosuppression, elevated LFT	Administer on an empty stomach. Metabolized via xanthine oxidase. Avoid concomitant xanthine oxidase inhibitors

(continued)

Drug Classification/ Subclassification/Agents	Mechanism of Action	Selected Toxicities	Other Pertinent Information
Nelarabine		Myelosuppression, neurotoxicity (somnolence, seizures, peripheral neuropathy), edema, fatigue, elevated LFT	Monitor closely for the development of neurotoxicity during the infusion
Pentostatin	Inhibits adenosine deaminase	Myelosuppression, fever, acute renal failure, elevated LFT, rash	Consider dose reduction for CrCl <60 mL/min. Do not use concomitantly with fludarabine due to increased pulmonary toxicity
6-Thioguanine		Myelosuppression, fluid retention, nausea, VOD	Take with or without food
Folate antagonists			
Methotrexate	Inhibits dihydrofolate reductase, which inhibits synthesis of thymidylate and purines	Myelosuppression, stomatitis, N/V, diarrhea, hepatotoxicity, nephrotoxicity, abnormal LFT, neurotoxicity	May be given intrathecally. High-dose therapy requires leucovorin administration and monitoring of methotrexate levels
Pemetrexed	Inhibits dihydrofolate reductase, thymidylate synthase, and glycinamide ribonucleotide formyltransferase, which are folate-dependent enzymes involved in the de novo biosynthesis of thymidine and purine nucleotides; G_1–S-phase specific	Myelosuppression, rash, chest pain, fatigue, N/V, neuropathy, nephrotoxicity, dyspnea	Premedicate with dexamethasone. Supplement with folic acid and vitamin B_{12} starting 1 wk prior to therapy and continuing for 21 d after last dose to reduce hematologic toxicity

TABLE 18-1   PHARMACOLOGIC AGENTS IN ONCOLOGY (Continued)

Drug	Mechanism	Toxicity	Notes
Pralatrexate	Additional inhibitor for polyglutamylation by folylpolyglutamyl synthetase	Myelosuppression, mucositis, N/V, fever, dehydration, SOB, nephrotoxicity, hepatotoxicity, fatigue, dermatologic reactions	Vitamin B_{12} and folic acid supplementation should be initiated 1 wk prior to the first pralatrexate and continued for 21 d after the last dose
Antitumor antibiotics			
Anthracyclines	Inhibits topoisomerase II, produces free radicals, and intercalates adjacent DNA base-pairs	Myelosuppression, alopecia, cardiotoxicity, mucositis, extravasation risk, secondary malignancies	
Daunorubicin			Recommended lifetime cumulative dose is 400–550 mg/m²
Daunorubicin liposomal	Daunorubicin encapsulated within liposomes	Infusion reaction	Infusion reaction generally occurs within the first 5 min and does not recur if resumed at a slower rate
Doxorubicin			Recommended lifetime cumulative dose is 450–550 mg/m²
Doxorubicin liposomal	Pegylated formulation of doxorubicin encapsulated within liposomes	Infusion reaction	
Epirubicin			Recommended lifetime cumulative dose is 750–900 mg/m²
Idarubicin			Recommended lifetime cumulative dose of 150 mg/m²
Mitoxantrone			

(*continued*)

TABLE 18-1 PHARMACOLOGIC AGENTS IN ONCOLOGY (Continued)

Drug Classification/ Subclassification/Agents	Mechanism of Action	Selected Toxicities	Other Pertinent Information
Other antitumor antibiotics			
Bleomycin	Inhibits DNA synthesis; S- and G_2-phase specific	Pulmonary fibrosis, stomatitis, fever, skin changes, hypersensitivity reactions, Raynaud phenomenon	A test dose is recommended, but may produce false-negative results. Concurrent use with filgrastim increases risk of pulmonary toxicity
Dactinomycin	Intercalates into DNA resulting in inhibition of DNA and RNA syntheses	Myelosuppression, N/V, pulmonary fibrosis, elevated LFT, alopecia, mucositis, diarrhea, fatigue	Orders commonly written in MICROgrams vs. MILLIgrams
Mitomycin C	Produces DNA crosslinks; noncell-cycle specific, but maximal effects in late G and early S phases	Myelosuppression, hemolytic uremic syndrome, acute bronchospasm, alopecia, CHF, nail banding, fever	May be given intravesically. Has been associated with development of TTP/HUS
Covalent DNA-binding agents			
Alkylating agents	Produce DNA–DNA crosslinks; noncell-cycle specific	Myelosuppression, N/V, secondary malignancies	
Bendamustine	Alkylating agent with purine analog ring leading to single- and double-strand DNA crosslinks	Infusion reactions/anaphylaxis, TLS, rash (SJS and TEN reported), stomatitis, peripheral edema	Monitor for drug interactions with inhibitors/inducers of CYP1A2 such as allopurinol. Contains mannitol—caution or avoid with hypersensitivity reactions

Drug	Toxicities	Comments
Busulfan	VOD, pulmonary fibrosis, seizures	Seizure prophylaxis should be used with high-dose regimens. Monitoring of levels may be important in high-dose regimens
Carmustine	Elevated LFT, VOD, alopecia, renal insufficiency	Diluent for intravenous preparation contains ethanol
Chlorambucil	Pulmonary fibrosis, rash, elevated LFT	Take on an empty stomach. Store tablets in the refrigerator
Cyclophosphamide	Hemorrhagic cystitis, SIADH, alopecia, cardiomyopathy, VOD, facial flushing, headache	The inactive metabolite, acrolein, may cause hemorrhagic cystitis. Consideration of mesna in high-dose therapy
Dacarbazine	Pain on infusion	
Estramustine	Edema, gynecomastia, nausea, diarrhea, dyspnea, CHF, MI	Take on an empty stomach. Moderate emetic potential
Ifosfamide	Hemorrhagic cystitis, nephrotoxicity, SIADH, alopecia, neurotoxicity (somnolence, confusion, and hallucinations)	The inactive metabolite, acrolein, may cause hemorrhagic cystitis. Use brisk hydration and mesna administration with all doses. Neurotoxicity may be reversed by administration of methylene blue
Lomustine		Do not dispense more than a single dose. Administer on an empty stomach with fluids
Mechlorethamine		Vesicant agent

(continued)

TABLE 18-1   PHARMACOLOGIC AGENTS IN ONCOLOGY (*Continued*)

Drug Classification/ Subclassification/Agents	Mechanism of Action	Selected Toxicities	Other Pertinent Information
Melphalan		Mucositis	IV or Oral. Administer oral on an empty stomach
Procarbazine		Neurotoxicity, hallucinations	Avoid tyramine-containing food/ beverages. Avoid concomitant use of SSRI, TCA due to inhibition of MAO
Streptozocin		Elevated LFT, nephrotoxicity, hypoalbuminemia, glucose intolerance, diarrhea	
Temozolomide		Lymphopenia, peripheral edema, headache, fever, fatigue, seizures	Take with or without food consistently. Consider PCP prophylaxis
Thiotepa		Rash	Cystitis may occur when given intravesically. High-dose thiotepa can be excreted through the skin via sweat. Encourage frequent bathing and minimum use of lotions
Platinum agents	Produce DNA–DNA adducts and crosslinks resulting in inhibition of DNA replication and synthesis; noncell-cycle specific	Nephrotoxicity, myelosuppression, peripheral neuropathy, hypomagnesemia, hypokalemia, hypocalcemia, hypophosphatemia, N/V, diarrhea, mucositis, alopecia	
Carboplatin			Dosed based on area under the curve (AUC)

Cisplatin		Ototoxicity	May induce acute and delayed N/V, which can be severe. Pre- and posthydration are necessary to minimize renal toxicity
Oxaliplatin		Acute/chronic neurotoxicity, cold sensitivity	Chronic toxicity is dose-dependent proprioception and neurosensory deficits
Differentiating agents			
Arsenic trioxide	Apoptosis of leukemia cells	QTc prolongation, tachycardia, fatigue, fever, electrolyte abnormalities, N/V, dyspnea, leukocytosis, APL differentiation syndrome	Use caution with any potential QTc prolonging medications. If QTc >500 ms during treatment, consider holding drug. ECG should be monitored at least weekly
Bexarotene	Binds to and activates retinoid X receptors which function as transcription factors to regulate expression of genes that control cellular differentiation and proliferation	Hepatotoxicity, hypothyroidism, myelosuppression, lipid abnormalities, pancreatitis, photosensitivity, visual disturbances, edema, rash	Hypothyroidism may occur quickly. Administer with meals. Monitor for drug interactions due to hepatic metabolism by CYP 3A4
Tretinoin	Terminal differentiation and apoptotic cell death	Headache, fever, weakness, fatigue, N/V, bleeding, leukocytosis, dyspnea, elevated cholesterol and triglycerides, APL differentiation syndrome, MI, DVT	Administer in two equally divided doses with a meal. Monitor for drug interactions due to hepatic metabolism by CYP 2A6, 2B6, 2C8, and 2C9

(continued)

TABLE 18-1 PHARMACOLOGIC AGENTS IN ONCOLOGY (Continued)

Drug Classification/ Subclassification/Agents	Mechanism of Action	Selected Toxicities	Other Pertinent Information
Epothilone B analog			
Ixabepilone	Bind to the beta-tubulin subunit of the microtubules and prevent their disassembly	Myelosuppression, peripheral and sensory neuropathy, hypersensitivity reaction, myalgia/arthralgia, N/V, mucositis, diarrhea, alopecia	Hypersensitivity reaction due to ixabepilone and/or its vehicle, Cremophor EL. Premedicate with H_1- and H_2-blockers; add corticosteroid if history of reaction. BSA is capped at 2.2 m^2 for dose calculation
Halichondrin B analog			
Eribulin	Nontaxane microtubule dynamics inhibitor that inhibits the growth phase of microtubules without affecting the shortening phase, sequesters tubulin	Myelosuppression, peripheral neuropathy, headache, fatigue, constipation, N/V, cough, arthralgia, elevated LFT	QTc prolongation possible; monitor closely in patients with CHF, on antiarrhythmics, or who have electrolyte abnormalities
Taxanes	Bind to microtubules and prevent their disassembly; G_2-M-phase specific	Myelosuppression, diarrhea, fatigue, peripheral neuropathy, alopecia, hypersensitivity reaction	
Cabazitaxel	Poor affinity for MDR proteins confers activity in taxane-resistant disease	N/V, weakness, hematuria	Hypersensitivity reaction due to cabazitaxel and/or its vehicle, Polysorbate 80. Premedicate with corticosteroids and H_1- and H_2-blockers. Often prescribed in combination with prednisone

Drug	Mechanism	Toxicities	Comments
Docetaxel		Elevated LFT, rash, stomatitis, fluid retention	Hypersensitivity reaction due to docetaxel or its vehicle, Polysorbate 80
Paclitaxel		HOTN, bradycardia, elevated LFTs	Hypersensitivity reaction due to paclitaxel or its vehicle, Cremophor EL. Premedicate with corticosteroids and H_1- and H_2-blockers. Irritant with vesicant-like properties—use with caution
Protein-bound Paclitaxel		Pneumonitis, ECG abnormality, peripheral edema, N/V, diarrhea, hepatotoxicity, visual disturbances	Lower incidence of neuropathy and less infusion reactions than paclitaxel
Topoisomerase inhibitors			
Topoisomerase I inhibitors	Active in the unwinding of DNA, causing DNA strand breaks; S-phase specific		
-Irinotecan		Myelosuppression, N/V, diarrhea, alopecia, elevated LFTs, dyspnea	
		Acute and delayed diarrhea, abdominal pain/cramping, other cholinergic effects	Acute diarrhea may be treated with atropine. A reduction in the starting dose by one dose level should be considered for known homozygosity for UGT1A1*28 allele
Topotecan		Rash, headache, stomatitis	

(continued)

TABLE 18-1 PHARMACOLOGIC AGENTS IN ONCOLOGY (Continued)

Drug Classification/ Subclassification/Agents	Mechanism of Action	Selected Toxicities	Other Pertinent Information
Topoisomerase II inhibitors			
Etoposide	Inhibits the ability to restore the structure of cleaved DNA, resulting in double-strand breaks; S- and G_2-phase specific	Myelosuppression, N/V, mucositis, anorexia, diarrhea, HOTN, disorientation, alopecia	Etoposide formulation contains ethanol, 30.3% (v/v). Etoposide phosphate 113.5 mg = etoposide 100 mg and dosages should always be calculated and expressed as the desired etoposide dose
Vinca alkaloids	Binds to tubulin and inhibits microtubule assembly; M- and S-phase specific		Fatal if given intrathecally
Vinblastine		Myelosuppression, stomatitis, alopecia, SIADH, pulmonary toxicity, extravasation risk	
Vincristine		Peripheral neuropathy, constipation, paralytic ileus, alopecia, extravasation risk	Doses may be capped at a max of 2 mg/dose
Vincristine Liposomal		Myelosuppression, fatigue, constipation, nausea, increased AST, peripheral neuropathy, cardiac arrest, extravasation risk	Do not substitute for vincristine. Dose based on actual body surface area and not capped. Extensive preparation time necessary, requiring ~90 min

Drug	Mechanism	Toxicity	Notes
Vinorelbine		Myelosuppression, peripheral neuropathy, constipation, stomatitis, elevated LFT, pulmonary toxicity, extravasation risk	
Immunomodulatory agents	Exact mechanism unclear; inhibits secretion of proinflammatory cytokines, enhances cell-mediated immunity, and directly induces cell death	Peripheral edema, fatigue, neuropathy, rash, N/V, thromboembolic events, rash	Thromboprophylaxis is recommended
Lenalidomide		Diarrhea, myelosuppression, hepatotoxicity	Give with or without food
Pomalidomide		Constipation	Give on an empty stomach, at least 2 h before or 2 h after a meal
Thalidomide		Hepatotoxicity, muscle weakness	Preferred to take at bedtime, at least 1 h after the evening meal. Doses >400 mg/d may be given in divided doses
Miscellaneous agents			
Hydroxyurea	Inhibits ribonucleotide reductase and DNA synthesis; S-phase specific	Myelosuppression, edema, rash, hepatotoxicity, peripheral neuropathy	Take with or without food. Larger doses may be given in divided doses
L-Asparaginase	Inhibits protein synthesis by converting asparagine to aspartic acid and ammonia; G_1-phase specific	Fever, chills, hyperglycemia, acute pancreatitis, hypofibrinogenemia, elevated LFT, hypersensitivity reactions, nephrotoxicity, thrombosis	A test dose is recommended

(*continued*)

TABLE 18-1 PHARMACOLOGIC AGENTS IN ONCOLOGY (Continued)

Drug Classification/ Subclassification/Agents	Mechanism of Action	Selected Toxicities	Other Pertinent Information
Mitotane	Adrenolytic agent that causes adrenal cortical atrophy due to mitochondrial changes and decrease production of cortisol	Drowsiness, rash, N/V, diarrhea, headache, neurotoxicity with long-term use	Monitoring of therapeutic drug levels is important. Give in divided doses to increase tolerability. Patients will develop adrenal insufficiency and require steroid replacement therapy starting with initiation of therapy
Omacetaxine	Reversible protein synthesis inhibitor binding to A-site cleft of ribosomal subunit to interfere with chain elongation	Myelosuppression, hyperglycemia, edema, fatigue, rash, diarrhea, N/V, injection-site reactions, weakness, epistaxis	Monitor for drug interactions due to hepatic metabolism by p-glycoprotein. Mechanism is independent of BCR-ABL kinase binding activity
Sipuleucel-T	Autologous cellular immunotherapy designed to stimulate an immune response against an antigen PAP which is expressed in most prostate cancers. CD54+ cells are activated with PAP-GM-CSF and cultured for ~40 h	Infusion reaction, DVT, stroke, MI, flu-like symptoms, back pain	Premedicate with acetaminophen and antihistamine. Patient must undergo leukapheresis for collection of CD54+ cells
Hormonal agents			
Selective estrogen receptor modulators (SERMs)			
Tamoxifen	SERM competitively binding to estrogen receptors on tumors and breast tissue	Hypertension, peripheral edema, hot flash, DVT, PE, arthralgia, ocular toxicity, endometrial thickening	Monitor for drug interactions due to hepatic metabolism by CYP 2D6, 3A4/5

Selective estrogen receptor down regulators (SERDs)

Fulvestrant	Estrogen receptor antagonist causing a dose-related downregulation of estrogen receptors	Hot flash, hepatotoxicity, injection-site pain, bone pain	Each 250 mg IM injection is 5-mL volume
Aromatase Inhibitors			
		Hypertension, fatigue, hot flash, nausea, arthralgia, osteoporosis	Monitor for the development of osteoporosis
Anastrozole	Nonsteroidal aromatase inhibitor	Skin rash	
Letrozole	Nonsteroidal aromatase inhibitor	Edema, headache, hypercholesterolemia	Monitor for drug interactions due to hepatic metabolism by CYP 2A6 and 3A4
Exemestane	Steroidal aromatase inhibitor		Administer with food. Monitor for drug interactions
Gonadotropin-releasing hormone (GNRH) agonist			
Goserelin	GnRH analog that causes an initial increase in LH and FSH followed by a sustained suppression of pituitary gonadotropins	Vasodilation, edema, headache, depression, pain, hot flash, tumor flare, decreased bone mineral density	Available in 1- or 3-mo formulation given SC
Leuprolide	GnRH analog that causes an initial increase in LH and FSH followed by a sustained suppression of pituitary gonadotropins	Edema, tumor flare, headache, injection-site reaction, hot flash, weight change, N/V	IM and SC products are available
Gonadotropin-releasing hormone (GNRH) antagonist			
Degarelix	GnRH antagonist	Fatigue, hot flash, hepatotoxicity, injection-site reactions, fever, hypertension	Does not cause tumor flare. Injection-site reactions more pronounced than with GnRH analogs

(continued)

TABLE 18-1 PHARMACOLOGIC AGENTS IN ONCOLOGY (Continued)

Drug Classification/ Subclassification/Agents	Mechanism of Action	Selected Toxicities	Other Pertinent Information
Inhibition of androgen synthesis			
Abiraterone	Selective and irreversible inhibition of CPY17 resulting in reduced androgen biosynthesis	Hepatotoxicity, hypertension, hypokalemia, fluid retention	Monitor for drug interactions. Concurrent administration with corticosteroids is required. Administer on an empty stomach
Antiandrogens		Peripheral edema, hypertension, fatigue, hot flash, constipation, arthralgia, osteoporosis	
Bicalutamide	Pure nonsteroidal antiandrogen	Hepatotoxicity, dizziness	Take with or without food. Monitor for drug interactions
Enzalutamide	Pure androgen receptor inhibitor with no agonistic properties	Neutropenia, seizure	Monitor for drug interactions. Avoid in patients with seizure history
Flutamide	Nonsteroidal antiandrogen	Galactorrhea, diarrhea, impotence, hepatotoxicity	Administer in three divided doses per day with or without food. Monitor for drug interactions
Nilutamide	Nonsteroidal antiandrogen	Insomnia, hepatotoxicity, ocular toxicity	Increased risk of hepatotoxicity and interstitial pneumonitis

Immunotherapy

CTLA-4 Inhibitor

Drug	Mechanism	Adverse effects	Comments
Ipilimumab	Binds to cytotoxic T-lymphocyte–associated antigen 4 (CTLA-4) to enhance T-cell activation and proliferation	Diarrhea, skin rash, immune-mediated toxicities (e.g., colitis, hypophysitis. hepatotoxicity. etc.)	Discontinue therapy and start high-dose corticosteroid treatment for severe immune-mediated adverse effects. May see a delayed response after an initial increase in tumor burden
Tremelimumab			

PD-1/PD-L1 Inhibitors

Drug	Mechanism	Adverse effects	Comments
Atezolizumab	Selectively inhibits programmed cell death-1 (PD-1) by blocking ligand binding activating an antitumor immune response	Diarrhea, pruritus, skin rash, fatigue, infusion reaction immune-mediated toxicities (e.g., colitis, hypophysitis. hepatotoxicity, etc.)	Discontinue therapy and start high-dose corticosteroid treatment for severe immune-mediated adverse effects. May see a delayed response after an initial increase in tumor burden
Avelumab			
Cemilimab			
Durvalumab			
Nivolumab			
Pembrolizumab			

Targeted therapy

ALK Inhibitors

Drug	Mechanism	Adverse effects	Comments
Alectinib	Inhibiting phosphorylation of ALK as well as c-MET preventing cell proliferation and leading to apoptosis	Fatigue, N/V, diarrhea	Administer with food
Brigatinib	IGF-1R, FLT-3, ROS1	Headache, cough	

(continued)

TABLE 18-1 PHARMACOLOGIC AGENTS IN ONCOLOGY (*Continued*)

Drug Classification/ Subclassification/Agents	Mechanism of Action	Selected Toxicities	Other Pertinent Information
Ceritinib	IGF-1R, InsR, ROS1	Neuropathy, skin rash, hyperglycemia, increased LFT, QTc prolongation, visual disturbances	Administer with food
Crizotinib		Edema, neuropathy, hypophosphatemia, neutropenia, hepatotoxicity, visual disturbances, PE, QTc prolongation	
Lorlatinib	ROS1	Cognitive effects	
BCR-ABL inhibitors			
Bosutinib	SRC, minimal c-KIT, and PDGFR. Overcomes most imatinib-resistant BCR-ABL mutations	Edema, fatigue, rash, hypophosphatemia, diarrhea, nausea, vomiting, arthralgia, QTc prolongation	Administer with food. Monitor for drug interactions due to hepatic metabolism by CYP 3A4
Dasatinib	SRC, c-KIT, PDGFRβ. Overcomes most imatinib-resistant BCR-ABL mutations	Myelosuppression, fluid retention/ edema, N/V, diarrhea, constipation, mucositis, rash, QTc prolongation, arrhythmia, elevated LFT, arthralgia/myalgia, neuropathy, infection, CHF, alopecia, photosensitivity	Monitor for drug interactions due to hepatic metabolism by CYP 3A4, UGT. Antacids, H₂-blockers, and PPIs may decrease dasatinib absorption
Imatinib	SCF/c-KIT, PDGFRα, PDGFRβ	N/V, diarrhea, dyspepsia, rash, fluid retention/edema, hepatotoxicity, hemorrhage, myelosuppression, arthralgia/myalgia, left ventricular, dysfunction, CHF, photosensitivity, SJS	Take with food and large glass of water. 800-mg dose should be divided twice daily. Monitor for drug interactions due to hepatic metabolism by CYP 3A4, 1A2, 2D6, 2C9, 2C19

Drug	Mechanism	Toxicities	Notes
Nilotinib	BCR-ABL TKI; also inhibits c-KIT and PDGFR; overcomes most imatinib-resistant BCR-ABL kinase mutations	Myelosuppression, QTc prolongation, pancreatitis, abnormal LFT, electrolyte abnormalities, N/V, abdominal pain, diarrhea, rash, myalgias/arthralgias, headache, constipation	Take on an empty stomach
Ponatinib	BCR-ABL TKI (including T315I); inhibitory effects on other receptor tyrosine kinases (VEGF, FGFR, PDGFR, SRC, KIT, RET, FLT3)	Arterial and venous thrombosis, hypertension, peripheral edema, arterial ischemia, CHF, fatigue, rash, constipation, nausea, myelosuppression, hepatotoxicity, arthralgia, pancreatitis, blurred vision	Monitor for drug interactions due to hepatic metabolism by CYP 3A4/5, 2C8, 2D6. Use caution in patients with preexisting cardiovascular disease or risk factors

EGFR inhibitors and monoclonal antibodies

Drug	Mechanism	Toxicities	Notes
Afatinib	EGFR TKI (irreversible binding)	Acneiform rash, erythematous rash, maculopapular dermatitis, dry skin, pruritus, paronychia, diarrhea, stomatitis, pulmonary toxicities	Monitor for drug interactions due to hepatic metabolism
Dacomitinib	EGFR TKI (irreversible binding)	Conjunctivitis	Administer on an empty stomach
Erlotinib	EGFR TKI	Edema, conjunctivitis, cardiovascular events, renal impairment	Administer on an empty stomach. Avoid concomitant use with PPIs. Take at least 10 h after H_2-blocker or 2 h before next dose
Gefitinib	EGFR TKI. Activity against wild-type and select (exon 19 deletion and exon 21 (L858R) substitution)	Ocular toxicity	

(continued)

TABLE 18-1 PHARMACOLOGIC AGENTS IN ONCOLOGY (*Continued*)

Drug Classification/ Subclassification/Agents	Mechanism of Action	Selected Toxicities	Other Pertinent Information
Osimertinib	EGFR TKI. Elective for sensitizing mutations and the T790M resistance mutation	Cardiovascular toxicity, aplastic anemia	
Cetuximab	Chimeric Mab	Hypomagnesemia, infusion reactions, peripheral edema, cardiopulmonary arrest (in combination with radiation therapy), photosensitivity	Risk of infusion-related reactions varies based on region. Premedicate with an H1 antagonist prior to the first dose and then as clinically indicated. A test dose may be utilized
Panitumumab	Human Mab	Fissures, peripheral edema, fatigue, hypomagnesemia, cough, eyelash growth, infusion reactions	Lower risk of infusion reactions since not chimeric antibody. Premedication not required
HER2 inhibitors and monoclonal antibodies			
Lapatinib	EGFR and HER2 TKI	Diarrhea, PPE, N/V, hepatotoxicity	Take on an empty stomach. Monitor for drug interactions due to hepatic metabolism by CYP 3A4/5, 2C19, 2C8
Pertuzumab	Binds to extracellular HER2 domain to inhibit dimerization and block HER downstream signaling initiating apoptosis. Binds to a different HER2 epitope than trastuzumab	CHF, decreased LVEF, fatigue, alopecia, rash, hand-foot syndrome, myelosuppression, myalgias/ arthralgias, hypersensitivity reactions	Evaluate LVEF prior to and during treatment in all patients

Drug	Mechanism	Adverse Effects	Notes
Trastuzumab	Binds to the HER2 co-receptor protein and inhibits HER-family receptor dimerization, inhibiting signal transduction; induces ADCC against cells that overproduce HER2; internalizes the HER2 receptor; downregulates surface HER2	Infusion-related reactions, diarrhea, CHF, left ventricular dysfunction, cardiomyopathy, myelosuppression, severe hypersensitivity reactions, pulmonary events	Do not substitute for ado-trastuzumab emtansine. Evaluate LVEF prior to and during treatment for all patients
VEGF inhibitors and monoclonal antibodies			
		Hypertension, fatigue, palmar-plantar erythrodysesthesia, diarrhea, nausea, stomatitis, proteinuria, PE, DVT, electrolyte changes, elevated LFTs, depigmentation of hair and skin, QTc prolongation, hypothyroidism, reversible posterior leukoencephalopathy	May impair wound healing, so use caution around surgical procedures Monitor for drug interactions due to hepatic metabolism
Axitinib	(VEGFR-1, VEGFR-2, VEGFR-3)		
Cabozantinib	Inhibitory effects on other receptor tyrosine kinases (Flt-3, KIT, MET, RET, VEGFR-1, 2, 3)	Hypothyroidism	Take on an empty stomach
Lenvatinib	Inhibitory effects on other receptor tyrosine kinases (FGFR, PDGFRα, KIT, RET)		
Pazopanib	Multi-TKI of VEGFR 1, VEGFR 2, VEGFR3, PDGFRα, PDGFRβ, FGFR1, FGFR 3, Kit, Itk, Lck, c-Fms TKI		Take on an empty stomach

(continued)

TABLE 18-1 PHARMACOLOGIC AGENTS IN ONCOLOGY (*Continued*)

Drug Classification/ Subclassification/Agents	Mechanism of Action	Selected Toxicities	Other Pertinent Information
Sunitinib	Effects on other receptor tyrosine kinases (SCF/c-KIT, PDGFRα, PDGFRβ, Flt-3)	Decreased LVEF, MI, peripheral neuropathy	
Vandetanib	Multikinase inhibitor including EGFR, VEGF, RET, BRK, SRC	CHF, interstitial lung disease, corneal changes, kidney toxicity	
Bevacizumab	Binds to and neutralizes VEGF	Nephrotic syndrome, GI perforations, intra-abdominal abscesses, CHF, infusion reactions	
Ramucirumab	Inhibits VEGF receptor 2	Intestinal obstruction, infusion-related reactions, GI perforations	
Ziv-Aflibercept	Recombinant fusion protein	Myelosuppression, fistula formation	
RAF inhibitors		HTN, diarrhea, PPE, hemorrhage, abdominal pains	
Regorafenib	Effects on other receptors (EGFR 1–3, PDGFRa, PDGFRb, RET, KIT, RET, FGFR1-2, and Abl)	Hyperbilirubinemia	Take with low-fat (<30% fat) meal
Sorafenib	Effects on other receptors (VEGFR 2, VEGFR 3, PDGFRβ, Flt-3, c-KIT)	Neuropathy, elevated amylase/ lipase, cardiac ischemia/ infarction	Take on an empty stomach
BRAF inhibitors		Dermatology toxicity, edema, QTc prolongation, diarrhea, arthralgias, hemorrhage, malignancy, ocular toxicity, hepatotoxicity	Use in combination with MEK inhibitors decreases occurrence of squamous cell carcinoma

Drug	Mechanism	Adverse effects	Notes
Dabrafenib			Take on an empty stomach
Encorafenib			
Vemurafenib		Cutaneous squamous cell carcinoma, uveitis, pancreatitis, photosensitivity	Frequent dermatology evaluation for cutaneous squamous cell carcinomas
MEK inhibitors			
Binimetinib			
Cobimetinib		Diarrhea, photosensitivity, acneiform reaction, N/V, pyrexia, decreased LVEF, hepatotoxicity, pulmonary toxicity, rhabdomyolysis	Take on an empty stomach. Refrigerated
Trametinib			
Mammalian target of rapamycin (m-TOR) inhibitors	Reduces protein synthesis and cell proliferation by binding to FK binding protein-12 to form a complex that inhibits activation of mTOR	Hyperglycemia, hypercholesterolemia, hyperlipidemia, hypophosphatemia, hypokalemia, mucositis, stomatitis, pneumonitis, rash, cough, secondary malignancy	
Everolimus		Myelosuppression, peripheral edema, elevated LFT, elevated creatinine, angioedema	Take consistently with or without food. Monitor for drug interaction
Temsirolimus		Chest pain	Premedicate with H_1-blocker to reduce incidence of infusion reaction. Monitor for drug interactions

(continued)

TABLE 18-1 PHARMACOLOGIC AGENTS IN ONCOLOGY (Continued)

Drug Classification/ Subclassification/Agents	Mechanism of Action	Selected Toxicities	Other Pertinent Information
BTK inhibitors		Myelosuppression, HTN, a.fib, diarrhea, bleeding/bruising, infections, arthralgia	Monitor for drug interactions
Acalabrutinib			
Ibrutinib			
Zanibruitinib			
Unconjugated monoclonal antibodies			
Alemtuzumab	Humanized Mab binds to CD52 resulting in complement-mediated and/or ADCC	HOTN, HTN, peripheral edema, tachycardia, fever, fatigue, rash, N/V, diarrhea, myelosuppression, rigors, myalgias, infection, serious and potentially fatal infusion-related reactions	Prophylactic therapy against PCP and herpes viruses needed; continue for at least 2 mo after completion. Premedicate with diphenhydramine and acetaminophen. Dose escalation is required at initiation and after therapy interruption for 7 d or more
BCL-2 inhibitors			
Venetoclax	Binds to BCL-2 to restore apoptotic process	Diarrhea, nausea, electrolyte disturbances, TLS, myelosuppression, infection	Titrations recommend to avoid TLS. Monitor for drug interactions. Administer with food

CC chemokine receptor 4 inhibitors

Drug	Target/Mechanism	Adverse effects	Notes
Mogamulizumab	Humanized MAb binds to CCR4 resulting in ADCC	Hyperglycemia, diarrhea, increased AST, skin rash, infusion-related reactions	Premedicate with diphenhydramine and acetaminophen. Hepatitis B reactivation possible

Hedgehog pathway inhibitors

Drug	Target/Mechanism	Adverse effects	Notes
Glasdegib		Fatigue, alopecia, nausea, arthralgia	Monitor for drug interactions
Sonidegib			Take on empty stomach
Vismodegib			

NTRK inhibitors

Drug	Target/Mechanism	Adverse effects	Notes
Entrectinib	Multiple TRK, ROS1 kinase, and ALK kinase	Fatigue, constipation, dizziness, nausea, arthralgias	Monitor for drug interactions
Larotectinib	Selectively to all TRK	Vision disturbances, cognitive impairment	

Fibroblast growth factor receptor (FGFR) Inhibitors

Drug	Target/Mechanism	Adverse effects	Notes
Ertafitinib	RET, CSF1R, PDGFRA, PDGFRB, FLT4, KIT, and VEGFR2	Increased LFTs, cough	

PI3K inhibitors

Drug	Target/Mechanism	Adverse effects	Notes
		Dermatologic toxicities, stomatitis, dry mouth, dry eyes, electrolyte imbalances, hepatotoxicity	
		Hepatotoxicity, pneumonitis, diarrhea, nausea, cough, myelosuppression	Monitor for drug interactions
Alpelisib	PI3K alpha	Hyperglycemia, lipase elevation, stomatitis	Take with food. Requires close monitor for glucose management
Copanlisib	PI3K alpha/delta		IV
Duvelisib	PI3K alpha/delta		

(continued)

TABLE 18-1 PHARMACOLOGIC AGENTS IN ONCOLOGY (*Continued*)

Drug Classification/ Subclassification/Agents	Mechanism of Action	Selected Toxicities	Other Pertinent Information
Idelalisib	PI3K-delta		
CD20 monoclonal antibodies	Binds to CD20; induces complement-dependent cytotoxicity and ADCC	Infusion-related reactions, CRS, infection, TLS, nausea, myelo-suppression, progressive multi-focal leukoencephalopathy (PML)	Screen all patients for HBV infection before initiation Premedications with acetamino-phen, an antihistamine, and a glucocorticoid and infusion rate titration are required
Obinutuzumab	Glycoengineered MAb	Elevated LFT, increased serum cre-atinine, electrolyte disturbances	DIC has occurred
Ofatumumab	Fully humanized MAb		
Rituximab	Chimeric murine/human MAb		
Conjugated monoclonal antibodies			
Ado-Trastuzumab Emtansine	HER2-antibody drug conjugate combining trastuzumab with the microtubule inhibitor DM1 (a maytansine derivative)	Hepatotoxicity, cardiotoxicity, fatigue, peripheral neuropathy, N/V, constipation, peripheral edema	Monitor LFTs prior to each dose. Withhold treatment for clinically significant decrease in LVEF. Do not interchange with other trastuzumab-like products
Fam-Trastuzumab Deruxtecan	HER2-antibody drug conjugate com-bining trastuzumab-like MAb with the topoisomerase I inhibitor	Myelosuppression, N/V/D, stomati-tis, cardiotoxicity, pulmonary tox-icity, alopecia, increased in LFTs	Do not interchange with other tras-tuzumab-like products. Withhold treatment for clinically significant decrease in LVEF

Drug	Mechanism	Toxicities	Notes
Sacituzumab Govitecan	Humanized antitrophoblast cell-surface antigen 2 (Trop-2) monoclonal antibody coupled to the topoisomerase 1 inhibitor SN-3	Myelosuppression, N/V/D, stomatitis, dyspepsia, alopecia, edema, electrolyte disturbances	Premedications with acetaminophen and an antihistamine
Proteasome inhibitors	26S proteasome inhibitor (enzyme complex that regulates cellular protein homeostasis)	Myelosuppression, N/V/D, rash, CHF, QTc prolongation, pulmonary toxicities, PML, hepatotoxicity	
Bortezomib		Peripheral neuropathy, edema, HOTN	Monitor for drug interactions. SC route may be associated with decreased peripheral neuropathy
Carfilzomib		Thromboembolic events, renal toxicity, infusion-related reactions	Premedicate with dexamethasone. Infusion reaction can occur in first 24 h after a dose
Ixazomib		Peripheral neuropathy, edema	Oral. Administer on empty stomach
Histone deacetylase (HDAC) inhibitors	HDAC inhibitor, induces cell-cycle arrest and apoptosis	QTc prolongation, electrolyte abnormalities, myelosuppression, N/V	
Belinostat		Diarrhea, hepatotoxicity, skin rash, pain at injection site	Dose reduction recommendation for patients with reduced UGT1A1 activity
Romidepsin		Dysgeusia, elevated LFT	Monitor for drug interactions
Panobinostat		Diarrhea, edema, elevated bilirubin	QTc must be <450 ms prior to starting therapy. Hold if ≥480 ms. Monitor for drug interactions
Vorinostat		Diarrhea, dysgeusia, xerostomia, PE, DVT, edema	Take with food

(continued)

TABLE 18-1 **PHARMACOLOGIC AGENTS IN ONCOLOGY (Continued)**

Drug Classification/ Subclassification/Agents	Mechanism of Action	Selected Toxicities	Other Pertinent Information
FLT3 inhibitors			
Gilteritinib		Eye disease, renal toxicity	Take with food
Midostaurin	Wild type FLT3, PDGFR, and KIT	QTc prolongation, electrolyte abnormalities, hepatotoxicity	
Cyclin-dependent kinase inhibitor (CDK4/6)	Block retinoblastoma hyperphosphorylation, thus regulating progression through the cell cycle at the G1/S phase	Myelosuppression, pulmonary toxicity, N/V/D, hepatotoxicity, headache	Monitor for drug interactions
Abemaciclib		Thromboembolism, increase Scr	
Palbociclib		Increases in LFTs	Capsules: Administer with food
Ribociclib		Dermatologic toxicity, QTc prolongation, hepatobiliary toxicity	
PARP inhibitor	Inhibitors of poly (ADP-ribose) polymerase (PARP), involved in DNA transcription, cell-cycle regulation, and DNA repair	Myelosuppression, peripheral edema, fatigue, N/V/D, myalgia, musculoskeletal pain, secondary malignancy, increase in Scr	Monitor for drug interactions
Olaparib		Pulmonary toxicity, thromboembolic events	
Niraparib		Cardiovascular effects	
Rucaparib		Increased LFTs	
Talazoparib		Increased LFTs	

JAK-STAT inhibitors

Ruxolitinib	JAK TKI	Dizziness, headache, fatigue, pruritus, increased cholesterol, hypertriglyceridemia, diarrhea, myelosuppression, hepatotoxicity, edema	May take with or without food. Monitor for drug interactions due to hepatic metabolism by CYP 3A4, 2C9

CD30 monoclonal antibodies

Brentuximab Vedotin	Antibody drug conjugate which delivers the microtubule-disrupting agent monomethyl auristatin (MMAE) to CD30-positive cells resulting in apoptosis	Peripheral edema, sensory/motor neuropathy, nausea, diarrhea, myelosuppression, arthralgias/myalgias, PML	Concurrent use with bleomycin is contraindicated due to risk for pulmonary injury

CD38 monoclonal antibodies

Daratumumab	Human MAb	Myelosuppression, infusion reactions, URTI, edema, neuropathy, N/V/D	Screen all patients for HBV infection before initiation. Premedications with acetaminophen, an antihistamine, and a glucocorticoid and infusion rate titration are required
Isatuximab	IgG1-derived MAb	Myelosuppression, infusion reaction, HTN, secondary malignancies, false-positive on indirect Coombs test	Premedications with a glucocorticoid and infusion rate titration are required

(continued)

TABLE 18-1 PHARMACOLOGIC AGENTS IN ONCOLOGY (Continued)

Drug Classification/ Subclassification/Agents	Mechanism of Action	Selected Toxicities	Other Pertinent Information
SLAM7 monoclonal antibodies			
Elotuzumab	Binds to SLAM7 interacting with NK cells leading to ADCC	Cardiac alterations, electrolyte disturbances, cough, hepatotoxicity, infusion reactions, secondary malignancies	Premedications with acetaminophen, an antihistamine, and a glucocorticoid and infusion rate titration are required
Bispecific T-cell engager (BiTE)			
Blinatumomab	BiTE targeting CD19 and CD3	CRS, neurotoxicity, leukoencephalopathy, infection, TLS, peripheral edema, rash, elevated LFT	Administered as a continuous infusion. Hospitalization recommended for first 9 d of cycle 1, and the first 2 d of cycle 2. Premedicate with dexamethasone prior to the first dose of each cycle and after a therapy interruption of ≥4 h
Epcoritamab	BiTE targeting CD3 and CD20	Cytopenias, CRS, ICANS, nausea, diarrhea, electrolyte disturbances, infections, increased LFTs	SC injection
Glofitamab	BiTE targeting CD3 and CD20	Cytopenias, CRS, neurotoxicity, electrolyte disturbances, infusion reactions, infections, tumor flare	Hospitalization recommended for first 2 doses. Premedications with acetaminophen, an antihistamine, and a glucocorticoid (at least cycle 1-3)

| Mosunetuzumab | BiTE targeting CD3 and CD20 | Cytopenias, CRS, edema, neuro-toxicity, infections, tumor flare, pruritus, electrolyte disturbances, peripheral neuropathy | Premedation with corticosteroids required for cycle 1 and 2 |

ADCC, antibody-dependent cell-mediated cytotoxicity; ALK, anaplastic lymphoma kinase; APL, acute promyelocytic leukemia; BCR-ABL, breakpoint cluster region-Abelson; BRAF, v-Raf murine sarcoma viral oncogene homolog B; BRK, protein tyrosine kinase 6; BSA, body surface area; CD, cluster of differentiation; c-Fms, macrophage colony–stimulating factor receptor; CHF, congestive heart failure; DVT, deep vein thrombosis; EGFR, epidermal growth factor receptor; FGFR, fibroblast growth factor receptor; Flt-3, FMS-like tyrosine kinase 3; FSH, follicle-stimulating hormone; GI, gastrointestinal; GnRH, gonadotropin-releasing hormone; H_1, histamine 1; H_2, histamine 2; HDAC, histone deacetylase inhibitor; HER2, human epidermal growth factor receptor 2; IGF-1R, insulin-like growth factor 1 receptor; IL-2, interleukin 2; INR, international ratio; InsR, insulin receptor; HTN, hypertension; JAK, Janus associated kinases; KRAS, V-Ki-ras2 Kirsten rat sarcoma viral oncogene homolog; Itk, IL2-inducible T-cell kinase; Lck, lymphocyte-specific protein tyrosine kinase; LFT, liver function tests; LH, luteinizing hormone; LVEF, left ventricular ejection fraction; MDR, multidrug resistance; MEK, mitogen-activated protein kinase; MET, hepatocyte growth factor receptor; MI, myocardial infarction/ischemia; m-TOR, mammalian target of rapamycin; MAb, monoclonal antibody; MAO, monoamine oxidase; N/V, nausea/vomiting; PAP, prostatic acid phosphatase; PAP-GM-CSF, prostatic acid phosphatase granulocyte macrophage colony–stimulating factor; PCP, pneumocystis pneumonia; PDGFR, platelet-derived growth factor receptor; PE, pulmonary embolism; PI-3K, phosphatidylinositol 3-kinase; PPIs, proton pump inhibitors; RET, rearranged during transfection; ROS1, v-ros avian UR2 sarcoma virus oncogene homolog 1; SCF, stem cell factor; SIADH, syndrome of inappropriate secretion of antidiuretic hormone; SJS, Stevens–Johnson syndrome; SOB, shortness of breath; SRC, sarcoma; TEN, toxic epidermal necrolysis; TKI, tyrosine kinase inhibitor; TLS, tumor lysis syndrome; TTP, thrombotic thrombocytopenia purpura; UGT, uridine diphosphate-glucuronosyltransferase; VEGF, vascular endothelial growth factor; VOD, veno-occlusive disease.

REFERENCES

1. DeVita VT, Rosenberg SA, Hellman S, eds. *Cancer: Principles and Practice of Oncology*. 12th ed. Lippincott Williams & Wilkins; 2022.
2. DiPiro J, Talbert R, Yee G, et al., eds. *Pharmacotherapy: A Pathophysiologic Approach*, 12th ed. McGraw Hill; 2023.
3. Lexicomp Online®. *Lexi-Drugs®*. Lexi-Comp, Inc; 2023.

Introduction to Radiation Oncology

19

Mustafaa Mahmood, Anthony Apicelli, Imran Zoberi, and Joanna C. Yang

R adiation oncology unifies the study of cancer with the therapeutic use of radiation therapy. At the highest level, radiation therapy is the use of ionizing radiation to kill cancer cells. The radiation oncologist is a physician with specialized training in the field of oncology who can help to decide when and how to best use radiation. Board certified radiation oncologists not only have residency training in clinical oncology but also Master's level knowledge of medical physics and radiation biology. Under the supervision of the radiation oncologist, an array of nonmedical specialists, including physicists, dosimetrists, and radiation therapists, assist in the planning and delivery of radiation to patients. This chapter introduces some of the basic principles of radiation oncology, some common treatment strategies, and an overview of the common reasons for referral to and consultation of a radiation oncologist in the clinical setting.

PHYSICAL AND BIOLOGIC PRINCIPLES

- **Ionizing radiation** is energy that causes the ejection of an orbital electron. It may be either electromagnetic (photons or gamma rays) or particulate (electrons, protons, or other atomic particles). **Radiation dose** is measured as energy per unit mass where 1 joule (J)/kg is 1 gray (Gy). The previously used term, **rad**, is equal to 1 centigray (cGy).
- Radiation causes DNA damage in both tumor cells and normal tissue. Healthy cells often have increased capacity to repair DNA damage compared to tumor cells, thus enhancing the therapeutic ratio in radiation delivery. In general, cells are most susceptible to radiation in the G2 and M phases of the cell cycle, while those in S phase are most radioresistant. Susceptible cells die most commonly via mitotic catastrophe, but can also die via apoptosis, necrosis, or other mechanisms. Hypoxic cells are thought to be less susceptible to radiation than well-oxygenated cells, as free radicals formed by ionizing radiation are more easily repaired in the absence of oxygen. **Fractionated radiation therapy** describes radiation given in multiple small doses over a given period instead of a single large dose and allows normal tissue to repair sublethal damage and repopulate while the tumor cells re-sort themselves in the cell cycle and become better oxygenated. A great deal of current research involves the cell cycle–signaling pathways involved in each aspect of the damage, repair, and reoxygenation pathways.[1]

RADIATION TREATMENT GOALS AND METHODS

- Radiation can be given by directing x-rays from a treatment machine such as a linear accelerator (linac) to the patient (**external-beam radiation therapy [EBRT]**) or by placing a radioactive source in close proximity to the tissue being treated using an instrument termed an applicator (**brachytherapy**). Brachytherapy (from Greek, meaning "short") is most often used in gynecologic cancers and prostate cancers. Sometimes both EBRT and brachytherapy are used to provide the optimal dose distribution.[2]
- Advances in imaging and external-beam delivery now allow for ablative radiation techniques (**stereotactic body radiation therapy [SBRT]**). These techniques require very

precise immobilization and deliver large doses of highly focused radiation in a few (i.e., 1–5) fractions. SBRT involves experienced physics and dosimetry support for accurate planning and delivery. SBRT works best for smaller, well-defined lesions such as limited brain/liver metastases, early-stage lung cancer, and oligometastases. SBRT is also increasingly being used in the reirradiation setting, as the dose heterogeneity inherent within SBRT treatment plans allows for rapid dose-falloff outside the treatment target (known as the planning target volume [PTV]).

- **Intensity-modulated radiation therapy** (IMRT) is now commonly used for a variety of tumor types to allow for more conformal treatment to the tumor while being able to better spare adjacent critical structures. The treating radiation oncologist outlines the target volume and organs-at-risk (OARs) and provides a list of dose objectives to the dosimetrist, who then optimizes the dose distribution to the target and OARs through an iterative process known as **inverse planning**. The resultant plan will use many different beam angles and many different beam apertures per angle to achieve this highly conformal dose distribution. Many linear accelerators across the country now allow for volumetric modulated arc therapy (VMAT), in which radiation treatment is delivered while the gantry of the linac is rotating around the patient. This technique has the advantage of faster dose delivery, which is particularly useful in treatment targets subject to respiratory motion as patients can be treated in the deep-inspiration-breath-hold position while maintaining patient comfort.
- Radiation can be given for curative or palliative intent. Often, it is combined with systemic therapy and surgery in the complete cancer care of the patient. It can be given before (neoadjuvant) or after (adjuvant) the surgery. Radiation therapy can also be used at the same time as chemotherapy (concurrent chemoradiation). Chemosensitization of the tumor cells can result in equivalent effect with reduced radiation dose, allowing the treating physician to better respect the tolerance of adjacent critical structures. Concurrent chemoradiotherapy regimens have become the mainstay of treatment for a number of solid malignancies as will be described briefly later.
- Accurate tumor **localization** is essential for optimum delivery of radiation. This can be done clinically (e.g., in palliative cases) or using radiographic studies. Clinical localizations, otherwise known as clinical setups, are quick and allow the patient to start treatment immediately but do not allow for conformal delivery of radiation. Clinical setup treatments often require hand calculations to determine linac output at the time of treatment. Alternatively, most radiotherapy treatments are planned using a computerized software known as a radiation therapy treatment planning system (TPS). Prior to treatment, the patient needs to have a **simulation** ("sim") in which they are brought to the radiation oncology department to obtain a simulation CT scan with the patient in the planned radiation therapy treatment position. Care must be taken to create a treatment position that is safe, comfortable, and reproducible. Treatment aids such as vaclock bags, alpha cradles, cushions, and masks can be used to help with immobilization. Increasingly, 4DCT scans are obtained to assess respiratory motion of structures in the thorax and upper abdomen. Once simulated, the patient's images are transferred to the TPS and the radiation oncologist, dosimetrist, and physicist work together to create a customized radiation plan for the patient. This plan will aid in delivering the maximal dose of radiation to tumor tissue while minimizing radiation exposure to healthy tissue. As the time between the initial consultation and the first treatment is often 2–3 weeks, patients are best served by early radiation oncology consultation, especially in settings where radiation therapy is to be initiated within certain time points of surgery or other treatments.
- In general, for external-beam radiotherapy, a patient will be placed on a flat, mobile treatment table each day during the course of radiation therapy. Marks on the patient's skin and any immobilization devices are used to align the patient in the same position as was used at time of simulation. Each treatment typically lasts approximately 30 minutes, with the majority of time spent in ensuring accurate and precise patient positioning. The total

course of radiation therapy can vary from 1 day (prostate brachytherapy, some stereotactic treatments) to several weeks (fractionated EBRT). Most fractionated treatments are given once a day, 5 days per week, although some treatments are given more frequently.

- **Proton-beam radiation therapy** is becoming increasingly common in centers across US and the world to help treat tumors that lie adjacent to critical dose-limiting structures. Due to unique properties of heavy charged particles, such as protons, nearly all of the ionizing energy is deposited in very narrow depth distribution (the **Bragg Peak**), resulting in little to no exit dose from the beam. The initial technique known as passive scatter is largely being replaced with pencil beam proton therapy, which utilizes magnets to steer the proton beam and deposit dose layer by layer, to allow for conformal dose delivery to the target. Proton therapy is most useful in pediatric malignancies, especially CNS malignancies, where nearby critical structures such as the brainstem, cochlea, optic apparatus, etc., may be difficult to spare with conventional techniques, or where one might want to limit dose to as low as reasonably achievable to prevent long-term complications from radiation therapy and decrease risk of secondary malignancy. Proton therapy is also useful in reirradiation cases where nearby OARs may be at or near tolerance dose from prior radiation treatments.

INDICATIONS FOR URGENT RADIATION THERAPY

Urgent radiation therapy is useful in certain oncologic emergencies. However, it is important to remember that in all settings, the effects of radiation therapy take time. Further, radiation therapy in the emergent setting must be considered carefully, as resource limitations can often affect treatment deliverability. Emergent radiotherapy is often performed using a clinical setup treatment approach, that is, without a simulation and computerized dose calculation using a TPS. Instead, hand calculations and portal images in the beam path are used for treatment setup. As such, care must be taken to ensure safe treatment delivery and clinical setups are never preferred as compared to simulation-based radiation plans. **Spinal cord compression** is an example of a radiation oncology emergency and is described further in Chapter 37. It is imperative that radiation oncology and surgical services are consulted early and that an MRI of the entire spine is obtained as soon as possible, preferably with and without contrast. **Brain metastases** can be treated with radiation therapy, with timing based on symptoms and performance status. **Uncontrolled bleeding** of tumors, which can be seen in gynecologic cancers, often responds well to radiation therapy. **Superior vena cava (SVC) syndrome**, in which the SVC is compressed by tumor (typically small-cell lung cancer), can be palliated by radiation, with resolution after weeks of therapy. In cases where SVC syndrome is causing immediate respiratory compromise, stenting is favored over radiotherapy due the inherent delay in radiotherapy treatment response.

LATE EFFECTS AND TISSUE TOLERANCE

Radiation therapy balances side effects to normal tissue with the need to deliver adequate doses to the tumor. Side effects are considered to be either **late** (months to years after completion of radiation therapy) or **acute** (during radiation therapy). The radiation tolerance of normal tissue varies from patient to patient and depends on dose, fractionation scheme, and exposed tissue volume. Radiation oncologists often reference the α/β ratio of a tissue, which is a unique metric that helps define the sensitivity of a particular tissue to different fractionation schemes. The most common fractionation scheme—otherwise known as conventional fractionation—typically delivers 1.8–2 Gy/day. Table 19-1 briefly summarizes the best available human data. These data represent only general parameters, and a radiation oncologist may elect to exceed these dose levels or be more conservative, based on individual patient considerations.

TABLE 19-1 NORMAL TISSUE TOLERANCE TO THERAPEUTIC IRRADIATION[a]

Critical Structure	Volume	Dose/Volume	Max Dose	Toxicity Rate	Toxicity Endpoint
Brain			<60 Gy	<3%	Symptomatic necrosis
Brain stem			<54 Gy	<5%	Neuropathy or necrosis
Optic nerve/chiasm			<55 Gy	<3%	Optic neuropathy
Spinal cord			50 Gy	0.2%	Myelopathy
Cochlea	Mean[b]	≤45 Gy		<30%	Sensory-neural hearing loss
Parotid, bilateral	Mean	≤25 Gy		<20%	Long-term salivary function <25%
Pharyngeal constrictors	Mean	≤50 Gy		<20%	Symptomatic dysphagia and aspiration
Larynx			<66 Gy	<20%	Vocal dysfunction
Larynx	Mean	<50 Gy		<30%	Aspiration
Lung	V20[c]	<30%		<20%	Symptomatic pneumonitis
Lung	Mean	7 Gy		5%	Symptomatic pneumonitis
Esophagus	Mean	<34 Gy		5–20%	Esophagitis
Pericardium	Mean	<26 Gy		<15%	Pericarditis
Heart	V25	<10%		<1%	Long-term cardiac events
Liver	Mean	<30–32 Gy		<5%	Radiation-induced liver disease
Kidney, bilateral	Mean	<15–18 Gy		<5%	Clinical dysfunction
Rectum	V50	<50%		<10%	Proctitis
Bladder[d]			<65 Gy	<6%	Cystitis

[a]Based upon data from older 3D conformal radiation techniques.
[b]Mean ≤5 Gy: The mean dose given to the whole organ should be ≤5 Gy.
[c]V20 ≤30%: The volume of tissue receiving >20 Gy should be ≤30% of the total volume.
[d]Variations in bladder size/shape/location during RT hampers the ability to generate accurate data.
Data adapted from Bentzen SM, Constine LS, Deasy JO, et al. Quantitative analyses of normal tissue effects in the clinic (QUANTEC). *Int J Radiat Oncol Biol Phys.* 2010;76(3 Suppl):S10–19.

COMMON TREATMENT GUIDELINES AND ASSOCIATED ACUTE EFFECTS

The following is a brief description of current commonly used treatment regimens. It must be emphasized that many patients are treated according to research protocols, which vary considerably. Common interests across the field of radiation oncology over the past decade have included a greater emphasis on hypofractionation and shorter treatment courses, largely due to improvements in imaging technology as well as for patient convenience as many radiation therapy centers are located in larger urban settings. Acute toxicities of radiation therapy typically result from direct tissue damage within the radiation path. Most radiation-alone acute effects can be managed on an outpatient basis. However, with higher doses of radiation, larger fields, and concurrent chemoradiation, acute effects increase substantially and may require inpatient management.

Palliative Therapy

Palliative treatment of brain and bone metastases is given at doses of 8–30 Gy over 1–10 fractions. This is a larger fraction size than used in most curative treatments because there is less concern about late effects and a greater interest in minimizing treatment time for patient convenience. A randomized trial from the Radiation Therapy Oncology Group (RTOG) has demonstrated that fraction sizes as large as 8 Gy in a single fraction can be used with equivalent rates of pain relief for noncomplicated bone metastases, especially for patients with poor performance status. The retreatment rates of these single-fraction regimens are higher than the 5–10 fraction courses, though.[3] During the COVID-19 pandemic, interest in minimizing patient visits led to the implementation of simulation-free RT for some palliative radiotherapy patients, an emerging paradigm.[4]

Bone Metastases

Bone metastases can be treated with 8–30 Gy over 1–10 fractions, depending on the number and location of lesions and the patient's life expectancy. Radiation therapy is very effective at decreasing pain, but its effects take time and typical time for a pain response is around 1 month. For this reason, it is important for oncologists to optimize a patient's pain management even if they are receiving palliative radiation therapy. For patients with multiple bone metastases and specific cancer types, an infusion of radioactive strontium, samarium, or yttrium can be used to decrease pain. Radium 223 chloride for bone-predominant castrate-resistant metastatic prostate cancer has been approved by the FDA and has shown a small overall survival advantage over best supportive care alone.[5] Recently, Lutetium-177-PSMA-617 has also shown a survival advantage in this population.[6] Recently, emerging data from a small phase II trial suggest that certain asymptomatic or minimally symptomatic high-risk bone metastases may benefit from prophylactic RT.[7]

Lung Cancer

Stereotactic radiation therapy has been shown to be promising for medically inoperable stage I and II lung cancer patients. Most studies that have evaluated surgery versus SBRT in the setting of medically operable early-stage lung cancer patient have been closed early due to low patient accrual, but the ongoing VALOR study being run the VA administration may give provide more insight on this topic in the coming decade. Stage III non–small-cell lung cancer is often treated with definitive radiotherapy, typically combined with chemotherapy and to a dose of 60 Gy. RTOG 0617 was a dose-escalation trial that showed that dose escalation beyond 70 Gy resulted in worse overall survival than 60 Gy.[8] Both chemotherapy and fractionated radiation therapy play a central role in the definitive management of limited-stage small-cell lung cancer.

In patients with lung cancer receiving concurrent or sequential chemotherapy and radiation therapy, one of the main acute toxicities is esophagitis. The subsequent odynophagia and dysphagia can lead to dehydration or significant weight loss, which may require inpatient management. Shortly after the completion of radiation therapy, radiation pneumonitis may occur. Anti-inflammatory steroid therapy is the mainstay of treatment for pneumonitis. In the long-term setting, intrathoracic radiotherapy dose to the heart may contribute to increased coronary artery disease events, a known late toxicity. In the modern era, IMRT and VMAT are increasingly being utilized to help deliver target dose while minimizing dose to normal tissues.

Esophageal Cancer

Radiation therapy with concurrent chemotherapy is used either as definitive treatment for esophageal/gastroesophageal junction tumors or as neoadjuvant treatment prior to surgery. Esophagitis is the major acute toxicity and this is typically managed symptomatically with narcotics as needed and intravenous fluids in the setting of decreased oral intake.

Central Nervous System Cancer

After maximal safe surgical resection, primary brain tumors may be treated to 50–60 Gy, depending on the area of the brain involved and the tumor histology. Brain metastases are traditionally treated with whole brain radiation therapy, most commonly 30 Gy in 10 fractions. Stereotactic radiosurgery (SRS) is increasingly being used for patients with limited brain metastases, as it can help spare the patient from neurocognitive side effects related to whole brain radiation therapy. Radiosurgery often involves just a single day of treatment, but sometimes treatments are fractionated, especially for larger tumors. Mild mental deterioration is seen in children and the elderly at standard palliative doses. Neurologic changes requiring hospitalization are uncommon. Hippocampal-avoidance whole brain radiation therapy and/or whole brain radiation therapy plus memantine can also be used to help mitigate neurocognitive decline.

Head and Neck Cancer

In general, early-stage head and neck cancers are treated equally well with surgery or radiation. Advanced head and neck cancers require surgery and postoperative adjuvant treatment, either with radiotherapy alone or concurrent chemoradiation, depending on the pathologic risk factors as well as institutional practice patterns. Unresectable tumors are treated with definitive chemoradiation. Doses are typically 60–70 Gy. Multiple treatments per day (hyperfractionation) can be used, but are associated with increased acute toxicity. Acute side effects include mucositis, xerostomia, loss of taste, esophagitis, odynophagia, dysphagia, and hoarseness. Acute toxicity often results in dehydration, which may require administration of IV fluids or placement of a temporary gastric tube for nutritional support. Chemotherapy has been shown to improve outcomes in the definitive radiotherapy of advanced head and neck cancers[9] at the cost of 1–3% treatment-associated mortality and 20–30% risk of hospitalization for dysphagia. Treatment-associated deaths are rare with radiotherapy alone, and the frequency of hospitalization for acute toxicity is generally ≤10%.

Breast Cancer

Radiation therapy is an important component of the management of breast cancer and is typically used after surgery. It is almost always indicated after breast conservation surgery (lumpectomy) as well as in postmastectomy patients with large initial tumors, positive lymph nodes, or positive resection margins. Hypofractionated courses have become standard in whole breast radiation therapy as part of breast conservation. This is feasible in light of the low α/β ratio for breast cancer and radiobiologic advantage for higher dose per fraction. For early-stage breast cancer treated with breast conservation, accelerated partial breast irradiation is an accepted standard for those patients with pathologic features meeting the 2016 ASTRO criteria as listed in consensus guidelines. Acute side effects are usually limited to skin reactions, but pneumonitis, lymphedema, and pericarditis can occur.

Prostate Cancer

Prostate cancer can be treated with either external-beam radiation therapy or prostate brachytherapy ("seeds"). External-beam radiation doses range from 70 to 80 Gy for high-risk disease. Hypofractionation is standard in low- and intermediate-risk disease, paradigms that have garnered significant interest due to the very low α/β ratio of prostate cancer cells. The most common side effects are urethritis, cystitis, and proctitis, which are managed on an outpatient basis in the vast majority of patients. Rates of impotence and cure are similar for external-beam radiation therapy, brachytherapy, and radical prostatectomy paradigms; as such, patients often benefit from meeting to discuss the advantages and disadvantages of each approach. Androgen-deprivation therapy is usually given on a neoadjuvant, concurrent, and adjuvant basis for patients who have either unfavorable intermediate- or high-risk prostate cancer. In patients with minimal urinary symptoms at baseline, brachytherapy boost may be preferred over external beam boost for those receiving pelvic nodal and prostate radiotherapy.[10]

Colon/Rectal Cancer

Radiation is not often used in colon cancers, except in those that are locally advanced (often fixed or perforated) and require preoperative radiation therapy, as dose is often limited by the presence of small bowel in the radiation field, which has a low tolerance to radiation. The confines of the pelvis make surgical resection of rectal cancer more challenging than that of colon cancer. Preoperative radiation therapy is used in most cases to facilitate surgical resection, for sphincter preservation, and to treat the poorly accessible presacral lymph nodes. Rectal cancer radiation therapy is often delivered as either short-course (25 Gy in 5 fractions) or long-course (50.4 Gy in 28 fractions). Total neoadjuvant therapy is supported by the consensus guidelines. Radiation therapy–induced proctitis is generally quite mild unless concurrent chemotherapy (generally 5-fluorouracil) is administered, in which case proctitis can be severe enough to cause dehydration leading to hospitalization. Patients may need nutritional support.

Anal Cancer

Most anal malignancies can be managed with definitive radiotherapy plus adjuvant chemotherapy, with surgery reserved for salvage. Although generally of squamous histology, anal cancers respond well to low doses of radiotherapy. IMRT is standard and doses are guided by RTOG 0529.[11] Classically, concurrent chemotherapy is mitomycin-C and 5-fluorouracil. Acute toxicities are mainly myelosuppression caused by mitomycin-C, proctitis, cystitis, hemorrhoid exacerbation, and dermatitis in the perineum. Hospitalization is sometimes required during the last week of treatment or the following week secondary to dehydration from diarrhea or pain control from proctitis or skin reactions.

Pediatric Cancer

Radiation is used in many pediatric tumors. Total-body irradiation and irradiation of sanctuary sites are used in leukemia, and many pediatric lymphoma protocols involve local irradiation. Many sarcomas are treated with radiation after or instead of surgery in an effort to pursue limb preservation. Most CNS tumors are treated in part with radiation. Treatment varies by site and long-term effects on development limit dose. Proton-beam radiation therapy (see Radiation Treatment Goals and Methods) may be especially useful for pediatric patients, so as to reduce the likelihood of secondary malignancy or other late effects of radiation.

Lymphoma

Lymphomas are very radioresponsive, and doses from 20 to 45 Gy are used, depending on the type of lymphoma and chemotherapy regimen. Most indolent lymphomas are treated with lower doses, 24–30 Gy, while chemorefractory diffuse large B-cell lymphomas may require higher doses of 40–45Gy. Treatment is normally very well tolerated, with some cytopenia and fatigue with a larger field, some nausea/vomiting when the abdomen is treated, and esophagitis when treating the neck and mediastinal nodes. The International Lymphoma Radiation Oncology Group (ILROG) provides guidelines for treatment.

Total-Body Irradiation

Total-body irradiation is used as part of the preparative scheme for peripheral blood stem cell transplant protocols. Treatment requires robust physics support and specialized treatment vaults due to the need to treat patients at farther distances away from the linac than used in typical radiation treatments. Treatment with fractionated total-body irradiation to doses around 1,200–1,400 cGy given BID or TID at a low dose rate is most common. This is normally well tolerated, except for self-limiting parotitis and occasionally, nausea and vomiting. More infrequently, pneumonitis may develop after treatment, requiring a course of high-dose steroids. For younger patients, fertility counseling is recommended.

Gynecologic Cancer

Cervical and uterine corpus cancers are often treated with radiation therapy. Most advanced cervical cancers are treated with definitive radiotherapy, and numerous phase III trials have demonstrated equivalent survival outcome between radical hysterectomy and radiotherapy for early cervical cancer. Radiation is generally used as adjuvant therapy in uterine corpus tumors. Radiotherapy for most gynecologic malignancies uses brachytherapy because it better delivers the dose to the at-risk tissues while sparing the bladder and rectum. Brachytherapy expertise is highly important and referral to a high-volume center is recommended. Doses are anywhere from 50 to 85 Gy. Patients can develop proctitis, enteritis, and urethritis/cystitis, depending on the dose and tumor location. As with other sites, the frequency of admission for acute toxicity increases with concurrent chemoradiation.

KEY POINTS TO REMEMBER

- Consult a radiation oncology specialist before starting therapeutic chemotherapy or surgery to allow for optimum multidisciplinary management of the malignancy. Evaluating patients in their presenting state is valuable to the radiation oncologist.
- When radiation toxicity is in the differential diagnosis, consult a radiation oncologist, who can help with diagnosis and management.
- Consider urgent radiation oncology consults when faced with oncologic emergencies such as cord compression, SVC syndrome, new brain metastases, or uncontrolled bleeding. However, it is important to remember that the effects of radiation therapy on the tumor take time and immediate symptom relief may not be seen.

REFERENCES

1. Tepper JE, Foote RL, Michalski JM, eds. *Gunderson & Tepper's Clinical Radiation Oncology.* 5th ed. Elsevier; 2020.
2. Halperin EC, Wazer DE, Perez CA, Brady LW, eds. *Principles and Practices of Radiation Oncology.* 7th ed. Lippincott Williams & Wilkins; 2018.
3. Hartsell WF, Scott CB, Bruner DW, et al. Randomized trial of short- versus long-course radiotherapy for palliation of painful bone metastases. *J Natl Cancer Inst.* 2005;97:798–804.

4. Schiff JP, Zhao T, Huang, Y, et al. Simulation-free radiation therapy: an emerging form of treatment planning to expedite plan generation for patients receiving palliative radiation therapy. *Adv Radiat Oncol.* 2023;8(1):101091.
5. Parker C, Nilsson S, Heinrich D, et al; ALSYMPCA Investigators. Alpha emitter radium-223 and survival in metastatic prostate cancer. *N Engl J Med.* 2013;369:213–223.
6. Sartor O, de Bono J, Chi KN, et al; VISION Investigators. Lutetium-177-PSMA-617 for metastatic castration-resistant prostate cancer. *N Engl J Med.* 2021;385(12):1091–1103.
7. Gillespie EF, Yang JC, Mathis NJ, et al. Prophylactic radiation therapy versus standard of care for patients with high-risk asymptomatic bone metastases: a multicenter, randomized phase II clinical trial. *J Clin Oncol.* 2024;42(1):38–46.
8. Bradley JD, Paulus R, Komaki R, et al. Standard-dose versus high-dose conformal radiotherapy with concurrent and consolidation carboplatin plus paclitaxel with or without cetuximab for patients with stage IIIA or IIIB non-small-cell lung cancer (RTOG 0617): a randomised, two-by-two factorial phase 3 study. *Lancet Oncol.* 2015;16:187–199.
9. Pignon JP, Le Maître A, Maillard E; MACH-NC Collaborative Group. Meta-analysis of chemotherapy in head and neck cancer (MACH-NC): an update on 93 randomised trials and 17,346 patients. *Radiother Oncol.* 2009;92:4–14.
10. Oh J, Tyldesley S, Pai H, et al. An updated analysis of the survival endpoints of ASCENDE-RT. *Int J Radiat Oncol Biol Phys.* 2023;115(5):1061–1070.
11. Kachnic LA, Winter KA, Myerson RJ, et al. Long-term outcomes of NRG Oncology/RTOG 0529: a phase 2 evaluation of dose-painted intensity modulated radiation therapy in combination with 5-fluorouracil and mitomycin-C for the reduction of acute morbidity in anal canal cancer. *Int J Radiat Oncol Biol Phys.* 2022;112(1):146–157.

Introduction to Immunotherapy

Brett H. Herzog, Tanner M. Johanns, and Jeffrey P. Ward

20

GENERAL PRINCIPLES

Cytotoxic chemotherapy and molecular targeted therapies have traditionally formed the backbone of standard-of-care interventions for patients with metastatic solid tumors. Common to both therapeutic modalities is that their mechanisms of action focus on processes required by tumor cells for growth and/or survival. An improved understanding of how the immune system generates and sustains systemic responses, while avoiding damage to healthy tissues, has led to the development of diverse classes of immunotherapeutics that serve to remove inhibitory constraints on T-cells as well as provide activating signals. Harnessing the immune system as a therapeutic agent has several advantages. T-cells exhibit exquisite specificity against their targets and can differentiate friend from foe by even a single amino acid change in a peptide presented by molecules of the major histocompatibility complex (MHC). The ability of the adaptive immune system to generate long-lasting memory can also be harnessed to prevent recurrence of disease. Recent studies have also shown the proliferation of adoptive cellular therapies that have dramatically changed the treatment landscape of hematologic malignancies.

Immunotherapy was the first therapeutic modality to be used to treat otherwise inoperable tumors. William Coley treated inoperable sarcomas with a crude form of immunotherapy in the early 1890s by injecting a mixture of bacterial products directly into tumors. This approach was based on several observed spontaneous remissions in cancer patients following severe bacterial infections.[1] Early interest in immunotherapy was tempered by inconsistent results and general lack of mechanistic insight, eventually being supplanted by the promise of radiation and chemotherapy. However, as a deeper appreciation for the important role of immunity in the treatment of cancer has evolved, a renewed interest in immunotherapies emerged.

This chapter will provide a brief overview of the various immunotherapeutic approaches currently being used in the treatment of cancer. Each section will give a brief description of the rationale or mechanism of action for each class of immunotherapy, the current status of development or FDA approval, as well as the important side effects with approaches to their management. Additional details, such as specific treatment regimens and indications for use can be found in the other disease-specific chapters of this manual.

CYTOKINES AND AGONISTS

Coley toxins are thought to act by eliciting an inflammatory response to nonspecifically activate an immune response via the release of cytokines. This ultimately leads to the recruitment of circulating innate (granulocytes and monocytes) and adaptive (predominantly T-cells) effector cells into the tumor tissue with the hope that a productive antitumor response is generated. The first immunotherapies acted similarly and included various cytokines and immunostimulatory molecules. While some of these agents are still used clinically, their overall use has decreased due to their side-effect profile and emergence of more specific immune-activating agents. This section will review those agents that remain in current clinical practice.

BCG

Bacillus Calmette-Guérin (BCG) is an avirulent strain of *Mycobacterium bovis* that is used as a preventative vaccine against *Mycobacterium tuberculosis*. The immunostimulatory effect of BCG is thought to be mediated by the activation of toll-like receptors (TLRs), specifically TLR2, TLR4, and TLR9. Agonism of TLRs leads to NF-κB activation and production of type I interferons (IFNs), IL-6, and IL-12. TLR activation also leads to the maturation of antigen-presenting cells, which facilitate the priming of antigen-specific T-cells. The antineoplastic properties of BCG were inferred from epidemiologic observations that noted a decreased incidence of cancer in patients with tuberculosis, and a lower incidence of leukemia among immunized neonates.[2] While the therapeutic utilization of BCG was trialed in various malignancies, its efficacy was most pronounced in bladder cancer. Intravesical BCG remains the standard of care for patients with high-risk, nonmuscle invasive bladder cancer (high-grade Ta, all T1) and bladder carcinoma in situ. Intravesical BCG is well tolerated with the exception of local bladder irritation; however, the development of local irritation is generally associated with a more favorable antitumor response. More severe side effects can occur in the setting of systemic dissemination of live BCG organisms, which typically occurs in immunocompromised hosts.

High-Dose IL-2

IL-2 is required for the proliferation of T-cells following stimulation of the T-cell receptor (TCR), and was the first FDA-approved immunotherapy to be used in patients with cancer. High-dose IL-2 has been given therapeutically in a wide range of malignancies, but its efficacy is largely limited to metastatic renal cell carcinoma and metastatic melanoma. While overall objective response rates are low (~15–20%), approximately one-third to one-half of responders will have a sustained complete remission (CR)[3] and IL-2 was the first systemic agent to yield effective cures of metastatic cancer.[4] Administration of high-dose IL-2 is complicated by serious associated toxicities, particularly capillary leak syndrome, which results in massive fluid extravasation into visceral organs and end organ dysfunction which limits its administration to the intensive care unit setting for close observation and management of hypotension with intravenous fluids and pressor support. These side effects are rapidly reversible following cessation of therapy and consensus guidelines for its use have been developed.[5]

Interferon-α

IFN-α is a pleiotropic cytokine that has been used in the treatment of more than 14 different malignancies, including both hematologic and solid tumors.[6] The therapeutic properties of IFN-α are thought to be multifactorial, and include the following: (i) an antiproliferative effect; (ii) upregulation of MHC class I molecules, thereby enhancing recognition of tumor cells by CD8+ T-cells; (iii) increasing the cytolytic activity of T-cells and NK cells; and (iv) stimulation of macrophage activity. The clinical activity of IFN-α was first demonstrated in patients with hairy cell leukemia and Kaposi sarcoma. In 1995, the FDA approved the use of adjuvant IFN-α in patients with locally advanced melanoma at high risk of disease recurrence following resection (node positive, stage IIB through IIIB), although its usage for this indication has been supplanted by the development of checkpoint inhibitors.[7] Similar to high-dose IL-2, the use of IFN-α is limited by its significant side-effect profile, which includes flu-like symptoms, fatigue, anorexia, weight loss, and depression, which can prevent administration of a full treatment course.

VACCINES

One of the most important medical discoveries in the past millennia is the advent of prophylactic vaccinations to treat infectious diseases. Unfortunately, success has been more tempered when it comes to the generation of therapeutic vaccines to treat chronic illnesses, such as the human immunodeficiency virus or malignancies. A number of novel agents are in early and late phases of development, and will be discussed below in further detail.

Sipuleucel-T

Sipuleucel-T, or Provenge, is a vaccine that generates a host immune response against the prostate cancer–associated antigen, prostatic acid phosphatase (PAP), and has been approved for the treatment of patients with asymptomatic, castrate-resistant, metastatic prostate cancer. The generation of this vaccine is a form of autologous cellular immunotherapy whereby peripheral blood mononuclear cells are removed from patients by leukopheresis, cultured ex vivo with a fusion protein of PAP and GM-CSF, then reinfused back into the patient at regular interval doses to prime and boost a tumor-specific immune response. This approach has been tested in the phase III setting, and despite a lack of a PSA biochemical response, it did demonstrate an increase in median overall survival of approximately 4 months compared to placebo.[8]

Personalized Vaccines

Genomic alterations that accumulate during cellular transformation lead to the expression of novel mutant peptides, that once bound to MHC class I and II molecules, can be recognized by the immune system as foreign. These tumor-specific mutant antigens, or neoantigens, can serve as the targets of the host immune response against cancer, and multiple groups have developed approaches to develop personalized neoantigen vaccines with the goal of either directly treating metastatic disease or preventing recurrence following surgical resection in the adjuvant setting. In an initial phase I study, neoantigens that were computationally selected from next-generation sequencing data and encoded into synthetic long peptides were utilized for vaccination of six patients with melanoma. No serious adverse events were seen. While four patients had no evidence of disease recurrence 25 months after vaccination, the remaining two patients went on to have complete responses when treated with anti–PD-1 antibody therapy at the time of recurrence.[9] In an independent first-in-human trial, RNA vaccines targeting neoantigens induced radiographic responses in two of five vaccinated melanoma patients.[10] Additional early-phase trials have been conducted that demonstrate the safety and feasibility of generating and administering personalized neoantigen peptide vaccines in melanoma, bladder cancer, and non–small-cell lung cancer,[11] even in a suitable timeframe to be included in standard-of-care first-line therapy.[12] Likewise, RNA-based vaccines have demonstrated preliminary evidence of efficacy in delaying recurrence of pancreatic cancer in the adjuvant setting.[13] Results from ongoing phase III studies of personalized neoantigen vaccines will ultimately determine if this treatment strategy will become a standard-of-care treatment option.

CHECKPOINT BLOCKADE

T-cells must integrate a combination of activating and inhibitory stimuli in order to recognize and ultimately destroy a tumor cell target. Engagement of the TCR by a complex of tumor-derived peptide presented by an HLA molecule gives each T-cell exacting specificity. However, a B7 family molecule on an antigen-presenting cell must deliver a second signal to CD28 in order to fully activate a T-cell's effector functions. In addition, once the T-cell's activating machinery has been engaged, inhibitory molecules are expressed in order to turn off the response and serve as a "checkpoint" to prevent collateral damage to normal tissue. Three of these inhibitory receptors have served as targetable molecules to "unleash" T-cells to kill tumor cell targets: (i) CTLA-4, which functions by attenuating costimulation through CD28 via direct competition for binding to B7 molecules, (ii) PD-1, which upon recognition of its ligand PD-L1 interferes with downstream signaling from the TCR, and (iii) LAG-3, which regulates stimuli delivered by its ligand, MHC class II.

CTLA-4 Blockade

Ipilimumab is a fully human antibody to CTLA-4 that prevents the dampening of T-cell responses soon after activation. In contrast to chemotherapy or targeted agents whose functions are directed at the tumor, ipilimumab instead targets the host's immune system. In two phase III trials, ipilimumab showed an overall survival benefit among patients with metastatic melanoma and became the first agent to dramatically improve the outcome of patients with this disease.[14,15] Although only 10–15% of patients with metastatic melanoma have an objective clinical response after receiving single-agent ipilimumab, these responses can be very durable and last many years.[16] More recently, tremelimumab, another CTLA-4 blocking antibody, has achieved FDA approval in combination with a PD-L1 blocking antibody in hepatocellular carcinoma. Notably, some patients treated with CTLA-4 blockade will first appear to have disease progression on imaging studies due to an immune infiltrate into areas of tumor, which can complicate disease assessment using conventional RECIST criteria. For this reason, responses are typically not measured until 12 weeks after initiating therapy, and the appearance of new subcentimeter lesions not associated with clinical deterioration should not prevent further treatment.

The side-effect profile of ipilimumab is dramatically different from that seen with traditional cytotoxic chemotherapy, and can essentially mimic autoimmunity due to breaking of self-tolerance against normal tissues. These immune-mediated adverse effects are common and a high degree of vigilance is necessary in order to diagnose and initiate treatment with corticosteroids in order to prevent serious or life-threatening complications.[17] Rash and pruritus typically occur 3–4 weeks after receiving the first dose of ipilimumab, and the development of vitiligo has been seen in a small percentage of patients. Severe diarrhea (at least six bowel movements daily) can be seen in nearly 20% of patients, typically beginning about 5 weeks after starting therapy, and this autoimmune colitis can lead to bowel obstruction or perforation. Hepatotoxicity, typically manifested as an asymptomatic rise in liver function tests, can be seen in <10% of patients, typically within 6–7 weeks of starting ipilimumab. Endocrinopathies, the most serious of which is hypophysitis, associated with headaches, nausea, and visual disturbances, are typically seen later (~9 weeks). Notably, patients should have blood tests to monitor pituitary, thyroid, adrenal, and gonadal hormones before and during therapy. It is stressed that these toxicities may be delayed, or may rarely occur after the first dose of ipilimumab, and close follow-up and good communication between patients and providers is necessary.

PD-1/PD-L1 Blockade

PD-1 is expressed on the surface of T-cells soon after activation and is triggered by its ligand PD-L1, which can be expressed on many different types of immune cells as well as endothelial cells and tumor cells. Numerous monoclonal antibodies targeting both PD-1 and PD-L1 have been developed that are either FDA approved or in clinical development for both hematologic and solid tumor malignancies. PD-1/PD-L1 blockade is now an essential treatment modality included into the standard of care of patients with metastatic, locally advanced, and early-stage melanoma and NSCLC as well as being indicated for multiple other genitourinary, gastrointestinal, gynecologic, cutaneous, head and neck and hematologic malignancies, and depending on the disease type may be given alone or in combination with cytotoxic chemotherapy, CTLA-4 antagonists, or kinase inhibitors. Additional discussion of these individual disease histologies can be found in disease-specific chapters of this manual.

The side-effect profiles of PD-1/PD-L1 blockade are more favorable than that of ipilimumab, with fewer patients experiencing serious adverse events. The most common side effects include fatigue, diarrhea, rash, pruritus, and hypothyroidism, with most being able to be managed in the outpatient setting. Of particular concern is the development of pneumonitis, which although uncommon, can become life threatening if not identified early and treated with corticosteroids.

LAG-3 Blockade

Lymphocyte-activation gene 3 (LAG-3) is an inhibitory cell-surface molecule expressed on T-cells, and host myeloid cells and can also be upregulated on tumor cells, including melanoma.[18] In a randomized phase 2–3 trial, the combination of relatlimab, a blocking antibody against LAG-3, and nivolumab, a PD-1 blocking antibody, improved progression-free survival of previously untreated patients with metastatic or unresectable melanoma compared to nivolumab alone (10.1 vs. 4.6 months).[19] Results of this trial led to FDA approval of the relatlimab/nivolumab combination as a standard-of-care frontline option in this population.

ADOPTIVE CELLULAR THERAPIES

While cytokine and checkpoint blockade immunotherapies are administered to patients and rely on the direct expansion and cytotoxicity of host T-cells, adoptive cellular therapy approaches utilize an ex vivo expansion step to generate large numbers of tumor-specific effector cells. The identification of IL-2 as a T-cell growth factor enabled the first clinical trials of tumor-infiltrating lymphocyte, or TIL, therapies by the Rosenberg group at the National Cancer Institute in the 1980s, spurring further innovations in cellular therapies leading to the development of chimeric antigen receptor (CAR) T-cell therapies.

Tumor-Infiltrating Lymphocytes (TIL)

The identification that metastatic tumor deposits are infiltrated with tumor-specific T-cells that could be expanded to large numbers ex vivo by repetitive rounds of stimulation in the presence of IL-2 led to the initial trials of TIL therapy for melanoma in the 1980s, with some patients demonstrating durable responses lasting decades.[20] In the largest phase 3 trial of TIL therapy, patients with metastatic melanoma, 86% of whom had disease refractory to anti–PD-1 therapies, were randomized to ipilimumab or a short course of lympho-depleting cyclophosphamide/fludarabine chemotherapy followed by a single infusion of 5×10^9–2×10^{11} TIL and a maximum of 15 doses of high-dose IL-2.[21] This study demonstrated an overall survival benefit from 18.9 months in the ipilimumab group to 25.8 months with TIL. A commercially generated autologous TIL product, lifileucel, recently demonstrated an overall response rate of 41% in patients with metastatic melanoma refractory to anti–PD-1 or anti–PD-L1-directed therapies.[22] Adverse events from TIL therapies are mostly related to the lymphodepleting chemotherapy and administration of high-dose IL-2, necessitating treatments at facilities with experience in their use. Based on these encouraging results multiple trials of TIL therapies are ongoing in melanoma, NSCLC, and cervical cancer, among other histologies, with expected FDA approval on the horizon.

Chimeric Antigen Receptors (CARs)

CAR T-cells are genetically modified autologous T-cells reengineered to express a fusion protein consisting of an intracellular T-cell activation domain linked to an extracellular antigen-recognition moiety. Target cells expressing the cognate antigen will activate CAR-expressing T-cells in a manner that bypasses HLA restriction. The initial clinical experience with CAR T-cells to gain FDA approval targeted the B-cell antigen CD19. When reengineered cells come into contact with a CD19-expressing target, they readily become activated and eliminate the target cell via direct cytotoxicity.

Early-phase clinical trials conducted in patients with both indolent B-cell malignancies (NHL or CLL) and aggressive high-grade disease (acute B-cell lymphoblastic leukemia, B-ALL) consistently reported a high response rate, including a number of CRs (reviewed by Ramos et al.[23]). In patients with relapsed or refractory B-ALL, the addition of anti-CD19 CAR T-cells to a standard salvage chemotherapy regimen resulted in a CR rate of 88% compared to 44% for those patients receiving salvage chemotherapy alone. Impressively, the majority of patients with a CR also had no evidence of minimal residual disease (MRD).[24] Consistently, a phase I study of patients with relapsed B-ALL treated with anti-CD19 CAR T-cells and a nonmyeloablative conditioning regimen reported a 70% CR rate with 60% of patients having no evidence of MRD.[25] While the long-term outcomes of CAR T-cell therapy in patients with relapsed or refractory B-ALL is confounded by the fact that many have undergone allogeneic stem cell transplantation after achieving CR, the high remission rate in an otherwise chemotherapy-resistant disease is impressive. Importantly, adoptively transferred CAR T-cells proliferate and can persist for >6 months after infusion.[26] A phase III trial of axicabtagene ciloleucel, a CD19-directed CAR, in patients with refractory diffuse large B-cell lymphoma demonstrated an improvement in event-free survival compared to salvage chemotherapy of (8.3 vs. 2.0 months, respectively).[27] There are currently FDA approvals for CD19-directed CAR T-cells for refractory lymphoma and ALL as well as BCMA-directed CAR T-cells in multiple myeloma, with a number of novel agents undergoing study in clinical trials.

Several unique complications related to CAR T-cell therapy have been reported in early trials and include cytokine release syndrome (CRS) and hypogammaglobulinemia. CRS generally develops within the first week after infusion of CAR T-cells but can be seen up to 2–3 weeks later. It is characterized by the development of persistent fevers, hypotensive shock, and respiratory collapse. This pattern displays similar clinical manifestations to hemophagocytic lymphohistiocytosis (HLH) and is related to the massive release of proinflammatory cytokines such as TNF-α, IFN-γ, IL-2, IL-10, and IL-6. The severity of clinical symptoms appears to be correlated with the degree in elevation of these cytokines, in particular, IL-6. In fact, CRP, which is highly correlated with IL-6 expression levels, is predictive of patients who will subsequently develop clinically significant CRS.[28] As such, CRS can be effectively treated with tocilizumab, an antibody against the IL-6 receptor, or siltuximab, an antibody against IL-6, often with rapid clinical improvement.

Due to the long-term persistence of CAR T-cells in treated patients and the normal expression of CD19 on all mature B-cells, patients develop B-cell aplasia, leading to a lack of antibody production. While the effects of hypogammaglobulinemia are not evident until months to years after treatment, it does result in an immunocompromised state, leading to increased susceptibility to infection or sepsis from encapsulated organisms and respiratory infections. In addition, immunity from prior vaccinations is often lost as well. Treatment involves monthly infusions with IVIG.

BISPECIFIC MOLECULES

Retargeting therapeutic approaches comprise a class of immunotherapies that attempt to enhance antitumor immunity by bringing host immune effector cells (i.e., T-cells or NK cells) into direct contact with tumor cells via an engineered fusion protein. These can take several forms, including engineered antibodies and scaffolds that include defined MHC class I molecules.

Bispecific T-cell Engagers (BiTEs®) refer to a molecule that combines two single-chain variable fragments (scFvs) into one molecule.[29] A variable fragment (Fv) refers to the minimal binding domain of a monoclonal antibody that determines its antigen specificity and generally consists of the third complementary determining region (CDR3) of the heavy and light chain linked covalently. In patients with refractory B-cell precursor ALL treated with blinatumomab, a CD19 × CD3 BiTE, the CR rate was 44%, enabling 24% of patients to undergo allogeneic stem cell transplant.[30] Blinatumomab is FDA approved for treatment of relapsed or refractory B-cell ALL.

An alternative method of constructing a retargeting molecule is to utilize the structure of a monoclonal antibody that is engineered to contain binding sites of interest. Mosunetuzumab-axgb is a humanized full-length IgG1 bispecific antibody with both CD20 and CD3 binding moieties in a 1:1 ratio. Mosunetuzumab simultaneously binds CD20 on a malignant B-cell and CD3 on a host T-cell, providing T-cell "signal one" and leading to TCR signaling. In a phase I–II trial, mosunetuzumab demonstrated a complete response rate of 60% in a cohort of relapsed or refractory follicular lymphoma patients who had received two or more prior therapies, leading to FDA approval in late 2022.[31] Glofitamab is a separate CD20 × CD3 bispecific antibody with two CD20 and one CD3 binding moieties, enabling binding to two separate malignant T-cells. In a phase I–II study of patients with relapsed or refractory DLBCL who had received at least two lines of therapy, glofitamab demonstrated an overall response rate of 39% and 12 months progression-free survival of 37%, with responses seen in patients refractory to prior CAR T-cell therapy.[27] Glofitamab achieved FDA approval in 2023. Effective T-cell–targeting bispecific antibodies are not only limited to lymphoma. Teclistamab and elranatamab are both BCMA × CD3 bispecific antibodies that are FDA approved for use in multiple myeloma, providing validation that the bispecific antibody approach is active in this disease.[32,33]

Bispecific antibodies are also in late-stage development for solid tumors. Identifying tumor-specific targets for bispecifics is a challenge in the solid tumor space, as expression in normal tissues can lead to on-target toxicity. Tarlatamab is a bispecific T-cell engager targeting delta-like ligand 3 (DLL3), which is commonly expressed in small-cell lung cancer, to CD3. In a phase I study, tarlatamab demonstrated an overall response rate of 23.4% in a population of relapsed/refractory small cell lung cancer, with an overall survival of 13.2 months.[34] Larger studies are ongoing to validate this finding and move toward FDA approval. There are a significant number of additional bispecific molecules in clinical development, many directly leading to CD3 engagement after targeting tumor-specific antigens, while others include moieties targeting CD28 or 4-1BB to provide costimulatory, or "signal two" signaling to T-cells. Forthcoming data from these studies may lead to additional FDA approvals in the future.

Antibodies are not the only molecules that can be utilized as tumor cell–targeting moieties in bispecifics. Tebentafusp is a bispecific molecule that includes a recombinant TCR specific for the gp100 peptide in complex with HLA-A*02:01 molecules and a CD3 engaging antibody. Unlike other bispecific molecules, tebentafusp is HLA-restricted to HLA-A*02:01 positive patients. In an open-label, randomized phase III trial of patients with previously untreated metastatic uveal melanoma, tebentafusp demonstrated an overall survival benefit at 1 year of 73% compared to 59% in the control group receiving the investigator choice of therapy.[35]

Due to their mechanism of action, CRS is a frequent complication of T-cell engaging bispecific antibodies, which can be severe. Management is similar to CRS developing during the course of CAR T-cell therapy.

CONCLUSION

Although immunotherapy is one of the oldest forms of cancer treatment, advances in our capacity to modulate immune responses have only recently brought multiple immuno-oncology agents into the standard of care. Since the first approval of a checkpoint inhibitor, the CTLA-4 antagonist ipilimumab, in 2010, and the first approvals of the PD-1 antagonists pembrolizumab and nivolumab in 2014, new agents have rapidly achieved regulatory approval with indications in both solid and hematologic tumors. Checkpoint inhibitors are now given as standard-of-care options in metastatic, locally advanced, and early-stage solid tumors, and knowledge of how to manage checkpoint-inhibitor–induced immune-related adverse events is now mandatory for the medical oncologist. Encouraging results from novel immuno-oncology approaches, including bispecific antibodies and cellular therapies, are a cause for optimism that even more advances are on the horizon.

REFERENCES

1. Coley WB II. Contribution to the knowledge of sarcoma. *Ann Surg.* 1891;14(3):199–220.
2. Gandhi NM, Morales A, Lamm DL. Bacillus Calmette-Guerin immunotherapy for genitourinary cancer. *BJU Int.* 2013;112(3):288–297.
3. Rosenberg SA. IL-2: the first effective immunotherapy for human cancer. *J Immunol.* 2014; 192(12):5451–5458.
4. Atkins MB, Lotze MT, Dutcher JP, et al. High-dose recombinant interleukin 2 therapy for patients with metastatic melanoma: analysis of 270 patients treated between 1985 and 1993. *J Clin Oncol.* 1999;17(7):2105–2116.
5. Dutcher JP, Schwartzentruber DJ, Kaufman HL, et al. High dose interleukin-2 (Aldesleukin)—expert consensus on best management practices-2014. *J Immunother Cancer.* 2014;2(1):26.
6. Kirkwood J. Cancer immunotherapy: the interferon-alpha experience. *Semin Oncol.* 2002;29(3 Suppl 7):18–26.
7. Kirkwood JM, Strawderman MH, Ernstoff MS, Smith TJ, Borden EC, Blum RH. Interferon alfa-2b adjuvant therapy of high-risk resected cutaneous melanoma: the Eastern Cooperative Oncology Group Trial EST 1684. *J Clin Oncol.* 1996;14(1):7–17.
8. Kantoff PW, Higano CS, Shore ND, et al; IMPACT Study Investigators. Sipuleucel-T immunotherapy for castration-resistant prostate cancer. *N Engl J Med.* 2010;363(5):411–422.
9. Ott PA, Hu Z, Keskin DB, et al. An immunogenic personal neoantigen vaccine for patients with melanoma. *Nature.* 2017;547(7662):217–221.
10. Sahin U, Derhovanessian E, Miller M, et al. Personalized RNA mutanome vaccines mobilize poly-specific therapeutic immunity against cancer. *Nature.* 2017;547(7662):222–226.
11. Ott PA, Hu-Lieskovan S, Chmielowski B, et al. A Phase Ib trial of personalized neoantigen therapy plus anti-PD-1 in patients with advanced melanoma, non-small cell lung cancer, or bladder cancer. *Cell.* 2020;183(2):347–362.e24.
12. Awad MM, Govindan R, Balogh KN, et al. Personalized neoantigen vaccine NEO-PV-01 with chemotherapy and anti-PD-1 as first-line treatment for non-squamous non-small cell lung cancer. *Cancer Cell.* 2022;40(9):1010–1026.e11.
13. Rojas LA, Sethna Z, Soares KC, et al. Personalized RNA neoantigen vaccines stimulate T cells in pancreatic cancer. *Nature.* 2023;618(7963):144–150.
14. Hodi FS, O'Day SJ, McDermott DF, et al. Improved survival with ipilimumab in patients with metastatic melanoma. *N Engl J Med.* 2010;363(8):711–723.
15. Robert C, Thomas L, Bondarenko I, et al. Ipilimumab plus dacarbazine for previously untreated metastatic melanoma. *N Engl J Med.* 2011;364(26):2517–2526.
16. Maio M, Grob JJ, Aamdal S, et al. Five-year survival rates for treatment-naive patients with advanced melanoma who received ipilimumab plus dacarbazine in a phase III trial. *J Clin Oncol.* 2015;33(10):1191–1196.
17. Weber JS, Kähler KC, Hauschild A. Management of immune-related adverse events and kinetics of response with ipilimumab. *J Clin Oncol.* 2012;30(21):2691–2697.
18. Hemon P, Jean-Louis F, Ramgolam K, et al. MHC class II engagement by its ligand LAG-3 (CD223) contributes to melanoma resistance to apoptosis. *J Immunol.* 2011;186(9):5173–5183.
19. Tawbi HA, Schadendorf D, Lipson EJ, et al. Relatlimab and nivolumab versus nivolumab in untreated advanced melanoma. *N Engl J Med.* 2022;386(1):24–34.
20. Rosenberg SA, Restifo NP, Yang JC, Morgan RA, Dudley ME. Adoptive cell transfer: a clinical path to effective cancer immunotherapy. *Nat Rev Cancer.* 2008;8(4):299–308.
21. Rohaan MW, Borch TH, van den Berg JH, et al. Tumor-infiltrating lymphocyte therapy or ipilimumab in advanced melanoma. *N Engl J Med.* 2022;387(23):2113–2125.
22. Sarnaik AA, Hamid O, Khushalani NI, et al. Lifileucel, a tumor-infiltrating lymphocyte therapy, in metastatic melanoma. *J Clin Oncol.* 2021;39(24):2656–2566.
23. Ramos CA, Savoldo B, Dotti G. CD19-CAR trials. *Cancer J.* 2014;20(2):112–118.
24. Davila ML, Riviere I, Wang X, et al. Efficacy and toxicity management of 19–28z CAR T cell therapy in B cell acute lymphoblastic leukemia. *Sci Transl Med.* 2014;6(224):224ra25.
25. Lee DW, Kochenderfer JN, Stetler-Stevenson M, et al. T cells expressing CD19 chimeric antigen receptors for acute lymphoblastic leukaemia in children and young adults: a phase 1 dose-escalation trial. *Lancet.* 2015;385(9967):517–528.

26. Maude SL, Frey N, Shaw PA, et al. Chimeric antigen receptor T cells for sustained remissions in leukemia. *N Engl J Med*. 2014;371(16):1507–1517.
27. Locke FL, Miklos DB, Jacobson CA, et al. Axicabtagene ciloleucel as second-line therapy for large B-cell lymphoma. *N Engl J Med*. 2022;386(7):640–654.
28. Maude SL, Barrett D, Teachey DT, Grupp SA. Managing cytokine release syndrome associated with novel T cell-engaging therapies. *Cancer J*. 2014;20(2):119–122.
29. Rader C. DARTs take aim at BiTEs. *Blood*. 2011;117(17):4403–4404.
30. Kantarjian H, Stein A, Gokbuget N, et al. Blinatumomab versus chemotherapy for advanced acute lymphoblastic leukemia. *N Engl J Med*. 2017;376(9):836–847.
31. Budde LE, Sehn LH, Matasar M, et al. Safety and efficacy of mosunetuzumab, a bispecific antibody, in patients with relapsed or refractory follicular lymphoma: a single-arm, multicentre, phase 2 study. *Lancet Oncol*. 2022;23(8):1055–1065.
32. Moreau P, Garfall AL, van de Donk N, et al. Teclistamab in relapsed or refractory multiple myeloma. *N Engl J Med*. 2022;387(6):495–505.
33. Lesokhin AM, Tomasson MH, Arnulf B, et al. Elranatamab in relapsed or refractory multiple myeloma: phase 2 MagnetisMM-3 trial results. *Nat Med*. 2023;29(9):2259–2267.
34. Paz-Ares L, Champiat S, Lai WV, et al. Tarlatamab, a first-in-class DLL3-targeted bispecific T-cell engager, in recurrent small-cell lung cancer: an open-label, phase I study. *J Clin Oncol*. 2023;41(16):2893–2903.
35. Nathan P, Hassel JC, Rutkowski P, et al. Overall survival benefit with tebentafusp in metastatic uveal melanoma. *N Engl J Med*. 2021;385(13):1196–1206.

Breast Cancer

21

Katherine Clifton

GENERAL PRINCIPLES

In US, an estimated 300,590 new cases of invasive breast cancer were expected to be diagnosed in 2023.[1] Breast cancer is second only to lung cancer as the leading cause of cancer deaths among women in US, with an estimated 43,700 deaths expected in 2023.[1] Breast cancer incidence has been increasing by approximately half a percent each year since the mid-2000s, potentially due to increased rates of obesity and decreasing fertility rates.[2] Despite this, breast cancer mortality appears to be declining, suggesting a benefit from screening, the withdrawal of hormone replacement therapy (HRT), and improved therapies.[1]

Definition

Breast cancers are neoplasms that originate from breast tissue. They most commonly arise from epithelium lining the milk ducts or the lobules.

Classification

- **Pathologic classification**
  - Most **invasive breast cancers** are adenocarcinomas that can be quite heterogeneous in histologic appearance. Infiltrating (invasive) ductal carcinoma accounts for about 80% of all breast cancers. Infiltrating ductal carcinomas metastasize predominantly to the bones, liver, lungs, and brain. Lobular carcinomas make up 10% of malignant breast cancers and are associated with bilateral tumors in up to 20% of cases. Lobular carcinomas also tend to be associated with multicentric disease within the same breast and have a predilection to metastasize to the meninges, serosal surfaces, and mediastinal and retroperitoneal lymph nodes. The loss of E-cadherin, which plays a role in cell adhesion, is a key event in the development of invasive lobular breast cancers. Less common subtypes of ductal carcinomas include mucinous and tubular, which may carry a more favorable prognosis. Another variant, with aggressive histologic appearance but a relatively good prognosis, is medullary carcinoma. Metaplastic carcinoma of the breast, a neoplasm with both epithelial and mesenchymal elements, is a rare (<1% of all breast cancers) but aggressive breast tumor.
  - **Noninvasive breast cancers**, which are characterized pathologically by the lack of penetration through the basement membrane into the surrounding stroma, include ductal carcinoma in situ (DCIS) and lobular carcinoma in situ (LCIS), which is not a true cancer, but may indicate an increased risk for future breast cancer. DCIS is most often identified with an abnormal mammogram showing clustered microcalcifications with or without a palpable mass. LCIS, on the other hand, is not detected on physical examination or mammography and is almost always an incidental finding in breast biopsies performed for other reasons.
  - **Paget disease of the nipple** is a specialized form of ductal carcinoma that arises from the main excretory ducts in the breasts and involves the skin of the nipple and areola.
  - **Inflammatory carcinomas** involve the lymphatic structures in the dermis and infiltrate widely throughout the breast tissue. Inflammatory carcinomas are not a special

morphologic pattern but are clinically diagnosed based on swelling, erythema, and tenderness in the involved breast and are associated with more aggressive disease.

- **Biomarker classification**
  - Breast cancer can be classified by biomarker expression, which provides basic prognostic information and predicts response to targeted therapies. Hormone receptor (HR)-positive breast cancers express the estrogen receptor (ER) and/or progesterone receptor (PR). HER2-positive breast cancers demonstrate overexpression or amplification of human epidermal growth factor receptor (EGFR) 2/homolog of the oncogene neu (HER2/neu), a member of the EGFR family. Triple-negative breast cancers (TNBCs) are negative for ER, PR, and HER2.
- **Intrinsic molecular subtypes**
  - More recently, gene expression profiling techniques were used to further classify breast cancer into distinctive molecular subtypes with prognostic significance: luminal A, luminal B, HER2 enriched, and basal.[3,4] Luminal A breast cancers are typically HR positive with low proliferation indices. Like luminal A breast cancers, luminal B breast cancers are also HR positive. However, luminal B breast cancers have higher proliferation indices and are associated with poorer outcomes compared to luminal A breast cancers. The HER2-enriched breast cancers are usually, but not always, HER2 positive. Basal-like breast cancers are usually triple negative, although the two terms are not synonymous. *BRCA1*-associated cancers are often basal-like. These molecular subtypes provide not only prognostic, but also predictive information about response to specific therapies; for instance, basal-like breast cancers are more responsive to DNA-damaging chemotherapy, such as platinum agents.

Epidemiology

An estimated 300,590 (2,800 men; 297,790 women) new cases of breast cancer will be diagnosed in 2023 and 43,700 deaths will occur.[1] Although most breast cancers occur in women, about 1% of new cases occur in men. The lifetime risk of developing breast cancer in women (assuming a life expectancy of 85 years) is 12.3% (~one in eight women).[1] The median age at diagnosis is in the sixth decade of life.

Risk Factors

- Identifiable risk factors for breast cancer include a history of breast cancer, female gender, increasing age, early menarche, late menopause, nulliparity, older age at first live childbirth, family history of breast cancer, genetic mutations (*BRCA1, BRCA2*), prolonged HRT, previous exposure to therapeutic chest wall irradiation, and benign proliferative breast disease such as atypical lobular or ductal hyperplasia.[5]
- Behavior factors also increase breast cancer risk. Obesity increases breast cancer risk in postmenopausal women while regular physical activity (4–7 hours per week) correlates with a 12–60% breast cancer risk reduction.[6] High intake of fruits and vegetables and adherence to diets such as the Mediterranean diet have been associated with decreased breast cancer incidence.[7,8] More than minimal alcohol intake (such as >7 drinks per week) has been associated with increased breast cancer risk.[9]
- The Modified Gail model is a statistical tool that calculates a woman's risk of developing breast cancer.[10] Variables in the model include age, age at menarche, age at first live birth, number of previous breast biopsies, history of atypical ductal hyperplasia, number of first-degree relatives with breast cancer, and race.
- While the majority of breast cancers are sporadic, inherited breast cancer is now well documented. *BRCA1* and *BRCA2* were identified as breast cancer susceptibility genes in the 1990s.[11,12] Mutations in *BRCA1* (chromosome 17q21) and *BRCA2* (chromosome 13q12–13), which are inherited in an autosomal dominant fashion, are responsible for ~90% of hereditary breast cancer diagnoses. Approximately 5–10% of all women with

breast cancer have a germline mutation of *BRCA1* or *BRCA2,* which is associated with younger age at diagnosis, bilateral disease, multiple affected family members, and an association with other cancers, especially ovarian cancer. Specific mutations of *BRCA1* and *BRCA2* are also more common in women of Ashkenazi Jewish descent. In a combined analysis of 22 studies, the average cumulative risk of developing breast cancer by the age of 70 years in *BRCA1* and *BRCA2* carriers were 65% (95% confidence interval of 44–78%) and 45% (31–56%), respectively.[13] The corresponding risk of developing ovarian cancer was 39% (18–54%) and 11% (2.4–19%) for *BRCA1* and *BRCA2* carriers, respectively.[13] Other less common but established hereditary causes for breast cancer include Li–Fraumeni syndrome (*p53* gene mutations), Cowden syndrome or multiple hamartoma syndrome (*PTEN* gene mutations), and Peutz–Jeghers syndrome (*STK11* gene mutations).[14]

Prevention

- **Risk-reducing surgery** can be considered for women at high risk of developing breast cancer (known genetic predisposition or significant family history). Risk-reducing bilateral salpingo-oophorectomy in women with *BRCA* mutations decreases risk of developing ovarian cancer and is associated with a lower all-cause mortality.[15] Bilateral risk-reducing mastectomy decreases the risk of developing breast cancer by more than 90% in *BRCA* mutation carriers.[16]
- **Chemoprevention** of breast cancer has been evaluated in multiple studies. Selective estrogen receptor modulators (SERMs) have been evaluated in the National Surgical Adjuvant Breast and Bowel Project (NSABP) Breast Cancer Prevention (BCPT) P-1 trial and the Study of Tamoxifen and Raloxifene (STAR) trial. The BPCT P-1 included women aged 35 and older who had either an absolute risk of at least 1.66% over a 5-year period on the basis of the Gail model or a history of LCIS.[17] In this trial, tamoxifen 20 mg daily for 5 years demonstrated a 49% reduction in the incidence of invasive breast cancer.[17] The STAR trial compared 5 years of raloxifene (60 mg daily) to tamoxifen (20 mg daily) in high-risk postmenopausal women. Raloxifene was equivalent to tamoxifen, but had a better side-effect profile, including a lower incidence of thromboembolic events and uterine hyperplasia.[18] Aromatase inhibitors (AIs) have also been studied for chemoprevention in breast cancer. The use of anastrozole for 5 years was associated with a reduction in invasive ER-positive breast cancer by 54% in the IBIS-II trial.[19] The MAP.3 study demonstrated a 65% relative reduction in the annual incidence of invasive breast cancer with the use of exemestane for chemoprevention.[20]

Screening

- **Monthly breast self-exam (BSE)** is frequently advocated as a screening tool for breast cancer, but there is little evidence showing its effectiveness in reducing mortality rates in breast cancer and it is no longer recommended.[21]
- **Regular mammographic screening** has a sensitivity and specificity of 77–95% and 94–97%, respectively.[22] Younger women have more false-positive mammograms and require additional imaging, but fewer biopsies than older women. According to the most recent draft United States Preventive Services Task Force (USPSTF) guidelines (released May 2023), women should undergo biennial screening mammography beginning at age 40 until age 74.[23]
- **Magnetic resonance imaging** (MRI) has also been found to be superior to mammograms and ultrasound (US) in young women and in women with *BRCA1* and *BRCA2* mutations, where mammography is less sensitive, and multicentric disease is more common.[24] USPSTF 2023 draft guidelines stated there is insufficient evidence for MRI in women identified to have dense breasts on an otherwise negative screening mammogram.[23]

DIAGNOSIS

Clinical Presentation

The majority of breast cancers are diagnosed as the result of an abnormal mammogram; however, any woman who presents with a new breast mass should be evaluated with a complete history and physical examination.

History

For patients presenting with a new breast mass, symptoms related to the new mass (including duration, tenderness, relationship to menstrual cycle, nipple changes, and discharge) should be elicited. A heightened concern for malignancy arises if nipple discharge is unilateral, spontaneous, or bloody, especially in a postmenopausal woman. A negative family history does not exclude malignancy, given that most women who develop breast cancer do not have a family history. Patients should be asked for a detailed history concerning any prior breast biopsies and personal and family history of breast, ovarian, and other malignancies, as well as any personal history of breast cancer or other malignancies. A full gynecologic history should be taken, including age at menarche, age at menopause, use of oral contraceptives or exogenous HRT (type and duration), age at first live birth, and number of pregnancies.

Physical Examination

The physical characteristics of a breast mass can be helpful in determining a diagnosis. One should begin with a careful inspection for breast symmetry, contours, and retraction of the skin. Other changes in the skin can include erythema, thickening, skin nodules, and peau d'orange appearance. Close inspection of the nipple can reveal rashes, ulceration, thickening, or discharge that may help identify an underlying malignancy or Paget disease of the breast. The characteristics of any palpable lumps in the breast should be noted, including the location, size, shape, consistency, demarcation, tenderness, and mobility. A complete examination for lymphadenopathy includes evaluation for axillary, supraclavicular, and infraclavicular lymph nodes. The final element of the breast examination is compression of the areola to try to elicit any nipple discharge. A nonmilky or bloody unilateral nipple discharge suggests underlying breast pathology and should be evaluated further. The most common source of nipple discharge is an intraductal papilloma, which is a benign lesion.

Differential Diagnosis

The individual risk of a primary breast cancer can be characterized as high or low based on the patient's age, presenting symptoms, history of breast pathology, and family history. For example, a new breast mass in a woman >40 years of age should be considered malignant until proven otherwise, whereas in women <35 years of age with a similar lesion, cancer is a possibility, and needs to be investigated further. The differential diagnosis of a breast mass can be broad, including malignant breast lesions (primary breast cancer, lymphoma, and sarcoma) and benign breast lesions (cysts, fibroadenomas, and fat necrosis). Skin conditions, such as sebaceous cysts, abscesses, or thrombophlebitis, may present with a palpable mass. The history and physical examination will help aid in the differential diagnosis, but ultimately a biopsy is required for confirmation.

Diagnostic Testing

Patients suspected of having breast cancer should undergo a biopsy to obtain tissue for diagnosis and biomarker evaluation. Imaging studies are useful in the staging of the cancer.

Laboratories

- Laboratory tests do not directly aid in the diagnosis or staging of breast cancer, but can allow the clinician to focus on possible metastatic sites of disease. Routine laboratory

studies obtained are complete blood count (bone marrow infiltration), liver function tests (liver metastasis), and alkaline phosphatase (bone metastasis). Abnormal blood tests can also give the physician an objective marker to assess for clinical response after therapy.
- Tumor markers (CA15–3, CA27–29, CEA), although not specific, may be elevated in patients with breast cancer. Tumor markers are not accurate for screening or diagnostic purposes; thus they are not indicated in the initial assessment of breast cancer. In the metastatic setting, however, tumor markers may be elevated, and the trend of elevation can assist in monitoring for response to therapy.

Imaging
- A solid mass is best evaluated with **diagnostic mammography**. Mammography allows the physician to assess the radiographic characteristics of the mass and the remainder of breast tissue in the ipsilateral and contralateral breast. **Ultrasound** (US) can be useful to determine whether a lesion is cystic or solid. In the evaluation of a patient with breast cancer, especially in the setting where neoadjuvant systemic therapy is contemplated, evaluation of the axillary lymph nodes with US is indicated. In select situations, **breast MRI** may be useful in identifying additional lesions or bilateral disease.
- In patients with locally advanced disease or suspected metastatic disease, computed tomography (CT) examination of the chest, abdomen, and pelvis and a nuclear medicine bone scan can be performed as clinically indicated and may be useful in identifying sites of metastatic disease. In patients with neurologic findings concerning brain metastases, a contrast-enhanced MRI of the brain will be helpful.

Diagnostic Procedures
- Any distinct breast mass should be considered for biopsy, even if the mammogram is negative. Aspiration of a cystic mass may be helpful. Cytology may reveal malignant cells, but the absence of malignant cells does not rule out a malignant lesion.
- After radiographic evaluation to determine the location and characteristics of the mass, a biopsy can be obtained using several different methods. Fine-needle aspiration (FNA) is a simple method for obtaining material for cytologic examination that can be performed in the clinician's office. False-negative rates for FNA can be as high as 10%, even among the most experienced technicians. FNA also cannot distinguish in situ disease from invasive carcinoma. If a negative result is obtained from FNA, a core-needle or excisional biopsy should be done to obtain appropriate tissue for pathologic review. The majority of these biopsies can also be performed in the outpatient setting. If the biopsy reveals only normal breast tissue, then further surgical biopsy is recommended if the lesion is suspicious for cancer. Needle localization or stereotactic biopsies may be helpful in this situation. Excisional biopsy is the gold standard, allowing complete histologic characterization with regard to biomarkers (ER, PR, HER2) as well as tumor grade. Excisional biopsy also may serve as the definitive lumpectomy in certain clinical situations. In patients who are slated to undergo neoadjuvant systemic therapy, a biopsy of an abnormal-appearing axillary lymph node is warranted for accurate staging.

TREATMENT

- The treatment of breast cancer utilizes a multidisciplinary approach, including local–regional treatment with surgery and/or radiation therapy and treatment of systemic disease with cytotoxic chemotherapy, endocrine therapy, target therapy, or a combination of these agents. The treatment plan for each patient is individualized based on the stage of disease, patient's age, comorbidities, menopausal status, and biomarker profile. The American Joint Committee on Cancer Eight Edition staging system is the current official staging guide.[25] The current staging system utilizes traditional TNM staging as well as tumor grade, HER2 status, and ER/PR status. In addition to the various prognostic and predictive factors, a patient's preference is also a major component of the decision-making process, especially when more than one option may provide similar benefits.

- Breast cancer treatment can be categorized into these general categories:
  - Noninvasive carcinoma, DCIS, and LCIS (stage 0)
  - Early-stage breast cancer (clinical stage I, stage II, stage III tumors)
  - Metastatic carcinoma (stage IV)

Noninvasive Carcinoma/Carcinoma In Situ

Lobular Carcinoma In Situ

LCIS is a misleading term, as it is not a premalignant lesion. It is noted as an incidental finding on breast biopsies performed for other reasons. It is a marker that identifies women at an increased risk (21% over 15 years) for the development of invasive breast cancer that may occur equally in either breast. Of note, the majority of subsequent cancers are infiltrating ductal rather than lobular carcinomas. LCIS can be managed by observation alone after biopsy. There is no evidence that re-excision after the initial biopsy to obtain histologically negative surgical margins is required. The increased risk of breast cancer persists beyond 20 years, so careful observation and diagnostic mammography should be performed indefinitely in these women. Bilateral prophylactic mastectomies are an alternate option for women who are uncomfortable with the increased risk of developing breast cancer, for patients with a strong family history of breast cancer, or for patients with known *BRCA1/BRCA2* mutations. Radiation therapy has no role in the management of LCIS.

Ductal Carcinoma In Situ

DCIS, also known as intraductal carcinoma, is being encountered more frequently with the increased use of screening mammography. Surgical treatments for DCIS range from local excision to total mastectomy. Total mastectomy results in a 98% long-term disease-free survival (DFS) rate for noninvasive cancer; however, it is now generally accepted that a lumpectomy followed by radiation therapy to the breast represents the optimal treatment option, as no difference in mortality has been found between lumpectomy and mastectomy.[26] Local chest wall irradiation reduces the rate of ipsilateral breast tumor recurrences by more than 50% compared to lumpectomy alone.[27] Contraindications for breast-conserving surgery followed by radiation include (1) inability to completely excise the underlying disease to negative surgical margins, (2) multifocal disease, and (3) patient contraindication to receive radiation. Routine axillary nodal dissection is not recommended, given a low (<5%) incidence of axillary nodal metastases in patients with DCIS. Chemotherapy or HER2-directed therapies are not recommended in the treatment of DCIS however adjuvant endocrine therapy with tamoxifen or anastrozole can be considered in patients with ER+ DCIS to reduce risk of subsequent breast cancers although they have not been shown to improve overall survival (OS).[28]

Early Breast Cancer

Surgery

The surgical options for the management of early breast cancer include breast-conserving therapy (BCT) followed by radiation therapy or total mastectomy. Randomized clinical trials have proven that OS is equivalent between BCT followed by radiation therapy and mastectomy in women with early breast cancer.[29] The selection of a surgical approach depends on the location and size of the tumor, other abnormalities present on the mammogram, the breast size, and the patient's attitude toward breast preservation. Multicentric disease (two or more primary tumors in separate quadrants), extensive malignant-appearing microcalcifications on imaging, pregnancy, and previous breast or mantle irradiation are contraindications for BCT. Relative contraindications for BCT include tumors >5 cm and active connective tissue disease involving the skin, such as scleroderma.

Axillary Lymph Node Dissection

Axillary lymph node dissection (ALND) remains an important part of the surgical approach, given the prognostic importance of lymph node involvement. In an effort to decrease the morbidity associated with ALND (especially lymphedema and pain), while maintaining accurate staging, a sentinel lymph node (SLN) biopsy can be obtained. The SLN (the first node in the lymphatic chain that receives lymphatic flow from the entire breast) is at the highest risk for harboring occult metastatic disease in breast cancer patients. Vital blue dye and/or technetium-labeled sulfur are injected in and around the tumor or biopsy site. The surgeon maps the dye or radioactive compound drainage to the axilla and identifies the SLN, which is then biopsied. The SLN can be identified in more than 90% of patients with breast cancer, with false-negative rates ranging from 0% to 10%.[30] No further axillary node dissection is needed if the SLN biopsy is negative. If the SLN is positive for malignancy, further treatment options include a full ALND, axillary radiation with no further surgery, and adjuvant chemotherapy. ACOSOG Z0011 trial revealed no benefit to ALND in patients with early-stage breast cancer with 1–2 SLN metastases who underwent breast-conserving surgery, whole breast radiation, and adjuvant systemic therapy.[31]

Adjuvant Radiation Therapy

Radiation therapy to the intact breast after BCT is the standard treatment based on several randomized trials that have shown higher local recurrence rates with BCT alone compared to BCT with radiation therapy.[32] A radiation boost to the tumor bed is often administered. Patients with positive axillary nodes may benefit from regional nodal irradiation in addition to irradiation of the intact breast. Postmastectomy adjuvant chest wall and axillary radiation is considered for the following: positive surgical margins, primary tumors >5 cm, and involvement of four or more lymph nodes.[33] Typically, adjuvant radiation is given following the completion of adjuvant chemotherapy.

Adjuvant Systemic Therapy

Predicting Benefits of Systemic Therapy

Given that not all patients with early-stage breast cancers recur, it is important to identify high-risk patients who will benefit the most and spare cytotoxic chemotherapy for the subset of patients with low-risk features. Selecting candidates for adjuvant systemic therapy of early breast cancers is thus based on clinicopathologic factors and, more recently, based on gene expression analysis. The development and validation of prognostic and predictive models is an area of active research and can be useful in the right clinical scenario for decision making. The clinical and pathologic prognostic determinants of adjuvant therapy are patient age, comorbidities, tumor size, histologic grade or differentiation, histologic type, number of involved axillary lymph nodes, dermal lymphatic invasion, markers of proliferation, HR status, and HER2 status. Several gene expression-based prognostic assays, such as Oncotype Dx and Mammaprint, are also commercially available. These multigene assays are mostly independent of clinicopathologic prognostic factors, and hence the treating oncologist has to familiarize the clinical contexts when these tests are applicable.

Hormone Receptor Positive (HR+) Disease

- **Chemotherapy**
  - Polychemotherapy in the adjuvant setting in early breast cancer reduces the annual breast cancer death rate by ~38% for women <50 years of age and by ~20% for those ages 50–69 years, largely irrespective of the use of tamoxifen, nodal status, tumor characteristics, and HR status.[34] Chemotherapy is recommended for patients with N2 (four or more positive lymph nodes). Patients with node-negative tumors <1 cm in size are often treated with endocrine therapy alone. In patients with node-negative disease and tumors >1 cm, the decision regarding adjuvant chemotherapy may be guided by multigene expression assays. The gene expression assay most commonly used as it has been

clinically validated for predicting benefit of adjuvant chemotherapy is the Oncotype DX. The TAILORx study revealed that endocrine therapy alone was noninferior to chemotherapy and endocrine therapy in patients older than 50 with a recurrence score <26.[35] Patients 50 years or younger with recurrence scores between 16 and 25 derived some benefit from chemotherapy.[35] Clinical-risk stratification, such as tumor size and grade, may help identify premenopausal patients who would benefit from chemotherapy.[36] RSClin is an online validated tool which incorporates tumor grade, size, age, and recurrence score to estimate the benefit of adjuvant chemotherapy and may be useful in these populations.[37] Patients with recurrence scores >25 are often treated with a taxane and/or anthracycline-containing regimen.[38]

○ In patients with one to three positive lymph nodes, postmenopausal patients with recurrence scores <26 did not benefit from the addition of chemotherapy to endocrine therapy.[39] Patients with N1 disease who were premenopausal benefitted from the addition of chemotherapy, regardless of recurrence score.[39] It is unclear if this benefit was from the ovarian function suppression that resulted from chemotherapy or the chemotherapy itself. Nevertheless, adjuvant chemotherapy is recommended in this population at this time, and trials to further assess the role of ovarian function suppression are ongoing.[40]

If adjuvant chemotherapy is recommended, the current standard of practice is to initiate adjuvant chemotherapy 4–5 weeks after surgery, before the initiation of radiation. Some of the adjuvant chemotherapy regimens are outlined in Table 21-1. Most modern and widely used chemotherapy regimens are taxanes and anthracycline-based regimens for four to six courses of treatment provide optimal benefit. For node-positive breast cancer, the addition of a taxane to anthracycline-containing chemotherapy improves DFS.[41]

- **Adjuvant endocrine therapy**
  ○ Patients with invasive breast cancer who are ER- or PR-positive should be considered for adjuvant endocrine therapy, regardless of the patient's age, menopausal status, or lymph node status, or whether or not adjuvant chemotherapy is to be administered. Adjuvant endocrine therapy should not be recommended in patients whose breast cancers are ER or PR negative because clinical trials have not shown any benefit in DFS or OS. A list of commonly used endocrine therapy agents are listed in Table 21-2.
  ○ **Tamoxifen**
    ▪ Tamoxifen is a SERM that inhibits the growth of breast cancer cells by competitive antagonism of estrogen at the ER.[42] Tamoxifen is a well-established form of endocrine therapy for both premenopausal and postmenopausal women. In women with ER-positive early breast cancer, adjuvant tamoxifen decreases the risk of recurrence by 40–50% and the risk of death by 30–40%, irrespective of the use of chemotherapy, age, menopausal status, or axillary lymph node status.[43] Tamoxifen also decreased the incidence of breast cancer in the contralateral breast by ~50%.[44] Prospective randomized trials have demonstrated that 10 years of tamoxifen therapy reduces the rate of recurrence and improves OS compared to 5 years of therapy, though the increased incidence of pulmonary embolism and endometrial cancer must be taken into consideration.[45] In patients requiring chemotherapy, tamoxifen is started after completion of chemotherapy.
  ○ **Aromatase inhibitors**
    ▪ In postmenopausal women, the primary source of estrogen is the peripheral conversion of androgens to estrogen by the enzyme aromatase, which is the target for AIs.[46] Numerous studies have utilized AIs in the treatment of postmenopausal women with early-stage breast cancer. These studies have utilized AI as upfront initial therapy for 5 years, as sequential therapy following 2–3 years of tamoxifen, or as extended therapy following 5 years of tamoxifen. Two upfront studies, BIG I-98, and ATAC,

TABLE 21-1	OVERVIEW OF COMMON NON–TRASTUZUMAB-CONTAINING AND TRASTUZUMAB-CONTAINING CHEMOTHERAPY REGIMENS FOR BREAST CANCER

Preferred non–trastuzumab-containing regimens

Docetaxel/cyclophosphamide (TC) × 4 cycles

Dose-dense adriamycin/cyclophosphamide (AC) × 4 cycles (with growth factor support) → dose-dense paclitaxel (T) × 4 cycles (with growth factor support)

Dose-dense adriamycin/cyclophosphamide (AC) × 4 cycles (with growth factor support) → weekly paclitaxel (T) × 12 wks

High-risk TNBC: preoperative pembrolizumab + carboplatin + paclitaxel followed by pembrolizumab + doxorubicin or epirubicin + cyclophosphamide followed by adjuvant pembrolizumab

TNBC with residual disease after preoperative therapy: capecitabine or olaparib if germline BRCA1/2 mutation

Useful in Certain Circumstances:

    Adriamycin/cyclophosphamide (AC) × 4 cycles

    Cyclophosphamide/methotrexate/fluorouracil (CMF) × 6 cycles

    Docetaxel/doxorubicin/cyclophosphamide (TAC) × 6 cycles (with growth factor support)

Trastuzumab-containing regimens

Preferred Regimens:

    Paclitaxel/trastuzumab (weekly paclitaxel × 12 wks; trastuzumab for 52 wks)

    Docetaxel/carboplatin/trastuzumab ± pertuzumab (TCH/TCHP) (docetaxel and carboplatin × 6 cycles; trastuzumab ± pertuzumab for 52 wks)

    If residual disease after preoperative therapy: Ado-trastuzumab emtansine

Useful in Certain Circumstances:

    AC × 4 cycles → paclitaxel/trastuzumab ± pertuzumab (paclitaxel × 4 cycles; trastuzumab ± pertuzumab for 52 wks)

    Docetaxel + cyclophosphamide + trastuzumab

    Paclitaxel + trastuzumab + pertuzumab

AC × 4 cycles → docetaxel/trastuzumab ± pertuzumab (docetaxel × 4 cycles; trastuzumab ± pertuzumab for 52 wks)

Neratinib (in adjuvant setting only)

have compared letrozole versus tamoxifen and anastrozole versus tamoxifen, respectively. Both studies have shown an improved DFS with the AI compared to tamoxifen when used in the upfront setting.[47,48] Several trials have also studied the use of sequential AI following either 2–3 years of tamoxifen or 5 years of tamoxifen. The NCIC CTG MA.[17] trial showed an improved DFS with continuation of letrozole versus placebo following 5 years of tamoxifen.[49] The Intergroup Exemestane Study showed an improved DFS, as well as a trend toward improved OS, with switching to exemestane following 2–3 years of tamoxifen versus continuation of tamoxifen.[50] Given the available data, AIs are now largely used as the treatment of choice for postmenopausal women with HR-positive early breast cancer.[51] In premenopausal women, there is evidence from the prospective SOFT and TEXT trials that AIs combined with ovarian suppression for 5 years may improve 5-year DFS compared to tamoxifen combined with ovarian suppression in patients with high-risk clinical features such as younger age at diagnosis, receipt of chemotherapy and node-positive disease.[52,53]

TABLE 21-2	ENDOCRINE THERAPY AGENTS COMMONLY USED IN BREAST CANCER

Nonsteroidal aromatase inhibitor
- Anastrozole (Arimidex) 1 mg PO daily
- Letrozole (Femara) 2.5 mg PO daily

Steroidal Aromatase inhibitor
- Exemestane (Aromasin) 25 mg PO daily

Selective estrogen receptor modulator (SERM)
- Tamoxifen 20 mg PO daily

Selective estrogen receptor downregulator (SERD)
- Fulvestrant (Faslodex) 500 mg IM on days 1, 15, and 29, then monthly
- Elacestrant 345 mg PO on days 1–28

Luteinizing hormone–releasing hormone (LHRH) analogs
- Goserelin (Zoladex) 3.6 mg subcutaneous monthly

- Risk of breast cancer recurrence has been found to continue to rise following 5 years of adjuvant endocrine therapy, raising the question of the need for extended adjuvant endocrine therapy beyond 5 years.[54] Although no trial has found an improvement in OS for extended adjuvant AIs beyond 5 years, it is recommended that higher-risk patients, such as patients with node-positive disease, be offered extended adjuvant AIs with the understanding that extended adjuvant endocrine therapy carries continued side effects and risks as discussed below.[51] The Breast Cancer Index is a gene expression-based signature that predicts the benefit of extended adjuvant endocrine therapy as well as provides a prognostic score of the risk of late distant recurrence and may be useful in decision making regarding extended adjuvant endocrine therapy.[55]
  - Side-effect profiles for tamoxifen and AIs
    - While both the agents can cause hot flashes, night sweats, and vaginal dryness, AIs are more commonly associated with musculoskeletal symptoms, osteoporosis, and an increased risk of bone fractures, whereas tamoxifen is associated with an increased risk of uterine cancer and deep vein thromboses.[56]
- Adjuvant CDK4/6 inhibitors
  Cyclin-dependent kinase inhibitors prevent progression through the cell cycle, leading to cell cycle arrest.[57] Given their success in the advanced breast cancer setting, CDK4/6 inhibitors have most recently been tested in the patients with early-stage, high-risk breast cancer. MonarchE trial demonstrated that 2 years of adjuvant abemaciclib improved invasive DFS in patients with high-risk HR+ node-positive breast cancer compared to endocrine therapy alone.[58,59] Similarly, 3 years of adjuvant ribociclib has also been shown to improve invasive DFS in high-risk patients.[60] A trial utilizing 2 years of adjuvant Palbociclib did not show improvement in outcomes.[61]

HER2-Positive Disease

Trastuzumab is a humanized, monoclonal antibody with specificity for the extracellular domain of HER2/neu.[62] A meta-analysis from five randomized trials of adjuvant trastuzumab in HER2-positive breast cancer has shown significant reduction in the mortality, recurrence, and metastases rate in patients receiving trastuzumab with or following chemotherapy.[63] A 33–52% reduction in the risk of recurrence was seen across these four important initial trials (NSABP B-31, NCCTG 9831, BCIRG 006, and HERA), with a 34–41% reduction in the risk of death.[64] These data are compelling to consider the use of 1 year of adjuvant trastuzumab in combination with anthracycline- and/or taxane-containing adjuvant chemotherapy regimens (outlined in Table 21-1) and should be offered to all patients with HER2-positive early breast cancer. The likelihood of cardiac toxicity was 2.4-fold higher in trastuzumab arms in the clinical trials, and therefore a non–anthracycline-containing regimen, which offers less cumulative cardiac toxicity, is often preferred.[65]

- **Neoadjuvant HER2-directed therapy**
  With the exception of small, node-negative tumors, neoadjuvant HER2-directed therapy is often used in early-stage breast cancer. In the NeoSphere trial, comparing patients who received docetaxel in combination with trastuzumab alone, pertuzumab alone, or both trastuzumab and pertuzumab, patients who received both trastuzumab and pertuzumab in combination with docetaxel achieved the highest pathologic complete response rate (39.3%) of all groups, leading to FDA approval of pertuzumab use in the neoadjuvant setting.[66] While pathologic response rates following neoadjuvant systemic therapy are prognostic, this modality of treatment has the advantage of testing in vivo sensitivity of the tumor to systemic therapy, and is an ideal setup to evaluate newer therapies and develop predictive biomarkers of response.

- **Adjuvant HER2-directed therapy**
  - In patients who received neoadjuvant HER2-directed therapy and had residual invasive disease at the time of surgery, adjuvant Ado-trastuzumab emtansine (T-DM1), an antibody–drug conjugate of trastuzumab and the cytotoxic agent DM1, has been shown to decrease risk of recurrence and death compared to trastuzumab alone.[67] Patients who achieve a pathologic complete response at the time of surgery continue on trastuzumab or trastuzumab and pertuzumab in combination to complete 1 year of HER2-directed therapy.
  - In patients with small (<3 cm), node-negative HER2-positive tumors, a 12-week course of adjuvant weekly paclitaxel combined with 1 year of trastuzumab was associated with excellent outcomes, resulting in a 3-year DFS of 98.7%., and thus is the preferred therapy. [68]
  - In patients with HR+ HER2+ disease with residual invasive disease at the time of surgery, 1 year of adjuvant neratinib, an oral tyrosine kinase inhibitor, post-trastuzumab or T-DM1 may be considered based on the ExteNET trial that demonstrated improvement in invasive DFS in patients with HR+ HER2+ disease with residual disease following neoadjuvant treatment.[69]

Triple-Negative Breast Cancer (TNBC)

Triple-negative breast cancers, which do not express ER, PR, or HER2, are often associated with a more aggressive biology as well as higher rates of recurrence and death.[70]

- **Neoadjuvant chemotherapy**
  Neoadjuvant chemotherapy has become the standard of care for the majority of early-stage TNBC, with the exception of small, node-negative tumors.[71] In HER2-positive disease, patients who achieve a pathologic complete response have improved disease-free and OS.[72] In the Keynote-522 Study, patients who received a neoadjuvant chemotherapy and immunotherapy regimen achieved higher rates of pathologic complete response compared to those who received chemotherapy alone.[73] This regimen, which consists of neoadjuvant carboplatin and paclitaxel with pembrolizumab followed by neoadjuvant anthracycline and cyclophosphamide with pembrolizumab with an additional nine cycles of adjuvant pembrolizumab after surgery, has become standard of care for early-stage, high-risk TNBC.[74]

- **Adjuvant therapy**
  In patients with residual disease following neoadjuvant therapy, adjuvant capecitabine has been found to improve disease-free and OS.[75] In patients with germline BRCA1/2 mutations and residual disease following neoadjuvant therapy, adjuvant olaparib, a PARP inhibitor, has been shown to also improve disease-free and OS.[76,77]

Inflammatory Breast Cancer

This subset of stage III breast cancer is one of the most aggressive forms of breast cancer. It is characterized by a triad of erythema, warmth, and edema of the skin (peau d'orange), secondary to involvement of dermal lymphatics.[78] While an underlying mass may or may not be palpable, the condition can be misdiagnosed for inflammatory or infectious condition. The biomarker profile is most often (not always) HR and HER2 negative, and they are characterized by rapid growth potential. Localized inflammatory breast cancers are treated similarly to noninflammatory breast cancer with the important exception that breast-conserving surgery and SLN biopsy alone are not offered in patients with inflammatory breast cancer, regardless of response to neoadjuvant therapy.[30] The overall prognosis is improving in recent years with a more aggressive multimodality approach compared to their historical dismal outcome.[79]

Metastatic Breast Cancer

Patients with metastatic breast cancer (MBC) are a heterogeneous group of patients with varied presentations and clinical courses. The disease can vary from clinically indolent disease to rapidly progressing disease with visceral involvement and resistance to therapy.[80] The primary goals of treatment for patients with metastatic disease are to control the disease, palliate symptoms, and prolong survival. The management of MBC depends on the site and extent of metastases, comorbid conditions, HR status, and HER2 overexpression.

Locoregional Recurrence

Patients who have had BCT or mastectomy and present with local recurrence are generally treated with mastectomy and local resection respectively (if obtaining clear surgical margins seems plausible) and radiation therapy if not received in the adjuvant setting. Unresectable chest wall recurrences should be treated with radiation therapy if the patient has not previously received this modality of treatment.[81] Regional lymph node recurrence is managed with surgical resection (or ALND, if not done before) and radiation therapy. Systemic therapy, with adjuvant chemotherapy or endocrine therapy, is considered for these patients as in the adjuvant setting. The CALOR trial found an improvement in DFS in patients with TNBC who underwent adjuvant chemotherapy following isolated local regional recurrence.[82] This improvement was not seen in patients with HR+ breast cancer however.[82]

Distant Metastatic Disease

With regard to distant metastatic disease, some of the important decisions regarding treatment are made based on risk categories. Patients in the low-risk group include those with a long disease-free interval, HR-positive tumors, and bone, soft tissue, or limited visceral organ involvement. High-risk groups include patients with rapidly progressing disease or extensive visceral involvement, as well as patients whose disease becomes refractory to endocrine therapy. At some point in the clinical course, the disease burden from MBC may interfere with the patient's ability to tolerate further treatment options and supportive or palliative care should be offered to the patient and family.[83] Failure to achieve response to three sequential chemotherapy regimens or an Eastern Cooperative Oncology Group (ECOG) performance status ≥3 may be indications for supportive therapy only.

- **Endocrine therapy**
  - In patients with ER+ MBC without rapidly progressive disease or visceral crisis, sequential endocrine therapy is the preferred initial management in both premenopausal and postmenopausal patients. In postmenopausal women with ER-positive tumors, CDK4/6 inhibitor, and an AI is the preferred first-line therapy.[84] Approved CDK4/6 inhibitors include palbociclib, abemaciclib and ribociclib. All three CDK4/6 inhibitors have shown similar PFS hazard ratios in the first-line setting, however the OS data from a clinical trial with palbociclib was not statistically significant.[85–89] Side effect profiles of the drugs also differs, with abemaciclib associated with higher rates of GI toxicity, palbociclib associated with higher rates of neutropenia, and ribociclib associated with rare increases in QTc prolongation.[90]
  - In premenopausal women, ovarian suppression with luteinizing-hormone–releasing hormone (LHRH) analogs in combination with ribociclib and an AI was found to improve overall survival and is the preferred therapy.[91]
  - For patients that progress on an AI or develop metastatic disease while on or within 1 year of adjuvant endocrine therapy, fulvestrant and a CDK4/6 inhibitor is the preferred line of therapy.[84] Fulvestrant is a selective estrogen receptor downregulator (SERD) that leads to ER degradation which has demonstrated efficacy in subsequent lines of therapy in disease refractory to AIs.[92]
  - Following progression on CDK4/6 inhibitors, alpelisib, a PIK3CA inhibitor, in combination with fulvestrant demonstrated improved progression-free survival and OS compared to fulvestrant alone in patients with a PIK3CA mutation.[93] In patients with an ESR1 mutation, single agent elacestrant, an oral SERD, is approved after progression on CDK4/6 inhibitors.[94] Other options for patients without PIK3CA or ESR1 mutations include single agent fulvestrant or the combination of everolimus, an mTOR inhibitor, with exemestane, which showed improvement in progression-free survival compared to exemestane alone.[95] With each subsequent endocrine therapy, the duration of a clinical response becomes shorter, and ultimately, the disease will become refractory to endocrine treatment. Systemic chemotherapy can be recommended in patients whose disease becomes refractory to multiple lines of endocrine therapy or patients with rapid progression or high burden of disease on early lines of endocrine therapy.
- **HER2-directed therapies**
  - Trastuzumab is approved for use in combination chemotherapy or as a single agent in HER2+ MBC. The response rate using trastuzumab as a single agent is approximately 25%.[96] Pertuzumab targets the extracellular domain of HER2 to block dimerization of HER2 and prevent ligand-dependent signaling. Pertuzumab in combination with trastuzumab and a taxane chemotherapy (THP regimen) has been shown to improve progression-free survival and OS compared to placebo with trastuzumab and chemotherapy, leading to FDA approval for its use in the first-line metastatic setting.[97]
  - Trastuzumab deruxtecan (T-DXd), an antibody–drug conjugate linking an anti-HER2 antibody with a topoisomerase I inhibitor payload, is now considered second-line therapy following progression on the THP regimen based on results from the DESTINY-Breast 03 trial which showed an improvement in progression-free survival and OS in patients who received T-DXd compared to T-DM1.[98–100] Options beyond progression on THP and T-DXd include T-DM1, which has shown to progression-free survival and OS versus lapatinib with capecitabine.[101] Tucatinib, an oral HER2 tyrosine kinase inhibitor, in combination with trastuzumab and capecitabine, improved progression-free survival and OS compared to trastuzumab and capecitabine alone.[102] This regimen also reduced risk of intracranial progression and may be a preferred option in patients with brain metastases.[103]
  - Other later-line options include neratinib, an irreversible pan-HER tyrosine kinase inhibitor, which in combination with capecitabine was shown to improve progression-free survival compared to lapatinib and capecitabine.[104] Lapatinib, an EGFR and

HER2 dual tyrosine kinase inhibitor, in combination with capecitabine, was shown to improve progression-free survival compared to capecitabine alone.[105] Margetuximab, a chimeric IgG monoclonal HER2 antibody, was found to improve progression-free survival, however not OS, in combination with chemotherapy when compared to trastuzumab and chemotherapy.[106,107] Other later-line options include trastuzumab in combination with traditional chemotherapy.

- **Immunotherapy**
  In the metastatic setting, immunotherapy is currently only approved in PD-L1 positive (combined positive score [CPS] ≥10) TNBC based on the Keynote-355 study which showed the combination of pembrolizumab and chemotherapy improved progression-free survival and OS compared to chemotherapy alone in patients with CPS of 10 or greater.[108,109] The combination of immunotherapy plus chemotherapy is now considered first-line standard of care for patients with metastatic TNBC who are PD-L1 positive. TNBC patients who are PD-L1 negative are recommended to proceed with chemotherapy alone first-line.

- **Antibody–drug conjugates**
  - There has been an increase in the number of antibody–drug conjugates approved for breast cancer. These drugs utilize a monoclonal antibody to target antigens expressed on cancer cells that subsequently deliver a cytotoxic payload.[109] In the advanced cancer setting, there are several antibody–drug conjugates approved for HR+ HER2- and TNBC in the later-line settings. T-DXd, which is also approved for HER2+ advanced breast cancer, is approved for patients with advanced HER2 low breast cancer who have received prior chemotherapy based on the DESTINY-Breast04 study. This study demonstrated a significant improvement in progression-free survival and OS when compared to chemotherapy.[110] HER2 low breast cancer is defined as breast cancers with HER2 1+ expression by IHC or 2+ by IHC and negative by FISH.[111] An important toxicity of this drug is interstitial lung disease, which occurred in 12% of patients in the DESINTY-Breast04 study and has the potential to be fatal.[110]
  - Sacituzumab govitecan is another antibody–drug conjugate approved for both metastatic TNBC and HR+ HER2- breast cancer. It is composed of a Trop-2 antibody linked to SN-38, a topoisomerase I inhibitor.[112] Sacituzumab govitecan showed improvement in progression-free survival and OS in patients with metastatic TNBC who had received two or more lines of previous chemotherapy when compared to chemotherapy alone.[113] In patients with advanced HR+ HER2- breast cancer, sacituzumab govitecan also showed improvement in progression-free survival and OS.[114]

- **PARP inhibitors.**
  The poly (ADP-ribose) polymerase is an enzyme used by cancer cells to repair DNA damage.[115] Tumors with *BRCA1/BRCA2* mutations lose a form of DNA repair and thus rely heavily on the PARP pathway. By blocking PARP in the already-compromised tumor cells, the PARP inhibitors can cause cell death through a synthetic lethality mechanism.[116] In patients with metastatic HER2-negative breast cancer with germline BRCA1/2 mutation, olaparib monotherapy was found to improve progression-free survival as well as OS when compared to chemotherapy.[117,118]

- **Chemotherapy**
  High-risk patients with rapidly progressive disease, extensive visceral involvement, or disease that becomes refractory to endocrine therapy may benefit from chemotherapy. Other indications for chemotherapy in advanced breast cancer are patients with TNBC who do not qualify for immunotherapy or PARP inhibitors, and those who have progressed antibody–drug conjugate therapies. Combination chemotherapy generally provides higher rates of objective responses and longer time to progression; however, these regimens are associated with increased toxicity without adding survival benefit.[119] Several chemotherapy agents produce objective responses in MBC; while there are overlapping toxicities of these agents, their specific toxicity profile and metabolism should be kept in

TABLE 21-3 CHEMOTHERAPY AGENTS USED IN METASTATIC BREAST CANCER (MBC)

Single agents that have shown activity in MBC
Anthracyclines: doxorubicin, liposomal doxorubicin, epirubicin
Taxanes: paclitaxel, docetaxel, albumin-bound nanoparticle paclitaxel
Alkylating agents: cyclophosphamide
Fluoropyrimidines: capecitabine
Antimetabolites: gemcitabine
Vinca alkaloids: vinorelbine
Platinum: carboplatin, cisplatin
Microtubule inhibitors: ixabepilone, eribulin

Combination regimens that have shown activity in MBC
AC: cyclophosphamide and doxorubicin
CAF: cyclophosphamide, doxorubicin, 5-fluorouracil
CMF: cyclophosphamide, methotrexate, 5-fluorouracil
FEC: fluorouracil, epirubicin, cyclophosphamide
Gemcitabine and paclitaxel
Gemcitabine and carboplatin
Docetaxel and capecitabine

mind, especially given the relatively higher frequency of renal and hepatic impairment in this patient population. Single-agent sequential therapies are preferred in patients who are candidates for chemotherapy but are relatively asymptomatic with no impending visceral crises.[120] The list of preferred chemotherapy options including sequential single agents and combination chemotherapy is shown in Table 21-3.

- **Bone metastases**
Although patients with bone-only metastatic disease have a better prognosis than those with visceral metastases, while bone metastases can lead to serious complications such as pain, fractures, spinal cord compression, and hypercalcemia.[121] Traditionally, treatment of symptomatic bone metastases has been with analgesics, localized radiation, or surgery. Since then, bisphosphonates and denosumab have further reduced the risk of skeletal-related events, and these agents should be given to all MBC patients with bone metastases, although neither therapy has been shown to improve OS.[122]

  ○ **Bisphosphonates**
  These agents improve bone health by inhibiting osteoclast-mediated bone resorption. Their use, alone or in combination with chemotherapy or endocrine therapy has been shown to reduce bone pain, improve quality of life, reduce the risk of developing a skeletal event, and increase the time to skeletal event.[123]

  ○ **Denosumab**
  Denosumab is a fully humanized antibody against receptor activator of nuclear factor κB (RANK) ligand, which has been shown to reduce skeletal-related events in patients with bone metastases and is another option for patients with MBC.[124]

MONITORING/FOLLOW-UP

Follow-up examinations should be individualized either to reflect the patient's risk of recurrence or to monitor treatment or disease progression. Patients with MBC are followed closely with imaging often every 3 months to monitor for concerns for progression. In patients with early-stage breast cancer who have completed treatment, posttreatment follow-up includes regular physical examination and mammography for patients with intact breast tissue. No randomized trials have demonstrated a benefit from routine laboratory or radiology testing compared to a careful history and physical examination.[125]

REFERENCES

1. Siegel RL, Miller KD, Wagle NS, Jemal A. Cancer statistics, 2023. *CA Cancer J Clin.* 2023; 73(1):17–48.
2. Pfeiffer RM, Webb-Vargas Y, Wheeler W, Gail MH. Proportion of U.S. trends in breast cancer incidence attributable to long-term changes in risk factor distributions. *Cancer Epidemiol Biomarkers Prev.* 2018;27(10):1214–1222.
3. Perou CM, Sørlie T, Eisen MB, et al. Molecular portraits of human breast tumours. *Nature.* 2000;406(6797):747–752.
4. Prat A, Perou CM. Deconstructing the molecular portraits of breast cancer. *Mol Oncol.* 2011; 5:5–23.
5. Amir E, Freedman OC, Seruga B, Evans DG. Assessing women at high risk of breast cancer: a review of risk assessment models. *J Natl Cancer Inst.* 2010;102(10):680–691.
6. Gammon MD, John EM, Britton JA. Recreational and occupational physical activities and risk of breast cancer. *J Natl Cancer Inst.* 1998;90(2):100–117.
7. Farvid MS, Chen WY, Rosner BA, Tamimi RM, Willett WC, Eliassen AH. Fruit and vegetable consumption and breast cancer incidence: repeated measures over 30 years of follow-up. *Int J Cancer.* 2019;144(7):1496–1510.
8. Turati F, Carioli G, Bravi F, et al. Mediterranean diet and breast cancer risk. *Nutrients.* 2018; 10(3):326.
9. McDonald JA, Goyal A, Terry MB. Alcohol intake and breast cancer risk: weighing the overall evidence. *Curr Breast Cancer Rep.* 2013;5(3):10.1007/s12609-013-0114-z.
10. Gail MH, Brinton LA, Byar DP, et al. Projecting individualized probabilities of developing breast cancer for white females who are being examined annually. *J Natl Cancer Inst.* 1989;81(24): 1879–1886.
11. Miki Y, Swensen J, Shattuck-Eidens D, et al. A strong candidate for the breast and ovarian cancer susceptibility gene BRCA1. *Science.* 1994;266(5182):66–71.
12. Wooster R, Bignell G, Lancaster J, et al. Identification of the breast cancer susceptibility gene BRCA2. *Nature.* 1995;378(6559):789–792.
13. Antoniou A, Pharoah PDP, Narod S, et al. Average risks of breast and ovarian cancer associated with BRCA1 or BRCA2 mutations detected in case series unselected for family history: a combined analysis of 22 studies. *Am J Hum Genet.* 2003;72(5):1117–1130.
14. Himes DO, Shuman HB. Hereditary cancer syndrome recognition and testing: beyond BRCA. *J Nurse Pract.* 2020;16:517–522.
15. Eleje GU, Eke AC, Ezebialu IU, et al. Risk-reducing bilateral salpingo-oophorectomy in women with BRCA1 or BRCA2 mutations. *Cochrane Database Syst Rev.* 2018;8(8):CD012464.
16. Rebbeck TR, Friebel T, Lynch HT, et al. Bilateral prophylactic mastectomy reduces breast cancer risk in BRCA1 and BRCA2 mutation carriers: the PROSE Study Group. *J Clin Oncol.* 2004;22(6):1055–1062.
17. Fisher B, Costantino JP, Wickerham DL, et al. Tamoxifen for prevention of breast cancer: report of the national surgical adjuvant breast and bowel project P-1 study. *J Natl Cancer Inst.* 1998;90(18):1371–1388.
18. Vogel VG, Costantino JP, Wickerham DL, et al; National Surgical Adjuvant Breast and Bowel Project (NSABP). Effects of tamoxifen vs raloxifene on the risk of developing invasive breast cancer and other disease outcomes: the NSABP Study of Tamoxifen and Raloxifene (STAR) P-2 trial. *JAMA.* 2006;295:2727–2741.
19. Cuzick J, Sestak I, Forbes JF, et al; IBIS-II investigators. Use of anastrozole for breast cancer prevention (IBIS-II): long-term results of a randomised controlled trial. *Lancet.* 2020;395:117–122.
20. Goss PE, Ingle JN, Alés-Martínez JE, et al; NCIC CTG MAP.3 Study Investigators. Exemestane for breast-cancer prevention in postmenopausal women. *N Engl J Med.* 2011;364(25): 2381–2391.
21. Oeffinger KC, Fontham ETH, Etzioni R, et al; American Cancer Society. Breast cancer screening for women at average risk: 2015 guideline update from the American Cancer Society. *JAMA.* 2015;314(15):1599–1614.

22. Nelson HD, Tyne K, Naik A, Bougatsos C, Chan BK, Humphrey L; U.S. Preventive Services Task Force. Screening for breast cancer: an update for the U.S. Preventive Services Task Force. *Ann Intern Med.* 2009;151(10):727–737, W237–W242.

23. US Preventive Services Task Force. Screening for breast cancer: US Preventive Services Task Force Recommendation Statement. *JAMA.* 2024;331(22):1918–1930.

24. Warner E, Plewes DB, Hill KA, et al. Surveillance of BRCA1 and BRCA2 mutation carriers with magnetic resonance imaging, ultrasound, mammography, and clinical breast examination. *JAMA.* 2004;292(11):1317–1325.

25. Giuliano AE, Connolly JL, Edge SB, et al. Breast Cancer—Major changes in the American Joint Committee on Cancer eighth edition cancer staging manual. *CA Cancer J Clin.* 2017;67(4): 290–303.

26. Schwartz GF, Solin LJ, Olivotto IA, Ernster VL, Pressman PI. Consensus conference on the treatment of in situ ductal carcinoma of the breast. April 22–25, 1999. *Cancer.* 2000;88(4):946–954.

27. Wapnir IL, Dignam JJ, Fisher B, et al. Long-term outcomes of invasive ipsilateral breast tumor recurrences after lumpectomy in NSABP B-17 and B-24 randomized clinical trials for DCIS. *J Natl Cancer Inst.* 2011;103(6):478–488.

28. Barrio AV, Van Zee KJ. Controversies in the treatment of ductal carcinoma in situ. *Annu Rev Med.* 2017;68:197–211.

29. Fisher B, Anderson S, Bryant J, et al. Twenty-year follow-up of a randomized trial comparing total mastectomy, lumpectomy, and lumpectomy plus irradiation for the treatment of invasive breast cancer. *N Engl J Med.* 2002;347(16):1233–1241.

30. Lyman GH, Giuliano AE, Somerfield MR, et al; American Society of Clinical Oncology. American Society of Clinical Oncology guideline recommendations for sentinel lymph node biopsy in early-stage breast cancer. *J Clin Oncol.* 2005;23(30):7703–7720.

31. Giuliano AE, Ballman KV, McCall L, et al. Effect of axillary dissection vs no axillary dissection on 10-year overall survival among women with invasive breast cancer and sentinel node metastasis: the ACOSOG Z0011 (Alliance) randomized clinical trial. *JAMA.* 2017;318(10):918–926.

32. Darby S, McGale P, Correa C, et al. Effect of radiotherapy after breast-conserving surgery on 10-year recurrence and 15-year breast cancer death: meta-analysis of individual patient data for 10,801 women in 17 randomised trials. *Lancet.* 2011;378(9804):1707–1716.

33. Recht A, Comen EA, Fine RE, et al. Postmastectomy radiotherapy: an American Society of Clinical Oncology, American Society for Radiation Oncology, and Society of Surgical Oncology focused guideline update. *J Clin Oncol.* 2016;34(36):4431–4442.

34. Early Breast Cancer Trialists' Collaborative Group (EBCTCG). Effects of chemotherapy and hormonal therapy for early breast cancer on recurrence and 15-year survival: an overview of the randomized trials. *Lancet.* 2005;365(9472):1687–1717.

35. Sparano JA, Gray RJ, Makower DF, et al. Adjuvant chemotherapy guided by a 21-gene expression assay in breast cancer. *N Engl J Med.* 2018;379(2):111–121.

36. Sparano JA, Gray RJ, Ravdin PM, et al. Clinical and genomic risk to guide the use of adjuvant therapy for breast cancer. *N Engl J Med.* 2019;380(25):2395–2405.

37. Sparano JA, Crager MR, Tang G, Gray RJ, Stemmer SM, Shak S. Development and validation of a tool integrating the 21-gene recurrence score and clinical-pathological features to individualize prognosis and prediction of chemotherapy benefit in early breast cancer. *J Clin Oncol.* 2021;39(6):557–564.

38. Sparano JA, Gray RJ, Makower DF, et al. Clinical outcomes in early breast cancer with a high 21-gene recurrence score of 26 to 100 assigned to adjuvant chemotherapy plus endocrine therapy: a secondary analysis of the TAILORx randomized clinical trial. *JAMA Oncol.* 2020;6(3):367–374.

39. Kalinsky K, Barlow WE, Gralow JR, et al. 21-Gene assay to inform chemotherapy benefit in node-positive breast cancer. *N Engl J Med.* 2021;385(25):2336–2347.

40. Vaz-Luis I, Francis PA, Di Meglio A, Stearns V. Challenges in adjuvant therapy for premenopausal women diagnosed with luminal breast cancers. *Am Soc Clin Oncol Educ Book.* 2021;41:1–15.

41. Blum JL, Flynn PJ, Yothers G, et al. Anthracyclines in early breast cancer: the ABC trials—USOR 06–090, NSABP B-46-I/USOR 07132, and NSABP B-49 (NRG oncology). *J Clin Oncol.* 2017; 35(23):2647–2655.

42. Dhingra K. Antiestrogens–tamoxifen, SERMs and beyond. *Invest New Drugs.* 1999;17(3):285–311.

43. Gray RG, Rea D, Handley K, et al. aTTom: Long-term effects of continuing adjuvant tamoxifen to 10 years versus stopping at 5 years in 6,953 women with early breast cancer. *J Clin Oncol.* 2013;31(Suppl 5).

44. Alkner S, Bendahl P-O, Fernö M, Nordenskjöld B, Rydén L; South Swedish and South-East Swedish Breast Cancer Groups. Tamoxifen reduces the risk of contralateral breast cancer in premenopausal women: results from a controlled randomised trial. *Eur J Cancer.* 2009;45(14): 2496–2502.

45. Davies C, Pan H, Godwin J, et al. Long-term effects of continuing adjuvant tamoxifen to 10 years versus stopping at 5 years after diagnosis of oestrogen receptor-positive breast cancer: ATLAS, a randomised trial. *Lancet.* 2013;381(9869):805–816.

46. Chumsri S, Howes T, Bao T, Sabnis G, Brodie A. Aromatase, aromatase inhibitors, and breast cancer. *J Steroid Biochem Mol Biol.* 2011;125(1–2):13–22.

47. BIG 1–98 Collaborative Group, Mouridsen H, Giobbie-Hurder A, Goldhirsch A, et al. Letrozole therapy alone or in sequence with tamoxifen in women with breast cancer. *N Engl J Med.* 2009;361(8):766–776.

48. Howell A, Cuzick J, Baum M, et al; ATAC Trialists' Group. Results of the ATAC (Arimidex, Tamoxifen, alone or in combination) trial after completion of 5 years adjuvant treatment for breast cancer. *Lancet.* 2005;365:60–62.

49. Jin H, Tu D, Zhao N, Shepherd LE, Goss PE. Longer-term outcomes of letrozole versus placebo after 5 years of tamoxifen in the NCIC CTG MA.17 trial: analysis adjusting for treatment crossover. *J Clin Oncol.* 2012;30(7):718–721.

50. Bliss JM, Kilburn LS, Coleman RE, et al. Disease-related outcomes with long-term follow-up: an updated analysis of the intergroup exemestane study. *J Clin Oncol.* 2012;30(7):709–717.

51. Burstein HJ, Lacchetti C, Griggs JJ. Adjuvant endocrine therapy for women with hormone receptor–positive breast cancer: ASCO clinical practice guideline focused update. *J Oncol Pract.* 2019;37(5):423–438.

52. Pagani O, Regan MM, Walley BA, et al; TEXT and SOFT Investigators; International Breast Cancer Study Group. Adjuvant exemestane with ovarian suppression in premenopausal breast cancer. *N Engl J Med.* 2014;371(2):107–118.

53. Francis PA, Pagani O, Fleming GF, et al; SOFT and TEXT Investigators and the International Breast Cancer Study Group. Tailoring adjuvant endocrine therapy for premenopausal breast cancer. *N Engl J Med.* 2018;379(2):122–137.

54. Pan H, Gray R, Braybrooke J, et al; EBCTCG. 20-year risks of breast-cancer recurrence after stopping endocrine therapy at 5 years. *N Engl J Med.* 2017;377(19):1836–1846.

55. Bartlett JMS, Sgroi DC, Treuner K, et al. Breast cancer Index and prediction of benefit from extended endocrine therapy in breast cancer patients treated in the Adjuvant Tamoxifen-To Offer More? (aTTom) trial. *Ann Oncol.* 2019;30(11):1776–1783.

56. Cella D, Fallowfield LJ. Recognition and management of treatment-related side effects for breast cancer patients receiving adjuvant endocrine therapy. *Breast Cancer Res Treat.* 2008;107(2):167–180.

57. Shah M, Nunes MR, Stearns V. CDK4/6 inhibitors: game changers in the management of hormone receptor–positive advanced breast cancer. *Oncology (Williston Park).* 2018;32(5):216–222.

58. Johnston SRD, Harbeck N, Hegg R, et al; monarchE Committee Members and Investigators. Abemaciclib combined with endocrine therapy for the adjuvant treatment of hr+, her2-, node-positive, high-risk, early breast cancer (monarchE). *J Clin Oncol.* 2020;38(34):3987–3998.

59. Johnston SRD, Toi M, O'Shaughnessy J, et al; monarchE Committee Members. Abemaciclib plus endocrine therapy for hormone receptor-positive, HER2-negative, node-positive, high-risk early breast cancer (monarchE): results from a preplanned interim analysis of a randomised, open-label, phase 3 trial. *Lancet Oncol.* 2023;24(1):77–90.

60. Slamon DJ, Stroyakovskiy D, Yardley DA, et al. Ribociclib and endocrine therapy as adjuvant treatment in patients with HR+/HER2– early breast cancer: primary results from the phase III NATALEE trial. *J Clin Oncol.* 2023;41(suppl 17):abstr LBA500.

61. Gnant M, Dueck AC, Frantal S, et al; PALLAS groups and investigators. Adjuvant palbociclib for early breast cancer: the PALLAS trial results (ABCSG-42/AFT-05/BIG-14-03). *J Clin Oncol.* 2022;40(3):282–293.

62. Baselga J, Carbonell X, Castañeda-Soto NJ, et al. Phase II study of efficacy, safety, and pharmacokinetics of trastuzumab monotherapy administered on a 3-weekly schedule. *J Clin Oncol.* 2005;23(10):2162–2171.

63. Viani GA, Afonso SL, Stefano EJ, De Fendi LI, Soares FV. Adjuvant trastuzumab in the treatment of HER-2-positive early breast cancer: a meta-analysis of published randomized trials. *BMC Cancer.* 2007;7:153.

64. Jahanzeb M. Adjuvant trastuzumab therapy for HER2-positive breast cancer. *Clin Breast Cancer.* 2008;8:324–333.

65. Shah AN, Gradishar WJ. Adjuvant anthracyclines in breast cancer: what is their role? *Oncologist.* 2018;23(10):1153–1161.

66. Gianni L, Pienkowski T, Im Y-H, et al. Efficacy and safety of neoadjuvant pertuzumab and trastuzumab in women with locally advanced, inflammatory, or early HER2-positive breast cancer (NeoSphere): a randomised multicenter, open-label, phase 2 trial. *Lancet Oncol.* 2012;13:25–32.

67. von Minckwitz G, Huang C-S, Mano MS, et al; KATHERINE Investigators. Trastuzumab emtansine for residual invasive HER2-positive breast cancer. *N Engl J Med.* 2019;380(7):617–628.

68. Tolaney SM, Barry WT, Dang CT, et al. Adjuvant paclitaxel and trastuzumab for node-negative, HER2-positive breast cancer. *N Engl J Med.* 2015;372(2):134–141.

69. Chan A, Moy B, Mansi J, et al; ExteNET Study Group. Final efficacy results of neratinib in HER2-positive hormone receptor-positive early-stage breast cancer from the phase III ExteNET trial. *Clin Breast Cancer.* 2021;21(1):80–91.e7.

70. Hudis CA, Gianni L. Triple-negative breast cancer: an unmet medical need. *Oncologist.* 2011; 16(Suppl 1):1–11.

71. Burstein HJ, Curigliano G, Loibl S, et al; Members of the St. Gallen International Consensus Panel on the Primary Therapy of Early Breast Cancer 2019. Estimating the benefits of therapy for early-stage breast cancer: the St. Gallen International Consensus Guidelines for the primary therapy of early breast cancer 2019. *Ann Oncol.* 2019;30(10):1541–1557.

72. Cortazar P, Zhang L, Untch M, et al. Pathological complete response and long-term clinical benefit in breast cancer: the CTNeoBC pooled analysis. *Lancet.* 2014;384(9938):164–172.

73. Schmid P, Cortes J, Pusztai L, et al; KEYNOTE-522 Investigators. Pembrolizumab for early triple-negative breast cancer. *N Engl J Med.* 2020;382(9):810–821.

74. Korde LA, Somerfield MR, Hershman DL; Neoadjuvant Chemotherapy, Endocrine Therapy, and Targeted Therapy for Breast Cancer Guideline Expert Panel. Use of immune checkpoint inhibitor pembrolizumab in the treatment of high-risk, early-stage triple-negative breast cancer: ASCO Guideline Rapid Recommendation Update. *J Clin Oncol.* 2022;40(15):1696–1698.

75. Masuda N, Lee S-J, Ohtani S, et al. Adjuvant capecitabine for breast cancer after preoperative chemotherapy. *N Engl J Med.* 2017;376(22):2147–2159.

76. Geyer CE Jr, Garber JE, Gelber RD, et al; OlympiA Clinical Trial Steering Committee and Investigators. Overall survival in the OlympiA phase III trial of adjuvant olaparib in patients with germline pathogenic variants in BRCA1/2 and high-risk, early breast cancer. *Ann Oncol.* 2022;33(12):1250–1268.

77. Tutt ANJ, Garber JE, Kaufman B, et al; OlympiA Clinical Trial Steering Committee and Investigators. Adjuvant olaparib for patients with BRCA1- or BRCA2-mutated breast cancer. *N Engl J Med.* 2021;384(25):2394–2405.

78. Anderson WF, Schairer C, Chen BE, Hance KW, Levine PH. Epidemiology of inflammatory breast cancer (IBC). *Breast Dis.* 2005;22:9–23.

79. Dawood S, Lei X, Dent R, et al. Survival of women with inflammatory breast cancer: a large population-based study. *Ann Oncol.* 2014;25(6):1143–1151.

80. Kida K, Olver I, Yennu S, Tripathy D, Ueno NT. Optimal supportive care for patients with metastatic breast cancer according to their disease progression phase. *JCO Oncol Pract.* 2021; 17(4):177–183.

81. Belkacemi Y, Hanna NE, Besnard C, Majdoul S, Gligorov J. Local and regional breast cancer recurrences: salvage therapy options in the new era of molecular subtypes. *Front Oncol.* 2018;8:112.

82. Wapnir IL, Price KN, Anderson SJ, et al; International Breast Cancer Study Group; NRG Oncology, GEICAM Spanish Breast Cancer Group, BOOG Dutch Breast Cancer Trialists' Group; Breast International Group. Efficacy of chemotherapy for ER-negative and ER-positive isolated locoregional recurrence of breast cancer: final analysis of the CALOR trial. *J Clin Oncol.* 2018;36(11):1073–1079.

83. Osoba D. Health-related quality of life as a treatment endpoint in metastatic breast cancer. *Can J Oncol.* 1995;5(Suppl 1):47–53.

84. Burstein HJ, Somerfield MR, Barton DL, et al. Endocrine treatment and targeted therapy for hormone receptor-positive, human epidermal growth factor receptor 2-negative metastatic breast cancer: ASCO guideline update. *J Clin Oncol.* 2021;39(35):3959–3977.

85. Finn RS, Martin M, Rugo HS, et al. Palbociclib and letrozole in advanced breast cancer. *N Engl J Med.* 2016;375(20):1925–1936.

86. Finn RS, Rugo HS, Dieras VC, et al. Overall survival (OS) with first-line palbociclib plus letrozole (PAL+LET) versus placebo plus letrozole (PBO+LET) in women with estrogen

receptor–positive/human epidermal growth factor receptor 2–negative advanced breast cancer (ER+/HER2– ABC): analyses from PALOMA-2. *J Clin Oncol.* 2022;40(17_suppl):LBA1003.

87. Hortobagyi GN, Stemmer SM, Burris HA, et al. Ribociclib as first-line therapy for HR-positive, advanced breast cancer. *N Engl J Med.* 2016;375(18):1738–1748.

88. Hortobagyi GN, Stemmer SM, Burris HA, et al. Overall survival with ribociclib plus letrozole in advanced breast cancer. *N Engl J Med.* 2022;386(10):942–950.

89. Johnston S, Martin M, Di Leo A, et al. MONARCH 3 final PFS: a randomized study of abemaciclib as initial therapy for advanced breast cancer. *NPJ Breast Cancer.* 2019;5:5.

90. Husinka L, Koerner PH, Miller RT, Trombatt W. Review of cyclin-dependent kinase 4/6 inhibitors in the treatment of advanced or metastatic breast cancer. *J Drug Assess.* 2020;10(1): 27–34.

91. Tripathy D, Im S-A, Colleoni M, et al. Ribociclib plus endocrine therapy for premenopausal women with hormone-receptor-positive, advanced breast cancer (MONALEESA-7): a randomised phase 3 trial. *Lancet Oncol.* 2018;19(7):904–915.

92. Chia S, Gradishar W, Mauriac L, et al. Double-blind, randomized placebo controlled trial of fulvestrant compared with exemestane after prior nonsteroidal aromatase inhibitor therapy in postmenopausal women with hormone receptor-positive, advanced breast cancer: results from EFECT. *J Clin Oncol.* 2008;26(10):1664–1670.

93. André F, Ciruelos EM, Juric D, et al. Alpelisib plus fulvestrant for PIK3CA-mutated, hormone receptor-positive, human epidermal growth factor receptor-2-negative advanced breast cancer: final overall survival results from SOLAR-1. *Ann Oncol.* 2021;32(2):208–217.

94. Bidard F-C, Kaklamani VG, Neven P, et al. Elacestrant (oral selective estrogen receptor degrader) versus standard endocrine therapy for estrogen receptor-positive, human epidermal growth factor receptor 2-negative advanced breast cancer: results from the randomized phase III EMERALD trial. *J Clin Oncol.* 2022;40(28):3246–3256.

95. Yardley DA, Noguchi S, Pritchard KI, et al. Everolimus plus exemestane in postmenopausal patients with HR(+) breast cancer: BOLERO-2 final progression-free survival analysis. *Adv Ther.* 2013;30(10):870–884.

96. Vogel CL, Cobleigh MA, Tripathy D, et al. Efficacy and safety of trastuzumab as a single agent in first-line treatment of HER2-overexpressing metastatic breast cancer. *J Clin Oncol.* 2002;20(3):719–726.

97. Swain SM, Baselga J, Kim SB, et al; CLEOPATRA Study Group. Pertuzumab, trastuzumab, and docetaxel in HER2-positive metastatic breast cancer. *N Engl J Med.* 2015;372:724–734.

98. Barok M, Joensuu H, Isola J. Trastuzumab emtansine: mechanisms of action and drug resistance. *Breast Cancer Res.* 2014;16(2):1–12.

99. Cortés J, Kim S-B, Chung W-P, et al; DESTINY-Breast03 Trial Investigators. Trastuzumab deruxtecan versus trastuzumab emtansine for breast cancer. *N Engl J Med.* 2022;386(12): 1143–1154.

100. Hurvitz SA, Hegg R, Chung WP, et al. Trastuzumab deruxtecan versus trastuzumab emtansine in patients with HER2-positive metastatic breast cancer: updated results from DESTINY-Breast03, a randomised, open-label, phase 3 trial. *Lancet.* 2023;401(10371):105–117.

101. Verma S, Miles D, Gianni L, et al; EMILIA Study Group. Trastuzumab emtansine for HER2-positive advanced breast cancer. *N Engl J Med.* 2012;367(19):1783–1791.

102. Murthy RK, Loi S, Okines A, et al. Tucatinib, trastuzumab, and capecitabine for HER2-positive metastatic breast cancer. *N Engl J Med.* 2020;382(7):597–609.

103. Lin NU, Borges V, Anders C, et al. Intracranial efficacy and survival with tucatinib plus trastuzumab and capecitabine for previously treated HER2-positive breast cancer with brain metastases in the HER2CLIMB trial. *J Clin Oncol.* 2020;38(23):2610–2619.

104. Saura C, Oliveira M, Feng YH, et al; NALA Investigators. Neratinib plus capecitabine versus lapatinib plus capecitabine in HER2-positive metastatic breast cancer previously treated with ≥ 2 HER2-directed regimens: phase III NALA trial. *J Clin Oncol.* 2020;38(27):3138–3149.

105. Geyer CE, Forster J, Lindquist D, et al. Lapatinib plus capecitabine for HER2-positive advanced breast cancer. *N Engl J Med.* 2006;355(26):2733–2743.

106. Rugo HS, Im S-A, Cardoso F, et al; SOPHIA Study Group. Efficacy of margetuximab vs trastuzumab in patients with pretreated ERBB2-positive advanced breast cancer: a phase 3 randomized clinical trial. *JAMA Oncol.* 2021;7(4):573–584.

107. Rugo HS, Im S-A, Cardoso F, et al; SOPHIA Study Group. Margetuximab versus trastuzumab in patients with previously treated HER2-positive advanced breast cancer (SOPHIA): final overall survival results from a randomized phase 3 trial. *J Clin Oncol.* 2023;41(2):198–205.

108. Cortes J, Rugo HS, Cescon DW, et al; KEYNOTE-355 Investigators. Pembrolizumab plus che-motherapy in advanced triple-negative breast cancer. *N Engl J Med.* 2022;387(3):217–226.
109. Hafeez U, Parakh S, Gan HK, Scott AM. Antibody-drug conjugates for cancer therapy. *Molecules.* 2020;25(20):4764.
110. Modi S, Jacot W, Yamashita T, et al; DESTINY-Breast04 Trial Investigators. Trastuzumab derux-tecan in previously treated HER2-low advanced breast cancer. *N Engl J Med.* 2022;387(1):9–20.
111. Tarantino P, Hamilton E, Tolaney SM, et al. HER2-low breast cancer: pathological and clinical landscape. *J Clin Oncol.* 2020;38(17):1951–1962.
112. Goldenberg DM, Cardillo TM, Govindan SV, Rossi EA, Sharkey RM. Trop-2 is a novel target for solid cancer therapy with sacituzumab govitecan (IMMU-132), an antibody-drug conjugate (ADC). *Oncotarget.* 2015;6(26):22496–22512.
113. Bardia A, Hurvitz SA, Tolaney SM, et al; ASCENT Clinical Trial Investigators. Sacituzumab govitecan in metastatic triple-negative breast cancer. *N Engl J Med.* 2021;384(16):1529–1541.
114. Rugo HS, Bardia A, Marmé F, et al. Sacituzumab govitecan in hormone receptor-positive/human epidermal growth factor receptor 2-negative metastatic breast cancer. *J Clin Oncol.* 2022;40(29): 3365–3376.
115. Jagtap P, Szabó C. Poly (ADP-ribose) polymerase and the therapeutic effects of its inhibitors. *Nat Rev Drug Discov.* 2005;4(5):421–440.
116. Rose M, Burgess JT, O'Byrne K, Richard DJ, Bolderson E. PARP inhibitors: clinical relevance, mechanisms of action and tumor resistance. *Front Cell Dev Biol.* 2020;8:564601.
117. Robson M, Im S-A, Senkus E, et al. Olaparib for metastatic breast cancer in patients with a germline BRCA mutation. *N Engl J Med.* 2017;377(6):523–533.
118. Robson ME, Tung N, Conte P, et al. OlympiAD final overall survival and tolerability results: Olaparib versus chemotherapy treatment of physician's choice in patients with a germline BRCA mutation and HER2-negative metastatic breast cancer. *Ann Oncol.* 2019;30(4):558–566.
119. Carrick S, Parker S, Thornton CE, Ghersi D, Simes J, Wilcken N. Single agent versus combi-nation chemotherapy for metastatic breast cancer. *Cochrane Database Syst Rev.* 2009;2009(2): CD003372.
120. Cardoso F, Paluch-Shimon S, Senkus E, et al. 5th ESO-ESMO international consensus guide-lines for advanced breast cancer (ABC 5). *Ann Oncol.* 2020;31(12):1623–1649.
121. Tsuzuki S, Park SH, Eber MR, Peters CM, Shiozawa Y. Skeletal complications in cancer patients with bone metastases. *Int J Urol.* 2016;23(10):825–832.
122. Van Poznak C, Somerfield MR, Barlow WE, et al. Role of bone-modifying agents in metastatic breast cancer: an American Society of Clinical Oncology–Cancer Care Ontario focused guideline update. *J Clin Oncol.* 2017;35(35):3978–3986.
123. O'Carrigan B, Wong MH, Willson ML, Stockler MR, Pavlakis N, Goodwin A. Bisphosphonates and other bone agents for breast cancer. *Cochrane Database Syst Rev.* 2017;10(10):CD003474.
124. Lipton A, Steger GG, Figueroa J, et al. Extended efficacy and safety of denosumab in breast cancer patients with bone metastases not receiving prior bisphosphonate therapy. *Clin Cancer Res.* 2008;14(20):6690–6696.
125. Runowicz CD, Leach CR, Henry NL, et al. American Cancer Society/American Society of Clin-ical Oncology Breast cancer survivorship care guideline. *J Clin Oncol.* 2016;34(6):611–635.

Lung Cancer

22

Christine Auberle and Saiama N. Waqar

GENERAL PRINCIPLES

Lung cancer is divided into two broad groups: small-cell lung cancer (SCLC) and non–small-cell lung cancer (NSCLC), based on histology. Their clinical behavior and management are different and, therefore, discussed separately.

Epidemiology

Lung cancer is the leading cause of cancer-related mortality in US, with an estimated 238,340 new cases and 127,070 deaths in 2023.[1] Due to improvements in therapies, earlier lung cancer detection, and advances in staging, the 3-year relative survival for all stages of NSCLC has increased from 22% to 33% for those diagnosed in 2004–2006 compared to those diagnosed in 2016–2018.[1]

Risk Factors

- **Tobacco smoke** is the major risk factor for lung cancer. There is a clear, dose-dependent relationship between tobacco use and lung cancer. Smoking reduction reduces the risk of lung cancer. Squamous cell lung cancers and SCLCs, in particular, are associated with tobacco smoking.
- Occupational exposures have also been associated with lung cancer, including asbestos, beryllium, cadmium, diesel fumes, coal smoke, silica, soot, radon, chromium, nickel, and arsenic compounds.
- Genetic predisposition is an important risk factor, and there are well-identified familial clusters of lung cancers. A lung cancer susceptibility locus has been reported to be within 6q23–25. Genes encoding for several subunits of the nicotinic acetylcholine receptor are localized to 15q24–25 and are associated with increased risk of lung cancer and nicotine dependence. Germline *EGFR* T790M mutations have also been associated with hereditary lung cancer especially in never smokers.[2]

Prevention and Screening

Current and former smokers have a significant risk of lung cancer, and **smoking cessation** should be encouraged. Low-dose CT chest is recommended for screening in patients ages 50 years and older with a 20-pack-year or more smoking history. Low-dose CT screening decreases mortality of lung cancer by 20%, based on the National Lung Screening Trial.[3] Current guidelines have extended eligibility for screening to include younger patients with less smoking history. Despite this, only 5.8% of individuals eligible for screening were screened as of 2022.

Non–Small-Cell Lung Cancer

GENERAL PRINCIPLES

NSCLC accounts for 80–85% of lung cancers in US. The most common pathologic subtypes include:

- **Squamous cell carcinoma** usually arises from the basal cells in proximal bronchi and can cause obstruction of the larger airways. It appears as malignant epithelial tumor with keratinization or intracellular bridges and immunohistochemistry that is often positive for p40 or p63.
- **Adenocarcinoma** is the most common subtype, representing 40% of lung cancers in North America. It usually arises from type II alveolar cells in the lung periphery with immunohistochemistry often positive for TTF-1 and napsin A. Adenocarcinoma in situ (formerly known as bronchioloalveolar carcinoma) grows along intact alveolar septa in a "lepidic" growth pattern.
- **Adenosquamous carcinoma** is a tumor comprised of both adenocarcinoma and squamous cell carcinoma with each subtype consisting of at least 10% of the tumor.
- **Large-cell carcinoma** is the least common subtype and must lack evidence of clear lineage with immunohistochemistry excluding adenocarcinoma or squamous cell.

DIAGNOSIS

Clinical Presentation

- Presenting signs and symptoms of lung cancer depend on the size, location, and degree of spread of the tumor. Lung cancer can present as an asymptomatic lung nodule found incidentally on imaging. Local symptoms can include cough, wheeze, hemoptysis, dyspnea, postobstructive pneumonia (due to tumors that occlude major bronchi), pain (particularly with pleural or chest wall involvement), dysphagia (due to esophageal compression by tumor or lymphadenopathy), and hoarseness (caused by recurrent laryngeal nerve involvement). Apical tumors that invade the lower brachial plexus can present with **Pancoast syndrome**, which is a brachial plexopathy, Horner syndrome, and shoulder pain. Mediastinal lymphadenopathy that compresses the superior vena cava (SVC) can cause **SVC syndrome**, which most commonly presents with dyspnea and facial swelling and is seen more in SCLC. Systemic symptoms usually accompany disease that is more advanced and can include weight loss, fatigue, and loss of appetite. Metastatic disease may cause symptoms specific to the involved organs. For example, patients may have pain from bone metastases or pathologic fractures, dyspnea from pericardial or pleural effusions, headache, seizures, and neurologic deficits from brain metastases. Although adrenal and liver metastases are common, they are usually asymptomatic.
- NSCLC has been associated with numerous paraneoplastic syndromes. Clubbing results from an increase in the soft tissue beneath the nail bed. Dermatomyositis, an autoimmune inflammatory myopathy, may present as proximal muscle weakness, a heliotrope rash on the eyelids, and erythematous papules on the hands. Hyponatremia from syndrome of inappropriate antidiuretic hormone secretion (SIADH) is seen more commonly in SCLC. Hypercalcemia may be due to ectopic parathyroid hormone production by the tumor and is seen most commonly in squamous cell carcinoma. **Pulmonary hypertrophic osteoarthropathy** is a syndrome consisting of bone and joint pain, clubbing, and increased alkaline phosphatase. It can be diagnosed by plain films (which show periosteal inflammation) or bone scans (which show increased uptake symmetrically in long bones).

Diagnostic Testing

The goal of the initial workup is to establish the diagnosis of malignancy and to determine accurately the clinical stage of the cancer so that candidates for potentially curable surgical resection are identified. Strategies for obtaining a pathologic diagnosis of a lung mass include percutaneous or transbronchial biopsy.

Imaging

CT of the chest and upper abdomen is crucial in evaluating the size of the tumor, mediastinal involvement, and the presence of liver or adrenal metastases. **Positron emission**

tomography (PET) scan is useful in detecting mediastinal lymph node involvement and distant metastases, especially bone metastases. MRI of the brain is needed to rule out intracranial metastases in asymptomatic patients with node-positive disease or patients with neurologic symptoms. For superior sulcus tumors with concern for involvement of the spine, subclavian vessels, or brachial plexus, an MRI with contrast of the spine and thoracic inlet should be considered.

Diagnostic Procedures

Potential lymph node metastases identified in imaging studies should be confirmed with direct biopsy. Endobronchial ultrasound (EBUS) has been utilized more to biopsy mediastinal lymph nodes as it is less invasive. Compared to transthoracic and endoscopic biopsy for mediastinal staging, **mediastinoscopy** has a higher negative predictive value and is the most accurate means of staging mediastinal lymph nodes. Cervical mediastinoscopy is beneficial for staging superior mediastinal lymph nodes and an extended or anterior (Chamberlain) approach is more appropriate for anterior mediastinal lymph nodes.

Staging

If tissue sampling confirms the diagnosis of NSCLC, the stage of disease should be determined using the tumor, node, metastasis (TNM) staging. Proposals for the ninth edition of TNM staging were developed by the International Association for the Study of Lung Cancer (IASLC).

The TNM classifications are then used to determine the stage grouping for the patient. A broad overview of each stage includes:

- Stage I disease consists of tumors ≤4 cm and node-negative disease.
- Stage II disease consists of either any tumor that is >4 cm and ≤7 cm or a small tumor with ipsilateral peribronchial, intrapulmonary, and/or hilar lymph nodes.
- Stage III disease consists of tumors larger than 7 cm, invading the mediastinum, with separate tumor nodules in a different ipsilateral lobe, or patients with mediastinal or supraclavicular lymph node involvement.
- Stage IV consists of metastatic disease.

TREATMENT

Early-Stage Node-Negative Disease

- Tumors are considered early-stage disease and **resectable**, if they have extended no further than adjacent resectable structures or first-level lymph nodes. The optimal treatment is surgical resection with lobectomy or pneumonectomy with curative intent. Preoperative workup includes spirometry to establish both that the FEV1 will be >1.2 L postresection and that the patient does not have hypercapnia or cor pulmonale. Patients with positive margins after resection should be considered for reresection or radiation therapy (RT).
- Patients who are not candidates for surgery because of poor lung function or comorbid conditions should be considered for **stereotactic body radiation therapy** (SBRT) administered with curative intent. Toxicities of SBRT include pneumonitis (shortness of breath, fever, nonproductive cough, and infiltrate on imaging), pulmonary fibrosis, acute esophagitis, pericarditis, and Lhermitte phenomenon or radiation myelitis (transient electric sensation radiating down the spine or into the limbs with neck flexion).

Early-Stage Node-Positive Disease

- Patients with early-stage disease with positive lymph nodes should be offered perioperative (adjuvant or neoadjuvant) therapy. Patients with node-negative early-stage disease should be considered for neoadjuvant or adjuvant therapy if high-risk features are present on resection such as tumors >4 cm, vascular invasion, wedge resection, visceral pleural involvement, and unknown lymph node status. For patients who are not eligible to receive cisplatin therapy, carboplatin may be substituted. Immunotherapy has now been integrated into perioperative therapy for eligible patients, and patients with tumors carrying *EGFR* mutations may be eligible for adjuvant osimertinib (Table 22-1).

Locally Advanced Disease

Treatment of patients with locally advanced disease requires a multidisciplinary approach, involving input from surgeons, medical oncologists, and radiation oncologists. Patients should be evaluated for resectability and if operable should receive neoadjuvant, perioperative, or adjuvant therapy as above. For inoperable locally advanced disease, definitive chemoradiation is recommended. Consolidation immunotherapy with durvalumab for 1 year is recommended following concurrent chemoradiation and has been shown to increase 5-year overall survival to 42.9% from 33.4% compared to placebo.[9] If patients are not candidates for consolidation immunotherapy, consolidation chemotherapy is an option. For patients with a resectable superior sulcus tumor, preoperative concurrent chemoradiation followed by surgical resection has been shown to increase overall survival.[10]

Metastatic Disease

- Patients with advanced or metastatic disease should have molecular testing to evaluate for actionable gene alterations and PD-L1 expression. For patients with tumors with actionable gene alterations, many options are available as first-line therapies including tumors with *EGFR* exon 19 deletions or exon 21 L858R mutations, *ALK* rearrangements, *ROS1* rearrangements, *BRAF* V600E mutations, *NTRK 1/2/3* gene fusions, *MET* exon 14 skipping mutations, and *RET* rearrangements. Patients with *KRAS* G12C mutations, *ERBB2* (*HER2*) mutations, or *EGFR* exon 20 insertions have molecularly targeted therapies approved starting as subsequent therapies (Table 22-2).
- For patients with tumors without actionable gene alterations and high PD-L1 expression (>50%), immunotherapy alone is preferred (Table 22-3), combination chemotherapy and immunotherapy are preferred for all other immunotherapy-eligible patients and has been shown to increase overall survival (Table 22-4).
- Oligometastatic disease, such as isolated single-brain metastasis or adrenal metastasis, may benefit from aggressive local therapy to the lung lesions in addition to systemic therapy combined with surgery or definitive radiation to metastatic sites.

MONITORING/FOLLOW-UP

According to the consensus guidelines, in patients with stage I–II disease after surgery with or without chemotherapy, a careful history and physical examination and CT of the chest with contrast should be performed every 6 months for 2–3 years followed by a low-dose noncontrast CT annually. For stage I–II disease treated primarily with radiation or stage III disease, surveillance should include a CT chest with contrast every 3 months for 3 years, then every 6 months for 2 years followed by a low-dose noncontrast CT annually. Further tests such as PET scan and MRI of the brain are not part of routine surveillance and should be obtained only if signs or symptoms suggest recurrent disease.

OUTCOME/PROGNOSIS

Prognosis varies by stage and presence of actionable molecular alteration, and there are patients with long-term responses even after completing immunotherapy. The 5-year survival rate for adenocarcinoma is 73.3% for localized disease, 46.4% for regional disease, and 11.0% for metastatic disease. For squamous cell, the 5-year survival rate was 48.7%, 27.9%,

TABLE 22-1	PERIOPERATIVE SYSTEMIC THERAPY FOR EARLY-STAGE RESECTABLE DISEASE		
Study	Regimen	Key Results	Notes
Neoadjuvant regimens			
CheckMate 816[4]	Nivolumab and platinum-doublet chemotherapy for three cycles	Compared to neoadjuvant chemotherapy alone, pathologic CR was 24% vs. 2.2% and median EFS was 31.6 vs. 20.8 mo	Resectable stage IB to IIIA (AJCC 7th ed.)
Neoadjuvant working group meta-analysis	Platinum-doublet chemotherapy for four cycles	Improvement of 5-y overall survival by 5% compared to surgery alone	Mainly resectable stage IB-IIIA (AJCC 7th ed.)
Perioperative regimens			
KEYNOTE-671	Pembrolizumab and platinum-doublet chemotherapy for four cycles prior to surgery and adjuvant pembrolizumab for 13 cycles	Compared to neoadjuvant chemotherapy alone, pathologic CR was 18.1% vs. 4.0% and median EFS was NR vs. 17.0 mo	Resectable stage II, IIIA, or IIIB (N2 stage) disease
Adjuvant regimens			
LACE Meta-analysis[5]	Platinum-doublet chemotherapy for four cycles	Improvement in 5-y overall survival by 5.4% compared to surgery alone	Node-positive disease
ADAURA[6]	Osimertinib for 3 y as monotherapy or following platinum-doublet for four cycles (chemotherapy not mandated)	Compared to placebo, median DFS was NR vs. 22.1 mo	Resectable IB-IIIA tumors positive for *EGFR* exon 19 deletion or *EGFR* exon 21 L858R mutation (AJCC 7th ed.)
Therapy following adjuvant chemotherapy			
IMpower010[7]	Atezolizumab for 1 y	Compared to supportive care, 3-y DFS was 60.0% vs. 48.2%	Resectable stage II-IIIA with PD-L1 of 1% or more (AJCC 7th ed.)
PEARLS/KEYNOTE-091[8]	Pembrolizumab for 1 y	Compared to placebo, 3-y DFS was 58% vs. 50%	Resectable IB-IIA irrespective of PD-L1 status (AJCC 7th ed.)

AJCC 7th ed, denotes studies performed using the American Joint Committee on Cancer 7th edition of staging; CR, complete response; DFS, disease-free survival; EFS, event-free survival; NR, not reached; PD-L1, programmed-death ligand 1.

TABLE 22-2	GENE ALTERATIONS IN METASTATIC NSCLC AND ASSOCIATED THERAPIES

Molecular Marker	Most Common Alteration	Therapies
First-line therapies		
EGFR	Exon 19 deletions Exon 21 L858R	Osimertinib[11] (preferred), erlotinib +/– bevacizumab or ramucirumab, gefitinib, afatinib, dacomitinib
ALK	EML4-ALK translocation	Alectinib[12], brigatinib, ceritinib, lorlatinib, crizotinib
ROS1	Rearrangements	Crizotinib, entrectinib, ceritinib
First-line or second-line therapies		
EGFR	Exon 19 deletions Exon 21 L858R	Osimertinib
ALK	EML4-ALK translocation	Alectinib, brigatinib, ceritinib, lorlatinib
ROS1	Rearrangements	Lorlatinib, entrectinib
BRAF	V600E	Dabrafenib in combination with trametinib
MET	Exon 14 skipping mutation	Capmatinib, tepotinib, crizotinib
NTRK	1/2/3 gene fusion	Larotrectinib, entrectinib
RET	Rearrangements	Selpercatinib or pralsetinib (preferred), cabozantinib, vandetanib
Second-line therapies		
EGFR	Exon 20 insertion	Mobocertinib, amivantamab-vmjw
KRAS	G12C	Sotorasib, adagrasib
ERBB2 (HER2)	Exon 20 insertion or duplication events	Ado-trastuzumab emansine, fam-trastuzumab deruxtecan-nxki

ALK, anaplastic lymphoma kinase; EGFR: epidermal growth factor receptor.

TABLE 22-3	IMMUNOTHERAPY REGIMENS FOR METASTATIC NSCLC WITH PD-L1 ≥50%

Study	Regimen	Key Results	Notes
IMpower110	Atezolizumab	Response rate: 38.3% Median PFS: 8.1 mo Median OS: 20.2 mo	Tumors with PD-L1 ≥50%
KEYNOTE-024[13]	Pembrolizumab	Response rate: 44.8% Median PFS: 10.3 mo Median OS: 30.0 mo	Tumors with PD-L1 ≥50%
EMPOWER-Lung 1	Cemiplimab	Response rate: 39% Median PFS: 8.2 mo Median OS: NR	Tumors with PD-L1 ≥50%

mo, months; NR, not reached; PD-L1, programmed-death ligand; PFS, progression-free survival.

TABLE 22-4 SYSTEMIC THERAPY REGIMENS FOR METASTATIC NSCLC WITH PD-L1 <50%

Study	Regimen	Notes	Key Results
KEYNOTE-189[14]	(Carboplatin or cisplatin), pemetrexed, and pembrolizumab for four cycles followed by maintenance pemetrexed and pembrolizumab up to 35 cycles	Nonsquamous histology, PD-L1 1-49%	Response rate: 48.3% vs. 19.9% Median PFS: 9.0 vs. 4.9 mo Median OS: 22.0 vs. 10.6 mo
KEYNOTE-407[15]	Carboplatin (paclitaxel or albumin-bound paclitaxel) and pembrolizumab for four cycles followed up by maintenance pembrolizumab up to 35 cycles	Squamous histology, PD-L1 1-49%	Response rate: 62.2% vs. 38.8% Median PFS: 8.0 vs. 5.1 mo Median OS: 17.2 vs. 11.6 mo
IMpower130[16]	Carboplatin, albumin-bound paclitaxel, and atezolizumab for four or six cycles followed by maintenance atezolizumab for up to 35 cycles	Nonsquamous histology, PD-L1 1-49%	Response rate: 49.2% vs. 31.9% Median PFS: 7.0 vs. 5.5 mo Median OS: 18.1 vs. 13.9 mo
IMpower150	Carboplatin, paclitaxel, bevacizumab, and atezolizumab for four or six cycles followed by maintenance atezolizumab and bevacizumab	Nonsquamous histology, PD-L1 1-49%	Response rate: 63.5% vs. 48% Median PFS: 8.3 vs. 6.8 mo Median OS: 19.0 vs. 14.7 mo
CheckMate 227[17]	Nivolumab and ipilimumab	Any histology, PD-L1 1-49%	Response rate: 45.3 vs. 26.9% Median PFS: 4.9 vs. 5.5 mo Median OS: 17.1 vs. 13.9 mo
CheckMate 9LA	Platinum-doublet chemotherapy, nivolumab, and ipilimumab for two cycles followed by maintenance nivolumab and ipilimumab for up to 35 cycles	Any histology, PD-L1 1-49%	Response rate: 38% vs. 25% Median PFS: 6.4 vs. 5.3 mo Median OS: 15.8 vs. 11 mo
EMPOWER-Lung 3[18]	Platinum-doublet chemotherapy and cemiplimab for four cycles followed by maintenance cemiplimab +/- pemetrexed up to 35 cycles	Any histology, PD-L1 1-49%	Response rate: 43.3% vs. 22.7% Median PFS: 8.2 vs. 5.0 mo Median OS: 21.9 vs. 13.0 mo
POSEIDON	Platinum-doublet chemotherapy, tremelimumab, and durvalumab for four cycles followed by maintenance durvalumab +/- pemetrexed	Any histology, PD-L1 1-49%	Response rate: 46.3% vs. 33.4% Median PFS: 6.2 vs. 4.8 mo Median OS: 14.0 vs. 11.7 mo

mo, months; NR: not reached; PD-L1, programmed-death ligand; PFS: progression free survival.

and 6.9% for localized, regional, and metastatic disease respectively. These trends have been increasing since 2015 with the advent of immunotherapy and molecularly targeted therapies.

Small-Cell Lung Cancer

GENERAL PRINCIPLES

SCLC accounts for 10–15% of lung cancers in US. Compared to NSCLC, SCLC grows more rapidly, is more often associated with diverse paraneoplastic syndromes, and is more chemosensitive initially. Most patients are current or previous heavy smokers.

DIAGNOSIS

Clinical Presentation

The presenting signs and symptoms of SCLC are similar to those of NSCLC. SCLCs are often centrally located and symptoms result from obstruction of the airway lumen. Common symptoms are cough, dyspnea, hemoptysis, wheezing, and postobstructive pneumonia. Patients with limited-stage disease may present with a small primary tumor or enlarged lymph nodes. Patients with extensive stage disease can often present with SIADH and 10% of patients have SVC syndrome at presentation.

- **Paraneoplastic syndromes** associated with SCLC include SIADH, Cushing syndrome from ectopic adrenocorticotropic hormone production, and neurologic paraneoplastic syndromes, including peripheral neuropathy and encephalomyelitis, and are thought to be due to the production of autoantibodies. Lambert–Eaton syndrome is caused by an autoantibody that impairs acetylcholine release at the neuromuscular junction, leading to proximal muscle weakness and hyporeflexia.

Diagnostic Testing

Initial workup should include a comprehensive history and physical examination. Initial studies include **CBC** and **complete metabolic profile (CMP)**. Tumor lysis syndrome may occur with bulky disease, so **lactate dehydrogenase** and **uric acid** should also be checked. **CT scan of the chest and abdomen** should be performed to define the extent of intrathoracic disease and to detect abdominal metastases. **Brain MRI** is needed whenever possible to rule out intracranial metastases. **PET-CT scan** is helpful in detecting distant metastases, especially if limited stage is suspected and the goal of treatment may be curative. Once the disease has been found outside of the thorax, workup for additional sites of metastasis is not necessary unless a metastasis requiring immediate intervention (e.g., to weight-bearing bone or CNS) is suspected.

Staging

The TNM staging system is not widely used to classify SCLC, although the IASLC has proposed the use of TNM staging.[19] Currently, SCLC is described either as **limited stage**, with disease confined to one hemithorax that is encompassed in a single radiation field, or as **extensive stage**, which describes all other patterns of disease. Approximately one-third of patients will have limited-stage disease when first diagnosed.

TREATMENT

- **Chemotherapy** is the primary modality used for the treatment of SCLC, as inferior results are obtained when RT is used alone. For patients with **limited-stage disease**, combined modality treatment with chemotherapy (cisplatin or carboplatin and etoposide for four cycles) and RT to the chest is standard of care.[20] **Extensive-stage disease** is treated with chemoimmunotherapy. The commonly used regimens for SCLC include combinations of four to six cycles of carboplatin, etoposide, and anti-PD-L1 therapy (atezolizumab or durvalumab) followed by maintenance immunotherapy. Both atezolizumab and durvalumab when added to chemotherapy have modestly improved OS to 12–13 months versus 10 months with chemotherapy alone.[21,22] For patients who respond to chemotherapy, consolidation thoracic radiation in combination with prophylactic cranial irradiation (PCI) has been shown to have a modest improvement in 2-year overall survival.[23] The role of consolidation radiation after chemoimmunotherapy is not yet defined.

- **Prophylactic cranial irradiation** (PCI) is recommended for patients with limited-stage SCLC who achieve complete response after initial chemoradiation to prevent intracranial metastases.[24] If patients do not undergo PCI with limited-stage disease then MRI surveillance should be performed. PCI can also be considered in patients with extensive-stage SCLC with response to treatment. However, it should not be administered to patients with poor performance status or impaired mental function. The benefit of very early-stage (I-IIA) SCLC is unclear.
- Patients with poor performance status or significant comorbidities may not be able to tolerate aggressive chemotherapy. These patients may receive only RT or attenuated schedules of chemotherapy, with the goal of palliating symptoms.
- Most patients with SCLC will experience relapse and unfortunately, the median survival in patients with relapse is 2–6 months despite additional therapy. Patients with tumor progression >90 days after primary treatment may be rechallenged with their primary treatment or lurbinectedin. For patients with progressive or resistant relapses (<90 days from their last day of treatment) treatment options include lurbinectedin, topotecan, irinotecan, paclitaxel, docetaxel, temozolomide, vinorelbine, gemcitabine, or immunotherapy if not given previously.

MONITORING/FOLLOW-UP

Patients usually develop relapsed SCLC in the first 2 years after diagnosis. Therefore, they should have close follow-up with a medical oncologist for the identification of symptoms and imaging. Patients with limited-stage disease should receive surveillance CT chest and/or abdomen and pelvis and Oncology visits every 3 months for the first 2 years, then 6 months during the third year, and then annually. Patients with extensive-stage disease should receive surveillance CT chest and/or abdomen and pelvis every 2 months during the first year, then every 3–4 months until year three, then every 6 months until year five, and then annually. Patients should receive a brain MRI for surveillance every 3–4 months during the first year, then every 6 months during the second year, then as clinically indicated. Patients should be counseled extensively on the importance of smoking cessation, as smokers can experience increased mortality and increased treatment toxicity. Patients with SCLC are also at a higher risk of developing additional primary malignancies due to smoking.

OUTCOME/PROGNOSIS

Stage (limited vs. extensive), performance status, and markers of disease burden, such as serum lactate dehydrogenase, are the factors that most reliably correlate with outcome. The median survival of limited-stage disease treated with chemotherapy and RT is 15–26 months. Approximately 60–70% of SCLC patients have extensive stage at diagnosis. The 3-year survival rate for extensive-stage disease is approximately 15%.

Other Malignant Tumors of the Lung

Malignant tumors of the lung, other than NSCLC and SCLC, are uncommon and include carcinoid tumors, mucoepidermoid carcinoma, and sarcomas. Carcinoid tumors account for 1% of lung malignancies and are derived from neuroendocrine cells. They arise in the bronchi, may cause bronchial obstruction, and may metastasize to the liver producing a variety of systemically active substances that cause the **carcinoid syndrome**: flushing, diarrhea, and wheezing. Typical carcinoid grows slowly and rarely spreads outside of the lungs accounting for approximately 90% of carcinoid tumors. Atypical carcinoid is less common, grows faster, and is more likely to metastasize. Management of symptoms of carcinoid syndrome includes long-acting somatostatin analogs such as octreotide long-acting repeatable or lanreotide. If disease is locoregional and resectable then surgery should be considered. For metastatic disease, treatment regimens include octreotide, everolimus, temozolomide ± capecitabine, or (cisplatin or carboplatin) with etoposide. Carcinoid tumors of the lung tend to grow slowly and are associated with a 5-year survival of 85–95%.

REFERENCES

1. Siegel RL, Miller KD, Wagle NS, Jemal A. Cancer statistics, 2023. *CA Cancer J Clin*. 2023;73(1):17–48.
2. Gazdar A, Robinson L, Oliver D, et al. Hereditary lung cancer syndrome targets never smokers with germline EGFR gene T790M mutations. *J Thorac Oncol*. 2014;9(4):456–463.
3. National Lung Screening Trial Research Team; Aberle DR, Adams AM, et al. Reduced lung-cancer mortality with low-dose computed tomographic screening. *N Engl J Med*. 2011;365(5):395–409.
4. Forde PM, Spicer J, Lu S, et al. Neoadjuvant nivolumab plus chemotherapy in resectable lung cancer. *N Engl J Med*. 2022;386(21):1973–1985.
5. Pignon J-P, Tribodet H, Scagliotti GV, et al. Lung adjuvant cisplatin evaluation: a pooled analysis by the LACE collaborative group. *J Clin Oncol*. 2008;26(21):3552–3559.
6. Wu Y-L, John T, Grohe C, et al. Postoperative chemotherapy use and outcomes from ADAURA: osimertinib as adjuvant therapy for resected EGFR-mutated NSCLC. *J Thorac Oncol*. 2022;17(3):423–433.
7. Felip E, Altorki N, Zhou C, et al. Adjuvant atezolizumab after adjuvant chemotherapy in resected stage IB–IIIA non-small-cell lung cancer (IMpower010): a randomised, multicentre, open-label, phase 3 trial. *Lancet*. 2021;398(10308):1344–1357.
8. O'Brien M, Paz-Ares L, Marreaud S, et al. Pembrolizumab versus placebo as adjuvant therapy for completely resected stage IB–IIIA non-small-cell lung cancer (PEARLS/KEYNOTE-091): an interim analysis of a randomised, triple-blind, phase 3 trial. *Lancet Oncol*. 2022;23(10):1274–1286.
9. Spigel DR, Faivre-Finn C, Gray JE, et al. Five-year survival outcomes from the PACIFIC trial: durvalumab after chemoradiotherapy in stage III non–small-cell lung cancer. *J Clin Oncol*. 2022;40(12):1301–1311.
10. Rusch VW, Giroux DJ, Kraut MJ, et al. Induction chemoradiation and surgical resection for superior sulcus non-small-cell lung carcinomas: long-term results of Southwest Oncology Group Trial 9416 (Intergroup Trial 0160). *J Clin Oncol*. 2007;25(3):313–318.
11. Soria J-C, Ohe Y, Vansteenkiste J, et al. Osimertinib in Untreated EGFR-mutated advanced non-small-cell lung cancer. *N Engl J Med*. 2018;378(2):113–125.
12. Mok T, Camidge DR, Gadgeel SM, et al. Updated overall survival and final progression-free survival data for patients with treatment-naive advanced ALK-positive non-small-cell lung cancer in the ALEX study. *Ann Oncol*. 2020;31(8):1056–1064.
13. Reck M, Rodríguez-Abreu D, Robinson AG, et al. Updated analysis of KEYNOTE-024: pembrolizumab versus platinum-based chemotherapy for advanced non–small-cell lung cancer with PD-L1 tumor proportion score of 50% or greater. *J Clin Oncol*. 2019;37(7):537–546.
14. Garassino MC, Gadgeel S, Speranza G, et al. Pembrolizumab plus pemetrexed and platinum in nonsquamous non–small-cell lung cancer: 5-year outcomes from the phase 3 KEYNOTE-189 study. *J Clin Oncol*. 2023;41(11):1992–1998.
15. Novello S, Kowalski DM, Luft A, et al. Pembrolizumab plus chemotherapy in squamous non–small-cell lung cancer: 5-year update of the phase III KEYNOTE-407 study. *J Clin Oncol*. 2023;41(11):1999–2006.

16. West H, McCleod M, Hussein M, et al. Atezolizumab in combination with carboplatin plus nab-paclitaxel chemotherapy compared with chemotherapy alone as first-line treatment for metastatic non-squamous non-small-cell lung cancer (IMpower130): a multicentre, randomised, open-label, phase 3 trial. *Lancet Oncol.* 2019;20(7):924–937.

17. Brahmer JR, Lee J-S, Ciuleanu T-E, et al. Five-year survival outcomes with nivolumab plus ipilimumab versus chemotherapy as first-line treatment for metastatic non–small-cell lung cancer in checkmate 227. *J Clin Oncol.* 2023;41(6):1200–1212.

18. Gogishvili M, Melkadze T, Makharadze T, et al. Cemiplimab plus chemotherapy versus chemotherapy alone in non-small cell lung cancer: a randomized, controlled, double-blind phase 3 trial. *Nat Med.* 2022;28(11):2374–2380.

19. Rami-Porta R, Nishimura KK, Giroux DJ, et al. The International Association for the Study of Lung Cancer Lung Cancer Staging Project: proposals for revision of the TNM stage groups in the forthcoming (ninth) edition of the TNM classification for lung cancer. *J Thorac Oncol.* 2024: S1556-0864(24)00079-0.

20. Faivre-Finn C, Snee M, Ashcroft L, et al. Concurrent once-daily versus twice-daily chemoradiotherapy in patients with limited-stage small-cell lung cancer (CONVERT): an open-label, phase 3, randomised, superiority trial. *Lancet Oncol.* 2017;18(8):1116–1125.

21. Liu SV, Reck M, Mansfield AS, et al. Updated overall survival and PD-L1 subgroup analysis of patients with extensive-stage small-cell lung cancer treated with atezolizumab, carboplatin, and etoposide (IMpower133). *J Clin Oncol.* 2021;39(6):619–630.

22. Paz-Ares L, Chen Y, Reinmuth N, et al. Durvalumab, with or without tremelimumab, plus platinum-etoposide in first-line treatment of extensive-stage small-cell lung cancer: 3-year overall survival update from CASPIAN. *ESMO Open.* 2022;7(2):100408.

23. Slotman BJ, van Tinteren H, Praag JO, et al. Use of thoracic radiotherapy for extensive stage small-cell lung cancer: a phase 3 randomised controlled trial. *Lancet.* 2015;385(9962):36–42.

24. Arriagada R, Le Chevalier T, Borie F, et al. Prophylactic cranial irradiation for patients with small-cell lung cancer in complete remission. *J Natl Cancer Inst.* 1995;87(3):183–190.

Colorectal Cancer

23

Patrick M. Grierson

Colorectal Cancer

GENERAL PRINCIPLES

Colorectal cancers (CRCs) are common and deadly malignancies. Early-stage disease may be cured, however, a significant proportion of patients will develop recurrent disease. Limited sites of metastatic disease may be successfully treated with local therapy (i.e., metastasectomy of a solitary hepatic lesion). While patients with metastatic disease may obtain long-term disease control with standard therapies, unfortunately the majority of patients will eventually develop progressive disease. This chapter gives an overview of colorectal and anal cancer presentation, pathophysiology, staging, and general principles of treatment.

Epidemiology

CRC is the estimated to be the third most frequently diagnosed cancer in men and women in 2023, as well as the third leading cause of cancer death in US. It accounts for approximately 9% of all cancer deaths. The incidence of CRC in the US has been rising in the population younger than 50, with an approximate 1.5% annual increase in incidence. The lifetime risk for CRC is approximately 4% for average-risk men and women living in the US.[1]

Pathophysiology

Most CRCs are thought to develop from adenomatous polyps that arise from the colonic mucosa. Studies have shown that adenomatous polyps can become malignant over a period of 5–20 years. The common histologies of a polyp are tubular, tubulovillous, and villous. Villous adenomas are most likely to become malignant. Other characteristic polyps to develop into malignancies are of size >1 cm in diameter and a high grade of dysplasia. Up to 5% of polyps are believed to become malignant over time. More than 95% of CRCs are adenocarcinomas. Of these, more than 80% are moderately differentiated. Other histologic types seen are undifferentiated, squamous, carcinoid, leiomyosarcomas, and lymphoid neoplasias. *Poor prognosis* is associated with colloid or signet-ring subtypes of adenocarcinoma, which together represent ~20% of tumors.

Risk Factors

Risk factors for CRC are listed below.

- First-degree relative with CRC
- Personal history of CRC
- History of other malignancies
- History of radiation therapy to the abdomen or pelvis
- Increasing age
- Ureterosigmoidostomies
- Inflammatory bowel disease, especially ulcerative colitis, but also Crohn disease
- Family history of a CRC syndrome

- **Familial adenomatous polyposis** (FAP) is an autosomal-dominant disease caused by a defect in the APC gene that leads to colon cancer in 100% of patients by the age of 40 years if they are left untreated. Affected persons will have up to thousands of adenomatous polyps with malignant potential in their bowel. Persons with FAP should have a prophylactic subtotal colectomy by the age of 30 years. Precolectomy screening for the development of cancer is also indicated. Other cancers such as medulloblastoma, papillary thyroid carcinoma, hepatoblastoma, pancreatic cancer, and gastric cancer are also associated with this syndrome.
- **Hereditary nonpolyposis colorectal cancer** (HNPCC) is inherited in an autosomal-dominant manner and often leads to malignancies with mucinous histology in the right side of the colon. Often these tumors may arise without going through a polyp phase and, therefore, are seen as flat adenomas. HNPCC is also associated with cancers of the endometrium, ovary, stomach, and hepatobiliary system. Prophylactic subtotal colectomy is also recommended for persons with HNPCC.
- Other inherited syndromes associated with an increased risk of CRC include MYH-associated polyposis, Gardner syndrome, Turcot syndrome, Muir–Torre syndrome, and Peutz–Jeghers syndrome.

Prevention/Screening

Screening methods and schedules are varied, and decisions are made based on the patient's risk of developing CRC. Early detection of precancerous polyps or early-stage malignancy improves survival. For patients with average CRC risk (age ≥45 years and no history of polyps, inflammatory bowel disease, CRC, or family history) screening options include colonoscopy (preferred modality) every 10 years, high-sensitivity guaiac-based or immunochemical-based testing annually, or flexible sigmoidoscopy every 3 years. Colonoscopy is recommended at shorter intervals for patients at increased risk of CRC. Several organizations publish screening guidelines, and variations exist between publications. Given the increased incidence of CSC in individuals younger than 50 years old, the US Preventative Services Task Force (USPSTF) now recommends colonoscopy screening beginning at age 45.

DIAGNOSIS

Diagnosis depends on tissue pathology consistent with invasive colon adenocarcinoma either via colonoscopy or biopsy of a distant metastatic site. Immunohistochemical markers consistent with colorectal origin are CK20, CDX2, and SATB2.[2]

Clinical Presentation

History
- CRC may present with symptoms such as fatigue, anorexia, failure to thrive, lower gastrointestinal bleeding, and right upper quadrant pain associated with liver metastasis, although it is often asymptomatic until the tumor is larger in size.
- Symptoms associated with CRC are often related to the location of the tumor within the bowel. ***Right-sided lesions*** often present with symptoms of anemia and, occasionally, of melena. ***Left-sided lesions*** more commonly cause obstruction, tenesmus, constipation, bright-red blood per rectum, and other changes in bowel habits. Patients often have an iron-deficiency anemia.
- Because CRC is a cause of anemia, it is important to evaluate any person who presents with unexplained anemia for CRC.
- CRC most often metastasizes to the liver, lung, adrenals, ovaries, and bone, so symptoms of organ compromise such as abdominal discomfort, shortness of breath, and bone pain may be present in metastatic disease.

Physical Examination

Signs of CRC on physical examination include gross blood or melanotic stool in the rectal vault, pallor in the conjunctivae and the nail beds, or a palpable mass in the abdomen or the rectum. If liver metastases are present, patients may have hepatomegaly and be tender to palpation in the right upper quadrant. On barium enema, an **apple core** lesion may be seen. Bacteremia or endocarditis with *Streptococcus bovis* is associated with CRC, and these findings should prompt an evaluation for underlying colon cancer.

Diagnostic Testing

Laboratories

- There is no diagnostic circulating biomarker currently available. Carcinoembryonic antigen (CEA) is not recommended as a screening test but may be used for disease monitoring.
- CBC, iron panel, and ferritin to evaluate for associated iron-deficiency anemia
- Chemistry and liver function tests to evaluate for liver involvement.

Imaging Studies

CT of the chest/abdomen/pelvis is used to evaluate for metastasis. CNS imaging is not standard in an asymptomatic patient.

Diagnostic Procedures

All patients should have the entire colon evaluated by colonoscopy or barium enema to rule out synchronous lesions. Up to 5% of patients have a second focus of CRC. Patients should have a tissue biopsy before therapy to confirm the diagnosis.

Staging

Surgery is critical for accurate staging of resectable CRC. The preferred staging system for CRC is the American Joint Committee on Cancer (AJCC) TNM (tumor, node, metastases) system. TNM uses the degree of tumor invasion (T), the presence of involved lymph nodes (N), and the presence of distant metastasis (M) to classify the disease into stages I, II, III, or IV. Current staging can be found online within the AJCC Cancer Staging Guidelines.

TREATMENT

The goals of therapy should be clearly communicated to the patient and re-evaluated throughout the patient's course. Colon cancer that has not metastasized is a potentially curable disease. Surgery and chemotherapy have standard roles in both curative and palliative treatment of CRC. Surgery is undertaken with the intent to cure or prevent obstruction, perforation, or bleeding. If the goal of surgical intent is palliation, a simple resection or diversion is used to lessen morbidity from the procedure. In selected patients with stage IV disease (predominantly lung or liver), resection of oligometastases and the primary tumor may be undertaken with curative intent using perioperative chemotherapy,[3] with 5-year survival rates of up to 40% have been obtained with resection of limited liver metastases.[4]

- **Adjuvant chemotherapy** is administered to patients who have undergone potentially curative resection of colon cancer with the goal of eradicating micrometastases, thereby reducing the likelihood of recurrence. For resected stage III disease, 6 months of adjuvant FOLFOX (5-Fluorouracil [5-FU], leucovorin, and oxaliplatin), CAPOX (capecitabine/oxaliplatin), or single-agent 5-FU/leucovorin or capecitabine has been standard of care.[5,6] Capecitabine is an oral prodrug that is converted to 5-FU in tumor tissues. Adjuvant chemotherapy has demonstrated an approximate 20% reduction in the risk of disease recurrence and mortality for stage III disease. In patients with stage II disease, the benefit to overall survival benefit with adjuvant chemotherapy is <5%,[6] thus these patients are risk stratified such that only those at highest risk of recurrence receive adjuvant therapy (those who present with a bowel obstruction or perforation, T4 tumors, poorly differentiated, lymphovascular/perineural invasion, positive surgical margins, or inadequately sampled nodes [<12 lymph nodes]).[7] In patients with stage II disease, microsatellite instability high (MSI-H) is associated with a more favorable outcome. Recent data demonstrates that for stage III, the optimal duration of adjuvant chemotherapy is dependent upon T and N stage, with 3 months of FOLFOX/CAPOX commonly used for tumors pT3N1, and 6 months of FOLFOX/CAPOX commonly used for tumors pT4 and/or ≥pN2 based on disease free survival (DFS) outcomes of the large international noninferiority study IDEA study.[8] However, for patients with intended 6 months of adjuvant FOLFOX/CAPOX, early stoppage of oxaliplatin (after ≥3 months) with continuation of 5-FU/LV for a total of 6 months is largely noninferior (regarding DFS and OS) to 6 months of adjuvant FOLFOX/CAPOX with a lower incidence of peripheral sensory neuropathy.[9] The nuances of the optimal duration of adjuvant chemotherapy are beyond the scope of this text.

• **Palliative therapy** without expectation of cure is given for metastatic disease and regimens depend on the performance status of the patient. Standard chemotherapy options are FOLFOX (5-FU, leucovorin, oxaliplatin) and FOLFIRI (5-FU, leucovorin, irinotecan)[10,11] or the triplet FOLFIRINOX/FOLFOXIRI.[12] These regimens may be combined with the antivascular endothelial growth factor (VEGF) antibody bevacizumab[13,14] or anti-EGFR antibodies cetuximab or panitumumab in patients with the wild-type KRAS/NRAS/BRAF and left-sided tumors.[15–18] Second-line therapy options include regimens not used in the first line as well as agents targeting BRAF V600E (encorafenib/panitumumab[19]) and Her2 (trastuzumab/pertuzumab,[20] trastuzumab/laptinib,[21] trastuzumab/tucatinib[22]). Patients with microsatellite instability may receive anti-CTLA4 (ipilimumab) with anti-PD1 (nivolumab, pembrolizumab, dostarlimab) or anti-PD1 immunotherapy alone in any line of treatment.[23,24] Other less common targets include NTRK and RET fusions. Given the emergence of molecularly targeted therapies, next-generation sequencing (NGS) is standard of care to identify targetable alterations. In the third line or later settings, regorafenib (an oral multikinase inhibitor) and trifluridine/tipiracil (TAS-102, an oral fluoropyrimidine analog) are both approved for patients with refractory metastatic CRC, and display approximately 6–7-week median survival benefit compared with placebo.[25,26] Rarely, patients with oligometastatic disease (most frequently to liver or lung) may be considered for curative-intent local therapies (resection, ablation, or stereotactic body radiation therapy [SBRT]) following multidisciplinary discussion. Patients at all stages of disease should be referred for clinical trials when possible.

Treatment of Rectal Cancer

The treatment landscape of locally advanced rectal cancer is rapidly changing. A multimodal approach (chemotherapy, radiation, surgery) is the current standard of care for most patients. Stage I tumors (T1–2, N0) may be surgically resected followed by surveillance. Historically, many patients with locally advanced rectal cancer (generally defined as node positive T2 or greater, or node positive for negative or T3 or T4) were treated with neoadjuvant long-course chemotherapy (5FU) with concurrent radiation over 28 fractions, followed by surgical resection and adjuvant FOLFOX. In recent years, treatment has shifted to a total neoadjuvant (TNT) approach. TNT may take the form of neoadjuvant short-course radiation therapy (SCRT) in five fractions followed by 12–16 weeks of FOLFOX (or CAPOX) or FOLFOX alone with selective use of neoadjuvant concurrent chemoradiation for nonresponders to FOLFOX. Following TNT, subsequent reassessment is by flexible sigmoidoscopy and pelvic MRI. Patients with no evidence of residual tumor at therapy completion may be offered nonoperative management (NOM) with close surveillance, avoiding the morbidity of surgery, while patients with persistent disease will undergo resection. Via different forms of TNT, patients may be able to avoid the toxicities of radiation as well as surgery with similar disease-free survival and overall survival rates.[27–29] For patients with MSI-high locally advanced rectal cancer, emerging data demonstrates high response rates (nearly 100% in small series) with neoadjuvant anti-PD1 immunotherapy alone,[30] however larger confirmatory studies are needed.

Recurrent and/or metastatic rectal cancer is treated similarly to metastatic colon cancer, as detailed above.

COMPLICATIONS

Tumor Related

Complications that can result from CRC include bleeding/anemia, bowel obstruction, perforation with peritonitis, and fistula formation. Complications can also result from sites of metastatic disease; liver metastases can lead to hyperbilirubinemia and hepatic impairment, while pulmonary metastases may result in cough or shortness of breath.

Treatment Related

Treatment-related complications can be a consequence of surgery, chemotherapy, or radiation. Postoperative mortality rates are 1–5%. Major morbidity includes bowel and bladder dysfunction, sexual dysfunction, anastomotic leaks, and bowel obstruction. Chemotherapy complications may include oxaliplatin-induced peripheral sensory neuropathy (possibly long term), nausea, diarrhea, and hand-foot syndrome. Radiation may cause local radiation dermatitis, fistula formation, or increased risk of fracture if osseous structures are in the radiation field.

MONITORING/FOLLOW-UP

For patients who have undergone curative resection, consensus guideline recommendations are for H&P and CEA every 3–6 months for 2 years, and then every 6–12 months until 5 years. Colonoscopy is recommended at 1-year postresection to assess for local recurrence and metachronous disease, with subsequent colonoscopies dependent upon findings. CT of the chest, abdomen, and pelvis should be repeated every 6–12 months for up to 5 years. Patients with resected stage I disease may only require surveillance colonoscopy.

OUTCOMES/PROGNOSIS

Stage and performance status have the greatest impact on prognosis and treatment options. In the US in 2023, based on the current online SEER database, the overall 5-year survival rate for all patients with CRC is 65%. The 5-year survival for stages I/II, III, and IV are 90.9%, 73.4%, and 15.6%, respectively.

Anal Cancer

GENERAL PRINCIPLES

Epidemiology

Anal cancer (anal squamous cell carcinoma) accounts for ~1.6% of all alimentary malignancies in US. Its incidence generally increases with age, with the peak incidence in the sixth and seventh decades of life. The incidence is increasing in men <40 years of age due to increased risk in the HIV+ population.

Risk Factors

- The risk factor most commonly associated with anal cancer is **human papilloma virus** (HPV) infection, particularly with serotypes 16 and 18. In women, increased anal cancers are seen with HPV-associated cervical cancer. In men, anal cancer is more frequently associated with receptive anal intercourse and HPV. As many as 70% of anal cancers are positive for HPV.
- Other risk factors include immunosuppression, such as post–solid organ transplant or HIV infection. Current cigarette smoking is also a risk factor for anal cancer, with a relative risk of seven- to ninefold for smokers.

DIAGNOSIS

Clinical Presentation

History

Anal cancers often present with bleeding, pain, mass, constipation, diarrhea, or/and pruritus. Often the symptoms are ascribed to hemorrhoids, which may delay diagnosis. Approximately 25% of people are asymptomatic when the cancer is discovered.

Physical Examination

Physical examination findings include an anal mass and lymphadenopathy. On palpation, an anal mass will often be firm and indurated. Anoscopy, proctoscopy, and transrectal ultrasonography are used to visualize the mass. Diagnosis is made by incisional biopsy of the mass and any suspicious inguinal lymphadenopathy.

Diagnostic Testing

Procedures

Digital rectal examination and **inguinal lymph node examination** should be accompanied by **anoscopy**. Notes should be made on the location of the mass, including its position relative to the dentate line. Anal cancers are divided into those of the anal margin and those of the anal canal. The line of demarcation is a zone approximately halfway between the dentate line and the anal verge. Women should have a pelvic examination for **cervical cancer screening** due to the association with HPV. Men and women should be tested for **HIV**, especially if any risk factors are present.

Imaging

Imaging may include chest/abdominal/pelvic CT or MRI, or PET scan to rule out metastatic disease.

Staging

Staging is based on the TNM system. Current staging can be seen online within the AJCC Cancer Staging Manual.

TREATMENT

Very small tumors at the anal margin may be treated with wide local excision. Larger (T2–T4) and node positive cancers should be treated with chemotherapy (5-FU/ Mitomycin C) concurrent with radiation with a 5-year locoregional recurrence rate of approximately 25–30%.[31,32] After treatment, close follow-up with physical examination is needed given that most recurrences are local.[32] For patients with metastatic recurrent disease or de novo metastatic disease, first-line preferred standard of care systemic therapy is carboplatin/paclitaxel,[33] while nivolumab[34] or pembrolizumab[35] are commonly used in the second-line setting.

OUTCOME/PROGNOSIS

Prognosis is related to the size of the primary tumor and the presence of lymph node involvement. The 5-year survival rates for anal squamous cell carcinoma are stage I (69.5%), stage II (59%), stage III (40.6%), and stage IV (18.7%).[36] Tumors in the anal margin have a more favorable prognosis than those in the canal.

REFERENCES

1. Siegel RL, Miller KD, Fuchs HE, Jemal A. Cancer statistics, 2022. *CA Cancer J Clin.* 2022;72(1):7–33.
2. Li Z, Rock JB, Roth R, et al. Dual stain with SATB2 and CK20/Villin is useful to distinguish colorectal carcinomas from other tumors. *Am J Clin Pathol.* 2018;149(3):241–246.
3. Gruenberger T, Bridgewater J, Chau I, et al. Bevacizumab plus mFOLFOX-6 or FOLFOXIRI in patients with initially unresectable liver metastases from colorectal cancer: the OLIVIA multinational randomised phase II trial. *Ann Oncol.* 2015;26(4):702–708.
4. Chandy ETJ, Saxby HJ, Pang JW, Sharma RA. The multidisciplinary management of oligometastases from colorectal cancer: a narrative review. *Ann Palliat Med.* 2021;10(5):5988–6001.
5. Andre T, Boni C, Mounedji-Boudiaf L, et al; Multicenter International Study of Oxaliplatin/5-Fluorouracil/Leucovorin in the Adjuvant Treatment of Colon Cancer (MOSAIC) Investigators. Oxaliplatin, fluorouracil, and leucovorin as adjuvant treatment for colon cancer. *N Engl J Med.* 2004; 350(23):2343–2351.
6. André T, Boni C, Navarro M, et al. Improved overall survival with oxaliplatin, fluorouracil, and leucovorin as adjuvant treatment in stage II or III colon cancer in the MOSAIC trial. *J Clin Oncol.* 2009;27(19):3109–3116.
7. Benson AB III, Schrag D, Somerfield MR, et al. American Society of Clinical Oncology recommendations on adjuvant chemotherapy for stage II colon cancer. *J Clin Oncol.* 2004;22(16):3408–3419.
8. Grothey A, Sobrero AF, Shields AF, et al. Duration of adjuvant chemotherapy for stage III colon cancer. *N Engl J Med.* 2018;378(13):1177–1188.
9. Gallois C, Shi Q, Meyers JP, et al. Prognostic impact of early treatment and oxaliplatin discontinuation in patients with stage iii colon cancer: an ACCENT/IDEA pooled analysis of 11 adjuvant trials. *J Clin Oncol.* 2023;41(4):803–815.
10. Saltz LB, Cox JV, Blanke C, et al. Irinotecan plus fluorouracil and leucovorin for metastatic colorectal cancer. Irinotecan Study Group. *N Engl J Med.* 2000;343(13):905–914.
11. de Gramont A, Figer A, Seymour M, et al. Leucovorin and fluorouracil with or without oxaliplatin as first-line treatment in advanced colorectal cancer. *J Clin Oncol.* 2000;18(16):2938–2947.
12. Loupakis F, Cremolini C, Masi G, et al. Initial therapy with FOLFOXIRI and bevacizumab for metastatic colorectal cancer. *N Engl J Med.* 2014;371(17):1609–1618.
13. Hurwitz H, Fehrenbacher L, Novotny W, et al. Bevacizumab plus irinotecan, fluorouracil, and leucovorin for metastatic colorectal cancer. *N Engl J Med.* 2004;350(23):2335–2342.
14. Saltz LB, Clarke S, Díaz-Rubio E, et al. Bevacizumab in combination with oxaliplatin-based chemotherapy as first-line therapy in metastatic colorectal cancer: a randomized phase III study. *J Clin Oncol.* 2008;26(12):2013–2019.
15. Van Cutsem E, Köhne C-H, Hitre E, et al. Cetuximab and chemotherapy as initial treatment for metastatic colorectal cancer. *N Engl J Med.* 2009;360(14):1408–1417.
16. Bokemeyer C, Bondarenko I, Makhson A, et al. Fluorouracil, leucovorin, and oxaliplatin with and without cetuximab in the first-line treatment of metastatic colorectal cancer. *J Clin Oncol.* 2009; 27(5):663–671.
17. Douillard JY, Siena S, Cassidy J, et al. Final results from PRIME: randomized phase III study of panitumumab with FOLFOX4 for first-line treatment of metastatic colorectal cancer. *Ann Oncol.* 2014;25(7):1346–1355.
18. Peeters M, Price TJ, Cervantes A, et al. Randomized phase III study of panitumumab with fluorouracil, leucovorin, and irinotecan (FOLFIRI) compared with FOLFIRI alone as second-line treatment in patients with metastatic colorectal cancer. *J Clin Oncol.* 2010;28(31):4706–4713.
19. Kopetz S, Grothey A, Yaeger R, et al. Encorafenib, binimetinib, and cetuximab in BRAF V600E-mutated colorectal cancer. *N Engl J Med.* 2019;381(17):1632–1643.
20. Meric-Bernstam F, Hurwitz H, Raghav KPS, et al. Pertuzumab plus trastuzumab for HER2-amplified metastatic colorectal cancer (MyPathway): an updated report from a multicentre, open-label, phase 2a, multiple basket study. *Lancet Oncol.* 2019;20(4):518–530.

21. Sartore-Bianchi A, Trusolino L, Martino C, et al. Dual-targeted therapy with trastuzumab and lapatinib in treatment-refractory, KRAS codon 12/13 wild-type, HER2-positive metastatic colorectal cancer (HERACLES): a proof-of-concept, multicentre, open-label, phase 2 trial. *Lancet Oncol.* 2016; 17(6):738–746.

22. Strickler JH, Cercek A, Siena S, et al; MOUNTAINEER investigators. Tucatinib plus trastuzumab for chemotherapy-refractory, HER2-positive, RAS wild-type unresectable or metastatic colorectal cancer (MOUNTAINEER): a multicentre, open-label, phase 2 study. *Lancet Oncol.* 2023;24(5):496–508.

23. Lenz H-J, Van Cutsem E, Luisa Limon M, et al. First-line nivolumab plus low-dose ipilimumab for microsatellite instability-high/mismatch repair-deficient metastatic colorectal cancer: the phase II CheckMate 142 study. *J Clin Oncol.* 2022;40(2):161–170.

24. Overman MJ, McDermott R, Leach JL, et al. Nivolumab in patients with metastatic DNA mismatch repair-deficient or microsatellite instability-high colorectal cancer (CheckMate 142): an open-label, multicentre, phase 2 study. *Lancet Oncol.* 2017;18(9):1182–1191.

25. Grothey A, Van Cutsem E, Sobrero A, et al; CORRECT Study Group. Regorafenib monotherapy for previously treated metastatic colorectal cancer (CORRECT): an international, multicentre, randomised, placebo-controlled, phase 3 trial. *Lancet.* 2013;381(9863):303–312.

26. Mayer RJ, Van Cutsem E, Falcone A, et al; RECOURSE Study Group. Randomized trial of TAS-102 for refractory metastatic colorectal cancer. *N Engl J Med.* 2015;372(20):1909–1919.

27. Schrag D, Shi Q, Weiser MR, et al. Preoperative treatment of locally advanced rectal cancer. *N Engl J Med.* 2023;389(4):322–334.

28. Bahadoer RR, Dijkstra EA, van Etten B, et al; RAPIDO collaborative investigators. Short-course radiotherapy followed by chemotherapy before total mesorectal excision (TME) versus preoperative chemoradiotherapy, TME, and optional adjuvant chemotherapy in locally advanced rectal cancer (RAPIDO): a randomised, open-label, phase 3 trial. *Lancet Oncol.* 2021;22(1):29–42.

29. Dijkstra EA, Nilsson PJ, Hospers GAP, et al; Collaborative Investigators. Locoregional failure during and after short-course radiotherapy followed by chemotherapy and surgery compared to long-course chemoradiotherapy and surgery: a five-year follow-up of the RAPIDO trial. *Ann Surg.* 2023; 278(4):e766–e772.

30. Cercek A, Lumish M, Sinopoli J, et al. PD-1 blockade in mismatch repair-deficient, locally advanced rectal cancer. *N Engl J Med.* 2022;386(25):2363–2376.

31. Ajani JA, Winter KA, Gunderson LL, et al. Fluorouracil, mitomycin, and radiotherapy vs fluorouracil, cisplatin, and radiotherapy for carcinoma of the anal canal: a randomized controlled trial. *JAMA.* 2008;299(16):1914–1921.

32. Northover J, Glynne-Jones R, Sebag-Montefiore D, et al. Chemoradiation for the treatment of epidermoid anal cancer: 13-year follow-up of the first randomised UKCCCR Anal Cancer Trial (ACT I). *Br J Cancer.* 2010;102(7):1123–1128.

33. Rao S, Sclafani F, Eng C, et al. International rare cancers initiative multicenter randomized phase II trial of cisplatin and fluorouracil versus carboplatin and paclitaxel in advanced anal cancer: InterAAct. *J Clin Oncol.* 2020;38(22):2510–2518.

34. Morris VK, Salem ME, Nimeiri H, et al. Nivolumab for previously treated unresectable metastatic anal cancer (NCI9673): a multicentre, single-arm, phase 2 study. *Lancet Oncol.* 2017;18(4):446–453.

35. Marabelle A, Cassier PA, Fakih M, et al. Pembrolizumab for previously treated advanced anal squamous cell carcinoma: results from the non-randomised, multicohort, multicentre, phase 2 KEYNOTE-158 study. *Lancet Gastroenterol Hepatol.* 2022;7(5):446–454.

36. Bilimoria KY, Bentrem DJ, Rock CE, Stewart AK, Ko CY, Halverson A. Outcomes and prognostic factors for squamous-cell carcinoma of the anal canal: analysis of patients from the National Cancer Data Base. *Dis Colon Rectum.* 2009;52(4):624–631.

Other Gastrointestinal Malignancies

24

Michael D. Iglesia

Esophageal Cancer

GENERAL PRINCIPLES

Definition

Primary carcinoma that arises from the cricopharyngeal sphincter to the gastroesophageal junction.

Classification

- Site: divided into upper, middle, and lower third
- Histology: most commonly adenocarcinoma (occurs predominantly at lower third of esophagus) and squamous cell carcinoma (occurs predominantly at middle and upper third); other less common types include mucoepidermoid carcinoma, small-cell carcinoma, sarcoma, leiomyosarcoma, and primary lymphoma

Epidemiology

- The incidence in US is approximately 5 per 100,000, although in African-American men it may be as high as 18 per 100,000. China and Iran have an incidence of 20 per 100,000.
- In US, 16,640 new cases and 14,500 deaths from this cancer were estimated in 2010. It is the seventh leading cause of cancer death in men.
- Age: sixth to seventh decades.
- Sex: M:F, 3:1–4:1.
- Race: In US, esophageal adenocarcinomas are more common in white males, whereas squamous cell carcinomas are more common in African Americans.
- Socioeconomic status: Lower socioeconomic status as defined by income, occupation, and education is associated with higher risk for squamous cell carcinoma.
- Histology: In US, squamous cell carcinoma was the more prominent type of cancer until the early 1990s, when it was surpassed by adenocarcinoma. Such shift is believed to be due to increased incidence of gastroesophageal reflux disease (GERD), Barrett esophagus, and obesity.

Etiology and Pathophysiology

The exact etiology of esophageal carcinoma remains unclear, but it is likely due to oncogenic changes within the esophageal epithelium, followed by chronic exposure to known carcinogens or chronic irritation by gastric acid in patients with GERD. Conversely, patients with chronic atrophic gastritis caused by cagA-positive *Helicobacter pylori* are associated with decreased risk of esophageal adenocarcinoma.

Risk Factors

- Alcohol, tobacco, nitrosamines, GERD, Barrett esophagus, obesity, Plummer–Vinson syndrome, history of head and neck cancer
- High-fat, low-calorie, and low-protein diets

Prevention
- Cessation from smoking and alcohol consumption
- Raw fruits and vegetables, fibers, selenium, as well as vitamins A, C, and E

Associated Conditions
Barrett esophagus (30- to 125-fold increased risk of developing adenocarcinoma), Howel–Evans syndrome.

DIAGNOSIS

Clinical Presentation
History
Due to the lack of initial symptoms, most cases are diagnosed at advanced stage. Typical presenting symptoms are dysphagia (95%), which typically progressed from solid to liquid, body weight loss (50%), odynophagia (20%), and gastric reflux (40%). Extraesophageal spread can cause pain, cough (20%), hoarseness (secondary to recurrent laryngeal nerve involvement), aspiration, tracheal narrowing, or tracheoesophageal fistula.

Physical Examination
Most patients lack obvious physical findings, but cervical or supraclavicular adenopathy may be appreciated in patients with nodal metastasis.

Diagnostic Criteria
Histopathologic diagnosis from endoscopic biopsy and/or transcutaneous lymph node biopsy (if applicable) is required.

Differential Diagnosis
Barrett esophagus, esophageal stricture, achalasia, gastric cancer.

Diagnostic Testing
Laboratories
Complete blood count (CBC), comprehensive metabolic panel (CMP), prothrombin time (PT), partial thromboplastin time (PTT), and iron studies.

Initial Diagnostic Test
- Upper endoscopy with directed biopsy is the current gold standard.
- Barium studies may show strictures or intraluminal lesions, but they are less sensitive and do not allow for biopsy.

Imaging Studies
- Once the diagnosis is established, an initial **CT scan of chest and abdomen with IV and oral contrast** should be obtained to assess extent of primary disease and nodal and distant organ metastasis.
- Bone scan is indicated in patients with bone pain or elevated alkaline phosphatase.
- If no distant metastasis is seen from the initial CT scan, more sensitive diagnostic tests should be performed to provide more accurate staging. A positron emission tomography (PET) or PET-CT scan (preferred by consensus guidelines) should be obtained. They have a higher sensitivity and specificity than conventional CT scan in detecting nodal and distant metastasis. In many medical centers, this PET scan has become part of the standard preoperative workup. If indicated, FDG-avid lymph nodes should be biopsied to confirm metastasis.

Diagnostic Procedures

- Once distant metastasis is excluded by PET scan, an **endoscopic ultrasonography** (EUS) should be performed. This procedure allows the most precise assessment of tumor depth, length of esophagus affected, and magnitude of lymph node metastases, particularly paraesophageal and celiac nodes. A fine-needle aspiration of suspicious lymph nodes can be done during the study.
- Patients presenting with cough, symptoms, or radiographic evidence of aspiration pneumonia, or tumor abutting/invading the trachea at or above carina should receive bronchoscopy to assess tracheal invasion or tracheoesophageal fistula.

TREATMENT

Treatment is based on TNM stage. Current staging guidelines are available online within the AJCC Cancer Staging Manual.

- **Stage 0**
  - Endoscopic mucosal resection followed by periodic surveillance.
- **Stage I**
  - Esophagectomy if patient is medically fit, with esophageal carcinoma at mid or lower third esophagus, or if patient has adenocarcinoma.
  - Concurrent chemoradiation is preferred for cancer in the upper third esophagus and is an alternative for patients who are not surgical candidates.
- **Stage II, III, or IVa**
  - Esophagectomy with regional lymphadenectomy is the main treatment, but surgery alone is inadequate.
  - Current consensus guidelines support the use of neoadjuvant chemoradiation in medically fit patients.
  - Perioperative chemotherapy may be considered for patients with gastroesophageal junction (GEJ) adenocarcinoma with fluorouracil, leucovorin, oxaliplatin and docetaxel (FLOT) (preferred), FOLFOX, or 5-FU and cisplatin.
  - One year of adjuvant nivolumab should be added for patients with residual disease after preoperative chemoradiation followed by R0 resection.
  - Patients with gross (R2 resection) or microscopic (R1 resection) residual disease following surgery may receive adjuvant combined chemoradiation.
  - Patients with localized unresectable disease or who are medically unfit for surgery should be considered for definitive chemoradiation. Regimens including carboplatin plus paclitaxel (preferred), cisplatin, 5-FU, or FOLFOX have been investigated combined with radiation.[1]
- **Stage IVb**
  Metastatic esophageal cancer is incurable and has a median survival of 9 months. Several chemotherapeutic agents including cisplatin, carboplatin, 5-FU, S-1, paclitaxel, docetaxel, vinorelbine, oxaliplatin, and irinotecan are commonly used. Additional testing for metastatic disease should include the tumor's Her-2-neu status, as Her-2-neu overexpressing adenocarcinomas may benefit from the addition of Trastuzumab to first-line chemotherapy.[2] Ramucirumab, a VEGFR2 antibody, has been approved for metastatic disease.[3]
  - In general, platinum-based combination regimens have the highest response rate, and FOLFOX is typically used as the backbone of first-line therapy.[4] Other acceptable chemotherapy-only regimens include cisplatin plus 5 fluorouracil, and epirubicin plus oxaliplatin plus capecitabine.[5]
  - First-line treatment of HER2 positive disease should include a backbone of fluoropyrimidine plus oxaliplatin plus trastuzumab, with or without the addition of pembrolizumab.
  - First-line treatment of HER2 negative disease should include a backbone of fluoropyrimidine plus oxaliplatin plus an immune checkpoint inhibitor, either nivolumab or

pembrolizumab. Evidence for addition of an immune checkpoint inhibitor is strongest for high PD-L1 immunohistochemical scores (combined positive score of ≥5 for nivolumab or ≥10 for pembrolizumab).

o Ramucirumab plus paclitaxel is preferred in the second-line setting for HER2-negative disease, while HER2-positive disease may be treated with fam-trastuzumab deruxtecan-nxki (T-dxd). HER2-negative squamous cell carcinoma with PD-L1 combined positive score of ≥10 should receive second-line pembrolizumab. Other acceptable second-line regimens include paclitaxel, irinotecan, docetaxel, or single-agent ramucirumab.

Other Nonpharmacologic Therapies

Palliative care in swallowing and nutritional support is especially important. This includes esophageal dilation, stent placement, brachytherapy, external-beam radiation, and laser therapy. Patients with metastatic esophageal cancer frequently require a gastrostomy tube.

Lifestyle/Risk Modification

All patients should be encouraged to **cease smoking and consuming alcohol**. Patients with gastroesophageal reflux should be managed by dietary modification, exercise, and, if necessary, treated medically with H2-blockers or proton pump inhibitors.

Diet
Increase consumption of fresh fruits and vegetables and dietary fibers, and abstain from alcohol and high-fat diet.

Activity
Overweight or obese patients should be encouraged to exercise and lose weight.

COMPLICATIONS

Hemorrhage, obstruction, tracheoesophageal fistula, aspiration pneumonia, and mediastinitis.

REFERRAL

Nutritional consult should be obtained for all patients undergoing treatment of esophageal cancer.

MONITORING/FOLLOW-UP

- Patients with Barrett metaplasia should receive surveillance endoscopy at least every 12 months with biopsy.
- After definitive treatment, asymptomatic patients should typically be evaluated by history and physical examination every 3 months for 2 years and then every 6 months for 3 additional years. CBC and CMP should be obtained during each routine follow-up, and imaging studies such as CT scan should be obtained at least every 6 months in the first 1–3 years or when clinically indicated.

OUTCOME/PROGNOSIS

- The most important prognostic factor is initial staging; others include age, performance status, and weight loss (>10%). Neither histology nor grade has been shown to affect prognosis. Molecular profiling of tumor cells is an area of active investigation.
- Five-year survival rates are >90% (stage 0), 70–80% (stage I), 10–30% (stage II), 5–10% (stage III), and rare in stage IV disease.

Gastric Cancer

GENERAL PRINCIPLES

Definition

Cancer that arises between the gastroesophageal junction and pylorus.

Classification

- Histology:
  - Adenocarcinoma (95%), primary lymphoma such as non-Hodgkin lymphoma, MALT lymphoma (MALToma), GI stromal tumor (GIST), leiomyosarcoma, squamous cell carcinoma, small-cell carcinoma, and carcinoid
- Lauren classification of gastric adenocarcinoma:
  - Intestinal type: more common in Japan, associated with diet and possibly *H. pylori* infection
  - Diffuse type: more common in US, not associated with diet, associated with poorer outcome
  - Mixed type
- Borrmann classification of gastric adenocarcinoma:
  - Type 1 (polypoid), II (ulcerated), III (ulcerated infiltrating), IV (diffusely infiltrating or *linitis plastica*)

Epidemiology

- Gastric cancer is a relatively less common cancer in US but much more common in eastern Asia, especially Japan. It is the second most common cause of cancer deaths in the world.
- In US, 21,000 new cases and 10,570 deaths from this cancer were estimated in 2010. Incidence and mortality of gastric cancer have been declining in US.
- Age: seventh decade.
- Sex: M:F, 2:1–3:1.
- Race: slightly more frequent in African Americans than Caucasians.

Etiology and Pathophysiology

- Oncogenic mutation of *K-Ras* and *H-Ras,* overexpression of *Her2/neu* and *c-met,* and loss of *p53* are among the common genetic changes found in gastric adenocarcinoma.
- *C-kit* (90–95%) or *PDGFR* (5%) mutations are found in most GISTs. MALTomas are frequently associated with *H. pylori* infection and can be cured with antibiotics alone.

Risk Factors

- History of atrophic gastritis or pernicious anemia, cigarette smoking, alcohol, *H. pylori* infection, chronic gastric ulcer, Barrett esophagitis, high salt, nitrate intake, smoked or pickled foods, family history of gastric cancer.
- Patients with germline E-cadherin (*CDH1* gene) mutation are at extremely high risk of developing diffuse-type gastric cancer at young age.

Prevention

Because **H. pylori infection** is associated with 40–50% of gastric adenocarcinomas, it **should be actively eradicated when diagnosed**. Patients diagnosed with gastric ulcer should undergo repeat endoscopic surveillance in 3–6 months.

DIAGNOSIS

Clinical Presentation

History

- Most gastric carcinomas are diagnosed at an advanced stage due to the lack of early warning symptoms. Most patients present with nonspecific constitutional symptoms such as weight loss, anorexia, fatigue, vague stomach pain, hematemesis, dysphagia (from gastroesophageal junction tumors), and vomiting (from gastric outlet obstruction).
- Patients with GIST typically present with bleeding such as hematemesis, tarry stools or melena, epigastric pain, and nausea.

Physical Examination

The physical findings in gastric carcinoma are typically manifestations of metastatic disease. **Virchow node** describes metastasis to the left supraclavicular node. **Sister Mary Joseph node** is a periumbilical lymph node metastasis. A **Krukenberg tumor** is a gastric cancer metastatic to the ovaries. **Blumer shelf** describes a "drop metastasis" into the perirectal pouch. Other common physical findings in patients with metastatic gastric cancer include cachexia, palpable abdominal masses, and malignant ascites.

Diagnostic Criteria

- Histopathologic diagnosis from endoscopic biopsy and/or transcutaneous lymph node biopsy (if applicable) is required.
- In the case of GIST, tumor size and mitotic index are important factors in risk stratification.

Differential Diagnosis

Gastric ulcer, gastritis, non-Hodgkin lymphoma, GIST, esophageal cancer

Diagnostic Testing

Laboratories

CBC, CMP, PT, PTT, CEA (carcinoma embryonic antigen), and iron studies

Initial Diagnostic Test

- **Upper endoscopy with directed biopsy** is the current gold standard.
- Barium studies with double contrast provide information on size of ulcerated lesion and gastric motility but are less sensitive and do not allow for biopsy.

Imaging

CT scans or PET/CT is frequently used to evaluate for extent of disease.

Diagnostic Procedures

- In the absence of metastasis by CT, endoscopic ultrasound can be used to gauge tumor depth and involvement of local lymph nodes.
- Metastatic peritoneal deposits may not be seen on routine imaging, and a diagnostic laparoscopy is necessary to rule this out before definitive resection.

TREATMENT

For gastric adenocarcinoma, treatment is based on TNM stage.

- **Stage 0 and Ia**
  - Endoscopic mucosal resection
- **Stage Ib**
  - Subtotal gastrectomy if at distal stomach, otherwise total gastrectomy with at least D1 resection

○ Chemotherapy or chemoradiation in combination with surgery should consider for T2 lesions
- **Stage II to III**
  ○ For potentially resectable disease and early-stage disease three approaches are considered standard of care: perioperative chemotherapy, postoperative chemoradiotherapy, or adjuvant chemotherapy following D2 resection. Phase II studies have supported the use of neoadjuvant chemoradiation.[6–9]
  ○ For medically unfit or unresectable localized gastric adenocarcinoma, 5-FU- or taxane-based chemoradiation (45–50 cGy) is the standard of care. Only a very small percentage of patients can be cured with chemoradiation alone.
- **Metastatic disease**
  ○ Metastatic gastric cancer is incurable, and systemic therapy offers improved quality and length of life.
  ○ As in esophageal cancer, first-line treatment depends on HER2 testing. For HER2-positive disease, a backbone of fluorouracil (5-FU or capecitabine) plus platinum (oxaliplatin or cisplatin) is combined with trastuzumab with or without pembrolizumab. HER2-negative disease is treated with the same chemotherapy backbone, with or without nivolumab.
  ○ In the second-line setting, patients with HER2-positive disease should receive T-dxd. There are several acceptable chemotherapy regimens for second-line treatment of HER2-negative disease, including ramucirumab plus paclitaxel (generally preferred), docetaxel, paclitaxel, irinotecan, or FOLFIRI.

Gastrointestinal Stromal Tumor (GIST)

- Surgical resection is the treatment of choice. Adjuvant imatinib for 3 years is recommended for patients with intermediate or high risk (based on tumor size and mitotic index). Neoadjuvant tyrosine kinase inhibitors may be considered in appropriate cases.
- For advanced or metastatic GIST, a tyrosine kinase inhibitor should be used until disease progression. Imatinib is generally preferred, except in the case of *PDGFRA* exon 18 mutations, which render the tumor insensitive to imatinib; avapritinib should be used in these instances.[10] For patients treated with first-line imatinib who experience disease progression, increased imatinib dosage and then switching to sunitinib can be considered. Regorafenib and ripretinib are options following failure of imatinib or sunitinib.[11,12] Dasatinib may be considered for patients with platelet-derived growth factor receptor alpha (PDGFRA) exon 18 mutations after progression on avapritinib.
- Rarely, GIST may lack both *KIT* and *PDGFRA* mutations and instead harbor an alteration resulting in succinate dehydrogenase (SDH) complex inactivation. These tumors are typically insensitive to imatinib, and alternate driver mutations should be evaluated with next-generation sequencing to guide targeted therapy.

SPECIAL CONSIDERATIONS

Given the rarity of gastric cancer in US, there is no justification for routine screening for esophageal or stomach cancer at this time. However, in countries of high incidence (e.g., Japan), screening for stomach cancer via endoscopy or upper gastrointestinal imaging is standard for those over 50 years of age.

COMPLICATIONS

- Hemorrhage, gastric obstruction, and malignant ascites.
- Disseminated intravascular coagulation (DIC) is a rare complication that may occur in patients with advanced gastric carcinoma and bone marrow metastasis. Mortality is high

at 1–4 weeks of onset and requires aggressive supportive management and, if possible, chemotherapy.
• Patients who underwent total gastrectomy often develop dumping syndrome, vitamin B_{12} deficiency, and reflux esophagitis.

MONITORING/FOLLOW-UP

After definitive treatment, asymptomatic patients should typically be evaluated by history and physical examination every 3 months for 2 years and then every 6 months for 3 additional years. CBC, CMP, and, if applicable, CEA should be obtained during each routine follow-up, and imaging studies such as CT scan should be obtained at least every 6 months in the first 1–3 years or when clinically indicated.

OUTCOME/PROGNOSIS

Five-year survival rates are 60–80% for stage I, 20–40% for stage II, and 10–20% for stage III.

Pancreatic Cancer

GENERAL PRINCIPLES

Definition
Cancer that arises from either the exocrine or the endocrine tissue of the pancreas.

Classification
• Site: Two-thirds of the cases originate from pancreatic head.
• Histology: 95% of pancreatic cancers are exocrine ductal carcinoma, with the rest being acinar carcinoma or neuroendocrine tumors.

Epidemiology
• Pancreatic cancer is the fourth leading cause of cancer death in US, with an annual incidence of approximately 12.3/100,000.
• Up to 64,050 new cases and 50,550 deaths were anticipated in 2023.
• Age: sixth to seventh decades
• Sex: slightly higher in males
• Race: higher in African Americans

Etiology and Pathophysiology
• Activation mutation of *K-Ras* and loss of tumor suppressor *INK4a* are found in >90% of pancreatic cancer. Recently, activation of Sonic hedgehog signaling pathway has been shown to be important in oncogenesis of pancreatic cancer.
• Chronic inflammation is believed to accelerate mutagenesis and cancer formation.

Risk Factors
Cigarette smoking, positive family history, chronic pancreatitis, obesity, diabetes mellitus

Associated Conditions
Lynch syndrome, ataxia-telangiectasia, *BRCA2* mutation, familial atypical mole melanoma syndrome, Peutz–Jeghers syndrome, hereditary nonpolyposis colorectal cancer (HNPCC)

DIAGNOSIS

Clinical Presentation

History

Most patients are asymptomatic until advanced stage. Presenting symptoms may include abdominal or back pain, weight loss, nausea, vomiting, painless jaundice, fatigue, and depression.

Physical Examination

- Palpable abdominal mass, jaundice, ascites, Courvoisier sign (painless palpable gallbladder), Virchow node, and Sister Mary Joseph node may occasionally be found.
- Paraneoplastic syndromes, such as Trousseau syndrome (migratory superficial phlebitis), idiopathic deep venous thrombosis, myositis syndromes, and Cushing syndrome, are rarely seen.

Diagnostic Testing

Laboratories

- CBC, CMP, PT, and PTT.
- CEA and CA19–9 levels should be obtained as a baseline and followed for response/recurrence.

Imaging

- Initial imaging studies are usually **abdominal CT scan** or **ultrasonography.**
- **Dynamic-phase spiral CT of the abdomen** ("pancreatic protocol") is the current most accurate imaging modality in assessing pancreatic tumor. It allows detailed evaluation of the pancreas, extent of local invasion, and common sites of metastasis such as peripancreatic lymph nodes and the liver. Magnetic resonance cholangiopancreatography (MRCP) may be used to supplement this imaging technique when masses are not easily visible on CT imaging.
- Patients with confirmed pancreatic cancer should complete staging workup with chest and pelvic CT scan.

Diagnostic Procedures

- Further tumor staging with an endoscopic ultrasound or endoscopic retrograde cholangiopancreatography (ERCP) may be necessary.
- **Tissue diagnosis** can be obtained by percutaneous ultrasound or CT-guided needle biopsy, laparoscopy, ERCP, or ascitic fluid cytology.
- Staging can be done by TNM system or, more commonly, by resectability (localized/resectable, borderline resectable, locally advanced/unresectable, and metastatic stages).

TREATMENT

- In the absence of metastatic disease, surgical consult should always be obtained to assess resectability, which is the basis for subsequent management.
- **Localized, resectable disease**
  - The standard procedure is a pancreaticoduodenectomy with choledochojejunostomy, cholecystectomy, and gastrojejunostomy (**Whipple procedure**). Surgical mortality is 1–4%, even at high-volume centers.
  - Tumors of the pancreatic tail are typically removed via distal pancreatectomy and splenectomy, which spares some of the morbidity of Whipple resection without a detriment to survival or disease control.
  - Adjuvant therapy is necessary after resection of the primary, since close to 80% of these patients later develop locoregional recurrence or distant metastases. The data are

not clear on the importance of radiation in the adjuvant setting; it may improve local disease control but no strong evidence exists to suggest it improves overall survival. Patients should be enrolled in clinical trials if available. Commonly used regimens include FOLFIRINOX, gemcitabine with capecitabine, or concurrent chemoradiation with 5-FU or capecitabine.

- **Borderline resectable disease**
  - This category is defined by certain radiographic features in which upfront surgery is likely to result in positive surgical margin.
  - Neoadjuvant chemotherapy with or without radiation has been proposed with hopes to downstage the tumor and improve the likelihood of complete resection, to exclude patients with rapidly progressive disease who may not benefit from surgery, and to avoid delay in chemoradiation due to prolonged postoperative recovery. While this approach is gaining popularity, its benefit has not been convincingly shown by large randomized controlled studies.
  - Neoadjuvant chemotherapy approaches are largely extrapolated from adjuvant and metastatic regimens. FOLFIRINOX or gemcitabine plus nab-paclitaxel are standard.
- **Locally advanced, unresectable disease**
  - While there is no clear standard approach, options include radiation, chemoradiation, or chemotherapy alone. Consensus guidelines suggest an initial course of chemotherapy (FOLFIRINOX, gemcitabine, gemcitabine, and albumin-bound paclitaxel, 5-FU, or FOLFOX). Chemoradiation may be considered, particularly in patients tolerating an initial course of chemotherapy without progression. A small minority of patients can become resectable using this approach.
- **Metastatic pancreatic cancer**
  - Metastatic pancreatic cancer is incurable. Chemotherapy improves quality of life and overall survival.
  - Clinical trials should be recommended if available.
  - Current recommended first-line chemotherapy is FOLFIRINOX or gemcitabine and albumin-bound paclitaxel. Alternative options include FOLFOX, gemcitabine, or gemcitabine combined with erlotinib.
  - Second-line chemotherapy largely depends on first-line treatment with either gemcitabine or 5-FU-based regimens recommended depending on prior exposure.

Lifestyle/Risk Modification

All patients should be encouraged to cease smoking and consuming alcohol.

Diet

Most patients undergoing treatment suffer from pancreatic insufficiency and, therefore, should be prescribed pancreatic enzymes and told to avoid high-fat diets.

SPECIAL CONSIDERATIONS

Routine **preoperative biliary stenting for obstructive jaundice** secondary to localized pancreatic head cancer is associated with higher postoperative complications compared to patients who received early surgery. Therefore, discussion should be made between hepatobiliary surgeon and gastroenterologist before stenting.

COMPLICATIONS

- **Pain management** is paramount in pancreatic cancer patients. In addition to standard analgesics, celiac plexus block may be an option in selected patients.

- **Biliary obstruction and subsequent cholangitis** should be relieved by stenting or draining procedures.
- Patients who undergo Whipple procedure will develop **diabetes**.

MONITORING/FOLLOW-UP

After definitive treatment, asymptomatic patients should typically be evaluated by history and physical examination every 3 months for 2 years and then every 6 months for 3 additional years. CBC, CMP, and, if applicable, CA19–9 or CEA and CT scan of chest/abdomen/pelvis should be obtained during each routine follow-up.

OUTCOME/PROGNOSIS

- Overall 5-year survival is 5%. Upon diagnosis, >50% of cases are metastatic, 25% locally advanced, and <20% are potentially resectable.
- The most important prognostic factors include surgical margin, lymph node status, and tumor size. However, even patients who underwent curative resection have a 15–20% 5-year survival rate.

Hepatocellular Carcinoma

GENERAL PRINCIPLES

Definition
Primary cancer that arises from hepatocytes.

Epidemiology
- Hepatocellular carcinoma (HCC) is the fifth most common cancer worldwide, but it is rare in US. Incidence in US is around 5 per 100,000, but this has been rising over the last few decades due to the increase in hepatitis B and C infections.
- Age: seventh decade.
- Sex: M:F, 3:1.
- Race: higher incidence in African Americans and Asians.

Etiology and Pathophysiology
- Chronic inflammation, necrosis, and liver regeneration likely predispose hepatocytes to acquire mutations.
- Integration of HBV DNA into the hepatocyte genome can contribute to cancer formation.

Risk Factors
- Hepatitis B, hepatitis C, and cirrhosis from any cause such as alcohol and nonalcoholic steatohepatitis, alpha1-antitrypsin deficiency, hemochromatosis.

Prevention
- Vaccination against hepatitis B.
- Treatment of chronic hepatitis B with lamivudine has been shown to decrease the risk of developing HCC.
- Treatment of hepatitis C may decrease the subsequent risk of HCC. Patients with hepatitis C should be screened with annual alpha-fetoprotein levels and liver ultrasound.
- Retinoids may have a role in secondary prevention of HCC.

Associated Conditions

Twenty percent to 30% of patients with untreated chronic hepatitis C eventually develop cirrhosis. Cirrhotic patients have a 2–6% per year risk of developing HCC.

DIAGNOSIS

Clinical Presentation

History

Patients may have nonspecific complaints of abdominal pain, malaise, weight loss, or fever. Most patients have history of liver cirrhosis.

Physical Examination

Patients may occasionally have a palpable liver mass. Most patients have physical **findings of cirrhosis** such as ascites, splenomegaly, spider angiomata, and collateral circulation muscle wasting.

Diagnostic Criteria

- **Imaging:** Lesions >1 cm in size that have characteristic imaging findings on MRI or CT meet a diagnosis of HCC.
- **Percutaneous needle biopsy** (FNA or core biopsy) should be performed in uncertain cases.

Differential Diagnosis

Adenoma, hemangioma, metastatic cancer

Diagnostic Testing

Laboratories

CBC, CMP, PT, PTT, and alpha fetoprotein (AFP) (elevated in 85% of cases)

Imaging Studies

- **Abdominal ultrasound** or **CT scan with contrast** is usually done initially.
- If primary hepatocellular cancer is strongly suspected, more detailed imaging studies including **triple-phase contrast-enhanced CT scan or MRI** are used to define anatomic relationships and vascular anatomy. Conventional angiography, CT, or MR-angiography is usually needed to completely reveal the anatomy and characteristics of the tumor vasculature.

TREATMENT

- Many staging systems have been proposed, which include the Okuda, CLIP, Barcelona Clinic Liver Cancer (BCLC), and TNM staging.
- The BCLC staging system integrates Okuda staging and Child–Pugh score and treatment recommendations, and is currently endorsed by the American Association for Study of Liver Disease.[13]
  - **Stage 0:** Solitary lesion <2 cm with preserved liver function. Surgical resection is the primary treatment. Unfortunately, <5% of patients are resectable because of advanced disease or cirrhosis at presentation. Recurrent local disease may also be treated surgically, with potential for cure.
  - **Stage A:** Patients who are not eligible for resection (primarily due to insufficient liver reserve) or who meet the Milan criteria (one tumor ≤5 cm or up to three tumors ≤3 cm, no extrahepatic manifestations, or vascular invasion). Liver transplantation is the treatment of choice, with 5-year survival up to 75%. Patients who are not transplant

candidates should be referred for percutaneous ethanol injection or radiofrequency ablation.

- **Stage B:** Patients typically have multinodular disease. Transarterial chemoembolization (TACE) is the treatment of choice. This therapy involves catheter-guided embolization of tumor-feeding hepatic artery using materials such as Lipiodol or Gelfoam with or without chemotherapeutic agents such as cisplatin or doxorubicin. It may provide a survival benefit. Due to risk of liver failure, TACE is contraindicated in patients with portal vein thrombosis and in most patients with Child C liver disease.
- **Stage C:** Palliative systemic therapy improves length and quality of life. Preferred front-line regimens include atezolizumab plus bevacizumab (for Child–Pugh A only) or durvalumab plus tremelimumab. These regimens are both associated with a median overall survival around 16.5 months. Other acceptable first-line regimens include sorafenib (Child–Pugh A or B7), lenvantinib (Child–Pugh A), durvalumab, or pembrolizumab. Clinical trials should be recommended if available.
- **Stage D:** Best supportive care.

COMPLICATIONS

- Liver decompensation is of major concern after surgical resection or TACE.
- Complications of liver cirrhosis such as ascites, jaundice, bleeding diathesis, and variceal bleed are commonly seen.

MONITORING/FOLLOW-UP

- Patients with chronic HCV or liver cirrhosis should be screened with AFP and liver ultrasonography every 6–12 months.
- Due to high risk of recurrence, patients should be followed closely. A repeat CT scan should be obtained 1 month after surgical resection or local therapy. CBC, CMP, PT, serum AFP, and abdominal CT/ultrasonography should be obtained every 3 months afterward.
- Patients who undergo liver transplantation should be followed by a liver transplant team regularly.

OUTCOME/PROGNOSIS

Overall 5-year survival for stage 0 and A is 50–70%, 3-year survival of stage B and C is 20–40%, and 1-year survival for stage D disease is <10%, with median survival of 6 months.

Gallbladder Cancer

GENERAL PRINCIPLES

Classification
Histology: 85% adenocarcinoma, the rest being squamous cell carcinoma or mixed type

Epidemiology
- Gallbladder cancer is a rare cancer of the biliary system, with approximately 5,000 cases diagnosed per year in North America.
- Age: Seventh decade.
- Sex: M:F, 1:1.7.

Risk Factors

Risk factors include chronic cholecystitis, cholelithiasis, and typhoid carriers. Seventy-five percent to 98% of patients with gallbladder cancer will have gall stones. Incidence of gallbladder cancer in patients with "Porcelain gallbladder" is up to 25%.

Prevention

Due to high risk of developing cancer, patients with porcelain gallbladder or gallbladder polyp >1 cm should be referred for surgery.

Associated Conditions

Gall stones, chronic cholecystitis, gallbladder polyp, typhoid carrier, inflammatory bowel disease

DIAGNOSIS

Clinical Presentation

History

These tumors may present with symptoms of acute or chronic cholecystitis, although jaundice and weight loss are more common. Many gallbladder cancer diagnoses are made incidentally on histologic review of cholecystectomy specimens.

Physical Examination

Scratch marks for pruritus, jaundice, hepatomegaly, right upper quadrant tenderness, or symptoms/signs of acute cholecystitis

Diagnostic Criteria

Histopathology diagnosis, usually after cholecystectomy, is required.

Differential Diagnosis

Cholecystitis, cholangitis, cholangiocarcinoma, biliary colic, choledocholithiasis, gallbladder polyp, primary HCC, metastatic cancer, primary sclerosing cholangitis

Diagnostic Testing

Laboratories

CBC, liver function tests (LFT), GGT, basic metabolic panel (BMP), PT, PTT, AFP, and CEA

Imaging

• **Right upper quadrant ultrasonography** is usually the first imaging modality to be ordered.
• When gallbladder tumor is suspected, further imaging modalities such as **liver MRI** or **abdominal CT** should be obtained. **MRCP** is recommended to delineate tumor extent and nodal status in more detail. Chest imaging should also be pursued to complete staging.

Diagnostic Procedures

Tissue diagnosis can be made by ERCP if the tumor is distal. However, diagnosis is often made at the time of surgery.

TREATMENT

• The only curative treatment for gallbladder cancer is **surgical resection**, but only <30% of patients have resectable disease at the time of presentation. Surgery typically involves cholecystectomy, en bloc hepatic resection, lymphadenectomy, and possible bile duct resection. Adjuvant therapy with capecitabine (preferred) or with 5-FU-based concurrent chemoradiation is recommended for most patients with resected gallbladder cancer, except for those with very small tumors (T1 N0).

- For patients with **unresectable but nonmetastatic gallbladder cancer**, therapy with gemcitabine/cisplatin combination therapy or 5-FU-based therapy, including 5-FU-based concurrent chemoradiation is recommended.
- For patients with **metastatic disease**, choices of chemotherapy include **cisplatin plus gemcitabine with or without durvalumab.**[14,15]
- Patients with metastatic disease should be evaluated for targetable alterations including microsatellite instability/mismatch repair deficiency, *FGFR2* fusions or rearrangements, *IDH1* mutations, HER2 overexpression or amplification, *RET* gene fusions, *NTRK* fusions, or *BRAF* V600E. In the second line and beyond, targeted therapy is preferred over chemotherapy.

COMPLICATIONS

Obstructive jaundice, cholecystitis, and cholangitis are commonly seen.

MONITORING/FOLLOW-UP

After definitive treatment, asymptomatic patients should typically be evaluated by history and physical examination every 3 months for 2 years, and then every 6 months for 3 additional years. CBC, CMP, and, if applicable, CA19–9 or CEA and CT scan of chest/abdomen/pelvis should be obtained during each routine follow-up.

OUTCOME/PROGNOSIS

Five-year survival rates for localized, regional, and distant disease are 40%, 15%, and <10%, respectively. The median survival for advanced disease is 2–4 months.

Cholangiocarcinoma

GENERAL PRINCIPLES

Definition

Cancers that arise from the biliary duct and before the ampulla of Vater

Classification

- Site: intrahepatic (<10%) and extrahepatic (>90%) origin. Intrahepatic cholangiocarcinomas arise in the small intrahepatic ductules or the large intrahepatic ducts proximal to the bifurcation of the right and left hepatic ducts. Extrahepatic cholangiocarcinomas originate in any of the major hepatic or biliary ducts. **Klatskin tumor** refers to extrahepatic cholangiocarcinoma that arises in the hilum of left and right hepatic duct.
- Histology: >95% adenocarcinoma, further subtyped into sclerosing, nodular, and papillary variants; <5% squamous cell carcinoma.

Epidemiology

- Cholangiocarcinoma is a rare cancer of the biliary tree, accounting for approximately 2,500 new cases each year in US.

- Age: Sixth decade.
- Sex: M:F, approximately 1:1.

Etiology and Pathophysiology

Largely unknown but chronic inflammation may result in accelerated mutagenesis and dysplastic change.

Risk Factors

Primary sclerosing cholangitis, hepatolithiasis, choledochal cysts, ulcerative colitis, and liver fluke infection

DIAGNOSIS

Clinical Presentation

History
Up to 98% of patients with cholangiocarcinomas present with jaundice, and quite frequently right upper quadrant pain, fever, pruritus, and body weight loss.

Physical Examination
Jaundice, hepatomegaly, or right upper quadrant mass.

Diagnostic Criteria

Histopathology diagnosis is required.

Differential Diagnosis

Cholecystitis, cholangitis, gallbladder cancer, primary HCC, pancreatic cancer, cancer of ampulla of Vater, metastatic cancer, primary sclerosing cholangitis

Diagnostic Testing

Laboratories
CBC, BMP, LFT, PT, PTT, CA19–9, and CEA

Imaging
- **Abdominal CT** and **ultrasonography** are usually the first imaging studies performed.
- When cholangiocarcinoma is suspected, further imaging modalities, such as liver MRI, should be obtained. MRCP is recommended to delineate tumor extent and nodal status in more detail. Chest imaging completes staging.

Diagnostic Procedures
Tissue diagnosis can be made by ERCP if the tumor is distal or by CT-guided biopsy if proximal or intrahepatic. Occasionally, diagnosis is often made at the time of surgery.

TREATMENT

- Complete surgical resection offers the only chance of cure. Overall management depends on location and stage of the disease.
- **Intrahepatic cholangiocarcinoma:** Resection is the primary approach to treatment when possible. If surgical margins are positive (R1 resection), adjuvant 5-FU-based chemoradiation or chemotherapy with a 5-FU- or gemcitabine-based regimen is recommended. Patients with negative margins may be observed or treated with 5-FU- or gemcitabine-based chemotherapy. For gross residual disease (R2 resection) treatment with gemcitabine or cisplatin should be pursued and radiofrequency ablation or repeat surgery should be considered.

- **Extrahepatic cholangiocarcinoma:** Resection is again a primary approach to treatment when possible. In some cases, hilar cholangiocarcinoma may be surgically treated with liver transplantation. Patients achieving complete resection with negative lymph nodes may be observed or treated with chemotherapy (capecitabine is preferred) or chemoradiation (5-FU- or gemcitabine-based). Positive margins, positive lymph nodes, or gross residual disease should be treated with systemic therapy (capecitabine is preferred) or 5-FU-based chemoradiation followed by additional 5-FU- or gemcitabine-based chemotherapy.
- **Metastatic or unresectable disease** is incurable and is managed along the principles outlined for gallbladder cancer in the previous section. Locoregional therapies including radiofrequency ablation, transarterial chemoembolization, radioembolization, or external beam radiation may complement systemic therapy for intrahepatic disease. Gemcitabine, cisplatin, and durvalumab is the preferred first-line systemic regimen.[15] Patients should be evaluated for clinical trials if available. Next-generation sequencing for evaluation of therapeutic targets is standard. Such targets include microsatellite instability/mismatch repair deficiency, *FGFR2* fusions or rearrangements, *IDH1* mutations, HER2 overexpression or amplification, *RET* gene fusions, *NTRK* fusions, and *BRAF* V600E.

COMPLICATIONS

Obstructive jaundice, cholecystitis, and cholangitis are commonly seen.

MONITORING/FOLLOW-UP

After definitive treatment, asymptomatic patients should typically be evaluated by history and physical examination every 3 months for 2 years, and then every 6 months for 3 additional years. CBC, CMP, and, if applicable, CA19–9 or CEA should be obtained. Imaging is suggested by consensus guidelines every 6 months for 2 years as clinically indicated.

OUTCOME/PROGNOSIS

- Prognosis depends on stage and performance status. However, >70% of patients present with advanced stage and <10% of patients are surgical candidates.
- Patients with distal extrahepatic tumors that are completely resected have a 5-year survival rate of up to 40%. Overall median survival duration in patients with localized disease who undergo resection and adjuvant chemoradiation is 17–27.5 months.
- Patients who are not surgical candidates and received chemoradiation alone have a median survival 7–17 months.
- Patients who can tolerate biliary stenting alone have median survival of a few months.

REFERENCES

1. Herskovic A, Martz K, Al-Sarraf M, et al. Combined chemotherapy and radiotherapy compared with radiotherapy alone in patients with cancer of the esophagus. *N Engl J Med.* 1992;326(24):1593–1598.
2. Bang Y-J, Van Cutsem E, Feyereislova A, et al; ToGA Trial Investigators. Trastuzumab in combination with chemotherapy versus chemotherapy alone for treatment of HER2-positive advanced gastric or gastro-oesophageal junction cancer (ToGA): a phase 3, open-label, randomised controlled trial. *Lancet.* 2010;376(9742):687–697.
3. Fuchs CS, Tomasek J, Yong CJ, et al; REGARD Trial Investigators. Ramucirumab monotherapy for previously treated advanced gastric or gastro-oesophageal junction adenocarcinoma (REGARD): an international, randomised, multicentre, placebo-controlled, phase 3 trial. *Lancet.* 2014;383(9911):31–39.
4. Mauer AM, Kraut EH, Krauss SA, et al. Phase II trial of oxaliplatin, leucovorin and fluorouracil in patients with advanced carcinoma of the esophagus. *Ann Oncol.* 2005;16(8):1320–1325.

5. Van Cutsem E, Moiseyenko VM, Tjulandin S, et al; V325 Study Group. Phase III study of docetaxel and cisplatin plus fluorouracil compared with cisplatin and fluorouracil as first-line therapy for advanced gastric cancer: a report of the V325 Study Group. *J Clin Oncol.* 2006;24(31):4991–4997.
6. Cunningham D, Allum WH, Stenning SP, et al; MAGIC Trial Participants. Perioperative chemotherapy versus surgery alone for resectable gastroesophageal cancer. *N Engl J Med.* 2006;355(1):11–20.
7. Macdonald JS, Smalley SR, Benedetti J, et al. Chemoradiotherapy after surgery compared with surgery alone for adenocarcinoma of the stomach or gastroesophageal junction. *N Engl J Med.* 2001; 345(10):725–730.
8. Sakuramoto S, Sasako M, Yamaguchi T, et al; ACTS-GC Group. Adjuvant chemotherapy for gastric cancer with S-1, an oral fluoropyrimidine. *N Engl J Med.* 2007;357(18):1810–1820.
9. Sasako M, Sakuramoto S, Katai H, et al. Five-year outcomes of a randomized phase III trial comparing adjuvant chemotherapy with S-1 versus surgery alone in stage II or III gastric cancer. *J Clin Oncol.* 2011;29(33):4387–4893.
10. Heinrich MC, Jones RL, von Mehren M, et al. Avapritinib in advanced PDGFRA D842V-mutant gastrointestinal stromal tumour (NAVIGATOR): a multicentre, open-label, phase 1 trial. *Lancet Oncol.* 2020;21(7):935–946.
11. Demetri GD, von Mehren M, Blanke CD, et al. Efficacy and safety of imatinib mesylate in advanced gastrointestinal stromal tumors. *N Engl J Med.* 2002;347(7):472–480.
12. Blay J-Y, Serrano C, Heinrich MC, et al. Ripretinib in patients with advanced gastrointestinal stromal tumours (INVICTUS): a double-blind, randomised, placebo-controlled, phase 3 trial. *Lancet Oncol.* 2020;21:923–934.
13. Llovet JM, Bru C, Bruix J. Prognosis of hepatocellular carcinoma: the BCLC staging classification. *Semin Liver Dis.* 1999;19(3):329–338.
14. Valle J, Wasan H, Palmer DH, et al; ABC-02 Trial Investigators. Cisplatin plus gemcitabine versus gemcitabine for biliary tract cancer. *N Engl J Med.* 2010;362(14):1273–1281.
15. Oh D-Y, He AR, Qin S, et al. Durvalumab plus gemcitabine and cisplatin in advanced biliary tract cancer. *NEJM Evid.* 2022;1(8):EVIDoa2200015.

Malignant Melanoma 25

Favour Ayomide Akinjiyan, Renee Morecroft, Alice Zhou, and George Ansstas

GENERAL PRINCIPLES

Definition

Malignant melanoma is an aggressive neoplasm that arises from melanocytes, which are long-lived pigment-producing cells. Melanocytes are located in the basal layer of the epidermis, hair bulb, and eyes. Melanoma most commonly arises in the skin; however, melanoma can also arise in noncutaneous sites as well, such as in mucosal and uveal tissue.[1]

Classification

Cutaneous malignant melanoma is traditionally classified into superficial spreading melanoma (SSM), nodular melanoma (NM), lentigo maligna melanoma (LMM), acral lentiginous melanoma, and desmoplastic melanoma. *SSM* accounts of about 50–75% of melanoma, and have pagetoid spread in the epidermis, with variations in pigmentation. *NM* (15–35%) can appear nodular, polypoid, or pedunculated. *LMM* (5–15%) affects the sun-exposed skin, face, and upper extremities of elderly patients. *Acral lentiginous melanoma* (5–10%) arises in the palmar, plantar, or ungual skin. *Mucosal melanoma* arises from mucosal tissue from the nasopharyngeal and oral cavity, vulva, vagina, and anus, and share histologic features of acral melanoma. *Uveal melanoma* arises in the eye and has a different biology and prognosis than cutaneous and mucosal melanoma.[1]

Epidemiology

The Surveillance, Epidemiology, and End Results Program (SEER) data demonstrate a steady rise in the incidence of melanoma since 1975 and a continued average of 1.5% year-over-year increase for the last 10 years (http://seer.cancer.gov). Death rates have fallen on average 2.5% each year from 2007 to 2016 in part of new effective therapies. The American Cancer Society estimates 97,610 new cases of melanoma in 2023. The lifetime risk of being diagnosed with melanoma in US is approximately 1 in 38 for Caucasian populations, 1 in 1,000 for African American populations, and 1 in 167 for Hispanic populations. Overall, melanoma is more common in men, but rates of melanoma are highest in women before the age of 50.

Risk Factors

- The most significant environmental risk factor for the development of melanoma is ultraviolet (UV) light exposure. UV exposure interacts with clinical and genetic risk factors, including fair skin, red hair (MC1R variants), and UV sensitivity syndromes such as xeroderma pigmentosum, all of which increases the risk for melanoma.[2] Other risk factors include increased number of nevi (>50), history of greater than five clinically atypical nevi, and large congenital nevi.[3] Organ-transplant patients on chronic immunosuppression have a higher risk of developing skin cancers, including melanoma.[4]
- The transformation of benign melanocytes to melanoma results from an accumulation of genetic changes. The majority of cases of melanoma are nonfamilial and are associated with environmental carcinogens such as UV exposure. Activating mutations in the *BRAF* gene are found in 50–60% of melanoma cases, often in younger patients, and with less

association to sun exposure. The *BRAF* gene encodes a serine/threonine protein kinase important in proliferation and is critical in the mitogen-activated protein kinase (MAPK) pathway. Dysregulated MAPK signaling promotes cell division.[5] Acral or mucosal melanoma had a significantly higher degree of chromosomal aberrations but less frequent mutations in *BRAF* and *NRAS,* two genes in the MAPK pathway, and instead can have activating mutations in *KIT.*[6] These genomic alterations have implications for the development of targeted therapies.

- Familial cases of melanoma typically account for approximately 10% of melanoma cases. Germline mutations in the cyclin-dependent kinase inhibitor 2A (*CDKN2A*) gene located on chromosome 9p21 conferred susceptibility to melanoma with high penetrance and in an autosomal-dominant manner and are found in about 20–40% of familial cases. Cyclin-dependent kinase 4 (*CDK4*) gene located on chromosome 12q14, is also a high-penetrant gene identified in some patients without *CDKN2A* mutations. Germline mutations in genes that maintenance telomere integrity, such as *POT1, ACD, TERF2IP, TERT, BAP1,* also confer high penetrance for the development of melanoma, although incidences are <1% for each gene.[2] In addition, the melanocortin-1-receptor (MC1R) and microphthalmia transcription factor (MITF), important in melanocyte biology, have also been implicated in familial melanoma, albeit at low to moderate penetrance.[7]

Prevention

Given the association between UV radiation and the development of melanoma, **avoiding UV rays** and using **sunscreen** are critical to reduce the risk of developing melanoma. For secondary prevention, patients at risk for developing melanoma might benefit from education on self-skin examinations, and to report any unusual or changing nevus.

DIAGNOSIS

Clinical Presentation

- The **"ABCDE" mnemonic** in melanoma diagnosis refers to **A**symmetry, **B**order irregularity, **C**olor variations, **D**imension, and **E**volution. The clinical history should review risk factors for melanoma. The physical exam should pay attention to any changes in lesions. Changes in the color or an increase in size of a new mole are usually the early signs noted by patients. Later changes include bleeding, itching, and tenderness. A global evaluation of the skin is necessary to assess the degree of sun damage, number of nevi, distribution of nevi, and the presence of atypical or dysplastic nevi. Full-body examination is essential, including scalp, hands and feet, genitalia, and oral cavity.
- When a lesion suspicious of melanoma is identified, the next key step is an appropriate biopsy. If melanoma is suspected, a **complete excisional removal** into adipose tissue, with a 1–3-mm margin of adjacent normal-appearing skin, is preferred. **Shave biopsies should be avoided** as they may not provide an accurate Breslow depth, which is an important part of melanoma staging. For large lesions that are not easily amenable to complete excision, such as large lesions or lesions on special sites like the palms, soles, face, or digits, an **incisional full-thickness biopsy** or multiple representative punch biopsies might be acceptable.
- Histologic diagnosis is made on the presence of melanoma-specific immunohistochemical (IHC) stains, including S100, MART-1, HMB-45, SOX10, which are not specific to melanoma but can identify cells of melanocytic lineage. Pathologic considerations should include the thickness, or Breslow depth, and ulceration. Additional testing including IHC stain for BRAFV600E mutation and PD-L1 expression is helpful for clinical management.
- Once a diagnosis of melanoma is made, a thorough history and physical examination will help guide further workup. Lymph nodes should be carefully examined, and patients

with clinically palpable suspicious lymph nodes should be referred for biopsy or imaging. Patients with symptoms suspicious of metastatic disease should be worked up as appropriate with a PET-CT or CT chest/abdomen/pelvis. Those with lymph node–positive disease should get a brain MRI to evaluate for brain metastasis. In patients with distant metastases, a serum lactate dehydrogenase (LDH) is of prognostic value.

Staging

- Staging of melanoma is based on the American Joint Committee on Cancer (AJCC) melanoma staging and classification, 8th edition, updated in 2017 is found online within consensus guidelines, using the tumor (T), nodal (N), and distant metastasis (M) system.[8] The most important prognostic factors in the staging of melanoma are the thickness of the primary lesion, the presence of ulceration on pathology, and involvement of regional lymph nodes. The thickness of the primary tumor (millimeters) is referred to as the Breslow thickness.
- Suspected regional metastatic disease should be evaluated by PET/CT or CT chest/abdomen/pelvis for clinical diagnosis. If there is disease on the leg below the thigh, then a whole-body PET/CT is required. Routine molecular testing for BRAF mutation is not recommended for stage I or II melanoma, but can be useful in the management of stage III and IV diseases. The consensus guidelines recommend sentinel lymph node biopsy (SLNB) patients with intermediate thickness melanomas (T2, or T3 tumors; >1–4 mm thick) and certainly for patients with thick melanomas (T4; >4.0 mm thick). SLNB is also an option for patients with T1b (0.8–1.0 mm thick, or <0.8 mm thick with ulceration) following a discussion regarding the potential risk of the procedure as those melanomas are associated with a ~10% risk of occult metastases in their SLNs. For patients who are ≥ stage IIB may consider a brain MRI at staging to rule out asymptomatic brain metastasis. Patients who have metastatic disease or neurologic symptoms should definitely have a brain MRI to complete staging.[8]

TREATMENT

Local and Locoregional Disease (Stage I–III)

- **Wide local excision (WLE)**, when feasible, is the primary treatment for localized melanoma. Margins of 0.5–1 cm is recommended for melanoma in situ; 1 cm for melanoma with a thickness of ≤1 mm, 1–2-cm margins for melanoma with a thickness >1–2 mm, and finally, margins of 2 cm for primary melanoma with a thickness >2 mm. Margins larger than 2 cm have not been demonstrated to improve survival.
- **Lymph node dissection.** Patients with a positive SLNB do not need a completion lymph node dissection (CLND), which carries significant morbidity without improvement in outcomes (DeCOG0SLT and MSLT-II).[9] In patients presenting with clinically involved lymph nodes without distant disease, therapeutic lymph node dissection (TLND) is recommended.
- **Neoadjuvant therapy**. While not yet in the consensus guidelines, two prospective phase II studies (PRADO and SWOG1801) demonstrated the consideration of neoadjuvant immunotherapy in stage III and resectable stage IV disease prior to surgery to improve outcomes. The SWOG1801 study randomized patients to receive either neoadjuvant pembrolizumab for 3 doses followed by surgery, then adjuvant pembrolizumab for an additional 15 doses or to up-front surgery followed by 18 doses of adjuvant pembrolizumab. All patients received a total of 18 doses of pembrolizumab and had surgery, but patients who received 3 doses of pembrolizumab neoadjuvantly had a higher 2-year event-free survival (EFS) compared to patients who received pembrolizumab only in the adjuvant setting. The PRADO study was a single-arm study where 99 patients with stage IIIB/C melanoma were treated with nivolumab at 3 mg/kg and ipilimumab at 1 mg/kg

for 2 cycles and then an index node was biopsied. After treatment with two doses of ipili-mumab and nivolumab, 61% of patients achieved a major pathologic remission on the index node biopsy and those patients had 93% EFS at 2 years. This study demonstrated the feasibility of a surgery-sparing protocol, which is relevant to patients who are not ideal surgical candidates. Despite the potential, there are reservations with neoadjuvant therapy as it would delay the time to surgical resection which is the current standard of care and primary method of achieving cure in localized disease.

- **Adjuvant systemic therapy** is recommended after definitive surgical resection on an individualized basis (taking into consideration the risk of recurrence and treatment tox-icity) with observation with close follow-up as an alternative. For patients with stage I/IIA melanoma, adjuvant systemic therapy is not indicated. Adjuvant immunotherapy is FDA approved for > stage IIB patients, although the decision to proceed with treatment should result from a discussion of the risks and benefits of therapy with the patient. Immunotherapies and BRAF-targeted therapies are used in the adjuvant setting.

- **Immunotherapies.** For patients with stage IIB or IIC melanoma, treatment with **pem-brolizumab** for 1 year after complete resection maintained nearly 76% recurrence-free survival (RFS) compared to 63% with placebo at 3 years. Rates of grade >3 adverse effects were 17% with treatment.[10] Despite the positive benefit, it is critical to discuss the risks and benefits given the relatively high rate of adverse events compared to the potential benefits to the patient. For stage III, and sometimes resected stage IV patients with melanoma, both pembrolizumab and nivolumab are approved for adjuvant therapy. **Pembrolizumab** treatment in patients with stage IIIA–IIIC resulted in a higher RFS at 55% compared to placebo at 38% at a median follow-up of 5 years.[11] Fourteen per-cent of patients discontinued pembrolizumab due to side effects. Adjuvant **nivolumab** shown in the CheckMate-238 study to be superior than ipilimumab with a significant improvement in RFS at 51.7% (vs. ipilimumab at 41.2%) at 4 years. Overall survival (OS) was similar in both groups but nivolumab was far better tolerated than ipilimumab (14.4% vs. 45.9% grade 3 or 4 adverse events).[12] Nivolumab and pembrolizumab are approved regardless of BRAF or PD-L1 status. The results from CheckMate-238 and KEYNOTE-054 suggest that these agents have similar efficacy and safety.

- **Targeted therapies. Dabrafenib and trametinib** can also be used to improve outcomes for patients with resected stage III melanoma that harbor a *BRAF* V600E or V600K mutation. In the COMBI-AD study, patients with stage III melanoma with a *BRAF* V600K or V600E mutation who received combination dabrafenib plus trametinib have an RFS of 52% compared to 36% with placebo at 5 years. The most common adverse reactions were pyrexia, fatigue, nausea, headache, rash, chills, diarrhea, vomiting, arthral-gia, and myalgia.[13]

Unresectable or Metastatic Disease (Stage IV)

For patients with unresectable or metastatic melanoma, workup should include LDH, imaging (including brain MRI on initial staging), and *BRAF* mutational testing. For those with oligometastatic disease, or limited metastatic disease amendable to surgery, surgical resection is an option, and cases should be discussed at multidisciplinary tumor boards. Prognosis is variable and depends significantly on the burden of disease, disease kinetics, sites of disease, and response to therapy. Those with brain and hepatic metastasis have the shortest survival, followed by lung metastasis; nodal and skin metastasis have the most favorable prognosis. Historically, metastatic melanoma was associated with poor out-comes, however, in the era of targeted therapies and immunotherapies, prognosis are much more improved. To date, multiple checkpoint inhibitors (ipilimumab, pembrolizumab, nivolumab, relatlimab) and targeted therapies (vemurafenib/cobimetinib, dabrafenib/trametinib, encorafenib/binimetinib) have received regulatory approval for unresectable or metastatic melanoma.

Targeted Therapies

The revolution in melanoma treatment began with the pivotal discovery of the B-Raf proto-oncogene mutation, with activating mutations in *BRAF* gene. Initial studies with single-agent BRAF or MEK inhibitors showed unfavorable side effects of increased rates of nonmelanoma skin cancer (with BRAF inhibitor monotherapy) and cardiomyopathy (with MEK inhibitor monotherapy) due to paradoxical signaling pathways. Combining BRAF and MEK inhibitors together greatly diminished those side effects, therefore, these agents are always used together in the clinical setting. Combination of **dabrafenib and trametinib** improved response rates (69% vs. 53%) and OS (25.1 vs. 18.7 months) when compared to dabrafenib alone.[14] Side effects of dabrafenib and trametinib were most notable for pyrexia leading to discontinuation or dose adjustment. Treatment with **vemurafenib and cobimetinib** led to an improved response rate (70% vs. 50%) and OS (22.3 vs 17.4 months) compared to treatment with vemurafenib and placebo.[15] Finally, the use of **encorafenib and binimetinib** resulted in superior median PFS (14.9 vs. 7.3 months) and OS (33.6 vs. 16.9 months) compared to vemurafenib.[16] The most common grade 3 or 4 side effects of encorafenib and binimetinib are increased gamma-glutamyl transferase (GGT), creatine kinase, and hypertension. While response rates are high with targeted therapies, disease remission is not durable and most patients will eventually relapse.

Immunotherapies

- **Anti–CTLA-4 therapy. Ipilimumab** is a human IgG1 monoclonal antibody that blocks cytotoxic T-lymphocyte antigen 4 (CTLA-4), which inhibits T-cell growth. Ipilimumab acts on T-cell priming, primary in the lymph nodes. Ipilimumab was the first checkpoint inhibitor that showed significant clinical benefit in cancer patients and the FDA-approved ipilimumab in 2011 for use in patients with melanoma.[17,18] However, ipilimumab can cause serious side effects leading to severe, and sometimes fatal, side effects. After the approval of safer and more effective immunotherapies, ipilimumab monotherapy is rarely, if ever, used in the clinical setting anymore.
- **Anti–PD-1 therapy.** PD-1 is expressed on antigen-stimulated T-cells and induces downstream signaling that inhibits T-cell proliferation and antitumor effector activity. PD-1 inhibitors block the interaction between the PD-1 receptor and its ligands PD-L1/2, releasing the PD-1–mediated inhibition of T-cell response. **Pembrolizumab** is a fully human monoclonal IgG4 antibody that targets PD-1 and was granted accelerated approval for the treatment of unresectable or metastatic melanoma by the FDA in 2014 as the KEYNOTE-006 study demonstrated the superiority of pembrolizumab over ipilimumab, prolonging OS to 32.7 months versus 15.9 months with ipilimumab.[19] Pembrolizumab was also found to be more tolerable, with 13.3% grade 3 or 4 adverse events as opposed to 19.9% experience with ipilimumab. **Nivolumab** is another fully human monoclonal IgG4 antibody against PD-1 and was demonstrated to be efficacious for metastatic melanoma in two large phase III clinical trials[20,21] where patients with melanoma treated with nivolumab had a superior overall response rate (ORR) and OS than the comparator. Similar to pembrolizumab, nivolumab was reasonably well tolerated with rates of grade 3 or 4 adverse effects occurring in 11.7% of patients.
- **Combination checkpoint inhibitor therapy.** The landmark randomized phase III CheckMate-067 study showed that combination **ipilimumab and nivolumab** is superior to nivolumab or ipilimumab monotherapy.[22] Combination nivolumab and ipilimumab resulted in the highest ORR at 57.6%, then 43.7% in the nivolumab-only group, and 19% in the ipilimumab-only group. Combination nivolumab and ipilimumab also resulted in the most durable remission; however, it was also the most toxic regimen, with grade 3 or 4 adverse events up to 59%, compared to 28% with nivolumab only, or 23% with ipilimumab only. Combination nivolumab and ipilimumab remains the most potent regimen and is commonly used in those with high burden of disease, brain metastasis, and *BRAF*-mutated disease. Alternative dosing

(flip dosing) decreases toxicity as shown by CheckMate-511 study but the study is not powered for efficacy.

- **Nivolumab and relatlimab** is the most recent combination immunotherapy approved for metastatic melanoma. Relatlimab is a fully human IgG4 monoclonal antibody against LAG-3, which is a checkpoint inhibitor relevant to T-cell activation. Patients with newly diagnosed unresectable stage III or IV melanoma treated with combination nivolumab had superior 12 months PFS at 47.7% compared with nivolumab at 36%.[23] The rate of grade 3 or 4 adverse events is 18.9% in the combination-treated group, compared to 9.7% in the monotherapy group. There is no head-to-head trial comparing the efficacy or tolerability of nivolumab and relatlimab to nivolumab and ipilimumab.

- For patients with *BRAF*-mutated disease, the DREAM-seq study showed that sequencing of therapies is important, with those who were treated with immunotherapy first had longer 2-year OS than those who were treated first with dabrafenib/trametinib (71.8% vs. 51.5%).[24] Therefore, regardless of *BRAF* mutational status, checkpoint inhibitors are recommended in the first-line setting for unresectable or metastatic melanoma.

SPECIAL SITUATIONS IN MELANOMA

- **In-transit disease**. For patients who cannot tolerate systemic therapies and have accessible disease, an intralesional treatment is available. **Talimogene laherparepvec (TVEC)** is a first-in-class oncolytic virus treatment that is injected intralesionally into cutaneous, subcutaneous, or accessible nodal disease sites. Patients who received TVEC had significantly longer median OS (23 months) compared to patients who received GM-CSF (19 months).[25]

- **Brain metastasis.** Melanoma has a propensity to metastasize to the brain, with poor prognosis. Surgery and stereotactic radiotherapy are highly effective for limited lesions. Whole-brain radiotherapy is reserved for large or multiple brain metastasis. Patients with a *BRAF* V600 mutation can be treated with dabrafenib and trametinib with 58% intracranial response and a median OS of 10.8 months.[26] Ipilimumab and nivolumab can induce a response in 55% of patients with asymptomatic brain metastasis (CheckMate-204). In real-life experience, intracranial response to checkpoint inhibitors is abysmal if the patient is symptomatic from their brain metastases, most likely due to the use of steroids for symptom management.

- **Mucosal and acral melanoma.** Cutaneous melanoma accounts for the majority of histologies. However, acral melanoma (occurring on the soles, palms, and ungula surfaces) and mucosal melanoma (occurring on oral, sinus, vaginal, vulva, or anal surfaces) are rarer histologies that present a challenge to treatment. While these melanoma histologies are included in many of the studies, the response rates are lower and remission shorter than cutaneous melanoma. While *BRAF* mutations can be seen in acral melanoma, the incidence is considerably less common. Collective response rate of acral melanoma to combination nivolumab and ipilimumab is approximately 40%. Mucosal melanoma also has a differential mutational profile than cutaneous melanoma and can harbor driver mutations in *c-KIT,* and off-label use of imatinib has sometimes demonstrated efficacy. Response rate of mucosal melanoma to checkpoint inhibitors is also lower than in cutaneous melanoma at approximately 30% with combination nivolumab and ipilimumab.[27]

- **Uveal melanoma.** Melanoma arising from the melanocytes in the uveal tract is the most common intraocular tumor in adults. Histologic considerations include Castle testing and also detection of PRAME antigen, which hold prognostic relevance. Patients with Castle class I and PRAME-negative uveal melanoma have a low rate of recurrence, with 1.1% risk of distant metastasis at 18 months. Patients with Castle class I and PRAME-positive melanoma have an intermediate risk of disease recurrence, at 38% at 5 years. Patients with Castle class II disease have the highest rate of disease recurrence, at

70% at 5 years. Disease limited to the eye is treated locally, with either radioactive plaque or enucleation. Recurrent disease occurs almost always in the liver, sometimes in the lungs, and very rarely elsewhere. Metastatic disease limited to the liver can be managed with liver-directed therapies. The only FDA-approved systemic treatment for metastatic uveal melanoma is the bispecific antibody tebentafusp, which demonstrated a 1-year OS benefit of 79% compared to investigator's choice at 50%.[28] Tebentafusp is only approved for patients who are HLA-A 02:01 positive, and treatment consists of weekly infusions until progression.

- **Tumor-infiltrating lymphocytes (TILs).** A promising novel therapy for melanoma is the use of cellular therapy product TILs. The premise of TILs is the resection of tumor and subsequent isolation, and ex vivo expansion and activation of the TILs. These autologous activated and expanded TILs are then transfused back into a patient after lymphodepletion therapy, under the rationale that these TILs which are in immunologically cold tumors are now primed and activated against the tumors they once resided in. In a group of patients who were refractory to PD-1 therapy, treatment with TILs resulted in 49% ORR compared to 21% with ipilimumab.[29] The majority of patients experience grade 3 or 4 side effects, mostly cytopenias related to lymphodepletion therapy and cytokine-release symptoms related to IL-2 administration. Importantly, this therapy does not appear to worsen toxicities from prior checkpoint inhibitor treatments. While not yet FDA approved for the treatment of melanoma, cellular therapies, specifically TILs, represent a novel therapy that meets a significant unmet need in the treatment of melanoma.

REFERENCES

1. Bandarchi B, Ma L, Navab R, Seth A, Rasty G. From melanocyte to metastatic malignant melanoma. *Dermatol Res Pract*. 2010;2010(1):583748.
2. Hawkes JE, Truong A, Meyer LJ. Genetic predisposition to melanoma. *Semin Oncol*. 2016;43(5):591–597.
3. Gandini S, Sera F, Cattaruzza MS, et al. Meta-analysis of risk factors for cutaneous melanoma: I. Common and atypical naevi. *Eur J Cancer*. 2005;41(1):28–44.
4. Christenson LJ. Malignant melanoma in organ transplant recipients. *Ski Dis Organ Transplant*. 2008; 147(7):182–189.
5. Curtin JA, Fridlyand J, Kageshita T, et al. Distinct sets of genetic alterations in melanoma. *N Engl J Med*. 2005;353(20):2135–2147.
6. Curtin JA, Busam K, Pinkel D, Bastian BC. Somatic activation of KIT in distinct subtypes of melanoma. *J Clin Oncol*. 2006;24(26):4340–4346.
7. Wendt J, Rauscher S, Burgstaller-Muehlbacher S, et al. Human determinants and the role of melanocortin-1 receptor variants in melanoma risk independent of UV radiation exposure. *JAMA Dermatol*. 2016;152(7):776–782.
8. Gershenwald JE, Scolyer RA, Hess KR, et al. Melanoma staging: evidence-based changes in the American Joint Committee on Cancer Eighth Edition Cancer Staging Manual. *CA Cancer J Clin*. 2017;67(6):472–492.
9. Faries MB, Thompson JF, Cochran AJ, et al. Completion dissection or observation for sentinel-node metastasis in melanoma. *N Engl J Med*. 2017;376:2211.
10. Luke JJ, Rutkowski P, Queirolo P, et al. Pembrolizumab versus placebo as adjuvant therapy in completely resected stage IIB or IIC melanoma (KEYNOTE-716): a randomised, double-blind, phase 3 trial. *Lancet*. 2022;399(10336):1718–1729.
11. Eggermont AMM, Blank CU, Mandala M, et al. Adjuvant pembrolizumab versus placebo in resected stage III melanoma. *N Engl J Med*. 2018;378(19):1789–1801.
12. Ascierto PA, Del Vecchio M, Mandalá M, et al. Adjuvant nivolumab versus ipilimumab in resected stage IIIB–C and stage IV melanoma (CheckMate 238): 4-year results from a multicentre, double-blind, randomised, controlled, phase 3 trial. *Lancet Oncol*. 2020;21(11):1465–1477.
13. Long GV, Hauschild A, Santinami M, et al. Adjuvant dabrafenib plus trametinib in stage III BRAF-mutated melanoma. *N Engl J Med*. 2017;377(19):1813–1823.
14. Long GV, Stroyakovskiy D, Gogas H, et al. Combined BRAF and MEK inhibition versus BRAF inhibition alone in melanoma. *N Engl J Med*. 2014;371(20):1877–1888.

15. Ascierto PA, McArthur GA, Dréno B, et al. Cobimetinib combined with vemurafenib in advanced BRAFV600-mutant melanoma (coBRIM): updated efficacy results from a randomised, double-blind, phase 3 trial. *Lancet Oncol.* 2016;17(9):1248–1260.

16. Dummer R, Ascierto PA, Gogas HJ, et al. Overall survival in patients with BRAF-mutant melanoma receiving encorafenib plus binimetinib versus vemurafenib or encorafenib (COLUMBUS): a multicentre, open-label, randomised, phase 3 trial. *Lancet Oncol.* 2018;19(10):1315–1327.

17. Hodi FS, O'Day SJ, McDermott DF, et al. Improved survival with ipilimumab in patients with metastatic melanoma. *N Engl J Med.* 2010;363:711.

18. Robert C, Thomas L, Bondarenko I, et al. Ipilimumab plus dacarbazine for previously untreated metastatic melanoma. *N Engl J Med.* 2011;364:2517–2526.

19. Schachter J, Ribas A, Long GV, et al. Pembrolizumab versus ipilimumab for advanced melanoma: final overall survival results of a multicentre, randomised, open-label phase 3 study (KEYNOTE-006). *Lancet.* 2017;390(10105):1853–1862.

20. Weber JS, D'Angelo SP, Minor D, et al. Nivolumab versus chemotherapy in patients with advanced melanoma who progressed after anti-CTLA-4 treatment (CheckMate 037): a randomised, controlled, open-label, phase 3 trial. *Lancet Oncol.* 2015;16(4):375–384.

21. Robert C, Long GV, Brady B, et al. Nivolumab in previously untreated melanoma without BRAF mutation. *N Engl J Med.* 2015;372(4):320–330.

22. Wolchok JD, Chiarion-Sileni V, Gonzalez R, et al, Long-term outcomes with nivolumab plus ipilimumab or nivolumab alone versus ipilimumab in patients with advanced melanoma. *J Clin Oncol.* 2022;40(2):127–137.

23. Tawbi HA, Schadendorf D, Lipson EJ, et al. Relatlimab and nivolumab versus nivolumab in untreated advanced melanoma. *N Engl J Med.* 2022;386(1):24–34.

24. Atkins MB, Lee SJ, Chmielowski B, et al. Combination dabrafenib and trametinib versus combination nivolumab and ipilimumab for patients with advanced BRAF-mutant melanoma: the DREAMseq trial—ECOG-ACRIN EA6134. *J Clin Oncol.* 2023;41(2):186–197.

25. Andtbacka RHI, Collichio F, Harrington KJ, et al. Final analyses of OPTiM: a randomized phase III trial of talimogene laherparepvec versus granulocyte-macrophage colony-stimulating factor in unresectable stage III-IV melanoma. *J Immunother Cancer.* 2019;7(1):145.

26. Davies MA, Saiag P, Robert C, et al. Dabrafenib plus trametinib in patients with BRAFV600-mutant melanoma brain metastases (COMBI-MB): a multicentre, multicohort, open-label, phase 2 trial. *Lancet Oncol.* 2017;18(7):863–873.

27. Mao L, Qi Z, Zhang L, Guo J, Si L. Immunotherapy in acral and mucosal melanoma: current status and future directions. *Front Immunol.* 2021;12:680407.

28. Nathan P, Hassel JC, Rutkowski P, et al; IMCgp100-202 Investigator. Overall survival benefit with tebentafusp in metastatic uveal melanoma. *N Engl J Med.* 2021;385(13):1196–1206.

29. Rohaan MW, Borch TH, van den Berg JH, et al. Tumor-infiltrating lymphocyte therapy or ipilimumab in advanced melanoma. *N Engl J Med.* 2022;387(23):2113–2125.

Head and Neck Cancer

26

Peter Oppelt

GENERAL PRINCIPLES

Malignancies of the head and neck are the sixth most common cancer in US with head and neck squamous cell carcinoma (HNSCC) as the leading histology. Each year there are approximately 65,000 new cases in US, accounting for 15,000 deaths.[1] While there are many similarities between head and neck cancers arising from different sites, there are key differences in anatomy, natural history, and functional consequences that present unique treatment challenges for each site.

Classification

Malignancies of the head and neck are classified by their anatomic location, which is divided into (a) lip and oral cavity, (b) pharynx (oropharynx, nasopharynx, and hypopharynx), (c) larynx (supraglottis, glottis, and subglottis), (d) nasal cavity and sinuses, and (e) salivary glands. Squamous cell carcinoma accounts for >90% of head and neck tumors; salivary gland tumors account for another 6–8%. Oropharyngeal squamous cell carcinoma is further classified by association with the human papilloma virus (HPV), as these cancers can be either HPV positive or negative. As nasopharyngeal cancer and neck masses with unknown primary have different epidemiology and/or management, they are discussed separately.

Squamous Cell Carcinoma of the Head and Neck

GENERAL PRINCIPLES

Epidemiology

Head and neck cancers have a significant male predominance, with a male-to-female ratio of 3:1. Incidence is highest in Caucasians. Average age at diagnosis is approximately 63 years with a trend toward younger age in HPV-related diseases.[2]

Pathophysiology

HNSCC is an example of the multistep process of carcinogenesis with accumulated genetic mutations that result in changes ranging from hyperplasia, to dysplasia, to carcinoma in situ, and finally to invasive cancer. Alterations in the tumor suppressor gene, *p53*, are implicated in the early steps of tumor development while later mutations are frequently identified in CDKN2A and the wnt signaling pathway.[3]

The epidermal growth factor receptor (EGFR) is overexpressed in a majority of squamous cell carcinoma of the head and neck (SCCHN), and EGFR signaling is a key pathway in HNSCC tumorigenesis. Activation of EGFR activates an intracellular signaling pathway via a tyrosine kinase, leading to inhibition of apoptosis, activation of cell proliferation, and angiogenesis.[4]

HPV infection is also implicated in a rising portion of oropharyngeal HNSCCs. HPV encodes for two oncogenes, E6 and E7. E6 binds to the tumor suppressor protein p53, leading to its destruction, causing increased cell proliferation. E7 interacts with Rb, another protein involved in regulating cell growth, promoting increased cell cycle activation.[5] Patients with HPV-associated HNSCC are less likely to have alterations in p53.

Risk Factors

- Historically, 80–90% of SCCHN were attributable to tobacco exposure. The other main risk factor for development of these malignancies is alcohol use. Tobacco and alcohol are sources of carcinogens that increase the risk of cancer in a dose-dependent fashion and are synergistic in their effects. Field cancerization is a key concept in the natural history of head and neck cancer. Exposure of the mucosa to carcinogens in tobacco is diffused across the aerodigestive tract. Consequently, tumors may be surrounded by areas of dysplasia or carcinoma in situ. Patients diagnosed with head and neck cancer are at an increased risk of developing new primary tumors in the head and neck, lung, and esophagus. The risk is estimated to be 3–4% per year. Sun exposure has been associated with an increased risk of carcinoma of the lip.
- However, ~20–30% of head and neck cancers occur in people without these established risk factors. A large subset of these cancers includes HPV-positive tumors of the oropharynx (tonsil, base of tongue, soft palate). HPV-positive oropharyngeal cancer has been steadily increasing over the years, and now ~70% of oropharyngeal cancers in US are associated with HPV; globally, the incidence varies widely geographically.[6] Risk factors for HPV-positive tumors of the oropharynx include an increasing number of sexual partners. As in cervical cancer, HPV-16 and HPV-18 are high-risk strains for the development of oropharyngeal cancer. The prognosis of HPV-positive oropharyngeal carcinoma is notably better than HPV-negative disease; AJCC staging differentiates between HPV-positive and HPV-negative disease to account for this difference. HPV vaccination provides a significantly lower risk of developing oropharyngeal squamous cell carcinoma.[7]

DIAGNOSIS

Clinical Presentation

- The clinical presentation of these malignancies varies depending on the anatomic location of the tumor. **Cancers of the lip and oral cavity** often present with nonhealing lesions in the mouth, pain in the mouth or ear, trismus, weight loss, and "hot potato speech." Leukoplakia and erythroplakia are premalignant lesions of the mucosa and are frequently seen in conjunction with dysplastic changes or invasive carcinoma.
- **Cancers of the nasal cavity** can present with epistaxis, nonhealing ulcers, or obstruction.
- **Cancers of the oropharynx** present with many of the features associated with cancers of the lip and oral cavity. Bleeding from the mouth, alterations in speech, dysphagia, odynophagia, otalgia, and weight loss can be symptoms of oropharyngeal cancers.
- **Cancers of the larynx and hypopharynx** can present challenges in management, as these anatomic structures are intricately associated with the key functions of speech and swallowing. Symptoms include dysphagia, odynophagia, weight loss, dyspnea (including dyspnea with speech), and hoarseness. Symptoms of aspiration should also be elucidated in the history. However, the time of presentation of these cancers varies greatly with their primary site. Supraglottic tumors or tumors in the pyriform sinus may be diagnosed only after cervical metastases occur because symptoms of dysphagia may not become significant until the tumors are quite advanced. On the other hand, glottic carcinomas are associated with symptoms of hoarseness even when they are small, which may lead to earlier detection.

Diagnostic Testing

- The initial workup of suspected head and neck cancers includes a detailed history and physical examination. Assessment should include a cranial nerve examination, dentition assessment, and palpation of the tongue, floor of mouth, and oropharynx. Lymph nodes in the neck should be carefully palpated and palpable nodes measured. Most patients will require assessment by an otolaryngologist as they will require a fiberoptic nasopharyngolaryngoscopy. Suspicious lesions should be biopsied for histologic confirmation and grading.

- Imaging studies should include a computed tomography (CT) or magnetic resonance imaging (MRI) of the neck to help further delineate disease extent at presentation. Positron emission tomography (PET) imaging is recommended for evaluation of metastatic disease; CT chest can also be considered. The staging for head and neck cancer is according to the American Joint Committee on Cancer TNM system.

- All patients with cancer of the oropharynx should have HPV testing performed on their tumor biopsy. This can be done with p16 immunohistochemistry (IHC), which is a surrogate marker for HPV. In equivocal cases, in situ hybridization (ISH) has demonstrated high specificity.[8]

- Approximately 4% of HNSCC will present as cervical node metastases without a clear primary site of origin. If imaging does not reveal a primary, then endoscopy with blind biopsy of potential sites in the nasopharynx, tonsils, base of tongue, and pyriform sinus should be performed. Testing for HPV and EBV is useful in narrowing the diagnosis.[9] The history should also include a search for invasive cutaneous squamous cell carcinomas.

TREATMENT

- Management of patients requires a multidisciplinary approach, including head and neck surgeons, radiation and medical oncologists, along with allied health professionals including speech-language pathologists and nutritionists. Radiation and surgery are the mainstays of treatment for head and neck cancers. Chemotherapy is reserved for patients with regionally advanced disease with adverse features (such as positive margins or extracapsular lymph node spread) or metastatic disease.

- Patients with T1/T2N0M0 as a group have survival rates of 70–80% with standard therapy, which includes either surgery or radiotherapy (RT) alone. Surgery is generally the preferred approach in operable patients because it is typically associated with less morbidity than RT. Definitive RT is reserved for patients who cannot tolerate surgery or for whom surgical resection would result in particularly significant functional loss.

- Unfortunately, patients often present with advanced locoregional disease and carry poor prognosis, with survival rates of 50–60% at 2 years with standard therapy.[10] HPV-positive oropharyngeal carcinoma, however, carries a far better overall prognosis; even with locally advanced disease, 5-year survival can exceed 80%.[11] Patients with tumors amenable to surgical resection undergo surgery followed by adjuvant therapy with postoperative radiation or concurrent chemoradiation. For patients with locally advanced, unresectable disease, the standard of care is definitive concurrent chemoradiation for patients who can tolerate such a therapy. A meta-analysis of more than 17,000 patients from 19 randomized trials showed a ~5% survival advantage at 5 years for patients undergoing concurrent chemoradiation compared to radiation alone, particularly with the use of platinum chemotherapy.[12] Cisplatin remains the gold standard radiosensitizing agent in the definitive setting given concurrently with a 7-week course of 66–70 Gy of radiation. Other agents, including cetuximab or combination carboplatin/5-FU, can be considered, but with less robust evidence.

- In patients with distant metastases, the prognosis is quite poor. Pembrolizumab has demonstrated improvement in overall survival, either as a single agent or in combination with platinum-based therapy.[13] While some patients can have durable responses to pembrolizumab, overall survival with metastatic disease is only ~13 months. The lungs represent the most common site of distant metastases followed by bone and liver.

COMPLICATIONS

- A multidisciplinary approach is essential to minimize the complications of the malignancy and treatment. Complications of the disease include weight loss, aspiration, and airway compromise. Nutritional support in the form of oral supplements or enteral feedings may be needed when caloric intake is inadequate. Tracheostomy may be needed in cases of airway compromise. Head and neck tumors may also invade into key structures, such as the carotid artery, leading to major bleeding, which may be a terminal event. Invasion into neural structures may lead to neuropathic pain syndromes. Amitriptyline or gabapentin may be helpful in such cases. The limitation to swallowing imposed by some head and neck cancers can make pain management difficult. In such cases, transdermal fentanyl patches or methadone elixir can be used in conjunction with concentrated opiate elixirs (breakthrough) for pain relief.
- Complications of treatment include complications from surgery, acute radiation toxicity, late radiation effects, and chemotherapy toxicities. Acute radiation toxicity may include severe mucositis, with resulting pain and difficulties in swallowing. Concurrent chemoradiation increases the risk of severe mucositis beyond radiation alone. Oral candidiasis complicating mucositis may be treated with topical or systemic antifungal agents. Many patients find a cocktail of equal volumes of diphenhydramine suspension, nystatin, viscous lidocaine, and aluminum hydroxide/magnesium hydroxide ("magic mouthwash") as a topical oral swish-and-swallow solution to be helpful. Opiates can also help in pain management, especially in severe cases. Skin toxicity should be treated with emollients. Late radiation effects include xerostomia, dental caries, osteoradionecrosis, and fibrosis of neck tissues resulting in trismus, lymphedema, and loss of range of motion. Xerostomia can be treated with cholinergic stimulants such as pilocarpine to improve salivary flow. Other measures, including topical lubricants, lozenges, coating agents, and artificial saliva, may provide some transient relief. The risk of dental caries should be minimized with good dental care. Osteoradionecrosis may be treated conservatively with antibiotics, hyperbaric oxygen therapy, or surgical debridement. Exercise may help in prevention of trismus associated with radiation therapy. With neck irradiation, hypothyroidism may occur, which can be treated with thyroid replacement therapy.
- The complications of chemotherapy are dependent on the agents used. Cisplatin is associated with nausea, nephrotoxicity, ototoxicity, myelosuppression, and peripheral neuropathy.

MONITORING/FOLLOW-UP

Patients should have close follow-up for evaluation of local recurrence as well as distant metastases, as well as physical therapy and speech pathology follow-up if needed. Posttreatment imaging with a PET scan is recommended 3–6 months after completion of therapy. Further imaging frequency can be individualized based on patient symptoms and physical exam findings. The majority of recurrences will occur within the first 2 years, although late recurrences are possible.

Nasopharyngeal Carcinoma

GENERAL PRINCIPLES

Epidemiology

Nasopharyngeal carcinoma is relatively rare globally with 129,000 cases diagnosed annually with only 2,000 cases diagnosed in US. However, the disease is much more prevented in Southeast Asia where it is considered endemic, with China alone accounting for almost 50% of all cases.[14]

Risk Factors

In Southeast Asia, nasopharyngeal cancer is almost universally associated with Epstein–Barr virus (EBV) infection. Histologically, EBV-related carcinoma has a nonkeratinizing appearance. Smoking and alcohol use are also causative factors and typically have a keratinizing appearance on histology.

DIAGNOSIS

Clinical Presentation

Nasopharyngeal cancer can present with a painless neck mass, but other symptoms include nasal obstruction, epistaxis, dysphagia, odynophagia, and eustachian tube obstruction with otitis media. Tumors may extend through the foramen ovale to access the middle cranial fossa and the cavernous sinus to involve the oculomotor, trochlear, trigeminal, and abducens nerves, leading to cranial neuropathy. In advanced cases, invasion of the optic nerve and orbital invasion can occur. Headaches, weight loss, trismus, and referred pain in the ear and neck can also be symptoms. Physical examination should include a thorough examination of the nares, oral cavity, and the cranial nerves. Proptosis suggests orbital invasion by the tumor.

Diagnostic Testing

Workup of patients with nasopharyngeal cancer should include a thorough physical evaluation and diagnostic imaging with CT or MRI from the skull down to the clavicles. A PET scan or chest CT should be performed to assess for metastatic disease. The staging for nasopharynx is according to the American Joint Committee on Cancer TNM system. Assessing for EBV status is recommended via ISH for EBV-encoded RNA (EBER) on pathologic specimens and EBV titers can be obtained in the plasma.

TREATMENT

Nasopharyngeal carcinoma is a radiation-sensitive disease with high cure rate with localized or locally advanced disease. The standard treatment for locally advanced nasopharyngeal carcinoma continues to evolve, but induction cisplatin and gemcitabine followed by concurrent cisplatin and radiation have demonstrated improvements in long-term cure rates.[15] In the metastatic setting, a range of systemic therapies have demonstrated efficacy including checkpoint inhibitors such as pembrolizumab or nivolumab.[16]

Salivary Gland Tumors

GENERAL PRINCIPLES

Salivary gland tumors are rare neoplasms and account for 6–8% of head and neck cancers. Salivary gland tumors may arise either in the major glands, namely, the parotid, submandibular, and sublingual glands, or in the minor glands located in the oral mucosa, palate, uvula, floor of the mouth, posterior tongue, retromolar area, peritonsillar area, pharynx, larynx, and paranasal sinuses. Salivary gland tumors consist of more than 20 different histologic subtypes, classified as either malignant or benign. Approximately 80% of salivary gland neoplasms arise from the parotid, although most of these are benign; common benign examples include pleomorphic adenoma and Warthin tumors. In contrast, more than 95% of tumors arising from the sublingual gland are malignant; mucoepidermoid carcinoma and adenoid cystic carcinoma are the most common malignant salivary gland tumors. Salivary gland tumors have a wide spectrum of behaviors and clinical courses. Adenoid cystic carcinomas can have a more indolent course, and late recurrences of even more than 10 years after "curative" therapy are characteristic of this histologic subtype. The median overall survival of patients who develop metastatic disease is 3 years, but some patients will survive more than 10 years, while others have rapidly progressive disease. Mucoepidermoid carcinoma is aggressive and often has local recurrence and metastasizes. Adenocarcinomas have a tendency to have a range of behaviors, from indolent to aggressive. Salivary duct carcinomas are rare, but they are an aggressive malignancy that usually arises in the parotid and has nodal involvement.

TREATMENT

The major therapeutic approach for salivary gland tumors is surgical resection. Radiation is used in the adjuvant setting for tumors with adverse features such as intermediate- or high-grade histologies, close or negative margins, perineural invasion, lymph node metastasis, or lymphovascular invasion, as well as for most malignant deep lobe parotid tumors. Efficacy for concurrent chemoradiation is limited as there are few published clinical trials.

Chemotherapy may be used for palliation in surgically unresectable or metastatic disease, but most have relatively poor response rates. Adenocarcinomas, mucoepidermoid carcinomas, and salivary duct carcinomas may overexpress potential therapeutic targets such as HER-2 and androgen receptors, which can be assessed through IHC.[17]

REFERENCES

1. Siegel RL, Miller KD, Wagle NS, Jemal A. Cancer statistics, 2023. *CA Cancer J Clin*. 2023;73(1):17–48.
2. Cline BJ, Simpson MC, Gropler M, et al. Change in age at diagnosis of oropharyngeal cancer in the United States, 1975–2016. *Cancers (Basel)*. 2020;12(11):3191.
3. Cancer Genome Atlas Network. Comprehensive genomic characterization of head and neck squamous cell carcinomas. *Nature*. 2015;517(7536):576–582.
4. Chung CH, Ely K, McGavran L, et al. Increased epidermal growth factor receptor gene copy number is associated with poor prognosis in head and neck squamous cell carcinomas. *J Clin Oncol*. 2006;24(25):4170–4176.
5. Palefsky JM, Holly EA. Molecular virology and epidemiology of human papillomavirus and cervical cancer. *Cancer Epidemiol Biomarkers Prev*. 1995;4(4):415–428.
6. Lechner M, Liu J, Masterson L, Fenton TR. HPV-associated oropharyngeal cancer: epidemiology, molecular biology and clinical management. *Nat Rev Clin Oncol*. 2022;19(5):306–327.
7. Nielsen KJ, Jakobsen KK, Jensen JS, Grønhøj C, Von Buchwald C. The effect of prophylactic HPV vaccines on oral and oropharyngeal HPV infection—a systematic review. *Viruses*. 2021;13(7):1339.
8. Cantley RL, Gabrielli E, Montebelli F, Cimbaluk D, Gattuso P, Petruzzelli G. Ancillary studies in determining human papillomavirus status of squamous cell carcinoma of the oropharynx: a review. *Patholog Res Int*. 2011;2011:138469.
9. Motz K, Qualliotine JR, Rettig E, Richmon JD, Eisele DW, Fakhry C. Changes in unknown primary squamous cell carcinoma of the head and neck at initial presentation in the era of human papillomavirus. *JAMA Otolaryngol Head Neck Surg*. 2016;142(3):223–228.
10. Forastiere AA, Goepfert H, Maor M, et al. Concurrent chemotherapy and radiotherapy for organ preservation in advanced laryngeal cancer. *N Engl J Med*. 2003;349(22):2091–2098.
11. Gillison ML, Trotti AM, Harris J, et al. Radiotherapy plus cetuximab or cisplatin in human papillomavirus-positive oropharyngeal cancer (NRG Oncology RTOG 1016): a randomised, multicentre, non-inferiority trial. *Lancet*. 2019;393(10166):40–50.
12. Pignon JP, le Maître A, Maillard E, Bourhis J; MACH-NC Collaborative Group. Meta-analysis of chemotherapy in head and neck cancer (MACH-NC): an update on 93 randomised trials and 17,346 patients. *Radiother Oncol*. 2009;92(1):4–14.

13. Burtness B, Harrington KJ, Greil R, et al. Pembrolizumab alone or with chemotherapy versus cetuximab with chemotherapy for recurrent or metastatic squamous cell carcinoma of the head and neck (KEYNOTE-048): a randomised, open-label, phase 3 study. *Lancet.* 2019;394(10212):1915–1928.

14. Chen Y-P, Chan ATC, Le QT, Blanchard P, Sun Y, Ma J. Nasopharyngeal carcinoma. *Lancet.* 2019;394(10192):64–80.

15. Zhang Y, Chen L, Hu G-Q, et al. Gemcitabine and cisplatin induction chemotherapy in nasopharyngeal carcinoma. *N Engl J Med.* 2019;381(12):1124–1135.

16. Hsu C, Lee S-H, Ejadi S, et al. Safety and antitumor activity of pembrolizumab in patients with programmed death-ligand 1-positive nasopharyngeal carcinoma: results of the KEYNOTE-028 study. *J Clin Oncol.* 2017;35(36):4050–4056.

17. Weaver AN, Lakritz S, Mandair D, Ulanja MB, Bowles DW. A molecular guide to systemic therapy in salivary gland carcinoma. *Head Neck.* 2023;45(5):1315–1326.

Sarcoma

27

Mia C. Weiss

GENERAL PRINCIPLES

Sarcomas (from the Greek *sarx* for flesh) are a rare group of malignancies of the connective tissue. They represent over 170 different histologies of tumors derived from the mesenchymal or ectodermal germ layers. The presenting signs and symptoms depend on the anatomic site of origin and can vary markedly. In general, sarcomas can be divided into two large groups: soft tissue tumors and bone tumors.

Epidemiology

Sarcomas are rare tumors, comprising 1% of adult malignancies and 7% of pediatric malignancies. Sarcomas occur with equal frequency in both genders.[1] In the US in 2023, the estimated incidence of soft tissue sarcomas (STSs) is 13,400 cases with 5,140 expected deaths. For bone sarcomas, the estimated incidence is 3,970 cases with 2,140 deaths.[2] Compared to other rare tumors, sarcomas carry a high mortality rate.

Risk Factors

Most cases of sarcoma are sporadic; however, a number of etiologic factors have been identified, as detailed below.

- **Radiation**
  Sarcomas have been found to originate in or near tissues that have received prior external-beam radiation therapy. They tend to develop at least 2 years after radiation therapy but can develop decades after radiation.[3,4] The majority of these lesions are high grade, and they are typically osteosarcomas, malignant fibrous histiocytomas, and angiosarcomas. The relative risk of radiation-induced sarcoma is 0.6 for patients who receive 10 Gy of radiation and 38.3 for patients who receive 60 Gy.[5]
- **Chemical exposure**
  Thorotrast, an IV contrast dye, has been found to cause hepatic angiosarcomas.[6] Other agents, such as vinyl chloride[7], arsenic, and dioxin in chemical workers and farmers but not in Vietnam Veterans (i.e., dioxin is in Agent Orange), have also been linked to sarcomas.[8] Alkylating chemotherapy, particularly when used to treat childhood malignancies, has also been associated with the development of sarcomas in adulthood.[9]
- **Genetic conditions**
  Patients with neurofibromatosis type I have a 10% risk of developing a malignant peripheral nerve sheath tumor.[10] Sarcomas also occurs in patients with Li–Fraumeni syndrome.[11] Familial retinoblastoma is linked to the development of osteosarcoma,[12] and Werner syndrome is a risk factor for multiple types of sarcomas.[13]
- **Other risks associated with sarcomas**
  Lymphangiosarcomas have been known to develop in a lymphedematous arm after mastectomy (Stewart–Treves syndrome).[14] Kaposi sarcoma is associated with coinfection with the HIV and the human herpes virus 8.[15] Paget disease of bone is a risk factor for the development of osteosarcoma or fibrosarcoma.[16]

SPECIAL CONSIDERATIONS

The treatment of sarcoma is complex because sarcoma is an ever-growing group of many very rare diseases that have been historically treated as a large group in clinical trials. Since many of the specific subtypes are driven by known translocations or other mutations, the treatment and understanding of each individual subtype is rapidly evolving.[17,18] Translocation or mutation-based treatment of sarcoma is the reason patients with **sarcomas should be evaluated and have a treatment plan formulated by physicians who specifically subspecialize in the treatment of sarcoma**.

Soft Tissue Sarcomas

DIAGNOSIS

Clinical Presentation

STSs represent >75% of all sarcomas diagnosed each year.[19] Patients typically present with an asymptomatic mass. Pain may be present if there is entrapment of neurovascular structures or involvement of bone. Sarcomas may grow quite large before they become obvious on physical examination.

- **Extremity sarcomas**
  Approximately half of all STSs arise in the extremities. The majority are first seen as a painless soft tissue mass.
- **Retroperitoneal sarcomas**
  Most patients have an abdominal mass and approximately half have abdominal pain that is vague and nonspecific. Weight loss is seen less frequently, with early satiety, nausea, and emesis occurring in <40% of patients. Neurologic symptoms, particularly paresthesias, occur in up to 30% of patients.[20]

Physical Examination
Physical examination of a patient presenting with a soft tissue mass should include an assessment of the size of the mass and its mobility with respect to the underlying tissue. If a mass is >5 cm and deep, it should be presumed to be sarcoma until proven otherwise. High-grade sarcomas may have significant necrosis and can be confused with a hematoma or abscess. A site-specific neurovascular examination should also be performed.

Differential Diagnosis

The differential diagnosis includes benign soft tissue tumors as well as carcinoma, lymphoma, and melanoma. The most common benign tumors include lipoma, desmoid tumor, neurofibroma, hemangioma, and schwannoma.

Diagnostic Testing

Imaging
Patients with masses suspicious of sarcoma should undergo **radiologic evaluation and biopsy**. The studies needed for adequate staging vary depending on the site of disease. Sarcoma of the head and neck or extremities should be evaluated with **plain films** and **MRI**. Plain films may reveal soft tissue mineralization (which is typical for synovial sarcoma) or may reveal skeletal reaction to the tumor. MRI is valuable for assessing fat and distinguishing it from surrounding tissues. This may assist in the diagnosis of the lesion and allows for planning of the biopsy and subsequent surgery.[21] For retroperitoneal and abdominal sarcomas, CT is the imaging modality of choice, as this provides the best anatomic definition of the tumor.[22]

| TABLE 27-1 | GUIDELINES TO THE HISTOLOGIC GRADING OF SARCOMAS |

Low-Grade Sarcomas	High-Grade Sarcomas
Good differentiation	Poor differentiation
Hypocellularity	Hypercellularity
Increased stroma	Minimal stroma
Hypovascularity	Hypervascularity
Minimal necrosis	Much necrosis
<5 mitoses per high-power field	>5 mitoses per high-power field

Adapted from Hajdu SI, Shiu MH, Brennan MF. The role of the pathologist in the management of soft tissue sarcomas. *World J Surg.* 1988;12:326–331, with permission.

In addition to evaluating the primary lesion with imaging, **distant metastatic disease** may also be assessed. STS spreads *hematogenously*, and the **lung** is the **most common site** of metastasis.[23] Lymph node metastases are not common in STS with exception of certain subtypes including but not limited to embryonal rhabdomyosarcoma (ERMS), clear cell sarcoma, angiosarcoma, and epithelioid sarcoma.[24] Chest x-ray may be sufficient for small, low-grade lesions, but in patients with high-grade tumors or tumors larger than 5 cm, a staging CT of the chest should be performed.

Diagnostic Procedures
• An accurate biopsy diagnosis is essential for STS. Any lesion >5 cm or any rapidly growing lesion should be biopsied. The placement of the biopsy tract is also critical, as it can be seeded with tumor and must be excised at the time of resection. Generally, the preferred technique is open incisional biopsy performed by a surgeon with experience in resection of STS. Hemostasis is also very important, as a hematoma may require enlarging radiation fields or may interfere with resection planning.
• **Histologic evaluation** should be performed at an experienced center, as **grade is critically important to determining prognosis**.[25] STSs are named for their tissue of origin based on light microscopy examination, and there are many possible histologic types. Tumors are also carefully evaluated for grade, which takes into account cellularity, mitotic activity, nuclear atypia, and necrosis (Table 27-1). In general, the *grade, size,* and *depth* are more important factors than the histologic type. Immunohistochemistry and FISH studies are used to subclassify STS. The three most common types of STS in adult patients are undifferentiated pleomorphic sarcoma, liposarcoma, and leiomyosarcoma. In children, rhabdomyosarcoma is the most common soft tissue sarcoma subtype in children.[26]

TREATMENT

Early-Stage Disease (Stages I–III)
• **Extremity STSs**
  ○ **Surgery**
    Surgery is the mainstay of therapy for early-stage STSs of the extremities. Sarcomas grow along planes and grossly appear to be well encapsulated. However, they usually extend into the pseudocapsule (an area around the tumor that is composed of tumor fimbriae and normal tissue), and "shelling-out" of lesions is associated with high local recurrence rates of 37–63%. In the past, radical excision and amputation were utilized to avoid this problem. Over the past 20 years, there has been a gradual shift in

the surgical management of extremity STSs away from radical ablative surgery toward limb-sparing surgery (LSS). Today, LSS is the standard of care, and amputation is only required in a small subset of patients today.[27]

○ **Radiation therapy**

Wide local excision alone is all that is necessary for small (T1), low-grade, STSs of the extremities, with a local recurrence rate of <10%. **Adjuvant radiation therapy**, however, is required in a number of situations: (a) virtually all high-grade extremity sarcomas, (b) lesions larger than 5 cm (T2), and (c) positive or equivocal surgical margins in patients for whom reexcision is impractical.[28] When adjuvant radiation is planned, metal clips should be placed at margins of resection to facilitate radiation field planning.[29] **Neoadjuvant radiation** may be needed prior to definitive resection. This is most commonly performed for tumors that are borderline resectable or for tumors located adjacent to the joint capsule. A phase III National Cancer Institute of Canada trial comparing adjuvant (postoperative) and neoadjuvant (preoperative) radiation demonstrated similar local control rates, metastatic outcomes, and overall survival rates between the two arms. However, patients receiving preoperative radiation had a significantly higher incidence of wound complications (35% vs. 17%).[30]

▪ **Radiation as definitive therapy** alone in the treatment of unresectable or medically inoperable STS patients yields a 5-year survival rate of 25–40% and a local control rate of 30%. Radiation doses should be at least 65 Gy, if feasible, given the site of the lesion.[31]

▪ **Brachytherapy** also has been used in treatment of sarcomas. Iridium-192 is the most commonly used agent. It has similar local control rates to adjuvant external-beam radiation and has the advantage of a decrease in the patient's entire treatment from 10 to 12 weeks to 10 to 12 days. In addition, smaller volumes of tissues are irradiated, which may be useful if important structures, such as joints, are nearby.

○ **Adjuvant chemotherapy**

The benefit of adjuvant chemotherapy for extremity STSs is controversial. The only exceptions to this are embryonal and alveolar rhabdomyosarcomas, in which adjuvant chemotherapy is accepted as standard of care.

▪ A formal meta-analysis of individual data from 1,568 patients who participated in 13 trials was performed by the Sarcoma Meta-Analysis Collaboration. The analysis demonstrated a significant reduction in the risk of local or distant recurrence in patients who received adjuvant chemotherapy. There also was a decrease in the risk of distant relapse (metastasis) by 30% in treated patients. Overall survival, however, did not meet criteria for statistical significance between the control group and adjuvant chemotherapy arm, with a hazard ratio of 0.89.[32] Most of the randomized trials examined in this meta-analysis were limited by patient numbers, inclusion of all subtypes of STS and of low-grade tumors, heterogeneous patient and disease characteristics, and varied chemotherapy regimens.

▪ Certain subgroups of patients, such as those with high-grade extremity lesions, may benefit from adjuvant chemotherapy,[33] but further studies are needed.

• **Retroperitoneal sarcomas (RPS)**

○ **Surgery**

As with other STSs, surgery is the primary treatment of RPS. Tumors that are <5 cm and that are not located close to adjacent viscera or critical neurovascular structures are considered resectable. If a tumor is thought to be a sarcoma and is resectable, a preoperative biopsy is not necessary. One should consider a preoperative CT-guided core biopsy if an incomplete resection is a reasonable possibility to allow neoadjuvant therapy to be considered.

▪ Unfortunately, only 50% of patients with early-stage RPS are able to undergo complete surgical resection. Of the tumors removed, approximately half will develop a local recurrence.[34] Despite high recurrence risk, adjuvant therapy is a controversial topic and ultimately needs to be individualized to the patient.

○ **Radiation therapy**
○ **Adjuvant radiation** therapy in RPS not routinely recommended. In the postoperative setting, it is often difficult to define treatment margins without significant risk for toxicity to surrounding organs. In a large single institution series including 121 patients, the 10-year complication rate was 20% versus 0% in patients receiving pre- versus postoperative RT demonstrating that specifically late toxicities remain a significant risk with this treatment modality.[35]
○ **Neoadjuvant radiation** therapy for RPS remains a debated topic. Data from the STRASS trial has brought into question the efficacy of preoperative RT in that it demonstrated no significant difference in intra-abdominal recurrence-free survival or overall survival in 266 patients who received preoperative radiation versus surgery alone.[36] While interpretation of this data remains controversial with regard to the endpoints used and concerns for statistical underpowering based on histology, it is agreed upon that preoperative RT should only be considered in the context of an expert multidisciplinary discussion.
○ **Management of unresectable, locally advanced RPS**
Unresectable RPS can be managed in a number of ways. Palliative surgery to reduce local symptoms can be performed. Novel radiation techniques, such as spatially fractionated radiation therapy (SFRT) can be utilized to safely target large, deep-seated tumors.[37] Chemotherapy can also be administered.

Stage IV Metastatic Soft Tissue Sarcomas

Metastatic STSs can be divided into limited metastasis and extensive metastasis. **Limited metastatic disease** is defined as resectable metastasis involving one organ system. The prognosis of these two subsets of patients is very different. **It is possible to cure limited metastatic disease**, whereas patients with extensive metastatic disease can only be palliated.

• **Management of limited metastatic disease**
For patients with a limited number of pulmonary metastases, metastasectomy has been performed with some improvement in survival compared with no surgery.[38] In patients with visceral sarcomas and limited liver metastasis, it is sometimes possible to perform a metastasectomy by surgery, chemoembolization, or radiofrequency ablation.
• **Management of extensive metastatic disease**
The goal of therapy for patients with metastatic sarcoma is palliation and prolongation of survival. Cure is not a viable goal. Systemic chemotherapy is the primary modality of treatment. Radiation and surgery may be used with a goal of palliation.

Numerous chemotherapy agents have been used as single agents or in combination for the treatment of STSs. These include epirubicin, doxorubicin, ifosfamide, cyclophosphamide, dacarbazine, gemcitabine, and taxanes, among others.

PROGNOSIS

• The most important prognostic factors for STS are **size, grade, depth**, and **relationship to fascial planes**. The American Joint Committee on Cancer (AJCC) staging system for STSs incorporates histologic grade (G), size of the primary (T), nodal involvement (N), and distant metastasis (M).[39]
• Grade of the tumor is the predominant feature predicting early metastatic recurrence and death. Beyond 2 years of follow-up, the size of the lesion becomes as important as the histologic grade.
• Nomograms exist for the relapse-free survival prediction by histology.[40]

Bone Sarcomas

GENERAL PRINCIPLES

Bone sarcoma may arise from any tissue within the bones. The most common bone sarcomas are osteosarcoma, chondrosarcoma, and Ewing sarcoma.

Classification

- **Osteosarcoma**
  Osteosarcoma is the most common primary bone tumor, accounting for 40–50% of bone sarcomas.[41] It usually presents with pain and swelling. Approximately 60% occur in adolescents and children. Ten percent may occur in the third decade. There is a second peak in the fifth and sixth decades, which is frequently due to radiation-associated osteosarcomas or transformation of existing lesions. They are spindle cell neoplasms that produce bone and are more common in long bones. Most osteosarcomas occur in the metaphyseal region, near the growth plate of skeletally immature long bones. The distal femur, proximal tibia, and proximal humerus are common sites. The majority are classified as "conventional osteosarcoma" and this type is more common between 10 and 20 years of age. Most of these lesions are high grade and highly vascular.
- **Chondrosarcoma**
  Chondrosarcoma is the second most frequent malignant primary bone tumor, representing ~20% of bone sarcomas. They generally occur between the fourth and the sixth decade. They tend to develop in flat bones, including the shoulder and pelvic girdles. They may arise de novo or from pre-existing lesions. They are indolent and are generally low grade. Chondrosarcoma may arise peripherally or centrally. Imaging studies may be bland, particularly in central lesions, which may make it difficult to distinguish between benign and malignant lesions. New pain, increasing size, and signs of inflammation point toward malignant lesions. In general, these malignancies are resistant to chemotherapy and radiation. A subset of chondrosarcomas harbor IDH 1 or 2 mutations.
- **Ewing sarcoma**
  Ewing sarcoma accounts for 10–15% of bone sarcomas, and incidence peaks in the second decade. It is the second most common malignant tumor of the bone in childhood and adolescence. It tends to occur in the diaphysis of long bones. The femoral diaphysis is the most common location. These are highly aggressive tumors and are best considered a systemic disease. A characteristic chromosomal translocation, $t(11:22)$, is associated with this sarcoma and with peripheral primitive neuroectodermal tumor (PNET), though there are many alternative translocations that have now been described. Ewing sarcoma is pathologically described as one of the small, round, blue cell tumors.

DIAGNOSIS

An accurate tissue biopsy is needed for diagnosis. Imaging studies may be suggestive of tumor type; however, it can be difficult to distinguish benign and malignant bone tumors. Biopsy specimens are used to determine the histologic type of tumor as well as the grade. **An open incisional biopsy is preferred for bone sarcomas.** The biopsy should be performed by a surgeon experienced in sarcoma so that it does not compromise the definitive surgical procedure.

Clinical Presentation

History
Localized pain and swelling are the hallmark clinical features of bone sarcomas. The pain is initially insidious but can become unremitting. Occasionally, a pathologic fracture will

bring the patient to medical attention. If the tumor arises in the lower extremities, the patient may have a limp. Constitutional symptoms are rare but can be observed in patients with Ewing sarcoma or patients with metastatic disease. A pertinent history should note how long a lesion has been present and any change in it. Rapid growth or change in a lesion favors a malignant etiology.

Physical Examination

Physical examination may reveal a palpable mass. A joint effusion may be observed, and range of motion of the joint may be limited, with stiffness or pain. Neurovascular and lymph node examinations are usually normal.

Diagnostic Testing

Imaging

- Patients who are suspected to have bone sarcoma should undergo imaging studies, including plain films and MRI.
- **Plain films** may demonstrate characteristic lesions for bone sarcoma. Osteosarcoma is associated with destructive lesions, showing a moth-eaten appearance. In addition, a spiculated periosteal reaction and cuff of periosteal new bone may be seen. Plain films in chondrosarcoma show lesions with a lobulated appearance with punctate or annular calcification of cartilage. Ewing sarcoma is associated with an "onion peel" periosteal reaction and soft tissue mass. Metastatic disease may be associated with either osteolytic or osteoblastic lesions, depending on the type of primary malignancy.
- **MRI** is the imaging modality of choice to evaluate the relationship of the tumor to surrounding structures and determine resectability. CT scan of the primary site may be considered in place of MRI to demonstrate cortical destruction more accurately and for evaluation of pelvic tumors. CT scan of the chest is used to evaluate for pulmonary metastases. **Bone scan** helps to evaluate the local extent of the tumor as well as to evaluate for other lesions.

Diagnostic Procedures

- Tissue biopsy, preferably open incisional biopsy, is essential for diagnosis.
- Bone sarcomas are staged using the American Joint Committee on Cancer staging system based on grade, tumor size, and metastatic disease. Adverse prognostic indicators include elevated lactate dehydrogenase (LDH), elevated alkaline phosphatase, and an axial primary. Patients with Ewing sarcoma should have bone marrow biopsies or screening MRI of the spine and pelvis as part of staging.[42]

TREATMENT

The treatment of bone sarcoma is dependent on histologic subtype.

- **General principles of local therapy**
  - **Surgical excision is the mainstay of treatment for patients with low-grade bone sarcomas. For high-grade tumors, multimodality therapy is indicated.** As an example, for high-grade osteosarcomas, preoperative multiagent chemotherapy is followed by surgical removal of the tumor and then further adjuvant chemotherapy. **Physical therapy** and **prosthetics** are of great importance to these patients because of the highly invasive nature of the treatment.
  - The Musculoskeletal Tumor Society and the leading cancer centers in the US recognize wide excision, either by amputation or by a limb-salvage procedure, as the recommended surgical approach for all high-grade bone sarcomas. This type of resection is predicated on complete tumor removal, effective skeletal reconstruction, and adequate soft tissue coverage.

- **Osteosarcoma therapy**

  The 5-year survival for osteosarcoma with surgery alone is <20%. This occurs because microscopic metastatic dissemination is likely to be present in 80% of patients at the time of diagnosis. The addition of adjuvant chemotherapy has improved survival for high-grade osteosarcoma, permitting long-term survival as high as 80% in selected patients.

  ○ **Neoadjuvant and adjuvant chemotherapy**

    Neoadjuvant chemotherapy began as a strategy to permit LSS, allowing time for creation of custom-made prosthetics. Since its acceptance, other advantages have been recognized with this approach. It permits earlier treatment of occult micrometastatic disease, preventing emergence of resistant clones and potentially allowing for the debulking of the primary to improve chances for LSS.

    ▪ Chemotherapeutic agents active in osteosarcomas include doxorubicin, cisplatin, ifosfamide, and high-dose methotrexate with leucovorin rescue. These agents are typically used in combination to improve response, although the optimal combination and duration of therapy remain controversial.

    ▪ Histologic response to preoperative therapy is recognized as a significant prognostic factor. Various systems have been developed for grading histologic response to chemotherapy, but >90% necrosis of tumor cells is associated with the best prognosis.[43] If the tumor has been resected to negative margins and had a good histologic response to chemotherapy, the patient continues on chemotherapy for an additional 2–12 cycles. If the tumor was fully resected but has <90% necrosis, salvage chemotherapy is attempted. Data from the Euramos-1 trial presented in 2014 suggested that adding ifosfamide and etoposide (IE) to standard postoperative chemotherapy does not improve event-free survival.[44] If the tumor margins are positive, additional local surgery should be attempted.

  ○ **Radiation therapy**

    Radiation is not routinely used in the therapy of osteosarcoma, with the exception of osteosarcoma of the jaw, but it may prove helpful in patients who refuse definitive resection or in palliation of patients with metastatic disease.

  ○ **Management of metastatic disease**

    Approximately 10–20% of patients with osteosarcoma have evidence of metastatic disease at presentation. Some of these patients may be candidates for the surgical resection of pulmonary metastases. For patients with more extensive metastatic disease, chemotherapy is used to provide control of disease and palliation of symptoms. More recently, use of targeted therapies such as cabozantinib and regorafenib which target vascular endothelial growth factors has shown response in metastatic osteosarcoma.

- **Ewing sarcoma**

  Therapy for Ewing sarcoma and the related primitive peripheral neuroectodermal tumors uses a combined modality approach.[45]

  ○ **Treatment of the primary tumor**

    The optimal treatment for local tumor control is not well defined. Historically, radiation therapy has been the mainstay of local therapy, but there has been a recent trend toward surgery. No prospective randomized trials have been performed to compare the two modalities, but retrospective data suggest improvements in local control and survival when surgery is done with a complete resection of the tumor. Patients with unresectable disease or positive margins require radiation therapy to improve local control.

  ○ **Chemotherapy**

    Before the availability of effective chemotherapeutic agents, <10% of patients with Ewing sarcoma survived beyond 5 years, despite the fact that only 15–35% of patients with Ewing sarcoma/primitive peripheral neuroectodermal tumors had evidence of metastatic disease at presentation. This suggests that many patients with Ewing sarcoma have occult microscopic dissemination of the disease at the time of diagnosis. The current standard regimen is to use vincristine, actinomycin D, and cyclophosphamide (VAC), alternating with IE.[46]

○ **Recurrent metastatic Ewing sarcoma**

In this setting, cure is not a realistic goal. Palliation and prolongation of survival are more realistic expectations. Fortunately, aggressive combination chemotherapy (VAC or IE) and radiation therapy can still lead to prolonged progression-free survival. Targeted therapies such as cabozantinib have also shown some improvement in progression free survival (PFS).

REFERENCES

1. NG VY, Scharschmidt TJ, Mayerson JL, Fisher JL. Incidence and survival in sarcoma in the United States: a focus on musculoskeletal lesions. *Anticancer Res.* 2013;33(6):2597–2604.
2. American Cancer Society. Facts & Figures 2023. Accessed May 22, 2023.
3. Pitcher ME, Davidson TI, Fisher C, Thomas JM. Post irradiation sarcoma of soft tissue and bone. *Eur J Surg Oncol.* 1994;20(1):53–56.
4. Laurino S, Omer LC, Albano F, et al. Radiation-induced sarcomas: a single referral cancer center experience and literature review. *Front Oncol.* 2022;12:986123.
5. Tucker MA, D'Angio GJ, Boice JD Jr, et al. Bone sarcomas linked to radiotherapy and chemotherapy in children. *N Engl J Med.* 1987;317(10):588–593.
6. van Kampen RJ, Erdkamp FL, Peters FP. Thorium dioxide-related haemangiosarcoma of the liver. *Neth J Med.* 2007;65(8):279–282.
7. Edwards D, Voronina A, Attwood K, et al. Association between occupational exposures and sarcoma incidence and mortality: systematic review and meta-analysis. *Syst Rev.* 2021;10(1):231.
8. Steenland K, Bertazzi P, Baccarelli A, et al. Dioxin revisited: developments since the 1997 IARC classification of dioxin as a human carcinogen. *Environ Health Perspect.* 2004;112(13):1265–1268.
9. Falk H, Caldwell GG, Ishak KG, Thomas LB, Popper H. Arsenic-related hepatic angiosarcoma. *Am J Ind Med.* 1981;2(1):43–50.
10. Hirbe AC, Gutmann DH. Neurofibromatosis type 1: a multidisciplinary approach to care. *Lancet Neurol.* 2014;13(8):834–843.
11. Upton B, Chu Q, Li BD. Li-Fraumeni syndrome: the genetics and treatment considerations for the sarcoma and associated neoplasms. *Surg Oncol Clin N Am.* 2009;18(1):145–156, ix.
12. Benedict WF, Fung YkT, Murphree AL. The gene responsible for the development of retinoblastoma and osteosarcoma. *Cancer.* 1988;62(S1):1691–1694.
13. Yu CE, Oshima J, Fu YH, et al. Positional cloning of the Werner's syndrome gene. *Science.* 1996; 272(5259):258–262.
14. Chung KC, Kim HJ, Jeffers LL. Lymphangiosarcoma (Stewart-Treves syndrome) in postmastectomy patients. *J Hand Surg Am.* 2000;25(6):1163–1168.
15. Mesri EA, Cesarman E, Boshoff C. Kaposi's sarcoma and its associated herpesvirus. *Nat Rev Cancer.* 2010;10(10):707–719.
16. Mankin HJ, Hornicek FJ. Paget's sarcoma: a historical and outcome review. *Clin Orthop Relat Res.* 2005;438:97–102.
17. Osuna D, de Alava E. Molecular pathology of sarcomas. *Rev Recent Clin Trials.* 2009;4(1):12–26.
18. Jain S, Xu R, Prieto VG, Lee P. Molecular classification of soft tissue sarcomas and its clinical applications. *Int J Clin Exp Pathol.* 2010;3(4):416–428.
19. Gamboa AC, Gronchi A, Cardona K. Soft-tissue sarcoma in adults: an update on the current state of histiotype-specific management in an era of personalized medicine. *CA Cancer J Clin.* 2020; 70(3):200–229.
20. Toulmonde M, Bonvalot S, Méeus P, et al. Retroperitoneal sarcomas: patterns of care at diagnosis, prognostic factors and focus on main histological subtypes: a multicenter analysis of the French Sarcoma Group. *Ann Oncol.* 2014;25(3):735–742.
21. Vibhakar AM, Cassels JA, Botchu R, Rennie WJ, Shah A. Imaging update on soft tissue sarcoma. *J Clin Orthop Trauma.* 2021;22:101568.
22. Messiou C, Morosi C. Imaging in retroperitoneal soft tissue sarcoma. *J Surg Oncol.* 2018;117(1): 25–32.
23. Billingsley KG, Burt ME, Jara E, et al. Pulmonary metastases from soft tissue sarcoma: analysis of patterns of diseases and postmetastasis survival. *Ann Surg.* 1999;229(5):602–610; discussion 610–602.

24. Fong Y, Coit DG, Woodruff JM, Brennan MF. Lymph node metastasis from soft tissue sarcoma in adults. Analysis of data from a prospective database of 1772 sarcoma patients. *Ann Surg.* 1993;217(1):72–77.

25. Hong JH, Jee W-H, Jung C-K, Chung Y-G. Tumor grade in soft-tissue sarcoma: prediction with magnetic resonance imaging texture analysis. *Medicine (Baltimore).* 2020;99(27):e20880.

26. Loeb DM, Thornton K, Shokek O. Pediatric soft tissue sarcomas. *Surg Clin North Am.* 2008; 88(3):615–627, vii.

27. Ferrone ML, Raut CP. Modern surgical therapy: limb salvage and the role of amputation for extremity soft-tissue sarcomas. *Surg Oncol Clin N Am.* 2012;21(2):201–213.

28. Gronchi A, Miah AB, Dei Tos AP, et al. Soft tissue and visceral sarcomas: ESMO-EURACAN-GENTURIS Clinical Practice Guidelines for diagnosis, treatment and follow-up(☆). *Ann Oncol.* 2021;32(11):1348–1365.

29. Cormier JN, Pollock RE. Soft tissue sarcomas. *CA Cancer J Clin.* 2004;54(2):94–109.

30. O'Sullivan B, Davis AM, Turcotte R, et al. Preoperative versus postoperative radiotherapy in soft-tissue sarcoma of the limbs: a randomised trial. *Lancet.* 2002;359(9325):2235–2241.

31. Roeder F. Radiation therapy in adult soft tissue sarcoma-current knowledge and future directions: a review and expert opinion. *Cancers (Basel).* 2020;12(11):3242.

32. Sarcoma Meta-analysis Collaboration (SMAC). Adjuvant chemotherapy for localised resectable soft-tissue sarcoma of adults: meta-analysis of individual data. Sarcoma Meta-analysis Collaboration. *Lancet.* 1997;350(9092):1647–1654.

33. Frustaci S, Gherlinzoni F, De Paoli A, et al. Adjuvant chemotherapy for adult soft tissue sarcomas of the extremities and girdles: results of the Italian randomized cooperative trial. *J Clin Oncol.* 2001;19(5):1238–1247.

34. Strauss DC, Hayes AJ, Thway K, Moskovic EC, Fisher C, Thomas JM. Surgical management of primary retroperitoneal sarcoma. *Br J Surg.* 2010;97(5):698–706.

35. Bishop AJ, Zagars GK, Torres KE, et al. Combined modality management of retroperitoneal sarcomas: a single-institution series of 121 patients. *Int J Radiat Oncol Biol Phys.* 2015;93(1):158–165.

36. Bonvalot S, Gronchi A, Le Péchoux C, et al. Preoperative radiotherapy plus surgery versus surgery alone for patients with primary retroperitoneal sarcoma (EORTC-62092: STRASS): a multicentre, open-label, randomised, phase 3 trial. *Lancet Oncol.* 2020;21(10):1366–1377.

37. Duriseti S, Kavanaugh J, Goddu S, et al. Spatially fractionated stereotactic body radiation therapy (Lattice) for large tumors. *Adv Radiat Oncol.* 2021;6(3):100639.

38. Schur S, Hoetzenecker K, Lamm W, et al. Pulmonary metastasectomy for soft tissue sarcoma–report from a dual institution experience at the Medical University of Vienna. *Eur J Cancer.* 2014; 50(13):2289–2297.

39. Amin MBES, Greene FL, Byrd DR, et al. *American Joint Committee on Cancer. Soft Tissue Sarcoma of the Trunk and Extremities.* 8th ed. Springer; 2017.

40. Eilber FC, Brennan MF, Eilber FR, Dry SM, Singer S, Kattan MW. Validation of the postoperative nomogram for 12-year sarcoma-specific mortality. *Cancer.* 2004;101(10):2270–2275.

41. Maki RG. Pediatric sarcomas occurring in adults. *J Surg Oncol.* 2008;97(4):360–368.

42. Kumar J, Seith A, Kumar A, et al. Whole-body MR imaging with the use of parallel imaging for detection of skeletal metastases in pediatric patients with small-cell neoplasms: comparison with skeletal scintigraphy and FDG PET/CT. *Pediatr Radiol.* 2008;38(9):953–962.

43. Bernthal NM, Federman N, Eilber FR, et al. Long-term results (>25 years) of a randomized, prospective clinical trial evaluating chemotherapy in patients with high-grade, operable osteosarcoma. *Cancer.* 2012;118(23):5888–5893.

44. Marina NM, Smeland S, Bielack SS, et al. Comparison of MAPIE versus MAP in patients with a poor response to preoperative chemotherapy for newly diagnosed high-grade osteosarcoma (EURAMOS-1): an open-label, international, randomised controlled trial. *Lancet Oncol.* 2016;17(10):1396–1408.

45. Schiffman JD, Wright J. Ewing's sarcoma and second malignancies. *Sarcoma.* 2011;2011:736841.

46. Brennan B, Kirton L, Marec-Bérard P, et al. Comparison of two chemotherapy regimens in patients with newly diagnosed Ewing sarcoma (EE2012): an open-label, randomised, phase 3 trial. *Lancet.* 2022;400(10362):1513–1521.

Endocrine Malignancies

28

Michael D. Iglesia, Peter Oppelt, and Nikolaos A. Trikalinos

GENERAL PRINCIPLES

In 1954, a family was described with hyperparathyroidism and tumors of the pituitary and pancreatic islet cells. Now known as multiple endocrine neoplasia type I (MEN I), it is one of the most well-known hereditary endocrine neoplastic syndromes. Since then, our knowledge about the genetics and pathology of endocrine tumors has grown tremendously and has led to various new diagnostic and therapeutic modalities. This chapter will cover the most common hereditary and sporadic endocrine neoplasm types, including pituitary, thyroid, parathyroid, adrenal, and gastroenteropancreatic.

Thyroid Carcinoma

GENERAL PRINCIPLES

Multiple histologic subtypes of thyroid cancer exist (Table 28-1), and together they account for >90% of all endocrine malignancies. The normal thyroid is composed of two main cell types. One is the follicular cell type that concentrates iodine and produces thyroid hormones. The other cell type is the parafollicular cell that produces calcitonin. Follicular cells give rise to differentiated cancers (papillary, follicular, and Hürthle) and anaplastic tumors. Parafollicular cells give rise to medullary thyroid carcinoma (MTC).

Epidemiology

Thyroid malignancies are relatively uncommon. Data from the Surveillance Epidemiology and End Results (SEER) program estimate 43,720 new thyroid cancer cases and 2,120 cancer deaths from the disease with a favorable 5-year relative survival of 98.5%.[1] This represents 2.2% of all new cancer cases and 0.3% of all cancer deaths.

Risk Factors

The main known risk factors for thyroid cancer include sex, radiation exposure, and family history. Thyroid cancer is nearly three times more common in women than in men.[2] Prior radiation exposure to the neck, especially during childhood, can increase the risk of thyroid neoplasms with a lag time of up to 24 years to cancer presentation. Some patients with familial cancer predisposing syndromes such as multiple endocrine neoplasia 2 (MEN2), familial polyposis (FAP), or Carney complex are also at increased risk.

DIAGNOSIS

Clinical Presentation

Initial presentation is typically a solitary thyroid nodule, discovered by palpation of the thyroid gland or noted incidentally on radiographic imaging. The majority of thyroid nodules (>90%) are benign, and history and physical examination assist in directing further

TABLE 28-1	THYROID CANCER HISTOLOGIC SUBTYPES AND KEY FEATURES	

Histologic Subtype	% of Thyroid Cancers	Characteristics
Differentiated		Younger patients, relatively benign, indolent course. Metastases occur late and to bone, lungs, cervical lymph nodes, and skin. Surgery and radioactive iodine are treatments of choice.
Papillary	80	Psammoma bodies present on histology in 50%.
Follicular	12–20	Hürthle cell variety (3%) is more aggressive form.
Anaplastic (spindle cell)	2	Older patients, aggressive tumors with local invasion common and always considered stage IV. Metastases to lung common and advanced diseases are uniformly fatal. External-beam radiation is marginally effective.
Medullary thyroid carcinoma	5–9	Neoplasia of the parafollicular/C cells. Sporadic and inherited forms exist. Secrete calcitonin and occasionally ACTH. May cause diarrhea in advanced disease. Metastases to inferior surface of liver capsule typical. Treatment is surgical.

investigations. Signs of aggressive disease can include rapid growth, subjective symptoms of hoarseness, dysphagia, or shortness of breath. The prevalence of malignancy is also higher if the nodule is found in children and adults <30 years of age, and in those with the aforementioned risk factors of family history and radiation exposure. The rare subtype of medullary thyroid cancer (MTC) can secrete calcitonin or ACTH and these patients present with diarrhea and flushing or hypercortisolism, respectively.

Physical Examination

Examination should evaluate nodule size, firmness, mobility, and local lymphadenopathy, but ultimately patients will receive an ultrasound (US) of neck and thyroid and serum testing (see below). The American College of Radiology has proposed the TIRADS system to identify nodules of different sizes for tissue sampling based on characteristics such as echogenicity, composition, and microcalcifications.[3]

Diagnostic Testing

- Thyroid-stimulating hormone (**TSH**): The workup of a thyroid nodule also involves obtaining a TSH level. A low TSH is suggestive of a hyperactive adenoma while a high TSH raises the concern for malignancy.

- **US of the thyroid** is recommended for initial evaluation of any thyroid nodule; there are several features that are suggestive of malignancy including hypoechoic appearance, central hypervascularity, irregular borders, and microcalcifications. US findings are not diagnostic of malignancy, but may be used to determine nodules that should undergo fine-needle aspiration (FNA).
- **FNA** is combined with US as the initial approach to obtain cells for pathologic review. FNA biopsy is generally used for solid nodules measuring >1–1.5 cm in a patient with no risk factor but suspicious sonographic findings. In patients with risk factors for thyroid cancer, the threshold for biopsy can be <1 cm. If malignancy cannot be excluded by FNA, a lobectomy may be performed to obtain adequate tissue for determining the correct diagnosis.[4] Alternatively, for indeterminate cytology, molecular sequencing can be used to assess for high-risk alterations (BRAF, TERT, RET, RAS); the presence of such alterations supports the need for surgery, while negative findings can allow for observation.[5]
- **Radioactive isotope scan** is performed to evaluate the functional status of a nodule. It should be performed when a patient has low TSH.
- **Laboratory markers:** Serum thyroglobulin (Tg) level is not useful in making the diagnosis of a thyroid malignancy. It may be helpful in the postoperative setting to monitor for disease recurrence, especially if a patient has undergone radioactive iodine (RAI) ablation of residual thyroid tissue. Patients with MTC can have elevations of calcitonin and carcinoembryonic antigen (CEA). These labs should be checked in both the preoperative and postoperative settings.
- **Genetic evaluation:** Germline testing and next-generation sequencing can identify familial syndromes and targetable mutations in select populations. This includes T4 or node-positive disease and patients with unresectable and iodine-resistant disease. Patients with MTC need to be evaluated for the *RET* proto-oncogene mutation as part of the MEN2 familial syndrome.

Imaging

Once a diagnosis of malignancy is made, all individuals should have a chest x-ray (CXR) to evaluate for metastases to the lungs. If not already done, a US of the central and lateral compartments of the neck is needed to evaluate for lymphadenopathy. A CT or MRI of the neck is helpful for surgical planning if the thyroid nodule is fixed, bulky, or extending into the substernal space. Note: if iodinated contrast is given with a CT scan this can delay the use of RAI for 1–3 months. Patients with anaplastic tumors can frequently have metastases and should receive complete imaging of the neck with US or MRI as well as contrast-enhanced CT scan of the chest, abdomen, and pelvis. An FDG PET/CT may also be considered to evaluate for metastasis.

Staging

The staging of thyroid cancer differs from other malignancies. In addition to tumor size, current prognostic stage groups consider tumor histology and the patient's age at presentation. For example, in patients <55 years old, differentiated papillary or follicular cell carcinomas are not classified as higher than stage II. On the other hand, all anaplastic tumors are classified as stage IV, regardless of anatomic extent, due to their aggressive nature and high potential for metastasis. In MTC, staging information follows more classical TNM rules and comes from evaluation of the total thyroidectomy and cervical lymph node dissection.

TREATMENT

Treatment of the three main types of thyroid cancer varies significantly. RAI, external-beam radiation, surgery, and systemic targeted therapy each have their role in comprehensive therapeutic regimens. Chemotherapy is not usually effective.

- **Differentiated thyroid carcinoma (i.e., papillary, follicular, and Hürthle)** is mainly treated by surgical resection in all stages. Patients younger than 40 years of age have an excellent prognosis with thyroidectomy alone. Patients without prior radiation exposure, no distant metastases, no cervical lymph node metastases, no extrathyroidal extension, and tumors <4 cm in diameter may be considered for unilateral lobectomy. If a patient is not a candidate for unilateral lobectomy, they should consider total thyroidectomy. A total thyroidectomy carries the risk of recurrent laryngeal nerve damage resulting in hoarseness and hypocalcemia from hypoparathyroidism. In more advanced diseases, dissection of the central and lateral cervical neck compartments should be considered.
  - **RAI therapy** with ^{131}I induces cytotoxicity and is a key therapeutic agent. There are two main indications for use of ^{131}I. The first indication is to ablate residual normal thyroid tissue post-total thyroidectomy to improve the sensitivity of subsequent surveillance tumor markers and ^{131}I scans in detecting a recurrence. The second indication is to treat metastatic disease or as adjuvant therapy to eliminate microscopic malignant foci. Follow-up imaging with ^{131}I can determine treatment efficacy by revealing residual normal tissue and/or carcinoma. RAI is generally recommended for patients with a higher risk of recurrence such as gross extrathyroidal extension, tumors >4 cm, or postoperative unstimulated Tg >5 ng/mL. Patients with a primary tumor size between 1 cm and 4 cm, poorly differentiated histology, lymphovascular invasion, cervical lymph node metastases, presence of anti-Tg antibodies, or postoperative unstimulated Tg between 1 and 10 ng/mL may be considered for RAI therapy. Treatment ends when there is no further RAI uptake present or when toxicity risk is too high. There is concern that patients treated with RAI have an increased risk of secondary malignancies such as leukemia and salivary gland malignancies. Therefore, RAI is not indicated for patients with a low risk of thyroid cancer recurrence.
  - **External-beam radiation therapy** has a rare role in the treatment of differentiated thyroid carcinomas. It may be considered a possible treatment for an isolated skeletal metastasis or in the case of palliative treatment of a symptomatic metastasis in RAI-refractory thyroid cancer.
  - **Adjuvant hormonal therapy** with exogenous thyroid hormone is also routinely used in differentiated thyroid carcinomas to suppress TSH, since both normal and neoplastic thyroid tissue depend on TSH for growth. In addition, thyroid hormone is also necessary to treat iatrogenic hypothyroidism after extensive thyroid resection. The optimal level of TSH suppression is not defined but is generally based on the patient's risk of recurrence. For patients with residual carcinoma or those at high risk for recurrence, the recommended TSH level is <0.1 mU/L. For patients with a low risk of recurrence, TSH suppression is a bit more liberalized, with TSH goals being slightly below or slightly above the reference range. Long-term supplementation can lead to bone loss and an increased incidence of atrial fibrillation. Suppression of TSH to undetectable levels for the initial 5–10 years is reasonable; afterward exogenous thyroid hormone supplementation may be decreased to allow TSH levels to rise to the lower limits of normal.[3]
  - **Traditional chemotherapy** has no established role in the treatment of differentiated thyroid cancer.
  - **Targeted agents,** sorafenib and lenvatinib, are tyrosine-kinase inhibitors (TKIs) that are FDA approved for the treatment of RAI-resistant, locally advanced, or metastatic differentiated thyroid cancer. The double-blind phase III DECISION trial randomized RAI-refractory locally advanced or metastatic differentiated thyroid cancer patients to sorafenib 400 mg orally twice daily versus placebo. The median progression-free survival (PFS) was 10.8 months in the sorafenib arm and 5.8 months in the placebo arm. The subjective response rate was 12% in the sorafenib group. Median overall survival (OS) was not reached at the time of publication in either group.[6] The most common side effects of sorafenib were hand-foot skin reaction, diarrhea, alopecia, and rash. In the SELECT trial, 392 patients with locally advanced or metastatic RAI-refractory

thyroid cancer were randomized to receive oral lenvatinib 24 mg by mouth daily or placebo. The median PFS was 18.3 months versus 3.6 months in the lenvatinib and placebo arms, respectively. Importantly, the objective response rate was 65% and benefits were seen in both TKI-naïve and nonnaïve patients and older patients (>65) seemed to benefit more.[7] It stands to reason that a patient with progressive, symptomatic RAI-refractory differentiated thyroid cancer may have more benefit from lenvatinib, given its superior response rate. A small percentage of patients have a targetable driver mutation such as NTRK, ALK, RET, or BRAF. TRK inhibitors such as larotrectinib of entrectinib have broad FDA approval for treatment regardless of tissue of origin and can be used in patients with DTC. Selpercatinib, a RET inhibitor, was tested in the open-label LIBRETTO-001 trial[8] in 19 patients with RAI refractory, nonmedullary RET fusion–positive DTC. A complete or partial response was seen in 79% of the patients. Another RET inhibitor, pralsetinib was tested in the open-label ARROW trial in 9 patients with response rate of 89%. Common side effects of RET inhibitors included hypertension, fatigue, and LFT abnormalities. For BRAF V600E mutated DTC, the BRAF inhibitors vemurafenib and dabrafenib or dabrafenib with trametinib (a MEK inhibitor) can be used.

- **MTC** is sporadic in most cases, but roughly 25% of cases are part of inherited tumor syndromes (MEN IIA, MEN IIB, and familial MTC). This possibility makes ruling out a germline *RET* proto-oncogene mutation essential to the initial preoperative management, along with calcitonin and CEA measurement.
  - **Total thyroidectomy with bilateral central neck dissection** is the mainstay of therapy for MTC because of the high frequency of bilateral disease. Although MTC is somewhat indolent in its progression, no effective systemic chemotherapy regimens exist, and MTC cells take up RAI poorly. For this reason, patients with genetic predisposition to the disease (i.e., *RET* mutations) should be highly encouraged to undergo prophylactic total thyroidectomy with the timing of surgery dependent on the aggressiveness of the *RET* mutation.[9] Complications of local MTC invasion mirror those of anaplastic tumors, yet progression is less rapid.
  - **Postoperative adjuvant EBRT** is rarely used, as MTC is radioresistant.
  - **Traditional chemotherapy** has not been shown to be useful in the treatment of MTC.
  - **Targeted agents:** For patients with a known RET mutation, selpercatinib is a selective RET inhibitor that has demonstrated high response rates and is an FDA-approved option.[8] For patients with progressive, symptomatic metastatic or locally advanced disease, the use of either vandetanib or cabozantinib improves progression-free survival and is a reasonable option in patients without a known RET mutation. Vandetanib is an oral kinase inhibitor against RET, VEGFR, and EGFR. In a phase III, randomized trial patients with advanced or metastatic MTC were randomized to either vandetanib 300 mg orally daily or placebo. Patients treated with vandetanib had an estimated median PFS of 30.5 months versus 19.3 months in the placebo group. The objective response rate was 45% versus 13% between the treatment and placebo groups.[10] Cabozantinib is a multitargeted TKI that inhibits RET, VEGFR2, and MET. The phase III EXAM trial randomized patients with progressive locally advanced or metastatic MTC to cabozantinib versus placebo. Patients on cabozantinib had an increased median PFS compared to those treated with placebo (11.2 months vs. 4 months) and a response rate of 28% for cabozantinib versus 0% for placebo.[11] It is important to select patients appropriately as these oral therapies have side effects that may worsen their quality of life and have a low but real risk of life-threatening complications such as hemorrhage, arterial thrombosis (myocardial infarction, stroke), or bowel perforation.
- **Anaplastic thyroid carcinoma** is poorly responsive to therapy and is often locally invasive, if not metastatic, at the time of presentation. Patients are thus always staged as IV regardless of size, grade, node involvement, or metastasis. The invasive nature makes tumor resection difficult or even impossible, as the tumor may encompass the carotid

arteries, esophagus, and/or trachea. Recurrent or superior laryngeal nerve damage may also occur. The complications of local invasion account for the major morbidity of this cancer, often leading patients to require gastrostomy tubes and/or a tracheostomy. Local control is the priority when at all possible.

- **Resection:** If imaging reveals limited disease, resection should be pursued for improved local control and delay of complications, although survival is not altered.
- **Radiation/Chemotherapy/Targeted agents:** RAI is rarely taken up by anaplastic carcinoma cells, so external-beam radiation therapy is commonly used concurrently with systemic radiosensitizing chemotherapy. Chemotherapy alone (e.g., with doxorubicin) has a poor track record. For patients with BRAF V600E mutations, dabrafenib and trametinib can be used with overall response rate of about 60% in one study.
- End-stage care typically includes managing local complications, with ~50% of patients dying from airway obstruction.

FOLLOW-UP

For routine follow-up of differentiated thyroid carcinoma, physical examination, TSH, thyroglobulin level, and CXR are recommended twice yearly for 4 years, then once yearly for 10 years. Thyroglobulin levels are expected to be <5 ng/mL if complete thyroid ablation has been successful. For MTC, serum calcitonin and CEA levels should initially be followed every 4 months postoperatively for a year, and then every 6–12 months. Abnormal serum markers should trigger diagnostic imaging evaluation but isolated marker increase is not a reason for treatment.

PROGNOSIS

Patients with differentiated thyroid carcinomas have an excellent prognosis. Cure rates reach nearly 100% at 10 years, even with capsular invasion, as long as there is no vascular involvement. The two most important predictors of mortality are age >55 years and tumor stage at the time of initial therapy. Relative survival at 10 years for papillary, follicular, and Hürthle cell carcinomas is 93%, 85%, and 76%, respectively. Anaplastic tumors carry a grim prognosis, often leading rapidly to death within the first few years after diagnosis, regardless of treatment. MTCs have 5-year survival rates of >80% in stage I and II disease but <40% in stage III or IV disease.

Parathyroid Carcinoma

GENERAL PRINCIPLES

Although adenomas of the parathyroid glands are a common cause of hyperparathyroidism, parathyroid carcinoma is quite uncommon, involving <1% of the cases of hormone hyperproduction. Unlike benign hyperparathyroidism, which is found primarily in the postmenopausal female population, parathyroid carcinoma is found equally in both genders at younger ages. With an incidence of only 0.015 in 100,000, parathyroid cancer is classified as one of the rarest human cancers.

DIAGNOSIS

Patients with parathyroid carcinoma often present with either **hypercalcemia** or a **neck mass**. On physical examination, 30–50% of patients with parathyroid carcinoma have palpable masses in the central neck region. A hyperfunctional parathyroid tumor leads to excessive production of parathyroid hormone and, ultimately, the clinical syndrome of primary hyperparathyroidism. Clinical signs and symptoms include fatigue, renal stones, bone disease, and neuromuscular/neuropsychiatric disturbances related to hypercalcemia. Grossly elevated calcium levels lead to nausea, vomiting, polyuria, and dehydration. Cytologic examination of a needle aspirate is considered an unreliable criterion for diagnosis of malignancy. Definitive diagnosis of parathyroid carcinoma is made in the operating room, where local invasion and metastasis can be assessed.

TREATMENT

- The mainstay of treatment is **surgical exploration of the neck and complete en bloc resection of the tumor along with the ipsilateral thyroid lobe and central cervical lymph nodes.**[11] There is no proven role for adjuvant chemotherapy or radiation therapy. Likewise, the only effective therapy for recurrent or metastatic disease is complete resection.
- The management of severe hypercalcemia includes saline hydration, furosemide diuresis, and bisphosphonates. Octreotide and calcimimetic agents are occasionally used to lower calcium in patients refractory to other therapeutic interventions.

PROGNOSIS

Hypercalcemia is the major cause of morbidity and mortality. The prognosis for parathyroid carcinoma depends on the adequacy of the initial en bloc resection. The most common site of recurrence is local, followed by lung, liver, and bone, in decreasing order of incidence. Early recurrence correlates with death from the disease. The OS is 85% at 5 years and 50–70% at 10 years.

Pituitary Neoplasms

GENERAL PRINCIPLES

Pituitary neoplasms are rare endocrine malignancies that arise from epithelial origin in the adenohypophysis. Pituitary adenomas account for 10–15% of intracranial tumors. Previously classified by histopathology (acidophilic, basophilic, chromophobic), pituitary adenomas are now classified by the hormones they secrete, that is, prolactin, growth hormone (GH), adrenocorticotropic hormone (ACTH), gonadotropins, and TSH. Tumors that do not secrete hormones above physiologic levels are termed nonfunctional adenomas.

Epidemiology

Incidence peaks in the third and fourth decades of life. In general, males and females are affected equally, with the exception of some subtypes, such as ACTH and prolactin-secreting adenomas, which are more common in females.

DIAGNOSIS

Clinical Presentation

Initial symptoms include headache, visual disturbance, and increased intracranial pressure, as well as syndromes related to the type of hormone secreted (Cushing syndrome, acromegaly, hirsutism, hyperprolactinemia, or hyperthyroidism).

Diagnostic Testing

Initial evaluation involves a dedicated gadolinium-enhanced MRI of the pituitary and laboratory evaluation for active adenomas with a panel consisting of GH, insulin-like growth factor 1 (IGF-1), prolactin (PRL), TSH, free T4, T3, ACTH, cortisol, luteinizing hormone (LH), follicle-stimulating hormone (FSH), and testosterone. Diagnosis is made on imaging, confirmed by hormone levels in active adenomas, and, when appropriate, pathologically by transsphenoidal biopsy or resection. No TNM staging classification exists for these rare tumors, and prognostic markers include levels of hormone secreted, size of tumor, and extent of suprasellar extension.

TREATMENT

Management of pituitary adenomas depends on the type, but in general, transsphenoidal surgical resection is the preferred curative approach. The exceptions are prolactin-secreting microadenomas, which are managed by dopamine agonists, or inactive adenomas, which remain stable in size on serial imaging. The goals of surgery are to alleviate mass effect while preserving pituitary function and abating endocrine hyperactivity. Postoperative management depends on the type of pituitary adenoma.

Prolactin-Secreting Adenomas

- Prolactin-secreting adenomas are the most commonly diagnosed pituitary tumor, representing ~30% of cases. Symptoms of hyperprolactinemia include galactorrhea and hypogonadism (oligomenorrhea or amenorrhea, dry vaginal mucosa, sterility, decreased libido, and impotence).[12] Prolactinomas are usually slow-growing microadenomas in premenopausal women, but can grow to a larger size (macroadenomas) in men and postmenopausal females. Macroadenomas can cause mass effect, classically manifested by visual disturbances (bitemporal hemianopsia) and headaches.
- The **differential diagnosis** of hyperprolactinemia includes pregnancy, prolactin-stimulating drugs, hypothyroidism, and renal failure. The definitive diagnosis requires radiographic evidence of an adenoma and a persistently elevated prolactin level (>200 ng/mL in females and >100 ng/mL in males), with the other etiologies of hyperprolactinemia having been ruled out.
- **Treatment** of prolactinomas is dependent on size. Microadenomas are treated medically, since most do not increase in size, and surgery is rarely curative. Medical treatment is achieved with dopamine agonists (e.g., bromocriptine), with response rates 70–80% for tumor shrinkage and 80–90% for restoration of ovulation. In cases where dopamine agonist therapy is not tolerated (~30% of cases) or fertility is not a concern, oral contraceptives containing estrogen and progesterone can be used to treat the symptoms of hypogonadism. In cases of macroadenomas with significant suprasellar involvement or in pregnancy (which stimulates growth of adenomas), surgery or radiation therapy can be used, often in combination with dopamine agonists.
- **Follow-up** should include yearly prolactin levels. If prolactin increases to >250 ng/mL or neurologic symptoms develop, repeat MRI is indicated. For patients with macroadenomas, visual field testing and MRI at 6 months after commencement of therapy should be performed. When prolactin levels are normalized for 2 years and at least 50% tumor reduction is observed, a trial of tapering the dopamine agonist may be considered.

Growth Hormone–Secreting Adenomas

- GH-secreting adenomas account for 30% of pituitary adenomas. GH excess results in acromegaly (coarse facial features, macroglossia, and acral growth). GH leads to an increase in IGF-1, which affects bone and tissue growth and can ultimately lead to organomegaly, hypertension, cardiomyopathy, arthropathies, and restrictive lung diseases. Symptoms include arthralgias, oily skin, hyperhidrosis, headaches, and fatigue.

- The **diagnosis** is suggested by a physical examination showing acromegaly, elevated IGF-1 levels (preferred over fasting GH because the levels are more stable), oral glucose suppression test failing to suppress IGF-1, elevated GH, and a pituitary adenoma evident on MRI.
- The **treatment** of choice is transsphenoidal resection. In patients not eligible for surgery, external-beam or gamma knife radiation may be used. Control of hormone overproduction is not immediate with radiation and may take up to 3 years to normalize. Medical treatment with dopamine agonists or somatostatin analogs (SSAs) such as octreotide are not curative but may be used for symptomatic control of acromegaly.
- **Follow-up** should include monitoring GH and IGF-1 levels. Monitoring for hypopituitarism after radiation is also essential.

Adrenal Corticotrophin Hormone–Secreting Adenomas

- These less common pituitary adenomas can secrete ACTH, resulting in adrenal hyperplasia and hypercortisolism. Hypercortisolism results in centripetal obesity, moon facies, buffalo hump, hirsutism, abdominal striae, and acne (i.e., Cushing syndrome). Clinical signs include hypertension, bone loss, myopathies, diabetes, and psychiatric disorders.
- **Diagnosis** is made by confirming hypercortisolism with a 24-hour urinary cortisol. The pituitary origin of cortisol is demonstrated by failure of the low-dose dexamethasone suppression test to suppress serum cortisol to <10 μg/dL. Finally, serum ACTH should be elevated to rule out an adrenal adenoma. Ectopic ACTH syndrome is excluded if the high-dose dexamethasone suppression test results in reduction of cortisol levels to <50% of baseline. If the above laboratory testing is inconclusive, inferior petrosal sinus sampling for ACTH can be performed to confirm the pituitary etiology. Imaging studies are less reliable, as 50% of ACTH-secreting adenomas may not be detectable by MRI; nonetheless, MRI remains essential to guiding therapy and is performed in all cases.
- **Treatment** of choice is transsphenoidal resection, with cure rates ranging from 76% to 94%. External-beam radiation or gamma knife radiation may be used for poor surgical candidates or as adjuvant therapy to surgery. Medical therapy with ketoconazole, metyrapone, or mitotane may be used for symptom control in those unable to tolerate surgery or in relapsed cases. Some patients might have to undergo bilateral adrenalectomy with long-term steroid supplementation.
- **Follow-up** requires replacement hormonal therapy for up to 1 year after surgery and monitoring for hypopituitarism after radiation.

Gonadotropin-Secreting Adenomas and Nonsecreting Pituitary Adenomas

- These adenomas account for 30% of pituitary tumors. They are more common in older patients. Most are nonsecretory, but demonstrate secretory granules containing FSH and LH.
- **Clinical presentation** typically presents secondary to a mass effect, with symptoms of headaches, visual changes, and hypopituitarism.
- **Diagnosis** is suggested by increased LH and FSH and by MRI findings of a macroadenoma. Postmenopausal women may have naturally elevated FSH and LH, and diagnosis relies on final surgical pathology.
- The **treatment** is primarily transsphenoidal resection. Adjuvant external-beam radiation or gamma knife radiation therapy may be considered in patients with residual tumor on imaging postoperatively. **Follow-up** several months postoperatively with repeat MRI is essential since most tumors are nonsecretory.

TSH-Secreting Adenomas

- TSH-secreting adenomas are the least common pituitary tumors, comprising ~1% of pituitary adenomas. Typical clinical presentation includes symptoms of hyperthyroidism (heat intolerance, diarrhea, weight loss, or exophthalmos) or mass effect.

- **Diagnosis** is made by demonstrating increased TSH despite elevated T4 and T3. MRI may confirm the presence of an adenoma.
- **Treatment** is primarily transsphenoidal resection. Adjuvant external-beam radiation or gamma knife radiation is used in refractory cases. Palliative medical therapy with octreotide has been used in refractory cases, with response rates of 90%.
- **Follow-up** requires monitoring of TSH, T4, and T3 levels.

Adrenal Tumors: Pheochromocytoma, Paraganglioma, and Adrenocortical Tumors

GENERAL PRINCIPLES

The majority of adrenal tumors are benign, nonfunctioning adenomas found incidentally on imaging. The size and radiographic features of these tumors guide timing of repeat imaging to confirm stability. A minority of adrenal masses are functioning adrenal tumors. A pheochromocytoma needs to be ruled out prior to an adrenal biopsy, as tissue manipulation without alpha blockade can trigger hormone release. Rarely, an adrenal mass may represent an adrenocortical carcinoma (ACC), a rare and aggressive malignancy.

DIAGNOSIS

Clinical Presentation

- Adrenal "incidentalomas" can be found on 1–3% of CT scans of the abdomen. The differential diagnosis includes benign adenomas and metastases. The chance of malignancy is directly related to the size of the mass (<3 cm, benign; >6 cm, malignant), with most carcinomas presenting as large masses.
- Adrenal adenomas can be nonfunctional or functional. Functional adenomas secrete cortisol, sex hormones, or aldosterone. The clinical presentation is dependent on the predominant hormone secreted. The most common clinical presentation is Cushing syndrome, which results from cortisol excess. Sex hormone excess can lead to acne, oligomenorrhea, and virilization/hirsutism in women and feminization in men. Rarely, these carcinomas may produce aldosterone, resulting in hypertension and hypokalemia.

Diagnostic Testing

- Initial evaluation involves staging with imaging with a **CT of the abdomen and pelvis** and determination of hormone levels, which are used to monitor for recurrence and progression.
- ACC should be suspected in nonfunctioning tumors >4 cm with irregular margins. A Hounsfield unit number >10 is suggestive of ACC.
- The definitive diagnosis is obtained by surgical pathology. High urinary-free cortisol and serum cortisol, low ACTH, and lack of suppression in a high-dose dexamethasone suppression test occur in the instance of cortisol-secreting carcinoma. Virilizing sex hormone–secreting carcinomas demonstrate high levels of testosterone, androstenedione, and dehydroepiandrosterone sulfate (DHEA-S), while feminizing tumors demonstrate high estradiol levels. Some tumors are nonsecretory, and definitive diagnosis relies on tissue sampling.
- The staging of adrenal carcinoma depends on tumor size, nodal involvement, and presence of distant metastasis. Tumors <5 cm with no nodal involvement are stage I; those >5 cm without nodal involvement, stage II; those with nodal involvement, stage III; and those with distant metastasis, stage IV.

TREATMENT

- **Surgical resection** is the treatment of choice, even in advanced disease. Debulking of the tumor and metastectomy are often considered. Repeat surgeries may be needed in some slow-growing, nonfuctional tumors.
  - The role of adjuvant chemotherapy in adrenocortical cancers is debated, but can be considered in some cases of advanced, high-grade disease. There is not enough evidence to support any single regimen at this point.

Adjuvant Therapy for Resected Disease

- **Adjuvant mitotane**, an oral adrenocorticolytic agent, may be considered if the patient is at high risk for local recurrence based on positive margins, ruptured capsule, large tumor size, or high grade. The optimal exposure time of adjuvant treatment with mitotane is not known, although the median duration of treatment was 29 months in retrospective data of an Italian cohort of 177 patients with ACC treated with adjuvant mitotane.[13] Based on the ADIUVO trial, adjuvant mitotane does not appear to offer benefit beyond observation in patients with ACC with low–intermediate risk of recurrence.[13]
- **Adjuvant external-beam radiation therapy** may also be effective for local control after resection or for symptomatic metastasis.

Systemic Treatment for Unresectable Disease

- In patients ineligible for surgery, most chemotherapeutic regimens will include **mitotane**, which targets the adrenal cortex and results in selective chemical ablation. The overall response rate to mitotane is 33%, but its effect on overall and disease-free survival has not been conclusively determined.[14] Mitotane requires titration to therapeutic levels which can take several weeks to attain and is usually continued for 3–5 years. It has a lot of drug interactions and can suppress the thyroid function. Moreover, given its adrenolytic properties, patients will require steroid supplementation to prevent adrenal insufficiency, more so in times of stress. The EDP (etoposide, doxorubicin, cisplatin) regimen, plus mitotane, is typically considered in the first-line setting in patients with aggressive disease.[15] Later-line options can include pembrolizumab with responses up to 23% in a phase II study of 39 patients.[16]

PROGNOSIS

The prognosis of adrenal carcinoma depends on initial stage and resectability, as well as degree of hormone production. For surgically resectable tumors, the median OS is almost 6 years, but with medical therapy alone, <10% of patients live to 6 years. Follow-up with repeat CT scans and hormone levels at 6-month intervals is recommended.

Pheochromocytoma

GENERAL PRINCIPLES

- Pheochromocytomas arise from the chromaffin cells primarily in the adrenal medulla in 80–90% of cases, although they can also arise from para-aortic sympathetic ganglia along the aorta, within the carotid body, or inside the heart. The "Rule of 10" is also useful in recognizing general features of pheochromocytomas: 10% are malignant, 10% are extra-adrenal, and 10% are bilateral. This widespread distribution reflects the location of chromaffin cells associated with the sympathetic ganglia. Pheochromocytoma is present in only 0.1% of hypertensive patients.

- The incidence of malignancy in pheochromocytomas ranges from 5% to 45% in several series. Extra-adrenal tumors are more commonly malignant. Pheochromocytomas are associated with several inherited disorders. Bilateral adrenal medullary pheochromocytomas are elements of the inherited MEN IIA and MEN IIB neuroendocrine syndromes. Although ~25% of patients with von Hippel–Lindau disease develop pheochromocytomas, <1% of patients with neurofibromatosis and von Recklinghausen disease are found to have the tumor. Most cases of familial paraganglioma are caused by pathogenic variants in the succinate dehydrogenase (SDH) subunit genes.

DIAGNOSIS

Clinical Presentation

The most common presenting complaint is severe hypertension unrelated to physical or emotional stress. The production of catecholamines results in the clinical symptoms of episodic or sustained hypertension and anxiety attacks. Pheochromocytomas have been known to produce other hormones, including ACTH, somatostatin, calcitonin, oxytocin, and vasopressin. Classically, patients describe spells of hypertension, palpitations, headaches, and diaphoresis. Other presenting findings include lactic acidosis, hypovolemia, and unexplained fever. Clinically, the cluster of symptoms can be recalled by remembering the five Ps: pain, pressure, palpitation, perspiration, and pallor. However, it should be appreciated that many patients do not exhibit these "classic" episodes and may have persistent hypertension rather than episodic.

Diagnostic Testing

- Traditionally, diagnosis has been based on a **24-hour measurement of catecholamines and metabolites** in the urine, including vanillylmandelic acid and metanephrines. New data suggest that a **random plasma metanephrine level** is extremely sensitive (~99%) in diagnosing pheochromocytoma and is an excellent choice for initial screening.
- Localization of a pheochromocytoma is accomplished by **chest and abdominal imaging with CT or MRI**. Nuclear scanning after the administration of labeled metaiodobenzylguanidine (MIBG) can be done if the tumor is not identified by CT or MRI. MIBG is structurally similar to norepinephrine and is selectively taken up by adrenergic tissue. Alternatively, somatostatin receptor PET (SSTR PET) can help localize the tumor.

TREATMENT

- After diagnosis, tumor localization and operative preparation are indicated, as **surgical resection** represents the mainstay of curative therapy.
- **Preoperative alpha-adrenergic blockade** is necessary for patients with pheochromocytomas. **This applies both to surgery, as well as biopsy of a suspicious lesion.** Traditionally, phenoxybenzamine has been used to control hypertension. Propranolol may be used to control tachycardia but must always follow alpha-adrenergic blockade to avoid hypertensive exacerbation due to unopposed vasoconstriction. Intraoperative hypertensive episodes are controlled with alpha-adrenergic blockers or sodium nitroprusside.
- **Malignant pheochromocytomas** are difficult to distinguish from benign pheochromocytomas by pathology alone. Natural history, secondary tumor sites, and recurrence help determine the nature of the pheochromocytoma. Aggressive disease may require combination chemotherapy with cyclophosphamide, vincristine, and dacarbazine.[17] Routine follow-up consists of blood pressure measurements and urinary catecholamines, in addition to regularly scheduled CT, MRI, or metaiodobenzylguanidine scanning, to monitor for recurrence.

Diffuse Endocrine System Tumors

Some biochemically active tumors are not localized to any one organ, but share the common embryonic origin of the neural crest and neuroectoderm. These include neuroendocrine tumors (NETs) as they develop sporadically or within the familial endocrine neoplasia syndromes (e.g., MEN, VHL, SDH).

Nonfunctioning Gastroenteropancreatic Neuroendocrine Tumors

GENERAL PRINCIPLES

As a whole, NETs are rare. The most common NETs arise from the lungs or bronchi, pancreas, small intestine, appendix, rectum, and thymus. Regardless of their location, NETs are broadly classified (Table 28-2) by grade (low, intermediate, and high) and degree of differentiation: (well-differentiated or poorly differentiated). Well-differentiated NETs are classified as either low or intermediate grade with a mitotic count of ≤20 mitoses per 10 high-power fields (HPFs) and Ki-67 index <20%. Well-differentiated high grade NETs are by definition well differentiated but with a mitotic count of >20 mitoses per 10 HPFs or Ki-67 index >20%. In contrast, neuroendocrine carcinoma (NEC) refers to poorly differentiated NETs that are high grade with a mitotic count >20 mitoses per 10 HPFs or a Ki-76 index >20%. NECs behave more aggressively and treatment strategies include chemotherapy, some regimens similar to those of small-cell carcinoma of the lung. Most NETs produce neurosecretory granules, as evidenced by diffuse staining of neuroendocrine markers such as synaptophysin and chromogranin. Some well-differentiated tumors, especially of the pancreas, may secrete specific hormones such as insulin, glucagon, somatostatin, vasoactive intestinal peptide (VIP), and gastrin.

TABLE 28-2	WHO CLASSIFICATION CRITERIA FOR GASTROENTEROPANCREATIC NETs			
Classification	Differentiation	Grade	Mitotic Count (mitoses/ 2 mm^2)	Ki-67 Index
G1 NET	Well differentiated	Low	<2	<3%
G2 NET	Well differentiated	Intermediate	2–20	3–20%
G3 Well-differentiated NET	Well differentiated	High	>20	>20%
NEC	Poorly differentiated	High	>20	>20%
MiNEN	Well or poorly differentiated	Variable	Variable	Variable

MiNEN, mixed neuroendocrine nonneuroendocrine neoplasm; NEC, neuronedocrine carcinoma; NET, neuroendocrine tumors.

DIAGNOSIS

Clinical Presentation

Gastroenteropancreatic NETs present in various ways. It is now more common to discover a NET incidentally during endoscopic or radiographic procedures. Prior to the routine clinical use of diagnostic imaging, patients were more often diagnosed as a result of symptoms from the secretion of hormones or mechanical complications from tumor size. Clinical symptoms depend on the hormones secreted and the site of disease and are discussed more fully below ("Functioning neuroendocrine tumors" section). Tumor localization is essential for successful management of limited disease. CT and MRI may detect larger tumors, but often scintigraphy or angiography with venous hormone sampling may be required to localize tumors. FDG PET-CT is useful in detecting high-grade disease. Well-differentiated NETs typically express somatostatin receptors, and thus, SSTR PET-CT (including ^{68}Ga-DOTATATE, ^{64}Cu-DOTATATE, and ^{68}Ga-DOTATOC radiotracers) is used for localizing sites of disease.

TREATMENT

Treatment of gastroenteropancreatic NETs depends on multiple factors, including the stage and extent of disease, classification by grade and differentiation, and the presence or absence of hormone-related syndromes.

- Some patients with low tumor burden and low-grade disease may be safely **observed** without therapy.
- **SSAs, including octreotide and lanreotide,** are commonly used in the treatment of well-differentiated gastroenteropancreatic NETs.[18,19] They have a direct inhibitory effect on tumor growth, and, in the case of functioning tumors, symptoms of hormone excess may be controlled with SSAs.
- Peptide receptor radionucleotide therapy (PRRT) with ^{177}lutetium-DOTATATE treats SSTR-positive grade 1–2 NETs via targeted radiation. A large phase III trial tested the efficacy of lutetium dotatate versus high-dose octreotide in 229 patients with SSTR-positive small-bowel NETs and showed 65.2% survival at month 20 in the ^{177}Lu-Dotatate group and 10.8% (95% CI, 3.5–23.0) in the control group.[20] More intense uptake on SSTR-PET, and less intense uptake on FDG-PET, predicts response to this therapy. Side effects can include cytopenias, as well as the potential for myelodysplasia/leukemia.
- **Chemotherapy** has variable activity depending on the type of gastroenteropancreatic tumor, and most commonly is used for patients with aggressive, high-grade disease. Typical agents used include platinum (cisplatin or carboplatin) plus etoposide or 5-FU–based regimens. The combination of capecitabine and temozolomide was shown to be effective in well-differentiated pancreatic NETs. A study randomized 144 patients to temozolomide or capecitabine and temozolomide, showing a median PFS of 14.4 months for temozolomide versus 22.7 months for capecitabine/temozolomide. In the final analysis (May 2021), the median OS was 53.8 months for temozolomide and 58.7 months for capecitabine/temozolomide.[21]
- The oral mammalian target of rapamycin (MTOR) inhibitor everolimus may be used as second- or later-line treatment for GI, pancreatic, or lung NETs based on multiple clinical trials.[22,23] Stomatitis is a frequent dose-limiting toxicity.
- Tyrosine kinase inhibitors are effective in NETs. Sunitinib was approved for treatment of pancreatic NETs based on a large phase III placebo-controlled trial.[24] Belzutifan, a HIF inhibitor, is being tested for treatment of pancreatic NETs in patients with germline VHL alterations (i.e., von Hippel–Lindau disease) based on results of a trial in patients with renal cell carcinoma, a percentage of which also harbored pancreatic NETs.[25] The responses in patients with pancreatic lesions reached 77%.

- Checkpoint inhibitor therapy should be considered for all advanced MSI-H/dMMR NETs, though this represents a rare subcategory of NET. Immunotherapy has also been explored in grade 3 NEC, and either single-agent checkpoint blockade or dual-agent therapy with ipilimumab plus nivolumab may be employed in later lines.

Functioning Neuroendocrine Tumors

GENERAL PRINCIPLES

Functioning neuroendocrine neoplasms, previously called carcinoid tumors, are the most common NETs, with a yearly incidence of 3.8 in 100,000 in United States.[26] They are capable of secreting various vasoactive substances, including histamine, serotonin, catecholamines, and prostaglandins. The small bowel is the most common location for these tumors, but they may occur in the appendix, colon, rectum, stomach, lung, or thymus.[27] Fortunately, nonmetastatic functional NETs in the GI tract rarely cause symptoms since the bioactive hormones are secreted into the portal circulation and inactivated by hepatic enzymes as they pass through the liver. In contrast, functional tumors that have metastasized to the liver can bypass the portal venous system and may cause clinical symptoms of carcinoid syndrome or other hormone hypersecretion syndromes.

DIAGNOSIS

Clinical Presentation
- Clinical presentation is highly variable depending on the hormone secreted.
- Approximately 40% of NETs are hormonally active, leading to **carcinoid syndrome** in 10% of cases. This syndrome rarely occurs without liver metastasis. Symptoms include facial flushing and edema, abdominal cramping, diarrhea, bronchospasm, hypotension, and cardiac valvular lesions (typically on the tricuspid and/or pulmonic valve). Alcohol, stress, or exercise may precipitate symptoms. Tumors may also cause mechanical issues due to tumor growth such as bowel obstruction, appendicitis, or painful liver metastases.

Diagnostic Testing
- An elevated **24-hour urinary 5-HIAA** is often used for diagnosis, but it is not useful for detecting functioning NETs at the early stages when it can be curable. Levels >25 mg/24 hours are the typical finding (normal value of excretion is <9 mg/24 hours). Patients should avoid excessive intake of nuts, bananas, avocados, and pineapples for at least 2 days before testing, as these may result in erroneously high levels.
- **Plasma chromogranin A level** may also be a useful test with a high sensitivity and without significant variability or need for a 24-hour urine collection. However, it can be affected by concomitant medication use and thus is not very sensitive nor specific.
- Routine blood tests, with attention to liver function tests, hepatic and upper gastrointestinal system imaging, a CXR, and tissue acquisition should all be part of the workup. If available, somatostatin receptor scintigraphy is a useful imaging test. There is no accepted staging system for carcinoid.
- Finally, pathologic diagnosis is confirmed with positive stains for markers such as chromogranin, synaptophysin, and neuron-specific enolase.

Laboratory evaluation of functioning NETs is dependent on the suspected hormone hypersecretion syndrome, and is outlined as follows:

- For patients with carcinoid syndrome (flushing/diarrhea/wheezing), consider testing serum serotonin, 5-hydroxyindoleacetic acid (HIAA) 24-hour urine, and chromogranin.

- For patients with peptic ulcer disease, test gastrin for <u>gastrinoma.</u>
- For patients with hypoglycemia, test proinsulin and C-peptide for <u>insulinoma.</u>
- For patients with watery diarrhea and hypokalemia, test VIP for <u>VIPoma or gastrinoma.</u>
- For patients with dermatitis/diabetes/deep vein thrombosis, test glucagon, serum glucose, CBC for a <u>glucagonoma.</u>
- For patients with cyclic hypertension, test metanephrines (plasma and urine) urine catecholamines for a <u>pheochromocytoma.</u>
- Other rarer islet cell tumors can produce pancreatic polypeptide, calcitonin, somatostatin, chromogranin A, or parathyroid hormone–related peptide.

TREATMENT

- In general, the treatment of functioning NETs is similar to that of nonfunctioning NETs, as described in the previous section.
- For localized disease, surgical resection is the standard curative modality, with a 5-year OS of 70–90%. In metastatic disease, median OS is 2 years, with the focus of therapy on palliating symptoms both surgically and medically. As survival with untreated low-grade functioning NETs can exceed 10 years, therapy is usually focused on controlling symptoms.
- The SSA **octreotide**, used at doses of 100–600 mcg SC/day in 2–4 divided doses, is effective at symptom alleviation in nearly 90% of patients. A depot formulation of octreotide available as monthly dosing has become standardized. Histamine blockers, prochlorperazine, and cyproheptadine may decrease flushing. Atropine, diphenoxylate, and cyproheptadine can be used for diarrhea. Monoamine oxidase inhibitors (MAOIs) are contraindicated.
- **Surgery** can be risky, as anesthesia can, in theory, precipitate carcinoid crises. However, resection is indicated and highly successful in localized functioning NETs. Perioperative administration of octreotide can help manage carcinoid crisis, although the usefulness of this intervention has been called into question more recently.
- Liver metastases may be treated with cytoreductive surgery or ablative therapies in select cases where near-complete or complete tumor debulking can be achieved. Ablative therapies include radiofrequency ablation (RFA) or cryoablation.
- **Hepatic-directed therapies** such as chemoembolization may be considered in patients with unresectable, hepatic-predominant metastatic disease.
- **Telotristat ethyl** is an oral inhibitor of tryptophan hydroxylase, the enzyme responsible for serotonin synthesis, and is approved for treatment of carcinoid syndrome diarrhea.

Genetic Predisposition Syndromes

Multiple genetic predisposition syndromes are specifically associated with certain neuroendocrine neoplasms and/or endocrine malignancies, most notably the multiple endocrine neoplasia (MEN) syndromes. These disorders differ by the underlying genetic cause and the principal malignancies that affected patients are at risk for developing (Table 28-3).

- **Multiple endocrine neoplasia I (Werner syndrome)**
  This syndrome has high penetrance, with **parathyroid glands** most frequently involved. One-third of gastrinomas are associated with MEN I, and pituitary adenomas can also be discovered. MEN1 is also associated with NETs of the lung and thymus, adrenal tumors, multiple lipomas, and cutaneous angiomas. The *MEN1* gene locus has been mapped to 11q13 and codes for a tumor suppressor protein, menin. Inheritance of the mutation is autosomal dominant. Morbidity and mortality are predominately related to the development of a pancreatic or thymic NET. Patients require close follow-up for evidence of additional sites of involvement in the pituitary, parathyroid, and pancreas.

TABLE 28-3 FEATURES OF GENETIC PREDISPOSITION SYNDROMES

Syndrome	Associated Tumors and Abnormalities
MEN I	Pituitary adenomas Pancreatic islet cell tumors or duodenal (35–75%) Parathyroid hyperplasia (90%)
MEN IIA	Medullary carcinoma of thyroid Pheochromocytoma (bilateral) Parathyroid hyperplasia
MEN IIB	Medullary carcinoma of thyroid Pheochromocytoma (bilateral) Multiple mucosal ganglioneuromas Colonic and skeletal abnormalities with marfanoid body habitus
FMTC	Medullary carcinoma of thyroid

FMTC, familial non-MEN medullary thyroid carcinoma.

- **Multiple endocrine neoplasia IIA (Sipple syndrome) and IIB**
  MEN II syndromes demonstrate an autosomal-dominant inheritance of an activating mutation of the *RET* proto-oncogene, located on chromosome 10. Nearly all patients develop MTC, which is typically multifocal and bilateral and occurs at a young age. Other features of these syndromes are expressed variably and are reported in Table 28-3. Treatment is directed by sites of tumor involvement. All patients presenting with MTC should be considered for genetic screening for *RET* proto-oncogene mutations. Furthermore, **all patients with MTC should be evaluated for possible pheochromocytoma** before undergoing thyroidectomy to avoid a life-threatening hypertensive crisis.
- **Von Hippel–Lindau syndrome**
  Von Hippel–Lindau syndrome is a disease associated with a pathogenic variant in the *VHL* gene. It is inherited in an autosomal dominant fashion. Patients with this syndrome are at increased risk of developing multiple tumor types, among them pheochromocytoma and pancreatic NET. Belzutifan, a small-molecule inhibitor of HIF-2α, is approved for the treatment of renal cell carcinoma, CNS hemangioblastoma, and pancreatic neuroendocrine neoplasms in patients with Von Hippel–Lindau syndrome.
- **Neurofibromatosis type 1**
  Neurofibromatosis type 1 (NF1) is an autosomal dominant disorder associated with pathogenic variants in the *NF1* gene. Patients with NF1 are at risk of development of many benign and malignant tumors, including pheochromocytoma and paraganglioma.
- **SDH and familial paraganglioma**
  Pathogenic variants in *SDHA*, *SDHB*, *SDHC*, and *SDHD*, the genes encoding the four subunits of the succinyl dehydrogenase enzyme, as well as the associated gene *SDHAF2*, are associated with increased risk of developing pheochromocytoma or paraganglioma. The associated syndrome is associated with an autosomal dominant inheritance pattern. All patients with paragangliomas should undergo genetic screening for germline variants in these and other genes associated with familial syndromes.
- **Familial nonmultiple endocrine neoplasia medullary thyroid carcinoma (FMTC)**
  Like the MEN1 and MEN2 syndromes, this disease is also associated with an autosomal-dominant inheritance of the *RET* proto-oncogene. However, these patients develop

MTC without other abnormalities associated with MEN II syndromes. **Patients with MEN IIA and FMTC almost invariably develop MTC at an early age, and therefore, prophylactic thyroidectomy should be considered in patients with a known mutation.**

REFERENCES

1. National Cancer Institute. Cancer Stat Facts: Thyroid Cancer. *SEER.* https://seer.cancer.gov/statfacts/html/thyro.html
2. Siegel RL, Miller KD, Jemal A. Cancer statistics, 2015. *CA Cancer J Clin.* 2015;65:5–29.
3. Middleton WD, Teefey SA, Reading CC, et al. Multiinstitutional analysis of thyroid nodule risk stratification using the American College of Radiology Thyroid Imaging Reporting and Data System. *AJR Am J Roentgenol.* 2017;208:1331–1341.
4. Cooper DS, Doherty GM, Haugen BR, et al; American Thyroid Association (ATA) Guidelines Taskforce on Thyroid Nodules and Differentiated Thyroid Cancer. Revised American Thyroid Association management guidelines for patients with thyroid nodules and differentiated thyroid cancer. *Thyroid.* 2009;19:1167–1214.
5. Steward DL, Carty SE, Sippel RS, et al. Performance of a multigene genomic classifier in thyroid nodules with indeterminate cytology: a prospective blinded multicenter study. *JAMA Oncol.* 2019;5:204–212.
6. Brose MS, Nutting CM, Jarzab B, et al. Sorafenib in radioactive iodine-refractory, locally advanced or metastatic differentiated thyroid cancer: a randomised, double-blind, phase 3 trial. *Lancet Lond Engl.* 2014;384:319–328.
7. Schlumberger M, Tahara M, Wirth LJ, et al. Lenvatinib versus placebo in radioiodine-refractory thyroid cancer. *N Engl J Med.* 2015;372:621–630.
8. Wirth LJ, Sherman E, Robinson B, et al. Efficacy of selpercatinib in RET-altered thyroid cancers. *N Engl J Med.* 2020;383:825–835.
9. Wells SA Jr, Asa SL, Dralle H, et al; American Thyroid Association Guidelines Task Force. Medullary thyroid cancer: management guidelines of the American Thyroid Association. *Thyroid.* 2009; 19:565–612.
10. Wells SA, Robinson BG, Gagel RF, et al. Vandetanib in patients with locally advanced or metastatic medullary thyroid cancer: a randomized, double-blind phase III trial. *J Clin Oncol.* 2012;30:134–141.
11. Elisei R, Schlumberger MJ, Müller SP, et al. Cabozantinib in progressive medullary thyroid cancer. *J Clin Oncol.* 2013;31:3639–3646.
12. Schlechte JA. Clinical practice. Prolactinoma. *N Engl J Med.* 2003;349:2035–2041.
13. Terzolo M, Angeli A, Fassnacht M, et al. Adjuvant mitotane treatment for adrenocortical carcinoma. *N Engl J Med.* 2007;356:2372–2380.
14. Veytsman I, Nieman L, Fojo T. Management of endocrine manifestations and the use of mitotane as a chemotherapeutic agent for adrenocortical carcinoma. *J Clin Oncol.* 2009;27:4619–4629.
15. Fassnacht M, Terzolo M, Allolio B, et al; FIRM-ACT Study Group. Combination chemotherapy in advanced adrenocortical carcinoma. *N Engl J Med.* 2012;366:2189–2197.
16. Raj N, Zheng Y, Kelly V, et al. PD-1 blockade in advanced adrenocortical carcinoma. *J Clin Oncol.* 2020;38:71–80.
17. Huang H, Abraham J, Hung E, et al. Treatment of malignant pheochromocytoma/paraganglioma with cyclophosphamide, vincristine, and dacarbazine: recommendation from a 22-year follow-up of 18 patients. *Cancer.* 2008;113:2020–2028.
18. Rinke A, Wittenberg M, Schade-Brittinger C, et al. Placebo-controlled, double-blind, prospective, randomized study on the effect of octreotide LAR in the control of tumor growth in patients with Metastatic Neuroendocrine Midgut Tumors (PROMID): results of long-term survival. *Neuroendocrinology.* 2017;104:26–32.
19. Caplin ME, Pavel M, Ćwikła JB, et al; CLARINET Investigators. Lanreotide in metastatic enteropancreatic neuroendocrine tumors. *N Engl J Med.* 2014;371:224–233.
20. Strosberg J, El-Haddad G, Wolin E, et al. Phase 3 trial of 177Lu-Dotatate for midgut neuroendocrine tumors. *N Engl J Med.* 2017;376:125–135.
21. Kunz PL, Graham NT, Catalano PJ, et al. Randomized study of temozolomide or temozolomide and capecitabine in patients with advanced pancreatic neuroendocrine tumors (ECOG-ACRIN E2211). *J Clin Oncol.* 2023;41:1359–1369.
22. Yao JC, Fazio N, Singh S, et al; RAD001 in Advanced Neuroendocrine Tumours; Fourth Trial (RADIANT-4) Study Group. Everolimus for the treatment of advanced, non-functional

neuroendocrine tumours of the lung or gastrointestinal tract (RADIANT-4): a randomised, placebo-controlled, phase 3 study. *Lancet*. 2016;387:968–977.

23. Yao JC, Shah MH, Ito T, et al; RAD001 in Advanced Neuroendocrine Tumors; Third Trial (RADIANT-3) Study Group. Everolimus for advanced pancreatic neuroendocrine tumors. *N Engl J Med*. 2011;364:514–523.

24. Raymond E, Dahan L, Raoul JL, et al. Sunitinib malate for the treatment of pancreatic neuroendocrine tumors. *N Engl J Med*. 2011;364:501–513.

25. Jonasch E, Donskov F, Iliopoulos O, et al; MK-6482-004 Investigators. Belzutifan for renal cell carcinoma in von Hippel–Lindau disease. *N Engl J Med*. 2021;385:2036–2046.

26. Maggard MA, O'Connell JB, Ko CY. Updated population-based review of carcinoid tumors. *Ann Surg*. 2004;240:117–122.

27. Kulke MH. Clinical presentation and management of carcinoid tumors. *Hematol Oncol Clin North Am*. 2007;21:433–455; vii–viii.

Urologic Malignancies

29

Melissa A. Reimers

Prostate Cancer

GENERAL PRINCIPLES

Prostate cancer is the most common noncutaneous cancer among men in the US and is the second leading cause of cancer death in men after lung cancer. The American Cancer Society (ACS) estimated that in 2023, there will be 288,300 new cases and 34,700 deaths from prostate cancer. In the majority of cases, patients are diagnosed with asymptomatic, prostate-confined disease.

Risk Factors

Age is the most significant risk factor. Two out of every three prostate cancers are found in men older than 65 years, as per the ACS. Increased risk is also conferred to patients with a **positive family history** and those of **African American descent**. **High-fat and red meat diets** appear to correlate positively with prostate cancer development. **Benign prostatic hypertrophy is not a risk factor.**

Prevention

No method of prostate cancer prevention has been found to be effective in clinical trials to date.

DIAGNOSIS

- **Screening guidelines for prostate cancer in asymptomatic patients are heterogeneous.** The ACS recommends discussion about prostate cancer screening for (1) men aged 50 with at least a 10-year life expectancy and at average risk of prostate cancer, (2) men aged 45 at high risk of developing prostate cancer (i.e., African Americans, men with first-degree relative diagnosed younger than 65), and (3) men aged 40 at even higher risk (more than one first-degree relative with prostate cancer at an early age). The US Preventive Services Task Force's most recent guidelines from 2018 recommends against PSA-based screening for men older than 70 (grade D, do not screen), and recommends shared decision making between patient and clinician for men aged 55–69 (grade C, individualized patient decision). As of 2023, the American Urological Association recommends shared decision making for men who consider PSA screening. In particular, clinicians are recommended to offer prostate cancer screening at ages 40–45 for patients at increased risk for prostate cancer (Black ancestry, germline mutations, and strong family history of prostate cancer).

Clinical Presentation

Localized prostate cancer is frequently asymptomatic. However, obstructive symptoms as well as dysuria, back pain, and hematuria can be initial presenting symptoms. In advanced cases, disease may become evident only after investigation of symptoms such as spinal cord compression or bone pain.

Physical Examination

Carcinoma of the prostate most commonly develops in the peripheral zone, which is palpable during the **digital rectal exam (DRE)**. Trials for detecting early disease suggest that the physical examination, or even an ultrasonography, is less sensitive than measurement of prostate specific antigen (PSA).[1] On occasion, extensive pelvic lymphadenopathy may cause scrotal or lower-extremity lymphedema.

Diagnostic Testing

Laboratories

Total serum PSA is the most commonly utilized diagnostic test for prostate cancer. A normal serum is typically considered to be <4 ng/mL. Of note, levels typically rise with age and following prostatic massage, and they can be elevated in patients with benign prostatic hypertrophy and prostatitis. On the other hand, men with high Gleason score tumors may have tumors so undifferentiated that they do not synthesize large amounts of PSA. In the general population, the sensitivity of PSA >4 has been estimated at 70–80%, while the specificity is estimated to be about 60–70%.[2] Perhaps the most important feature of PSA testing is the ability to follow its change over time (PSA velocity).

Imaging

Although **transrectal ultrasound** has been used for screening and staging in some situations, its greatest use is to guide prostatic biopsies. **Prostate MRI** has become a valuable tool to assess local extent of disease prior to offering definitive therapy. **Technetium bone scan** is useful in identifying bone metastasis and is recommended for men with PSA >20, and **CT** of the chest, abdomen, and pelvis is utilized for lymph node and visceral disease evaluation. Most recently, **prostate-specific membrane antigen (PSMA) PET** imaging is increasingly utilized in conjunction with, or in lieu of, standard CT and bone scans.

Diagnostic Procedures

Biopsy is essential for diagnosis. Prostate core needle biopsy is performed either via transrectal ultrasound or a transperineal approach, with 8–12 cores typically obtained. **Histologic grade** is an important determinant of disease course and patient survival. Adenocarcinomas represent >95% of prostate cancers and are graded histologically using the **Gleason scoring system**. This system takes the two most predominant histologic patterns in the area of the tumor and assigns each a number from one to five. These numbers are then added together to give the total score. *Higher scores* correlate with more poorly differentiated tumors and worse prognoses. Squamous and transitional cell tumors make up the majority of the remaining prostate tumors, with another important subset being the high-grade neuroendocrine or small-cell tumors.

TREATMENT

The key determinants in considering the optimal treatment of prostate cancer are estimates of life expectancy and risk of cancer progression. The risk of cancer progression is estimated using the **pathologic stage**, which is determined by the clinical stage (based on DRE), preoperative PSA, and biopsy Gleason score. Patients with prostate cancer can be divided into three groups for the purpose of guiding treatment: localized prostate cancer, locally advanced prostate cancer, and metastatic prostate cancer.

- **Localized prostate cancer.** By definition, the cancer is confined to the prostate. These patients are further subdivided into three risk categories:
  - Low risk (T1–T2a, Gleason score ≤6, PSA <10): Expectant management, radical prostatectomy (RP), external-beam radiation therapy (EBRT), or brachytherapy are all reasonable options for treatment. If expectant management is chosen, PSA should be

checked at least every 6 months and DRE at least once a year. Curative therapy is initiated at onset of disease progression. No clinical trials have compared expectant management with immediate treatment. Choice of therapy otherwise is based on patient preferences, as no clinical trials have found any treatment modality to be superior.

- ○ **Intermediate risk** (T2b–T2c or GS 7 or PSA 10–20): Unless expected survival is <10 years, expectant management is not acceptable in this category. Otherwise, RP, EBRT, or brachytherapy are equivalent management options.
- ○ **High risk** (T3a or GS 8–10 or PSA >20): These patients are treated with either RP with pelvic lymph node dissection or EBRT combined with at least 2–3 years of androgen deprivation therapy.[3]
- **Locally advanced prostate cancer (T3b–T4).** Similar to patients with high-risk localized disease, these patients are treated with either RP with pelvic lymph node dissection or EBRT combined with 2–3 years of androgen deprivation therapy (ADT). High-risk or very high–risk and locally advanced prostate cancer patients being treated with RT may also receive abiraterone acetate, a CYP17 inhibitor, in conjunction with long-term ADT.[4]
- **PSA-only recurrence.** These patients have a "biochemical recurrence" that occurs after either radiation therapy or surgical resection, and no source of recurrence other than elevated PSA can be found clinically or through imaging. Treatment options include watchful waiting, radiation therapy if the patient had previously had RP, ADT, or occasionally salvage RP if they were originally treated with radiation therapy. With modern PSMA PET imaging, these patients are now sometimes found to have metastatic disease.
- **Androgen deprivation therapy.** Prostate cancer is testosterone dependent, and androgen deprivation is the backbone of treatment for localized and advanced disease. Castration can be achieved either surgically through orchiectomy or medically through hormonal suppression. GnRH agonists (leuprolide) induce LH suppression with subsequent decrement in testosterone production. A transient "flare" of testosterone production necessitates the concurrent transient use of second-generation antiandrogen therapy such as bicalutamide during the first several weeks of treatment. Direct GnRH antagonists (degarelix, subc; relugolix, oral) do not require antiandrogen therapy and lead to more rapid testosterone suppression. The main **adverse effects** of ADT include hot flashes, decreases in libido, and loss of muscle mass. Osteoporosis also occurs at a higher rate with long-term androgen deprivation. A baseline bone density screen is therefore recommended prior to initiation of ADT. Patients should be supplemented with calcium and vitamin D and bisphosphonate therapy should also be offered to men who are found to be osteopenic or osteoporotic.
- **Metastatic hormone–sensitive prostate cancer (mHSPC).** All patients with either relapsed (prior RP or RT) or de novo metastatic prostate cancer require continuous ADT. Upfront **docetaxel** chemotherapy has demonstrated a survival advantage in patients with high-volume disease or visceral metastases per the CHAARTED trial.[5] Most recently, the addition of either darolutamide (ARASENS) or abiraterone (PEACE-1) to docetaxel has demonstrated further benefit in this population.[6] Moreover, in patients who are not felt to be candidates for chemotherapy or who have lower volume disease, abiraterone acetate, and the **androgen-receptor targeting agents (ARTAs)** apalutamide and enzalutamide in conjunction with ADT have all been associated with an improvement in overall survival compared with ADT alone.[1–3,7,8]
- **Metastatic castration–resistant prostate cancer (mCRPC).** The majority of patients receiving long-term ADT eventually develop castration or hormone resistance, defined as a rising PSA and/or development of progressive radiographic metastatic disease in the setting of castrate testosterone levels (≤50 ng/dL). The optimal treatment of mCRPC is rapidly evolving. Both abiraterone and enzalutamide are approved in this population,[9,10] but are likely to be less useful over time as more patients receive upfront ARTAs for mHSPC.[11] Docetaxel is approved for mCRPC[11] for patients who did not receive it in the mHSPC setting, and docetaxel refractory patients may benefit from cabazitaxel, sometimes in combination with carboplatin.[12,13] **Sipuleucel-T**, an autologous cellular vaccine,

was FDA approved in 2010, as it has shown improved survival for those with minimally symptomatic mCRPC without having a significant effect on PSA or progression-free survival.[14] Molecular testing in advanced prostate cancer is critical to undertake early in the course of metastatic disease, as up to 20–30% of these patients may harbor deleterious DNA repair defect alterations.[15–17] Poly(ADP-ribose) polymerase 1 **(PARP1) inhibitors** have now been approved (or have accelerated FDA approval) both as monotherapy and in combination with mCRPC.[18–21] The greatest benefit from PARPi currently is in patients with *BRCA1/2* alterations, but the optimal strategy for utilizing this drug class in mCRPC is still been elucidated. Additional treatment options for mCRPC include bone-targeted therapy such as the alpha-emitter **radium-223**, which showed improved overall survival in patients with symptomatic bone metastases,[22] and most recently the radioligand therapeutic agent **lutetium Lu^{177} vipivotide tetraxetan**, which demonstrated improved PFS and OS in mCRPC after disease progression on prior ARTA and taxane chemotherapy.[23]

Renal Cell Carcinoma

GENERAL PRINCIPLES

Primary cancers of the kidney can be divided into cancers of the renal parenchyma and cancers of the renal pelvis which are generally upper tract urothelial carcinoma (UTUC). This section focuses on cancers of the renal parenchyma, which are generally renal cell carcinoma (RCC). Clear cell RCC is the most common histologic subtype and accounts for ~70% of cases. Non–clear cell RCC comprises the remaining 30%, with papillary RCC accounting for approximately 10%, followed by chromophobe RCC and collecting duct RCC. Medullary (SMARCB1/INI1 loss) RCC, which has an association with sickle cell trait, is uncommon, but can present with a very aggressive course in young patients and has a poor prognosis.

Epidemiology

The ACS estimates 81,800 new cases of RCC and 14,890 cancer deaths in 2023. RCC is more common in men and slightly more common in Blacks.

Risk Factors

As with prostate cancer, age is the major risk factor for RCC. Accordingly, the disease predominantly presents in the sixth to eighth decades of life. Other risk factors include cigarette smoking, obesity, hypertension, acquired cystic kidney disease associated with dialysis, polycystic kidney disease, and occupational exposure to heavy metals, asbestos, or petroleum products. Hereditary RCC syndromes such as von Hippel–Lindau syndrome are uncommon but confer an elevated risk of developing RCC.

DIAGNOSIS

Clinical Presentation

- Many patients are asymptomatic until advanced stages of disease; however, the increased use of abdominal imaging has led to an increased detection rate of incidental renal masses.[24] Hematuria, abdominal pain, and a palpable flank or abdominal mass are the classic triad of RCC diagnosis but occur in combination only 10% of the time.[15]
- **Hematuria** is the most common clinical finding in RCC. Other symptoms include fever, night sweats, malaise, and weight loss. Paraneoplastic syndromes are rare but include erythrocytosis and hypercalcemia from overproduction of erythropoietin or parathyroid

hormone–related protein, respectively. Stauffer syndrome consists of hepatic dysfunction in the absence of liver metastasis. This dysfunction may be due to production of tumor cytokines.

Diagnostic Testing

Imaging

The best initial imaging modality for a suspected RCC is an **ultrasound**. It is inexpensive, without radiation, and has a high sensitivity. It is also very useful for distinguishing simple cysts from complex and malignant masses. If a suspicious mass is found, ultrasound is typically followed by **abdominal CT or MR** to further characterize lymph node and regional involvement. Role of **PET** in initial diagnosis is unclear.

Diagnostic Procedures

Despite the sensitivity of imaging studies, **biopsy** of suspected metastatic lesions or nephrectomy is needed to definitely establish RCC diagnosis, as well as to delineate histologic subtype. Needle biopsy of the renal mass is not recommended due to concern for seeding of the peritoneum, as well as sampling errors that result in a negative biopsy.

TREATMENT

Localized disease is comprised of stages I–III, determined by tumor size, extent of local invasion, and regional lymph node involvement.

- **Resectable disease.** Surgical resection can be curative and is the treatment of choice in patients with stage I, II, and III diseases. This even includes patients with tumor thrombus involving the inferior vena cava (IVC). Either radical nephrectomy or partial nephrectomy is performed, depending on the size of mass and the patient's reliance on the affected kidney for total renal function.
  - **Adjuvant therapy.** Despite multiple prior negative adjuvant trials utilizing various tyrosine kinase inhibitors, the checkpoint inhibitor pembrolizumab has now been shown to provide a disease-free survival compared with placebo benefit in clear cell RCC patients with a high risk of recurrence.[25,26] At this time, overall survival data is still immature.
  - After surgical resection, patients should be followed with repeat imaging for evidence of recurrence, with frequency of imaging determined by national guidelines and stage at diagnosis. Solitary locally recurrent or metastatic lesions may be treated with metastasectomy or focal radiation therapy in the context of multidisciplinary discussion.
- **Metastatic clear cell RCC.** There are now four FDA-approved frontline combination regimens that have demonstrated an overall survival benefit in patients with advanced clear cell RCC. International Metastatic RCC Database Consortium (IMDC) favorable risk patients appear to benefit from combination therapy with checkpoint inhibitor immunotherapy (CPI) and a TKI. Approved regimens include axitinib/pembrolizumab, cabozantinib/nivolumab, and lenvatinib/pembrolizumab.[27–32] These regimens have also demonstrated an overall survival benefit in patients with IMDC intermediate/poor risk disease, as has doublet CPI therapy with ipilimumab/nivolumab.[33,34] Multiple second-line regimens are now available, including cabozantinib monotherapy, lenvatinib/everolimus combination therapy, and many clinical trials are currently ongoing.
- **Metastatic non–clear cell RCC.** Given the heterogeneity of non–clear cell RCC, there is no one single optimal regimen for each subtype. When feasible, patients should preferentially be offered enrollment in clinical trials. The SWOG1500 clinical trial did demonstrate a longer progression-free survival in patients with metastatic papillary RCC compared with other MET inhibitors.[35] Lenvatinib/pembrolizumab was evaluated in the basket non–clear cell RCC KEYNOTE-B61 trial, with activity in most histologic

subtypes.[36] Cabozantinib/nivolumab has also demonstrated activity in non–clear cell RCC, with the exception of the chromophobe subtype, which had overall lower activity.[37]

Testicular Cancer

GENERAL PRINCIPLES

Due to remarkable advances in treatment, testicular cancer is now one of the most curable solid organ cancers. This is especially important since it affects a much younger population than most neoplasms. The 5-year survival rate is now over 95%.

Classification

Testicular tumors are divided into **seminoma** and **nonseminoma tumors**. The nonseminoma tumors include embryonal carcinomas, teratomas, choriocarcinomas, and mixed germ cell types. Leydig, granulosa, and Sertoli cell tumors occur rarely. Nonseminomas are clinically more aggressive tumors. If elements of both seminoma and nonseminoma are found on biopsy, management follows that of nonseminoma, which is the more aggressive tumor type.

Epidemiology

According to the ACS, 9,190 new cases of testicular cancer are anticipated in 2023. Although these tumors represent only 2% of all human malignancies, it remains the most common cancer among men aged 15–35 years.

Risk Factors

Although it can affect men of any age, 9 out of 10 cases are in men between 20 and 54 years of age. For unclear reasons, white men have five times the risk of Black men and three times the risk of Asian Americans. Other risk factors include cryptorchidism, Klinefelter syndrome, and family history.

DIAGNOSIS

Clinical Presentation

A **painless testicular mass** is the classic presenting symptom. Testicular pain or swelling can be present, but typically suggests epididymitis or orchitis, and an initial course of antibiotics may be appropriate in this situation. **Gynecomastia** as the first sign of testicular cancer is seen in ~10% of patients. It is due to tumor production of human chorionic gonadotropin (hCG).

Physical Examination

A thorough physical examination is essential in patients with suspected testicular cancer. Examination should focus on the testicles, lymphadenopathy (particularly supraclavicular), scrotal edema, and evaluation for gynecomastia. Early metastases to bone are rare but possible, and back pain can result from bulky retroperitoneal lymphadenopathy.

Laboratories

Three serum markers have roles in testicular cancer: **alpha fetoprotein** (AFP), β-**hCG**, and **lactate dehydrogenase** (LDH). These tumor markers are useful for diagnosis, prognosis, and assessment of treatment. Although nondiagnostic by themselves, it is important to know that pure seminomas do not produce AFP, and β-hCG is elevated in only

15–20% of these cancers. By contrast, AFP and/or β-hCG are elevated in more than 80% of nonseminomas.

Imaging

Testicular ultrasound is the initial test of choice in suspected testicular cancer. Subsequent tests include a **chest x-ray** to rule out pulmonary metastasis and **abdominal and pelvic CT** examination with oral and intravenous contrast to assess nodal enlargement and staging. **Chest CT** should be included if any retroperitoneal lymphadenopathy is present or if there is high suspicion of pulmonary metastasis. Other imaging options, such as bone scan or brain imaging, are guided by the patient's symptoms.

Diagnostic Procedures

Biopsy of a testicular mass should be avoided due to concern for seeding and dissemination of an otherwise curable cancer. A radical inguinal orchiectomy is therefore recommended when workup, including imaging and laboratories, indicates testicular cancer. Transscrotal orchiectomy has an increased risk of seeding. In addition, retroperitoneal lymph node dissection is frequently used in patients with low-stage nonseminomas for staging and curative purposes and to remove remaining viable tumor tissue in the lymph nodes.

TREATMENT

Treatment is **based on histology type and stage**. In general, stage I disease is localized to the testis, stage II disease has spread to retroperitoneal lymph nodes, and stage III disease is metastatic or has spread to nonregional lymph nodes. Prognosis is generally very favorable, with >90% of patients being cured with therapy, including 70–80% of patients with advanced tumors. Sperm banking should be discussed before initiation of any therapy.

- **Seminomas** are radiation and chemotherapy sensitive. Stage I tumors have historically been treated with either adjuvant radiation therapy or single-agent carboplatin for one to two cycles. However, active surveillance is now the preferred option in motivated patients due to its favorable prognosis.[38] Stage II seminomas are treated with radiation therapy in nonbulky disease and cisplatin-based combination chemotherapy, such as BEP (bleomycin, etoposide, cisplatin) in bulky disease. Stage III seminomas are treated similarly to bulky stage II with chemotherapy.
- **Nonseminomas** are less radiosensitive, and patients often require additional surgical therapies following orchiectomy. However, similar to seminomas, active surveillance is the preferred option for stage I tumors in patients who can comply with regular follow-ups. Patients with more extensive disease will often undergo retroperitoneal lymph node dissection for either diagnostic or therapeutic purposes. The major morbidity of this surgery is retrograde ejaculation with resulting infertility, which occurs in ~10% of cases using an open nerve dissection technique. Chemotherapy is recommended if the surgical resection reveals lymph node involvement or in patients with advanced disease. Etoposide and cisplatin with or without bleomycin is the chemotherapeutic regimen of choice.

MONITORING/FOLLOW-UP

Patients with testicular cancer should have close follow-up after diagnosis and treatment. This includes serial chest x-rays, CT scanning of the abdomen and pelvis, and blood work for relevant tumor markers, in addition to a detailed clinical examination. Consensus guidelines recommend tumor markers and chest x-ray monthly for the first year and every 2 months for the second year, as well as abdominal and pelvic CT every 3 months in the first 2 years. PET scan may have a role in surveillance, but this has yet to be fully determined. Screening for **late effects** of platinum-based chemotherapy, most commonly dyslipidemias, cardiovascular disease, and cerebrovascular diseases, should be included in follow-up as well.

Bladder Cancer

GENERAL PRINCIPLES

Bladder cancer is primarily a malignancy of the epithelium. Urothelial (transitional cell) carcinomas are the most common histologic subtype and account for >97% of bladder tumors. Other histologic subtypes include squamous cell carcinoma, adenocarcinoma, and small-cell tumors.

Epidemiology

The ACS estimates that 82,290 new cases of bladder cancer will be diagnosed in 2023, with 16,710 deaths. Similar to prostate cancer, the median age at presentation is late in life (65 years of age). Medical comorbidities and life expectancy play key roles in management decisions.

Risk Factors

Bladder cancer affects men almost threefold more than women. The most important risk factor is **cigarette smoking**, with smokers twice as likely to get bladder cancer as nonsmokers. Other known risk factors include occupational exposure to aromatic amines in the dye industry and work in certain other industries such as rubber, leather, textile, paint, printing, and hairdressing industries. Although uncommon in US, squamous cell carcinoma is a prevalent subtype in areas endemic to *Schistosoma haematobium*.

DIAGNOSIS

Clinical Presentation

Symptoms are not always appreciated by patients, but **hematuria** is present in ~90% of individuals with bladder cancer. This may be intermittent or constant, frank or microscopic, and is occasionally associated with symptoms of urinary frequency or urgency. Any episode of gross hematuria should result in urgent evaluation with prompt urology consultation and cystoscopic evaluation as warranted.

Diagnostic Testing
Laboratories
Urinalysis, including microscopic and gross examination, should be performed to detect the presence and degree of hematuria. **Urine cytology** generally has low sensitivity, but it is usually sent as a noninvasive adjunctive test that may yield the diagnosis.

Imaging
Imaging studies are performed to determine extent of disease involvement, usually after bladder cancer is already confirmed by cystoscopy and transurethral resection of bladder tumor (TURBT). **Abdominal and pelvic CT**, with and without IV contrast, is typically the initial staging test of choice. MRI of the pelvis with bladder protocol may also be utilized. FDG PET scan can be utilized to assess for distant metastatic disease.

Diagnostic Procedures
Cystoscopy is the diagnostic test of choice for evaluation and initial staging of suspected localized bladder cancer. If a suspicious lesion is found on office cystoscopy, cystoscopy is usually repeated under anesthesia for biopsy TURBT.

TREATMENT

For purposes of treatment, bladder cancer is divided into three categories: non–muscle-invasive bladder cancer (NMIBC), muscle-invasive bladder cancer (MIBC), and metastatic urothelial carcinoma.

- **Non–muscle-invasive bladder cancer (NMIBC).** Up to 75% of bladder cancers are noninvasive at presentation. Most can be completely resected by TURBT. Recurrences can occur; therefore, it is recommended that patients undergo cystoscopy every 3 months after initial resection and, depending on level of progression, be considered for intravesical therapy. Intravesical Bacillus Calmette-Guérin (BCG) therapy is still most commonly utilized as first-line therapy for high-risk disease. Intravesical gemcitabine/docetaxel has demonstrated benefit in the BCG refractory setting, and multiple other novel agents are in development and evaluation in clinical trials.
- **Muscle-invasive bladder cancer (MIBC).** The primary treatment modality for curative intent therapy for MIBC is still neoadjuvant cisplatin-based chemotherapy followed by radical cystectomy. The VESPER trial has demonstrated benefit of both neoadjuvant dose-dense MVAC (methotrexate, vinblastine, doxorubicin, and cisplatin with growth factor support) and doublet chemotherapy with cisplatin/gemcitabine, but a modest increase in pathologic complete response rate and trend towards improved overall survival with ddMVAC. Thus, patients who are fit for ddMVAC should be offered this treatment regimen, and all cisplatin-eligible patients should be offered neoadjuvant chemotherapy.[39,40] The ABC meta-analysis has now also demonstrated a 6% overall survival benefit at 5 years for patients receiving adjuvant cisplatin-based chemotherapy; thus, in patients who are still fit for cisplatin after cystectomy, adjuvant therapy should be offered.[41] For high-risk patients with significant residual disease either with or without prior platinum-based neoadjuvant chemotherapy, adjuvant nivolumab demonstrated improved disease-free survival versus placebo in the CheckMate-274 trial.[42] Although overall survival data is still maturing, this is now guideline-approved adjuvant therapy for eligible patients. For patients who are good candidates for bladder preservation with relatively small or unifocal tumors, absence of hydronephrosis, and good baseline bladder function, or are too frail for cystectomy, trimodality therapy (TMT) may be pursued. TMT consists of maximal TURBT followed by concurrent chemotherapy and radiation therapy. Multiple systemic therapy regimens may be utilized depending on patient factors, including cisplatin-based regimens, mitomycin C/5-fluorouracil, or twice-weekly gemcitabine.
- **Metastatic bladder cancer.** Treatment decision making for patients with metastatic disease is centered firstly around eligibility for cisplatin-based chemotherapy, contingent on factors such as performance status, renal function, and comorbidities including peripheral neuropathy, hearing loss, and symptomatic heart failure. In cisplatin-eligible patients, patients should be offered either ddMVAC or cisplatin/gemcitabine.[43,44] Cisplatin-ineligible patients may be treated with frontline carboplatin and gemcitabine.[45] Regarding which platinum agent is used, responding patients after four to six cycles of chemotherapy (complete or partial response or stable disease), should be offered maintenance CPI with avelumab, as this has demonstrated an overall survival benefit compared with placebo.[46] Pembrolizumab monotherapy may also be utilized in cisplatin-ineligible patients, although the objective response rate is only 28% in the overall population.[47] Most recently, combination therapy with the nectin-4 antibody-drug conjugative enfortumab vedotin in conjunction with pembrolizumab has been granted accelerated approval in locally advanced or metastatic urothelial carcinoma as frontline therapy for cisplatin-ineligible patients, with an objective response rate of 64%.[48]

Multiple treatment modalities are now available in the third-line setting and beyond. Enfortumab vedotin monotherapy is associated with an overall survival benefit in the third-line setting postplatinum and after checkpoint inhibitor therapy, and may also be used in the second-line setting.[49,50] The Trop-2 direct antibody–drug conjugate sacituzumab govitecan has also demonstrated activity in the pretreated advanced bladder cancer setting.[51] Molecular testing should be performed for all advanced bladder cancer patients. Approximately 25% of patients with advanced urothelial carcinoma harbor *FGFR3/2* genomic alterations that can be targeted with the FGFR inhibitor erdafitinib, which is approved for patients with susceptible *FGFR3/2* alterations and prior progression on platinum-containing chemotherapy.[52] Both frontline and subsequent treatment paradigms for metastatic urothelial carcinoma continue to advance rapidly.

REFERENCES

1. James ND, De Bono JS, Spears MR, et al. Abiraterone for prostate cancer not previously treated with hormone therapy. *N Engl J Med.* 2017;377(4):338–351.
2. Armstrong AJ, Szmulewitz RZ, Petrylak DP, et al. ARCHES: a randomized, phase iii study of androgen deprivation therapy with enzalutamide or placebo in men with metastatic hormone-sensitive prostate cancer. *J Clin Oncol.* 2019;37(32):2974–2986.
3. Davis ID, Martin AJ, Stockler MR, et al. Enzalutamide with standard first-line therapy in metastatic prostate cancer. *N Engl J Med.* 2019;381(2):121–131.
4. Attard G, Murphy L, Clarke NW, et al. Abiraterone acetate and prednisolone with or without enzalutamide for high-risk non-metastatic prostate cancer: a meta-analysis of primary results from two randomised controlled phase 3 trials of the STAMPEDE platform protocol. *Lancet.* 2022;399(10323): 447–460.
5. Sweeney CJ, Chen Y-H, Carducci M, et al. Chemohormonal therapy in metastatic hormone-sensitive prostate cancer. *N Engl J Med.* 2015;373(8):737–746.
6. Smith MR, Hussain M, Saad F, et al. Darolutamide and survival in metastatic, hormone-sensitive prostate cancer. *N Engl J Med.* 2022;386(12):1132–1142.
7. Fizazi K, Tran N, Fein L, et al. Abiraterone plus prednisone in metastatic, castration-sensitive prostate cancer. *N Engl J Med.* 2017;377(4):352–360.
8. Chi KN, Agarwal N, Bjartell A, et al. Apalutamide for metastatic, castration-sensitive prostate cancer. *N Engl J Med.* 2019;381:13–24.
9. Ryan CJ, Smith MR, De Bono JS, et al. Abiraterone in metastatic prostate cancer without previous chemotherapy. *N Engl J Med.* 2013;368(2):138–148.
10. Beer TM, Armstrong AJ, Rathkopf DE, et al. Enzalutamide in metastatic prostate cancer before chemotherapy. *N Engl J Med.* 2014;371(5):424–433.
11. De Wit R, De Bono J, Sternberg CN, et al. Cabazitaxel versus abiraterone or enzalutamide in metastatic prostate cancer. *N Engl J Med.* 2019;381(26):2506–2518.
12. De Bono JS, Oudard S, Ozguroglu M, et al. Prednisone plus cabazitaxel or mitoxantrone for metastatic castration-resistant prostate cancer progressing after docetaxel treatment: a randomised open-label trial. *Lancet.* 2010;376(9747):1147–1154.
13. Corn PG, Heath EI, Zurita A, et al. Cabazitaxel plus carboplatin for the treatment of men with metastatic castration-resistant prostate cancers: a randomised, open-label, phase 1-2 trial. *Lancet Oncol.* 2019;20(10):1432–1443.
14. Kantoff PW, Higano CS, Shore ND, et al. Sipuleucel-T immunotherapy for castration-resistant prostate cancer. *N Engl J Med.* 2010;363(5):411–422.
15. Abida W, Armenia J, Gopalan A, et al. Prospective genomic profiling of prostate cancer across disease states reveals germline and somatic alterations that may affect clinical decision making. *JCO Precis Oncol.* 2017;2017:PO.17.00029.
16. Robinson D, Van Allen EM, Wu Y-M, et al. Integrative clinical genomics of advanced prostate cancer. *Cell.* 2015;162(2):454.
17. Pritchard CC, Mateo J, Walsh MF, et al. Inherited DNA-repair gene mutations in men with metastatic prostate cancer. *N Engl J Med.* 2016;375(5):443–453.
18. de Bono J, Mateo J, Fizazi K, et al. Olaparib for metastatic castration-resistant prostate cancer. *N Engl J Med.* 2020;382(22):2091–2102.
19. Abida W, Campbell D, Patnaik A, et al. Rucaparib for the treatment of metastatic castration-resistant prostate cancer associated with a DNA damage repair gene alteration: final results from the phase 2 TRITON2 study. *Eur Urol.* 2023;84(3):321–330.

20. Agarwal N, Azad AA, Carles J, et al. Talazoparib plus enzalutamide in men with first-line metastatic castration-resistant prostate cancer (TALAPRO-2): a randomised, placebo-controlled, phase 3 trial. *Lancet.* 2023;402(10398):291–303.
21. Clarke NW, Armstrong AJ, Thiery-Vuillemin A, et al. Abiraterone and olaparib for metastatic castration-resistant prostate cancer. *NEJM Evid.* 2022;1(9):EVIDoa2200043.
22. Parker C, Nilsson S, Heinrich D, et al. Alpha emitter radium-223 and survival in metastatic prostate cancer. *N Engl J Med.* 2013;369(3):213–223.
23. Sartor O, de Bono J, Chi KN, et al. Lutetium-177-PSMA-617 for metastatic castration-resistant prostate cancer. *N Engl J Med.* 2021;385(12):1091–1103.
24. Silverman SG, Israel GM, Trinh Q-D, et al. Incompletely characterized incidental renal masses: emerging data support conservative management. *Radiology.* 2015;275:28–42.
25. Choueiri TK, Tomczak P, Park SH, et al. Adjuvant pembrolizumab after nephrectomy in renal-cell carcinoma. *N Engl J Med.* 2021;385(8):683–694.
26. Powles T, Tomczak P, Park SH, et al. Pembrolizumab versus placebo as post-nephrectomy adjuvant therapy for clear cell renal cell carcinoma (KEYNOTE-564): 30-month follow-up analysis of a multicentre, randomised, double-blind, placebo-controlled, phase 3 trial. *Lancet Oncol.* 2022;23(9):1133–1144.
27. Powles T, Plimack ER, Soulières D, et al. Pembrolizumab plus axitinib versus sunitinib monotherapy as first-line treatment of advanced renal cell carcinoma (KEYNOTE-426): extended follow-up from a randomised, open-label, phase 3 trial. *Lancet Oncol.* 2020;21(12):1563–1573.
28. Rini BI, Plimack ER, Stus V, et al. Pembrolizumab plus axitinib versus sunitinib for advanced renal-cell carcinoma. *N Engl J Med.* 2019;380(12):1116–1127.
29. Motzer R, Alekseev B, Rha S-Y, et al. Lenvatinib plus pembrolizumab or everolimus for advanced renal cell carcinoma. *N Engl J Med.* 2021;384(14):1289–1300.
30. Choueiri TK, Eto M, Motzer R, et al. Lenvatinib plus pembrolizumab versus sunitinib as first-line treatment of patients with advanced renal cell carcinoma (CLEAR): extended follow-up from the phase 3, randomised, open-label study. *Lancet Oncol.* 2023;24(3):228–238.
31. Motzer RJ, Powles T, Burotto M, et al. Nivolumab plus cabozantinib versus sunitinib in first-line treatment for advanced renal cell carcinoma (CheckMate 9ER): long-term follow-up results from an open-label, randomised, phase 3 trial. *Lancet Oncol.* 2022;23(7):888–898.
32. Choueiri TK, Powles T, Burotto M, et al. Nivolumab plus cabozantinib versus sunitinib for advanced renal-cell carcinoma. *N Engl J Med.* 2021;384(9):829–841.
33. Motzer RJ, Tannir NM, Mcdermott DF, et al. Nivolumab plus ipilimumab versus sunitinib in advanced renal-cell carcinoma. *N Engl J Med.* 2018;378(4):1277–1290.
34. Albiges L, Tannir NM, Burotto M, et al. Nivolumab plus ipilimumab versus sunitinib for first-line treatment of advanced renal cell carcinoma: extended 4-year follow-up of the phase III CheckMate 214 trial. *ESMO Open.* 2020;5(6):e001079.
35. Pal SK, Tangen C, Thompson IM, et al. A comparison of sunitinib with cabozantinib, crizotinib, and savolitinib for treatment of advanced papillary renal cell carcinoma: a randomised, open-label, phase 2 trial. *Lancet.* 2021;397(10275):695–703.
36. Albiges L, Gurney H, Atduev V, et al. Pembrolizumab plus lenvatinib as first-line therapy for advanced non-clear-cell renal cell carcinoma (KEYNOTE-B61): a single-arm, multicentre, phase 2 trial. *Lancet Oncol.* 2023;24(8):881–891.
37. Lee C-H, Voss MH, Carlo MI, et al. Phase II trial of cabozantinib plus nivolumab in patients with non-clear-cell renal cell carcinoma and genomic correlates. *J Clin Oncol.* 2022;40(21):2333–2341.
38. Nichols CR, Roth B, Albers P, et al. Active surveillance is the preferred approach to clinical stage I testicular cancer. *J Clin Oncol.* 2013;31(28):3490–3493.
39. Pfister C, Gravis G, Fléchon A, et al. Dose-dense methotrexate, vinblastine, doxorubicin, and cisplatin or gemcitabine and cisplatin as perioperative chemotherapy for patients with nonmetastatic muscle-invasive bladder cancer: results of the GETUG-AFU V05 VESPER trial. *J Clin Oncol.* 2022;40(18):2013–2022.
40. Pfister C, Gravis G, Flechon A, et al. Randomized phase III trial of dose-dense methotrexate, vinblastine, doxorubicin, and cisplatin, or gemcitabine and cisplatin as perioperative chemotherapy for patients with muscle-invasive bladder cancer. analysis of the GETUG/AFU V05 VESPER trial secondary endpoints: chemotherapy toxicity and pathological responses. *Eur Urol.* 2021;79(2):214–221.
41. Burdett S, Fisher DJ, Vale CL, et al. Adjuvant chemotherapy for muscle-invasive bladder cancer: a systematic review and meta-analysis of individual participant data from randomised controlled trials. *Eur Urol.* 2022;81:50–61.
42. Bajorin DF, Witjes JA, Gschwend JE, et al. Adjuvant nivolumab versus placebo in muscle-invasive urothelial carcinoma. *N Engl J Med.* 2021;384(22):2102–2114.

43. von der Maase H, Sengelov L, Roberts JT, et al. Long-term survival results of a randomized trial comparing gemcitabine plus cisplatin, with methotrexate, vinblastine, doxorubicin, plus cisplatin in patients with bladder cancer. *J Clin Oncol.* 2005;23(21):4602–4608.

44. Sternberg CN, de Mulder PH, Schornagel JH, et al. Randomized phase III trial of high-dose-intensity methotrexate, vinblastine, doxorubicin, and cisplatin (MVAC) chemotherapy and recombinant human granulocyte colony-stimulating factor versus classic MVAC in advanced urothelial tract tumors: European Organization for Research and Treatment of Cancer Protocol no. 30924. *J Clin Oncol.* 2001;19(10):2638–2646.

45. De Santis M, Bellmunt J, Mead G, et al. Randomized phase II/III trial assessing gemcitabine/carboplatin and methotrexate/carboplatin/vinblastine in patients with advanced urothelial cancer who are unfit for cisplatin-based chemotherapy: EORTC study 30986. *J Clin Oncol.* 2012;30(2):191–199.

46. Powles T, Park SH, Voog E, et al. Avelumab maintenance therapy for advanced or metastatic urothelial carcinoma. *N Engl J Med.* 2020;383(13):1218–1230.

47. Balar AV, Castellano DE, Grivas P, et al. Efficacy and safety of pembrolizumab in metastatic urothelial carcinoma: results from KEYNOTE-045 and KEYNOTE-052 after up to 5 years of follow-up. *Ann Oncol.* 2023;34(3):289–299.

48. O'donnell PH, Milowsky MI, Petrylak DP, et al. Enfortumab vedotin with or without pembrolizumab in cisplatin-ineligible patients with previously untreated locally advanced or metastatic urothelial cancer. *J Clin Oncol.* 2023;41(25):4107–4117.

49. Powles T, Rosenberg JE, Sonpavde GP, et al. Enfortumab vedotin in previously treated advanced urothelial carcinoma. *N Engl J Med.* 2021;384:1125–1135.

50. Yu EY, Petrylak DP, O'donnell PH, et al. Enfortumab vedotin after PD-1 or PD-L1 inhibitors in cisplatin-ineligible patients with advanced urothelial carcinoma (EV-201): a multicentre, single-arm, phase 2 trial. *Lancet Oncol.* 2021;22(6):872–882.

51. Tagawa ST, Balar AV, Petrylak DP, et al. TROPHY-U-01: a phase II open-label study of sacituzumab govitecan in patients with metastatic urothelial carcinoma progressing after platinum-based chemotherapy and checkpoint inhibitors. *J Clin Oncol.* 2021;39(22):2474–2485.

52. Siefker-Radtke AO, Necchi A, Park SH, et al. Efficacy and safety of erdafitinib in patients with locally advanced or metastatic urothelial carcinoma: long-term follow-up of a phase 2 study. *Lancet Oncol.* 2022;23(2):248–258.

Gynecologic Oncology

Andrea R. Hagemann

30

T umors of the female reproductive tract are often diagnosed and managed by the combined efforts of the primary care physician, gynecologist, gynecologic oncologist, medical oncologist, and radiation oncologist. This chapter describes the approach to common gynecologic oncology evaluations and briefly discusses selected gynecologic tumors.

Vaginal Bleeding

GENERAL PRINCIPLES

Vaginal bleeding can be caused by a wide range of etiologies that may include medical, iatrogenic, gynecologic, or idiopathic reasons. In 2011, Federation of Gynecology and Obstetrics (FIGO) approved a classification system for abnormal uterine bleeding (AUB), referred to as PALM-COEIN (polyp, adenomyosis, leiomyoma, malignancy and hyperplasia; coagulopathy; ovulatory dysfunction; endometrial, iatrogenic; and not yet classified) in order to standardize nomenclature and classification of AUB in order to assist in research, treatment, and prognostication regarding AUB (see Table 30-1). Generally, those etiologies of the PALM group are structural entities that can be measured with imaging techniques and/or histopathology. The COEIN group refers to nonstructural entities not defined by imaging or histopathology. The term dysfunctional uterine bleeding (DUB), previously used as a description of bleeding when there was no systemic or locally definable structural cause, should be abandoned, as most women who previously fit this description generally encompassed various diagnoses that are better described by the PALM-COEIN system. Iatrogenic AUB is defined as bleeding associated with the use of exogenous steroids, intrauterine devices, or other systemic or local agents, while the "not yet classified" category refers to etiologies that are poorly defined or rarely encountered.

DIAGNOSIS

Clinical Presentation

History

A thorough medical and gynecologic history, with careful attention to last menstrual period and amount and duration of bleeding, should be obtained.

Physical Examination

A careful gynecologic exam, including a **speculum exam and pelvic exam,** should be performed. A **Papanicolaou (Pap) smear** should be obtained, and any suspicious cervical or vulvar lesions should be biopsied. A **rectal exam with stool guaiac** should also be performed.

TABLE 30-1	ABNORMAL UTERINE BLEEDING
PALM: Structural Causes	**COEIN: Nonstructural Causes**
Polyp	Coagulopathy
Adenomyosis	Ovulatory dysfunction
Leiomyoma	Endometrial
Malignancy/hyperplasia	Iatrogenic
	Not yet classified

Diagnostic Testing

Laboratories

Appropriate laboratory studies include a **complete blood count** to detect anemia or thrombocytopenia and a pregnancy test in reproductive-age women. In certain individuals, **thyroid-stimulating hormone** and screening **coagulation studies** may be appropriate to rule out thyroid dysfunction and a primary coagulation problem, respectively. Von Willebrand disease is a common cause of heavy menses, especially in adolescent women.

Diagnostic Procedures

Women with chronic anovulation, women with obesity, and those older than 35 years of age require further evaluation. A **transvaginal ultrasound** can be helpful in evaluating for anatomic abnormalities, and assessment of endometrial stripe thickness may prove useful in postmenopausal women. **Endometrial sampling,** accomplished in the office using disposable plastic cannulae, should be performed in these women, as they are at risk for polyps, hyperplasia, or carcinoma of the endometrium.

TREATMENT

Medications

In most cases, abnormal bleeding can be managed medically. Acute, profound vaginal bleeding should first be managed by assessing for a primary coagulation disorder. If anovulatory bleeding is established as the working diagnosis, **hormonal therapy** with oral or intravenous estrogen will usually control bleeding. If hormonal management fails, a structural cause of bleeding is more likely. Hormonal management, including oral contraceptives, can be used to significantly reduce blood flow. When estrogen is contraindicated, progestins can be used, including cyclic oral medroxyprogesterone acetate, depot forms of medroxyprogesterone acetate, and the levonorgestrel-containing intrauterine device, which has been shown to decrease menstrual blood loss by 80–90%.

Surgical Management

Options range from dilatation and curettage (D&C), hysteroscopy with resection of uterine polyps or leiomyomas, myomectomy, uterine artery embolization, magnetic resonance-guided focused ultrasonography (US) ablation, and, most definitively, hysterectomy.

Pelvic Masses

A variety of entities may result in the development of a pelvic mass. These may be gynecologic in origin or, alternatively, may arise from the urinary or gastrointestinal (GI) tracts. Gynecologic causes of a pelvic mass may be uterine, adnexal, or, more specifically, ovarian. Age is an important determinant of the likelihood of malignancy.

- **Ovarian masses**

  These can be functional or neoplastic; neoplastic masses can be either benign or malignant.

  ○ **Ovarian cysts.** Functional ovarian cysts include follicular cysts, corpus luteum cysts, and theca lutein cysts. Women with endometriosis can develop ovarian endometriomas. Follicular cysts, defined by a diameter >3 cm, are most common, and are most often <8 cm. They usually resolve spontaneously and only require expectant management. Corpus luteum cysts can rupture, leading to hemoperitoneum, which may occasionally require surgical management. Theca lutein cysts are usually bilateral and occur with pregnancy due to ovarian stimulation by human chorionic gonadotropin (hCG). These cysts may be prominent in certain conditions such as multiple and molar pregnancies. Combination monophasic oral contraceptives can reduce the incidence of these functional cysts.

  ○ **Neoplastic masses.** The most common benign ovarian neoplasm is the mucinous cystadenoma. Eighty percent of cystic teratomas (dermoid cysts) occur during the reproductive years. Epithelial tumors of the ovary increase with age, and benign tumors of this type include serous and mucinous cystadenomas, fibromas, and Brenner tumors. Malignant ovarian neoplasms are discussed in the following section.

  ○ **Other masses.** Adnexal masses arising from the fallopian tube are primarily related to inflammatory causes in the reproductive age group. Examples of masses in this category include ectopic pregnancy, tubo-ovarian abscesses, and paraovarian or paratubal cysts.

- **Uterine masses**

  Uterine leiomyomas, commonly referred to as fibroids, are the most common benign uterine tumors. Asymptomatic fibroids are present in up to 50% of women older than age 35 years. Degenerative changes can occur in these tumors. Smooth muscle tumors of the uterus rather represent a continuum that ranges from benign lesions (leiomyoma or fibroid) to malignant neoplasms (uterine leiomyosarcoma). Smooth muscle tumors of uncertain malignant potential have 5–9 mitoses per 10 high-power fields (hpf) and do not demonstrate nuclear atypia or giant cells. Leiomyosarcomas (LMS) have ≥10 or more mitoses/hpf and demonstrate nuclear atypia.

DIAGNOSIS

Clinical Presentation

History

History should include any history of urinary or GI symptoms, pelvic pain, or vaginal bleeding.

Physical Exam

A complete pelvic exam, including a rectovaginal exam and Pap test, should be performed. Evidence of ascites or a pleural effusion heightens the suspicion of a malignant ovarian tumor.

Diagnostic Testing

Laboratory and Diagnostic Procedures

Workup usually includes **cervical cytology, complete blood count,** testing of **stool for occult blood,** and a **pregnancy test** in reproductive-age women. **CA-125** is a nonspecific tumor marker that may be obtained, but be aware that a number of benign conditions, including leiomyomas, pelvic inflammatory disease, pregnancy, and endometriosis, to name a few, can cause elevations of this marker. **Endometrial sampling** with an endometrial biopsy or D&C is necessary if both a pelvic mass and abnormal bleeding are present.

Imaging

Pelvic US, usually done transvaginally, will help to clarify the origin and characteristics of gynecologic masses. Additional imaging by means of computed tomography and/or magnetic resonance can be used in selected cases to further delineate the anatomy or evaluate concurrently other anatomic sites. A barium enema or endoscopic study of the lower GI tract may be indicated to exclude a GI etiology.

TREATMENT

- Once a nongynecologic problem is excluded, **management depends on the location and size of the mass as well as the age of the patient.** Premenopausal women with an adnexal mass <8 cm, with predominantly cystic features, can be followed with close observation and/or hormonal suppression. Women with a mass >8 cm, those with complex, solid, or suspicious features on ultrasound, and those whose masses persist or progress with close follow-up should be managed surgically by a gynecologist or a gynecologic oncologist.
- The American College of Obstetrics and Gynecologists, along with the Society of Gynecologic Oncologists, released guidelines for referral to a gynecologic oncologist for a pelvic mass. In these guidelines, they state that premenopausal women with any of the following should be referred: CA-125 >200 U/mL, ascites, evidence of abdominal or distant metastasis (by imaging or exam), or family history of breast or ovarian cancer in a first-degree relative. The criteria for referral for postmenopausal women are slightly different: CA-125 >35 U/mL, ascites, evidence of abdominal or distant metastasis (by imaging or exam), and family history of breast or ovarian cancer in a first-degree relative. Surgery can be done laparoscopically or by laparotomy depending on the size of the mass and concern for malignancy.
- Most postmenopausal women with an adnexal mass should undergo surgery to rule out an ovarian malignancy.
- The resection of benign uterine masses can be undertaken by various surgical approaches. Endocervical or endometrial polyps, as well as uterine leiomyomas protruding into the uterine cavity, may be removed under hysteroscopic guidance. The surgical treatment of leiomyomas may also be addressed via open or laparoscopic myomectomy, involving resection of only leiomyomatous tissue with uterine conservation, or total/supracervical hysterectomy. An open versus minimally invasive surgical approach depends upon many factors, including surgeon experience, size, and location of the leiomyomas, and several patient-related factors, including surgical history, body mass index, comorbidities, and desire for uterine retention and/or future fertility. In the minimally invasive surgical approach whether during myomectomy, total laparoscopic hysterectomy, or supracervical laparoscopic hysterectomy, tissue morcellation has previously been employed to remove large pieces of leiomyoma from the uterine cavity. However, given the concern of undiagnosed uterine malignancy, especially leiomyosarcoma, in women undergoing tissue morcellation, the use of morcellation should be surgically confined (within a bag) in order to minimize the risk of dissemination of malignant tissue.

Cervical Cancer

GENERAL PRINCIPLES

Classification

The most common histologic types identified in cases of invasive cervical cancer are squamous cell carcinoma (85%) and adenocarcinoma (5%). Less common histologies include neuroendocrine carcinoma, melanoma, and sarcomas (embryonal rhabdomyosarcoma in children and young adults).

Epidemiology

In 2023, there were an estimated 13,960 new cases of invasive cervical cancer in the US, resulting in 4,310 deaths. Even though screening programs are well established, cervical cancer is still the leading cause of death from cancer among women in developing countries and second only to breast cancer worldwide.

Risk Factors

Invasive cancer of the cervix is considered a preventable disease. There is a long preinvasive state (cervical dysplasia), and cytologic screening programs as well as effective treatments are readily available. Cervical intraepithelial neoplasia is a precancerous lesion of the cervix.

Several risk factors for cervical cancer have been identified. These include young age at first intercourse (<16 years), multiple sexual partners, cigarette smoking, immunosuppression, African American or Hispanic ethnicity, high parity, and lower socioeconomic status. **Human papillomavirus (HPV) infection** is considered to play a causal role and can be detected in up to 99% of women with cervical cancer.

Prevention

- Cervical cancer can be prevented by detecting and treating cervical dysplasia, thus avoiding progression from the preinvasive into the invasive state. The **Pap smear** has previously been the standard screening test for cervical cancer, however, given an increased understanding of the association between HPV and cervical cancer risk, the development of molecular tests for HPV have allowed for the potential for increased disease detection and increased length of screening intervals when used independently or alongside cytology.
- Cervical cytology screening should begin no earlier than 21 years, and women aged 21–29 years should undergo screening with cytology alone every 3 years. Women aged 30–65 years should undergo HPV and cytology contesting every 5 years (preferred screening method) or cytology alone every 3 years (acceptable screening method). For those women >65 years of age, no cervical cancer screening is necessary following adequate negative prior screening, although women with a history of CIN2 or a more severe diagnosis should continue routine screening for at least 20 years. For women without a history of CIN2 or a more severe diagnosis in the past 20 years who have undergone a hysterectomy, no cervical cancer screening is necessary.
- A quadrivalent **vaccine** against HPV types 6, 11, 16, and 18 (Gardasil®), is now approved for females and males aged 9–26 years. A bivalent vaccine (types 16 and 18) is also approved (Cervarix®) for girls 10–25 years of age. A 9-valent vaccine against HPV types 6, 11, 16, and 18, as well as types 31, 33, 45, 52, and 58 (Gardasil 9®) has recently been approved for girls ages 9–26 and males ages 9–15. Age-appropriate cervical cancer screening is still recommended for those receiving the vaccine. There has been a 65% drop in cervical cancer incidence from 2012 through 2019 among women in their early 20s, the first cohort to receive the HPV vaccine.

DIAGNOSIS

Clinical Presentation

The most common symptom in women with cancer of the cervix is **vaginal bleeding**, which can often be postcoital. Asymptomatic women are usually diagnosed on the basis of abnormal cytology. Advanced disease may present with symptoms of malodorous discharge, weight loss, or obstructive uropathy. Physical exam may reveal a palpable cervical mass, and palpation of the inguinal and supraclavicular nodes may reveal lymphadenopathy.

Diagnostic Testing

If a gross lesion is present, **cervical biopsy** should be performed. Abnormal cytologic screening should be evaluated as indicated with colposcopy and directed biopsies, along with endocervical curettage. Cervical cancer is a clinically staged disease, often via an exam under anesthesia to yield the most accurate assessment. Cystoscopy, proctoscopy, chest radiographs, and intravenous pyelograms may be used for staging purposes. CT, MRI, and PET scans are commonly used in the evaluation of disease extension and for treatment planning. However, such imaging modalities should not alter the clinical stage.

TREATMENT

The treatment of cervical cancer is **determined by the clinical stage of disease,** with the underlying principle that therapy should ideally consist of either radiation or surgery alone in order to prevent increased morbidity that results when the two are combined. Stage by stage, these modalities are equivalent in terms of survival outcomes.

Radiation Therapy

Radiation therapy can be classified as either primary or adjuvant therapy. **Primary therapy** combines external radiotherapy to treat parametria and regional lymph nodes and to lessen tumor volume with brachytherapy to target the central tumor. Brachytherapy is delivered by intracavitary or interstitial implants. Intensity-modulated radiotherapy utilizes computer algorithms to distinguish between normal and diseased tissues in order to optimize the delivery of radiation to the affected area while minimizing radiation complications. **Adjuvant radiotherapy** is often used postoperatively for patients with metastases to pelvic lymph nodes or channels, invasion of paracervical tissue, deep cervical invasion, or positive surgical margins. Adjuvant radiotherapy has been shown to decrease pelvic recurrence, but not necessarily to improve 5-year survival rates. Complications of radiation therapy include vasculitis and fibrosis of the bowel and bladder, as well as bowel and bladder fistulas.

Chemotherapy

Randomized trials have shown that the addition of chemotherapy to radiation therapy (known as chemoradiation) improves survival in patients with locally advanced cervical cancer. Chemotherapy allows for systemic treatment as well as sensitization of cancer cells to radiation therapy to improve local and regional control. **Cisplatin-based adjuvant chemotherapy** is the treatment of choice for patients with locally advanced cervical cancer. Single-agent platinum or multiagent chemotherapy with platinum in combination with topotecan or paclitaxel is usually prescribed in cases of advanced or recurrent cervical cancer. Multiagent chemotherapy may offer improved response rates and modest survival benefits at the expense of increased toxicity.[1] Pembrolizumab in combination with chemotherapy has been shown to be efficacious for advanced cervical tumors expressing programmed death ligand 1 (PDL1).

Surgical Management

Surgical management is **generally limited to patients with disease limited to the cervix or with limited involvement of the upper vagina.** Depending on the clinical stage, fertility goals, and physical condition of the patient, surgical treatment ranges from cone excision of the cervix to simple hysterectomy, to radical trachelectomy (where the cervix and parametria are removed with preservation of the uterine corpus), to radical hysterectomy. The removal of the ovaries is not part of the surgical therapy and should be considered on an individual basis. In fact, surgery, when feasible, represents an attractive option for younger women as it has the potential to preserve ovarian function and maximize quality of life.

Treatment for Recurrent Disease

Pelvic recurrences in patients initially treated by surgery are usually treated with radiation therapy. Cases of isolated central recurrences after radiation may be salvaged by radical or ultraradical (exenterative) surgical procedures. Systemic recurrences are most often treated with platinum-based chemotherapy typically in conjunction with bevacizumab, a vascular endothelial growth factor (VEGF) inhibitor, which is a first-line treatment for persistent, recurrent, or metastatic cervical cancer, with or without pembrolizumab (depending on PDL1 status).

MONITORING/FOLLOW-UP

Patients treated for cervical cancer require careful follow-up with clinical exams, cytology screening, and various imaging modalities, as indicated. Positron emission tomography at the completion of treatment appears to have important prognostic potential. Similarly, this modality is also capable of identifying localized and potentially salvageable recurrences.

OUTCOME/PROGNOSIS

The 5-year survival rate for early-stage cervical cancer is ~85% with either radiation therapy or radical hysterectomy. For patients with locoregional extension, 5-year survival falls to ≤40%.

Ovarian Cancer

GENERAL PRINCIPLES

Classification

Malignant ovarian tumors can arise from the germinal epithelium, the germ cells, or the sex-cord stroma. The World Health Organization (WHO) has developed and maintained a complex classification schema for ovarian tumors. Most malignant epithelial tumors are high-grade serous adenocarcinomas. Other histologies include the mucinous, endometrioid, clear cell, and transitional cell types. Mixed varieties and other rare variants also exist (squamous cell, undifferentiated, and neuroendocrine). The following discussion concentrates on epithelial ovarian cancer.

Epidemiology

In the US, 1 in 70 women will develop ovarian cancer in their lifetime (lifetime risk, ~1.4%). In 2023, it is estimated that 19,710 new cases of ovarian cancer will be diagnosed in the US, and 13,270 deaths will be expected to occur as a result of ovarian cancer. Epithelial ovarian cancer, which accounts for ~90% of all ovarian cancers, remains the leading cause of death from gynecologic cancer in the US. This type of cancer is often diagnosed at an advanced stage, as patients usually remain asymptomatic until metastasis occurs. The peak incidence of invasive epithelial ovarian cancer is 56–60 years of age. Germ cell and sex-cord stromal tumors are less common and typically occur in adolescents and younger women.

Risk Factors

Ovarian cancer has been associated with low parity and infertility; risk factors include early menarche and late menopause. Oral contraceptive use for ≥5 years has been shown to reduce the likelihood of ovarian cancer by 50%. Mutations in BRCA1 and BRCA2, moderate penetrance genes such as *RAD51C, RAD51D, BRIP1*, and Lynch or hereditary nonpolyposis colorectal cancer syndrome (HNPCC), are important genetic susceptibility factors for developing ovarian cancer. Women found to carry any of these genes should seek age- and fertility-appropriate care and counseling with a gynecologic oncologist to discuss risk-reduction strategies.

Prevention

There is considerable public controversy regarding ovarian cancer screening, but unfortunately, the value of tumor markers and US to screen for epithelial ovarian cancer has not been clearly established by prospective studies. The tumor marker CA-125 has played an important role in the diagnosis, management, and follow-up of patients with ovarian cancer. Particularly in premenopausal women, **CA-125 testing and transvaginal US have not been shown to be cost-effective and should not be used routinely to screen for ovarian cancer in the general population.** Different screening strategies are an active area of study in ovarian cancer research. Many ovarian cancers may in fact arise from the fallopian tubes. Salpingectomy reduces the risk of ovarian cancer in the general population and is an option for patients with hereditary cancer risk who are not yet ready for oophorectomy.

DIAGNOSIS

Clinical Presentation

- Symptoms from ovarian cancer can be vague and nonspecific, and many women remain asymptomatic for long periods of time. Abdominal distention, nausea, vomiting, early satiety, and increased abdominal girth may be reported.
- In premenopausal women, irregular or heavy menses may be noted. The Society of Gynecologic Oncologists has presented the Ovarian Cancer Symptoms Consensus Statement in an attempt to educate the general public about the signs and symptoms of ovarian cancer. The document states that women who have certain symptoms (bloating, pelvic and abdominal pain, difficulty eating, and early satiety as well as urinary urgency or frequency) on a daily basis for more than a few weeks should be specifically evaluated to rule out the possibility of ovarian cancer by means of a skillful pelvic exam, ultrasound examination, and CA-125 determination, as indicated. However, the value of screening for symptoms to diagnose ovarian cancer remains highly controversial.
- The most important sign on physical exam is the presence of a pelvic mass, abdominal mass, or ascites. Pleural effusions are not uncommon.

Diagnostic Testing

The diagnosis of ovarian cancer is most often made by surgical exploration and pathologic confirmation. Prior to exploratory laparotomy, a **CA-125 level** should be drawn, and other primary cancers metastatic to the ovaries should be excluded, specifically colon, gastric, or breast (via barium enema or colonoscopy, upper GI, and mammogram, respectively). Preoperative evaluation may also include a **CT of the chest, abdomen, and pelvis** to assess for extra-abdominal disease and parenchymal liver lesions. In certain circumstances, a preoperative pathologic diagnosis can be obtained by **cytologic study of pleural/ascitic fluid** or percutaneous biopsy.

TREATMENT

Surgical Management

Treatment of ovarian cancer has historically begun with surgical staging and cytoreduction. Thorough surgical staging is essential, as subsequent treatment will be based directly on the surgical stage. Cytoreduction, or debulking, refers to removing as much gross tumor as technically feasible. Surgical cytoreduction to no gross visible residual disease has been found to confer a significant survival advantage and remains the goal of surgery in the adjuvant or neoadjuvant setting.

Chemotherapy and Biologics

After cytoreductive surgery, adjuvant chemotherapy with a taxane- and platinum-containing compound is used unless precluded by toxicity. Multiple studies have evaluated the role of intraperitoneal (IP) chemotherapy in patients with ovarian cancer. While a randomized prospective Gynecologic Oncology Group (GOG172) study showed that IP cisplatin with intravenous paclitaxel improves disease-free and overall survival compared to intravenous cisplatin and paclitaxel in patients with optimally cytoreduced ovarian cancer, IP chemotherapy has significant toxicity, and has fallen out of favor in lieu of advances in combination chemotherapy with drugs that treat the microenvironment. The addition of bevacizumab to intravenous carboplatinum and paclitaxel followed by bevacizumab maintenance is associated with improvement in progression-free survival.[2]

Up to 18% of epithelial ovarian cancers are secondary to germline BRCA1/2 mutations, and a further 5–10% are secondary to other associated pathogenic mutations (Minion, Zhang). Results of genetic testing may have profound implications for family members, who can choose to undergo closer surveillance or risk-reducing measures should they also be found to carry a mutation. Testing results can also impact patient treatment, as there now exist multiple FDA-approved anticancer agents for BRCA mutation carriers. Given the high incidence of germline mutations in these patients, and the implications of a mutation for both patients and family, current national guidelines, including the 2014 SGO Clinical Practice Statement, recommend that all patients with ovarian, fallopian, or peritoneal cancer should be offered germline genetic testing.

Over the last decade, several poly(ADP-ribose) polymerase (PARP) inhibitors have been developed for therapeutic use in ovarian cancer, with particular benefit being demonstrated in patients with BRCA1/2 mutations. PARP is an enzyme involved in single-strand DNA repair. Defects in this enzymatic mechanism ultimately lead to single-strand breaks, which in turn lead to double-strand DNA breaks. In an homologous recombination deficiency (HRD)-deficient cell, such as a BRCA-mutated cell, the double-strand break cannot be repaired and cell death ensues. Multiple clinical trials have proved the efficacy of PARP inhibitors (PARPis) in improving progression-free survival in patients with BRCA1 and BRCA2 mutations and a diagnosis of ovarian cancer (15-21). Based on the success of these clinical trials, the current standard of care is to use PARPis as maintenance therapy after adjuvant chemotherapy, especially in the population of patients with HR-deficiency mutations.

Given the approval of PARPis use in patients with BRCA1 and BRCA2 and HR-deficient tumors, there is an increasing utilization of somatic tumor testing at time of diagnosis or initial surgery in patients with epithelial ovarian cancer. Approximately 3–9% of patients will have somatic alterations in BRCA1 or BRCA2 despite being germline negative. However, it is important to note that somatic testing does not obviate the need for germline testing, as it remains possible for a tumor to be BRCA1 or BRCA2 negative even if the patient does harbor a pathogenic germline variant.

Neoadjuvant and Maintenance Chemotherapy

- A multinational Phase III study recently demonstrated noninferiority of neoadjuvant chemotherapy followed by interval cytoreduction compared to up-front surgery followed by intravenous chemotherapy. Neoadjuvant chemotherapy must be considered in patients with obvious unresectable disease and medical comorbidities precluding up-front surgical cytoreduction.[3]
- The use of staging laparoscopy has become a common approach to describe intra-abdominal diffusion of advanced ovarian cancer and to determine which patients may be candidates for neoadjuvant chemotherapy. The Fagotti laparoscopic score assesses the

degree of omental caking, peritoneal carcinomatosis, diaphragmatic carcinomatosis, mesenteric retraction, bowel infiltration, stomach infiltration, and spleen/liver metastases to predict resectability of disease. Those patients with a high Fagotti score are considered candidates for neoadjuvant chemotherapy rather than upfront resection of disease.

Treatment for Recurrent Disease

Treatment in the recurrent setting usually consists of chemotherapy. Selected patients will undergo secondary cytoreductive surgery. In general, patients who present with recurrence or progression more than 6 months after platinum-based chemotherapy are **"platinum sensitive"** and therefore treated with combination chemotherapy including platinum compounds. Those who have recurrences within 6 months of platinum-based therapy are considered **platinum resistant**. These patients are treated with second-line chemotherapy agents such as pegylated liposomal doxorubicin, topotecan, and gemcitabine, among others. Biologic and/or hormonal agents are used in selected cases, alone or in combination with cytotoxic chemotherapy. Mirvetuximab soravtansine, an antibody–drug conjugate that targets folate receptor alpha-expressing ovarian cancer cells, is the most recent drug approved by the FDA for platinum-resistant ovarian cancer.

MONITORING/FOLLOW-UP

After completion of adjuvant therapy, patients are typically followed with clinical exams, Ca-125 levels, and imaging studies if clinically or biochemically indicated. Recent randomized data have called into question the benefits derived from routine surveillance using Ca-125. There appears to be no survival benefit derived from biochemical screening followed by "earlier" therapeutic intervention when compared to clinical follow-up.

OUTCOME/PROGNOSIS

Surgical staging is the most important prognostic variable for patients with ovarian cancer. Five-year survival rates are estimated to be 75–95% for patients with disease limited to the ovaries and 10–25% for those with extensive peritoneal disease or extraperitoneal metastases at diagnosis. Other independent prognostic variables include extent of residual disease after primary surgery, histologic grade, volume of ascites, patient age, performance status, and platinum-free interval before recurrence. Surgical management by a gynecologic oncologist experienced in the management of this disease has consistently been associated with better outcomes.

Endometrial Cancer

GENERAL PRINCIPLES

Classification and Risk Factors

Patients with endometrial carcinomas can be generally classified into two groups. The largest group is represented by **estrogen-dependent or type I tumors**. These patients tend to be younger at diagnosis. Unopposed estrogenic stimulation of the endometrium in these cases is thought to cause endometrial hyperplasia and well- to moderately differentiated endometrioid carcinomas. Tumors of this type usually carry an overall better prognosis. Risk factors for type I endometrial cancer (EC) include iatrogenic unopposed stimulation of estrogenic receptors in the uterus (estrogens or selective estrogen receptor modulators such as tamoxifen), chronic anovulation, truncal obesity, diabetes mellitus, hypertension, nulliparity, and late menopause. **Type II** patients are on average older at diagnosis and lack evidence of sustained unopposed estrogenic endometrial exposure as their main risk factor. Tumors in this group tend to be poorly differentiated and include more uncommon and aggressive histologic subtypes such as clear cell, papillary serous carcinoma, and carcinosarcoma (malignant mixed mullerian tumor).

Recently, consensus guidelines have been updated, incorporating the Proactive Molecular risk classifier for Endometrial Cancer (ProMisE), a validated molecular profiling algorithm to stratify treatment and prognosis for women with early-stage EC. Testing for *POLE*, MMR, and p53 may be more predictive of EC outcomes; traditional histologic and pathologic criteria for reporting EC may not be fully reproducible or predictive of prognosis.[4]

Epidemiology

EC is the most common gynecologic malignancy diagnosed in developed countries and accounts for more than 90% of malignancies affecting the uterine corpus. It is estimated that in 2023, 66,200 new cases of uterine cancer would be diagnosed and 13,030 women would die of this disease in the US. The median age at diagnosis is 63 years. Most women present at early stage, yet incidence and mortality rates continue to rise.[2,5] Racial and socioeconomic disparities in EC outcomes have been elucidated and continue to widen.[3]

Prevention

- Since <50% of cases of EC will have abnormalities on a Pap smear, evaluation of the endometrial cavity to rule out malignancy requires histologic evaluation. Several biopsy devices are currently available and allow for endometrial sampling to be performed in the office setting with a sensitivity >90%. However, screening for EC at the general population level is currently not recommended.
- Biopsy of the endometrium for screening purposes should be reserved for women at high risk. This includes postmenopausal women who have been treated with unopposed estrogen replacement therapy, premenopausal women with prolonged untreated chronic anovulation, and patients with estrogen-producing tumors. Tamoxifen use does not represent an indication for endometrial surveillance with ultrasound or biopsy in asymptomatic patients.
- EC is associated with Lynch syndrome (HNPCC) as well as other familial cancer syndromes. Women diagnosed with Lynch syndrome have a 40% lifetime risk of developing EC. Prophylactic hysterectomy with bilateral salpingo-oophorectomy is an effective strategy for preventing endometrial and ovarian cancer in these women.

DIAGNOSIS

Clinical Presentation

- More than 90% of cases will initially present with **abnormal uterine bleeding**. Therefore, the presence of abnormal peri- or postmenopausal bleeding should prompt immediate and thorough evaluation to rule out the presence of a gynecologic malignancy. If cervical stenosis is present, pyometra or hematometra may develop. Physical exam is usually unremarkable. Slight uterine enlargement may occasionally be present.
- A detailed history and physical examination should be performed. Physical examination may offer evidence of chronic anovulation. Pelvic and rectal exams will allow a complete evaluation of the genital tract and pelvic structures. This will assist in ruling out other diagnoses and assessing the presence of extrauterine extension.

Diagnostic Testing

Office **endometrial biopsy** is very accurate (>90% sensitive) in detecting endometrial carcinoma. Patients with a nondiagnostic office biopsy or negative biopsies in the context of high clinical suspicion should be further evaluated with hysteroscopy and D&C.

Initial evaluation usually includes investigation of blood counts, liver and renal function, and radiologic imaging as needed to evaluate for suspected advanced disease. This should include, at a minimum, a chest radiograph. When elevated, CA-125 may suggest extrauterine disease and assist in evaluating response to treatment.

TREATMENT

Surgical Management

All patients who are medically fit should undergo surgical exploration with complete staging. The surgical staging procedure includes pelvic washings for cytologic evaluation, evaluation of peritoneal surfaces with directed biopsies as indicated, extrafascial hysterectomy with bilateral salpingo-oophorectomy, and pelvic and para-aortic lymph node dissection. Nodal dissection can be omitted in cases of well-differentiated adenocarcinoma without myometrial invasion. Sentinel lymph node biopsies, done via injection of dye into the cervix preoperatively and with near-infrared technology with minimally invasive surgeries, have now become commonplace. The majority of initial surgical staging and treatment of EC is done by minimally invasive laparoscopy or robotic surgery.

Radiation Therapy

- Adjuvant treatment with radiation and/or cytotoxic chemotherapy is indicated for extrauterine disease or those with high-risk clinicopathologic features (high-grade, deep myometrial invasion, and/or lymph-vascular space invasion).
- The use of adjuvant radiotherapy in patients with early-stage EC has not been proven to improve survival, but may play a role in preventing local recurrences that can have an important impact on the quality of life for these patients. Radiation modalities include the use of vaginal brachytherapy, external radiotherapy, and intensity-modulated radiotherapy.

Chemotherapy and Biologics

- Many cytotoxic chemotherapeutic agents have been evaluated in patients with EC.[6] The objective response rates to several cytotoxic agents have varied widely. **Platinum compounds** (cisplatin and carboplatin), **taxanes** (paclitaxel), and **doxorubicin** are among the most active agents and are commonly used alone or in combination for the treatment of advanced cases, with response rates ranging from 20% to >40%. Other cytotoxic agents such as topotecan, pegylated liposomal doxorubicin, and gemcitabine are also used in the advanced and recurrent setting.
- Growing understanding of genetic alterations caused by DNA mismatch repair deficiencies (dMMR) or presence of microsatellite instability (MSI-H) has been actively explored to guide drug development in EC. Nearly 30% of endometrial tumors present with increased numbers of somatic mutations attributable to deficiencies in MMR and express a large number of neoantigens, potentially rendering them more susceptible to immunotherapy. Understanding the mutational profile has now become critical in guiding treatment for advanced and recurrent EC.

   In the adjuvant advanced disease setting, platinum/taxane combined with either pembrolizumab or dostarlimab has been shown to improve progression-free survival.
- The combination of oral Lenvatinib and pembrolizumab is FDA-approved for use in patients with advanced EC that is not MSI-H or dMMR, and have disease progression following prior systemic therapy, and are not candidates for curative surgery or radiation.
- Pembrolizumab and dostarlimab are now approved for use in patients with unresectable or metastatic, MSI-H/dMMR solid tumors that have progressed following prior treatment and who have no satisfactory alternative treatment options.

   Hormonal manipulation with high-dose progestins approaches response rates of 20% in the presence of estrogen and progesterone receptors. This approach is often used for patients with advanced or recurrent disease whose tumors tested positive for these receptors (most commonly well-differentiated or moderately differentiated tumors) or in those with contraindication for cytotoxic chemotherapy or radiation.

Treatment for Recurrent Disease

Vaginal recurrences can often be salvaged with radiation therapy. Single-site recurrences may be amenable to surgical resection and/or radiation. Distant failures are typically treated with chemotherapy as previously discussed.

MONITORING/FOLLOW-UP

Patients are followed with periodic clinical exams and imaging studies if clinically indicated.

OUTCOME/PROGNOSIS

Early diagnosis in patients presenting with early symptoms accounts for high cure rates in patients with EC. In general, long-term survivorship exceeds 75%. Patients with localized disease and well-differentiated tumors are usually cured by hysterectomy and bilateral salpingo-oophorectomy alone.

Several factors are associated with prognosis in patients with EC. These include histologic type, age at diagnosis, tumor grade and stage, depth of myometrial invasion, and presence of lymph-vascular invasion. Overall, the survival by FIGO stage in EC approaches 85% for stage I, 75% for stage II, 45% for stage III, and 25% for stage IV disease. However, these figures can vary considerably depending on tumor grade, histologic type, and other clinicopathologic variables.

Uterine Sarcomas

GENERAL PRINCIPLES

Uterine sarcomas are a heterologous group of rare malignancies that arise from the myometrium or connective tissue elements within the endometrium. They are typically more aggressive and carry a worse prognosis.

Classification and Risk Factors

Uterine sarcomas fall into two broad categories histologically: mesenchymal tumors and mixed mesenchymal and epithelial tumors. Mesenchymal tumors include LMS, endometrial stromal sarcomas (ESS), and smooth muscle tumors of uncertain potential (STUMP), as well as mixed endometrial stromal and smooth muscle tumors. ESS have been previously described as either low or high grade; however, the term endometrial stromal sarcoma now refers to the low-grade variant, whereas high-grade ESS is now known as high-grade uterine sarcoma (HGUS). A uterine smooth muscle tumor that cannot be diagnosed unequivocally as benign or malignant should be termed as a STUMP, per WHO classification. As of FIGO 2009 staging, carcinosarcomas are now considered metaplastic epithelial carcinomas and are treated similarly to high-grade epithelial carcinomas, rather than based on their sarcomatous elements.

Epidemiology

Uterine sarcomas are rare and comprise approximately 3–10% of all uterine malignancies.

- Uterine LMS represent approximately 1% of all uterine malignancies, and are the most common uterine sarcomas.

- ESS account for 0.2–1% of all uterine malignancies, and approximately 20% of all uterine sarcomas.

Prevention

Given the concern of undiagnosed uterine malignancy, especially LMS, the use of morcellation in postmenopausal women or in women in whom a diagnosis of uterine sarcoma is confirmed or suspected is discouraged.

DIAGNOSIS

In most cases, the diagnosis of uterine sarcomas, especially LMS, cannot be made with certainty preoperatively. Office **endometrial biopsy** may diagnose uterine sarcoma; however, patients with a nondiagnostic office biopsy or negative biopsies in the context of high clinical suspicion should be further evaluated with hysteroscopy and D&C.

Initial evaluation usually includes investigation of blood counts, liver and renal function, and radiologic imaging as needed to evaluate for suspected advanced disease.

Clinical Presentation

- Uterine sarcomas typically present in peri- or postmenopausal women who present with AUB, pelvic pain/pressure, and/or a uterine mass.
- Although a rapidly enlarging uterine mass or large uterine size has been implicated in the diagnosis of uterine sarcoma in the past, these findings may also be present in women with benign disease.
- A detailed history and physical examination should be performed. Pelvic and rectal exams will allow complete evaluation of the genital tract and pelvic structures. Uterine enlargement or the presence of extrauterine disease may be noted on exam.

Diagnostic Testing

- The appearance of LMS on US typically includes a nonhomogeneous appearance and internal echo pattern, central necrosis, and irregular vessel distribution within the tumor. MRI/PET may allow for more specificity, as many findings on US may resemble those of benign leiomyomas.
- Preoperative imaging can be instrumental in surgical planning for ESS, as the tumor has been known to metastasize via the lymphatic and vascular system, as well as along the peritoneum.

TREATMENT

Gynecologic sarcomas in general are viewed as having very aggressive tumor biology, and local and distant relapse is common even after optimal tumor debulking.

Surgical Management

The standard approach to surgical treatment for uterine sarcomas remains total hysterectomy and bilateral salpingo-oophorectomy, with additional surgery as necessary to achieve cytoreduction. The utility of lymphadenectomy for both LMS and ESS may be employed as a cytoreductive technique, however, lymphadenectomy has not been shown to improve survival outcomes.

Radiation Therapy

- For patients with completely resected stage I or II LMS, radiation therapy has not been shown to improve progression-free survival or overall survival.

Chemotherapy and Biologics

- For LMS, no randomized, prospective trial has shown survival benefit to adjuvant chemotherapy. However, doxorubicin has shown activity alone and in combination, as well as gemcitabine and docetaxel.
- Hormonal treatment for uterine LMS, based on the finding that LMS has been shown to express estrogen and progesterone receptors, has been shown to exert only a modest response rate. Consideration for hormonal treatment for LMS may be given to those patients whose tumors strongly and diffusely express ER/PR positivity.
- At this time, with a paucity of clinical evidence regarding cytotoxic treatment, patients diagnosed with HGUS should be encouraged to enroll in clinical trials for soft tissue sarcomas.

Treatment for Advanced/Recurrent Disease

Due to the rarity of uterine sarcomas, there have been few clinical trials dedicated to the chemotherapeutic approach to advanced and/or recurrent disease. Women diagnosed with advanced/recurrent uterine sarcoma should be encouraged to enroll in clinical trials.

- LMS that presents with advanced or recurrent disease may be given consideration for resection of gross disease.
- Doxorubicin has been a standard, first-line treatment for advanced soft tissue sarcoma, and has shown activity in LMS when combined with ifosfamide. Ifosfamide, gemcitabine, and the combination of gemcitabine and docetaxel have also shown activity in advanced and/or recurrent LMS.
- Given the propensity of late recurrence in ESS, consideration of repeated cytoreductions may be given; however, it is unclear at this time how successful repeated cytoreductions may be.
- For ESS, in the event of progression while receiving hormonal treatment, in the absence of hormonal receptors, or when a high-grade variant is noted, cytotoxic chemotherapy in the form of doxorubicin and ifosfamide or gemcitabine plus docetaxel and doxorubicin has been noted to show activity in ESS.
- Although uncommon, STUMPs have been known to recur after resection. Often, a delayed recurrence, but prolonged survival, is noted, necessitating long-term surveillance.

MONITORING/FOLLOW-UP

After completion of adjuvant therapy, patients are typically followed with clinical exams and imaging studies if clinically or biochemically indicated.

OUTCOME/PROGNOSIS

- For LMS patients that present with disease limited to the uterus (~60%), cure rates vary from 20% to 60% based upon the extent of residual disease at the time of primary resection (Gadducci et al., 2008; Major et al., 1993; Ramondetta LM, 2006). There is a 70% rate of recurrence for stage I and II, with the sites of recurrence often noted in the lungs or the liver, evidenced by the aggressive biology of the disease and its hematogenous spread. Generally, uterine LMS is associated with a poor prognosis and 5-year OS rates vary from 25% to 75%. Diagnostic stage is the most important prognostic indicator in LMS.
- Recurrence is common in ESS, with relapse rates between 36% and 56%; however, the median time to recurrence has been shown to be up to 65 months, necessitating long-term oncologic follow-up for these patients (Chang et al., 1990).

Gestational Trophoblastic Disease

This entity encompasses a spectrum of pathologic conditions derived from placental tissues.

GENERAL PRINCIPLES

Classification

- **Complete hydatidiform moles** are tumors characterized by edematous chorionic villi with variable degrees of trophoblastic proliferation. No fetal tissue is identified. Most commonly, they have a 46,XX karyotype resulting from duplication of the paternal haploid chromosomal complement. Approximately 5% of cases have a Y chromosome (46,XY) derived from double sperm fertilization. The uterine size is typically greater than expected for gestational age. It is often possible to identify ovarian theca lutein cysts as a result of ovarian stimulation by large amounts of hCG. The risk of postmolar gestational trophoblastic neoplasia (GTN) in cases of complete moles is ~15–20%.
- **Partial or incomplete moles** have variable and usually just focal villous edema. Trophoblastic proliferation is mild and usually coexists with a fetus or fetal tissues. Most commonly they have a triploid (69,XXX or XXY) chromosomal complement derived from one maternal and two paternal haploid sets of chromosomes. Most cases present as a missed abortion, with uterine size less than that expected for gestational age. The risk of postmolar GTN in cases of partial moles is generally <5%.

Epidemiology

In the US, these conditions are rare and diagnosed in ~1 in 1,500 pregnancies.

DIAGNOSIS

Clinical Presentation

- Patients with **complete moles** usually present in early pregnancy with an **abnormally elevated hCG**. Clinical presentation also includes first-trimester bleeding (95%), excessive uterine enlargement (50%), and medical complications (10–25%) such as hyperemesis gravidarum, early-onset preeclampsia, and hyperthyroidism. These systemic manifestations are mainly seen in cases with uterine enlargement >14- to 16-week size.
- **Incomplete moles** often present as **missed or incomplete abortions** and incidental diagnosis is made upon histologic evaluation of products of conception. With the increased use of ultrasound and measurement of hCG levels in early pregnancy, this condition is usually diagnosed in the first trimester.

Diagnostic Testing

Once the diagnosis of molar pregnancy is suspected, **pelvic ultrasound is the imaging test of choice**. The classic **"snow storm pattern" sonographic appearance** is highly suggestive of molar pregnancy. Patients should be thoroughly evaluated with complete blood counts, coagulation studies, renal and liver function tests, blood type and antibody screen, determination of serum hCG level, and chest radiograph.

TREATMENT

Treatment consists of evacuation of the uterine cavity in the operating room by means of dilatation and suction curettage. High-dose uterotonics are usually administered after evacuation to prevent postevacuation hemorrhage.

MONITORING/FOLLOW-UP

- After evacuation, patients should be monitored with **periodic determinations of serum quantitative hCG levels**. These should be obtained weekly while hCG is elevated and then monthly for 6 months. The objective of this surveillance program is to identify patients who will develop postmolar GTNs. The hCG curve in these patients will usually demonstrate rising or plateaued levels.
- A normal pregnancy during the surveillance period would make identification of GTN by means of hCG follow-up virtually impossible. Therefore, effective contraception should be prescribed to these patients during this surveillance period. Oral contraceptives represent a highly desirable method for the motivated patient. This method does not increase the incidence of postmolar GTN and is usually associated with a cyclic and predictable uterine bleeding pattern.

OUTCOME/PROGNOSIS

- In general, the prognosis associated with this disease is excellent. However, ~20% of patients with complete moles and 5% of those with incomplete moles will go on to develop persistent GTN.
- After a mole, the vast majority of patients will have subsequent normal pregnancies. However, there is a 10-fold increased risk of a second hydatidiform mole (1–2%). Therefore, early obstetric ultrasound should be recommended in all subsequent pregnancies.

Gestational Trophoblastic Neoplasia

GENERAL PRINCIPLES

Classification

The term GTN or gestational trophoblastic tumor (GTT) refers to various histologic entities that have the ability to invade locally and/or metastasize. These conditions include persistent or invasive hydatidiform moles, placental site trophoblastic tumors, and choriocarcinomas.[7] GTN may develop after a normal pregnancy, after a molar pregnancy, or after an abortion or, alternatively, may present primarily.

DIAGNOSIS

Clinical Presentation

Most cases will be diagnosed as a result of **routine hCG level surveillance** after uterine evacuation following a molar pregnancy or a missed/incomplete abortion (plateau or rise in hCG levels). Patients with locally invasive persistent or recurrent disease often report **vaginal bleeding**. Diagnosis in these cases is usually clinical. D&C is generally avoided to prevent potential uterine perforations. Most patients with metastatic disease will have pulmonary involvement (80%). Other relatively common metastatic sites include the vagina (30%), liver, brain, spleen, and/or kidneys (≤10%). Biopsy of metastatic lesions should be avoided to avoid risk of uncontrollable hemorrhage.

Diagnostic Testing

Evaluation should include complete blood counts, coagulation studies, renal and liver function tests, pretreatment determination of serum hCG level, and radiographic survey to assess for metastatic disease in the head, chest, abdomen, and pelvis (usually CT scan and/or MRI).

TABLE 30-2	FIGO ANATOMICAL STAGING FOR GTN

Stage

I	Disease confined to the uterus
II	Disease extends outside of the uterus but is limited to genital structures
III	Disease extends to lungs, with or without known genital tract involvement
IV	All other metastatic sites

TREATMENT

After radiographic studies and clinical determination of risk category (based on age, type of antecedent pregnancy, time interval from index pregnancy, hCG levels, largest tumor size, site and number of metastases, and history of previous failed chemotherapy), patients are assigned a FIGO stage and a WHO risk score (Tables 30-2 and 30-3). A WHO risk score of 0–6 suggests a low risk of resistance to single-agent chemotherapy, while a score of ≥7 predicts a high risk of resistance to monotherapy and requires combination therapy.

Surgical Management

Almost all patients with nonmetastatic GTN can be cured without hysterectomy. These cases are usually treated with single-agent chemotherapy (methotrexate or, less commonly, actinomycin D). In patients without a desire for future fertility, pretreatment hysterectomy will reduce the amount of chemotherapy required to induce remission.

TABLE 30-3	MODIFIED WHO PROGNOSTIC SCORING SYSTEM AS ADAPTED BY FIGO

	Score			
	0	1	2	4
Age	<40	≥40	—	—
Antecedent pregnancy	Mole	Abortion	Term	—
Interval months from index pregnancy	<4	4–6	7–12	>12
Pretreatment serum HCG (IU/L)	$<10^3$	10^3–10^4	10^4–10^5	$>10^5$
Largest tumor size (including uterus)	<3	3–4 cm	≥5	—
Site of metastases	Lung	Spleen/kidney	Gastrointestinal	Liver/brain
Number of metastases	—	1–4	5–8	>8
Previous failed chemotherapy	—	—	Single drug	≥2 drugs

Chemotherapy

- Patients with **nonmetastatic or low-risk metastatic GTN** can be treated with single-agent chemotherapy (methotrexate or actinomycin D). A switch from methotrexate to actinomycin D or vice versa is made if the serum hCG levels plateau or rise.
- The Gynecology Oncology Group is currently investigating how effective methotrexate is compared to actinomycin D in treating patients with low-risk GTN in a phase III randomized trial (GOG 275). A multiday methotrexate regimen (5-day or 8-day regimen) is being evaluated against actinomycin D rather than a standard dose of 50 mg/m^2 that has been previously used.
- Patients with **high-risk metastatic disease** or those who have **failed single-agent treatment** will require multiagent chemotherapy. The most effective and frequently used multiagent regimen involves weekly administration of etoposide, methotrexate, and actinomycin D, alternating with cyclophosphamide and vincristine (EMA/CO). Therapy with methotrexate, actinomycin D, and chlorambucil or cyclophosphamide (MAC) was the standard of care for many years before widespread use of EMA/CO. Salvage regimens usually include combinations with etoposide, cisplatin, and other agents. Occasionally, patients with high-risk metastatic disease will require multimodal treatment, incorporating surgical excision of metastatic lesions and radiotherapy.

MONITORING/FOLLOW-UP

Weekly surveillance of hCG is required during treatment. Chemotherapy is usually continued for approximately 6 weeks after normalization of hCG levels. Additional serum hCG levels are required monthly for 1 year after normalization of hCG levels. Once complete remission is achieved, contraception is recommended and periodic physical exams and hCG levels should be followed strictly for 12 months. Imaging tests are used as necessary.

OUTCOME/PROGNOSIS

GTN is exquisitely sensitive to chemotherapy, and even patients with widespread disease can be cured. Cure rates exceed 95% in patients with nonmetastatic disease. Even in high-risk metastatic cases, multimodal treatment results in cure rates up to 75%.

REFERENCES

1. Long HJ III. Management of metastatic cervical cancer: review of the literature. *J Clin Oncol.* 2007; 25(20):2966–2974.
2. Burger RA, Brady MF, Bookman MA, et al. Phase III trial of bevacizumab (BEV) in the primary treatment of epithelial ovarian cancer (EOC), primary peritoneal cancer (PPC), or fallopian tube cancer: a Gynecologic Oncology Group study. *J Clin Oncol.* 2010;28:946.
3. Vergote I, Tropé CG, Amant F, et al. Neoadjuvant chemotherapy or primary surgery in stage IIIC or IV ovarian cancer. *N Engl J Med.* 2010;363(10):943–953.
4. Siegel RL, Miller KD, Wagle NS, Jemal A. Cancer statistics, 2023. *CA Cancer J Clin.* 2023;73(1):17–48.
5. Rao G, Crispens M, Rothenberg ML. Intraperitoneal chemotherapy for ovarian cancer: overview and perspective. *J Clin Oncol.* 2007;25:2867–2872.
6. Fleming GF. Systemic chemotherapy for uterine carcinoma: metastatic and adjuvant. *J Clin Oncol.* 2007;25(20):2883–2990.
7. Garner EIO, Goldstein DP, Feltmate CM, Berkowitz RS. Gestational trophoblastic disease. *Clin Obstet Gynecol.* 2007;50(1):112–122.

Primary Brain Tumors

31

Kaiden Barozinsky, Kaleigh Roberts, and Omar Hameed Butt

GENERAL PRINCIPLES

Brain tumors encompass a variety of diseases including neoplasms originating in cells of the central nervous system (CNS) (primary) and neoplasms that arise from a malignancy that has metastasized to the CNS (secondary). Here we will focus on primary brain tumors.

Epidemiology

The majority of CNS tumors are nonmalignant (70.3%). Of nonmalignant tumors, meningiomas are the most common (53.9%). Malignant tumors make up 29.7% of all CNS tumors. The most common being glioblastoma (GBM) (48.6%).[1] As age increases, incidence of brain tumors increases and the 5-year survival rate decreases.[1]

Risk Factors

Ionizing radiation and rare genetic predisposition syndromes are known to increase the risk of developing primary brain tumors. Notable syndromes with high risk of CNS tumor development involve alterations in MMR genes (Lynch), NF1, TP53 (Li–Fraumeni), and RB1 (retinoblastoma), among others. Smoking, low-frequency electromagnetic fields (e.g., radio, microwave, TV, radar, cell phones), diet, and BMI are not associated with brain tumor incidence. Notably, history of atopy has been shown to decrease risk of a brain tumor by ~30%.[2]

Grade 4 Gliomas

GENERAL PRINCIPLES

Imaging

MRI is the preferred imaging modality for all brain tumors including high-grade gliomas. Grade 4 gliomas classically have avid T1 post–contrast enhancement and significant vasogenic edema as indicated by hyperintensity on T2 sequences (e.g., FLAIR) with local CNS architectural loss/distortion. The presence of intra- and peritumoral blood products as seen on susceptibility-weighted imaging (SWI) and other heme imaging sequences (GRE/T2*/heme) are also commonly observed. Note that while enhancement and edema are hyperintense compared to surrounding tissue on their respective sequences, blood products are hypointense (black) on heme sequences. The presence of multifocal (ipsilateral multiple lesions), multicentric (bilateral multiple lesions or supra/infra tentorial lesions), or leptomeningeal spread may also be seen and portend poor outcomes.[3]

Classification

In 2021, the Word Health Organization (WHO) revised the classification for gliomas using an integrated method based on histologic and molecular features, building on experience from 2016.[4,5] Classic histologic characteristics associated with high-grade tumors include frequent mitoses, extensive microvascular proliferation, and prominent necrosis. While histologic traits are adequate for accurate diagnosis in many scenarios, select molecular features can also reflect more aggressive tumor phenotypes. In other words, certain molecular alterations (discussed below) can increase the grade of a brain tumor even without the presence of classical high-grade histologic characteristics. Today, there are five major types of grade 4 glioma: (1) GBM, IDH-wild type, (2) astrocytoma, IDH-mutant, (3) diffuse midline glioma, H3 K27-altered, (4) diffuse hemispheric glioma, H3 G34-mutant, and (5) diffuse pediatric-type high-grade glioma, IDH-wild type and H3-wild type. The first two belong to the category of adult-type diffuse gliomas and the latter three are classified as pediatric-type diffuse high-grade gliomas, although they can be seen in adults. Tumors that do not fit into a specific diagnostic category either through incomplete workup or exhaustive workup that is incongruent with known entities are termed glioma, not otherwise specific (NOS) or not elsewhere classified (NEC) respectively.[4]

Key Molecular Features

Adopting a major change from prior versions, the WHO 2021 dissolved the entity of GBM, IDH-mutant. Diffuse astrocytic gliomas with IDH-mutation and high-grade histologic features are now called astrocytoma, IDH-mutant, WHO grade 4.[4,5] In addition, an astrocytic glioma may meet criteria for grade 4 designation based on homozygous deletion of CDKN2A/B even in the absence of microvascular proliferation or necrosis.

GBM is the prototypical IDH-wild type high-grade glioma and often has the classic histologic features discussed above. However, when these histologic features are absent, GBM may still be defined molecularly by TERT promoter mutation, EGFR-amplification, and/or polysomy chromosome 7 with monosomy chromosome 10.[4,5] Histone-altered gliomas include H3 G34 mutant diffuse hemispheric glioma and H3 K27M-altered diffuse midline glioma. Diffuse hemispheric gliomas are often associated with ATRX loss and p53 overexpression. H3K27M mutant gliomas often present in adolescents and young adults and are associated with very poor survival even compared to other grade 4 gliomas. As a result, all gliomas with midline location, regardless of histologic appearance, should be evaluated for this alteration.

In addition to markers notable for classification, O6-methylguanine-DNA methyltransferase (MGMT) promotor status is vital in determining the treatment response and prognosis for grade 4 gliomas. Gliomas with methylated MGMT promoters are associated with a greater response to chemotherapy.[6] The majority of IDH-mutant gliomas are MGMT promoter methylated.[7] Conversely, the majority of H3 K27M gliomas are MGMT promoter unmethylated.[8] Finally, next-generation sequencing is essential in the identification of the mutations described in the 2021 WHO classification guidelines for CNS tumors, as well as for identifying potential therapeutically targetable alterations.

TREATMENT

First-line therapy for brain lesions suspicious for malignancy is a maximum-safe resection; when amenable by size, location, and number of lesions, a gross-total resection has the best survival outcome.[9] After max-safe resection, standard-of-care treatment remains concurrent radiation therapy (RT) and temozolomide (TMZ) per EORTC 26981.[10] A total of approximately 60 Gy is administered in 30 fractions over 6 weeks (5 days/week), though dosing over 20 fractions is under active investigation.[11] TMZ is concurrently dosed at 75 mg/m² daily from the start to the end of radiation.[12] In patients ≥60 years of age, short-course RT is reasonable, administering 40 Gy in 15 fractions over the course of 3 weeks.[13] Even with short-course RT, concurrent TMZ is beneficial (EORTC 26062-22061[14]). After concurrent radiochemotherapy, adjuvant therapy includes six cycles of 200 mg/m² TMZ taken on days 1–5 of a 28-day cycle.[12] To date, there is no known clinical benefit of extending beyond six cycles of TMZ in grade 4 gliomas.[15] Along with adjuvant TMZ, use of tumor-treating fields (TTF) in patients with supratentorial lesions and preserved functional status is strongly recommended[16]: as of 2023, TTF are the preferred category 1 recommendation for GBM. Finally, consideration for clinical trial is essential for all grade 4 tumors. This is particularly important for H3 K27M midline gliomas, where overall survival is poor and targeted and cellular therapies are showing marked promise.[17]

Other notable treatments include bevacizumab, which can improve clinical status by addressing vasogenic edema, but it does not improve overall survival.[18] In addition, it may be used as an alternative for steroid-refractory severe vasogenic edema. Unfortunately, the majority of immunotherapies have failed to date. Future treatment considerations include next-generation targeted therapies such as regorafenib. Use of regorafenib is best under consultation with a neuro-oncologist or on a trial basis, as it may affect future trial enrollment.

PROGNOSIS

Grade 4 gliomas have an overall 5-year survival rate of 6.8%, which generally decreases with age.[1] As mentioned earlier, MGMT promoter methylation status is associated with greater response to chemotherapy. As a result, patients with MGMT-methylated tumors tend to have the longest overall survival. Conversely, the presence of multifocal, multicentric, or leptomeningeal spread is associated with poorer outcomes.[3]

Grade 2–3 Gliomas

GENERAL PRINCIPLES

Classification

According to the updated WHO 2021 classification, nearly all grade 2–3 diffuse gliomas in adults are IDH-mutant, with mutations occurring at either codon 132 of *IDH1* or codon 172 of *IDH2*. The presence of an IDH mutation and 1p/19q codeletion defines oligodendroglioma.[4,5] Alternatively, IDH mutation with ATRX loss and p53 mutation and retained 1p/19q defines astrocytoma. Oligodendroglioma, IDH-mutant, and 1p/19q-codeleted may be either grade 2 or 3. High-grade histologic features or brisk mitotic activity (≥6/10 HPF) will upgrade an oligodendroglioma to grade 3. Astrocytoma, IDH-mutant may be grade 2, 3, or 4. High-grade histology or homozygous CDKN2A deletion results in grade 4. Increased mitotic activity (≥2/specimen) or anaplasia can upgrade to grade 3. Given astrocytomas harboring low-grade appearance can be molecularly defined as grade 4, it is important to evaluate CDKN2A/B status in all of these tumors.[3,4]

Imaging

Grade 2 and 3 gliomas are often solitary lesions with poorly demarcated borders. As they are comparatively slow growing, the magnitude and distribution of T2 hyperintensity is highly variable and may appear significantly worse on imaging than clinical exam. T1 post–contrast enhancement is highly variable, but more often seen with anaplastic tumors or transformed low-grade tumors. Calcifications are more common with oligodendrogliomas. Blood products are very uncommon although calcifications may appear similar to blood products on susceptibility-weighted artifacts.

TREATMENT

As with grade 4 gliomas, maximum-safe resection is the first-line therapy. After max-safe resection, further treatment depends on several key factors. For patients with grade 2 tumors, if a gross total resection was achieved, who are <40 years of age, and have high functional status, observation is reasonable versus adjuvant treatment. For patients who are on observation after surgery with high functional status, recent results suggest monotherapy with the IDH-inhibitor vorasidenib may be considered. The INDIGO trial revealed monotherapy with vorasidenib prolongs progression-free survival and the time to the next intervention versus observation alone (NCT04164901[19]). As of this writing, vorasidenib is under fast-track status at the FDA and should be considered in the near future for patients on observation. Alternatively, if one of the criteria above is not met, the standard of care remains RT and chemotherapy. Typically chemotherapy is given over the course of 12 cycles. As of this writing, it remains unknown if concurrent then adjuvant chemotherapy provides any benefit beyond adjuvant chemotherapy after RT monotherapy. Standard-of-care chemotherapy for grades 2–3 gliomas remains TMZ for astrocytoma and combination of procarbazine, lomustine, and vincristine (PCV) for oligodendroglioma. It remains unclear if PCV is superior to TMZ in terms of survival, and is currently being studied in the CODEL trial (NCT00887146[25]). As highlighted by the INDIGO and CODEL trials, clinical trials remain key for lower-grade gliomas to provide additional treatment options beyond standard of care.

PROGNOSIS

Oligodendrogliomas tend to have better outcomes than astrocytomas. Low-grade oligodendrogliomas have a median survival time of 10–12 years, decreasing to 3.5 years for grade 3 oligodendroglioma. Grade 2 astrocytomas have a median survival of 4.8 years while grade 3 astrocytomas have a median survival of 2 years.[20]

Meningiomas

GENERAL PRINCIPLES

Imaging

Meningiomas are often found incidentally on MRI, as they are asymptomatic the vast majority of the time. When symptomatic, the most common symptoms include headaches and seizures. These tumors are homogeneously enhancing and have well-defined borders, always located extra-axially though invasion into brain parenchyma, sinuses, and other structures is possible over time. Meningiomas often present with an attachment to the adjacent dura known as a "dural tail." Mass effect and peritumoral edema are also common.

Pathology/Classification

- Meningiomas originate from arachnoid cap cells and have a diverse molecular and histologic profile spanning over 15 subtypes. Mutations causing meningiomas fall into two main categories: deletion or inactivation of NF2 on chromosome 22 (transitional fibroblastic) and non-NF2 mutants with mutations in SHH (meningothelial), PI3K/AKT (meningothelial/transitional, KLF4 (secretory, skull-base variants), TRAF7, SMO (olfactory variants), POLR2A (skull-base meningothelial tumors), AKT1 (median skull-base tumors), and more. The non-NF2 mutations are mutually exclusive and associated with low-grade meningiomas. Some mutations are associated with poorer outcomes, such as TERTp and CDKN2A, as well as overall hypermutation.[21,22] Conversely, meningiomas with intact Merlin tend to have the best outcome.[22]
- Meningiomas can be grade 1 meningioma, grade 2 atypical meningioma, or grade 3 anaplastic meningioma. Grading is dependent on mitotic activity with grade 1 having

<4 mitoses/10 HPF, grade 2 having 4–19 mitoses/10 HPF, and grade 3 having ≥20 mitoses/10 HPF. Additional ways of reaching a grade 2 designation include (1) brain invasion, (2) clear cell or chordoid morphology, and (3) presence of at least three of the five atypical histologic features which include spontaneous necrosis, macronucleoli, sheeting architecture, small cell change, and hypercellularity. Besides the mitotic threshold, a meningioma may reach grade 3 by frank anaplasia, TERT promoter mutation, or homozygous loss of CDKN2A/B.

TREATMENT

Treatment of a lesion suspected to be a meningioma depends on the size, location, and associated symptoms. For small, nonenlarging lesions that are asymptomatic, close observation with serial imaging is reasonable. If a patient is symptomatic, surgical intervention is indicated. After the resection, the available tissue makes it possible to determine the grade of the meningioma, which determines further treatment. Grade 1 meningiomas resected with good margins can be observed with serial imaging, as the risk of recurrence is low. For incomplete resections and higher-grade meningiomas, RT is indicated followed by serial imaging. MRIs should occur at 3 months, 6 months, and 1 year. Then, MRIs typically occur every 6–12 months for the next 5 years, then as clinically indicated. At the time of recurrence, a second resection is recommended followed by RT, and possibly chemotherapy.

PROGNOSIS

A gross total resection with good margins for a low-grade meningioma is considered curative. Higher-grade meningiomas are more likely to recur after the initial resection. Grade 2 meningiomas have a median survival time of 14 years while grade 3 meningiomas have a survival time of 6 years.[23]

Other Tumor Types

Rarer tumor types in adults include medullobastomas, ependymomas, and a cohort of rare CNS malignancies. Management should be in concert with a neuro-oncologist and radiation oncologist as the utility of adjuvant chemotherapy can vary widely (e.g., medulloblastomas can benefit greatly while ependymomas tend to be more resistant as a class[24]).

REFERENCES

1. Miller KD, Ostrom QT, Kruchko C, et al. Brain and other central nervous system tumor statistics, 2021. *CA Cancer J Clin*. 2021;71(5):381–406.
2. Ostrom QT, Fahmideh MA, Cote DJ, et al. Risk factors for childhood and adult primary brain tumors. *Neuro Oncol*. 2019;21(11):1357–1375.
3. Shakur SF, Bit-Ivan E, Watkin WG, Merrell RT, Farhat HI. Multifocal and multicentric glioblastoma with leptomeningeal gliomatosis: a case report and review of the literature. *Case Rep Med*. 2013; 2013:132679.
4. WHO Classification of Tumours Editorial Board. *World Health Organization Classification of Tumours of the Central Nervous System*. 5th ed. International Agency for Research on Cancer; 2021.
5. Louis DN, Perry A, Wesseling P, et al. The 2021 WHO classification of tumors of the central nervous system: a summary. *Neuro Oncol*. 2021;23(8):1231–1251.
6. Hegi ME, Diserens A-C, Gorlia T, et al. MGMT gene silencing and benefit from temozolomide in glioblastoma. *N Engl J Med*. 2005;352(10):997–1003.
7. Kinslow CJ, Mercurio A, Kumar P, et al. Association of MGMT promoter methylation with survival in low-grade and anaplastic gliomas after alkylating chemotherapy. *JAMA Oncol*. 2023;9(7):919–927.

8. Abe H, Natsumeda M, Okada M, et al. MGMT expression contributes to temozolomide resistance in h3k27m-mutant diffuse midline gliomas. *Front Oncol.* 2020;9:1568.

9. Sanai N, Polley M-Y, McDermott MW, Parsa AT, Berger MS. An extent of resection threshold for newly diagnosed glioblastomas. *J Neurosurg.* 2011;115(1):3–8.

10. Mirimanoff R-O, Gorlia T, Mason W, et al. Radiotherapy and temozolomide for newly diagnosed glioblastoma: recursive partitioning analysis of the EORTC 26981/22981-NCIC CE3 phase III randomized trial. *J Clin Oncol.* 2006;24(16):2563–2569.

11. Mallick S, Kunhiparambath H, Gupta S, et al. Hypofractionated accelerated radiotherapy (HART) with concurrent and adjuvant temozolomide in newly diagnosed glioblastoma: a phase II randomized trial (HART-GBM trial). *J Neurooncol.* 2018;140(1):75–82.

12. Stupp R, Mason WP, van den Bent MJ, et al; European Organisation for Research and Treatment of Cancer Brain Tumor and Radiotherapy Groups; National Cancer Institute of Canada Clinical Trials Group. Radiotherapy plus concomitant and adjuvant temozolomide for glioblastoma. *N Engl J Med.* 2005;352(10):987–996.

13. Roa W, Brasher PM, Bauman G, et al. Abbreviated course of radiation therapy in older patients with glioblastoma multiforme: a prospective randomized clinical trial. *J Clin Oncol.* 2004;22(9):1583–1588.

14. Perry JR, Laperriere N, O'Callaghan CJ, et al; Trial Investigators. Short-course radiation plus temozolomide in elderly patients with glioblastoma. *N Engl J Med.* 2017;376(11):1027–1037.

15. Alimohammadi E, Bagheri SR, Taheri S, Dayani M, Abdi A. The impact of extended adjuvant temozolomide in newly diagnosed glioblastoma multiforme: a meta-analysis and systematic review. *Oncol Rev.* 2020;14(1):461.

16. Stupp R, Taillibert S, Kanner A, et al. Effect of tumor-treating fields plus maintenance temozolomide vs maintenance temozolomide alone on survival in patients with glioblastoma: a randomized clinical trial. *JAMA.* 2017;318(23):2306–2316.

17. Chi AS, Tarapore RS, Hall MD, et al. Pediatric and adult H3 K27M-mutant diffuse midline glioma treated with the selective DRD2 antagonist ONC201. *J Neurooncol.* 2019;145(1):97–105.

18. Kaka N, Hafazalla K, Samawi H, et al. Progression-free but no overall survival benefit for adult patients with bevacizumab therapy for the treatment of newly diagnosed glioblastoma: a systematic review and meta-analysis. *Cancers (Basel).* 2019;11(11):1723.

19. Mellinghoff IK, van den Bent MJ, Blumenthal DT, et al; INDIGO Trial Investigators. Vorasidenib in IDH1- or IDH2-mutant low-grade glioma. *N Engl J Med.* 2023;389(7):589–601.

20. Dong X, Noorbakhsh A, Hirshman BR, et al. Survival trends of grade I, II, and III astrocytoma patients and associated clinical practice patterns between 1999 and 2010: a SEER-based analysis. *Neurooncol Pract.* 2016;3(1):29–38.

21. Patel B, Desai R, Pugazenthi S, Butt OH, Huang J, Kim AH. Identification and management of aggressive meningiomas. *Front Oncol.* 2022;12:851758.

22. Choudhury A, Magill ST, Eaton CD, et al. Meningioma DNA methylation groups identify biological drivers and therapeutic vulnerabilities. *Nat Genet.* 2022;54(5):649–659.

23. Wang Y-C, Chuang C-C, Wei K-C, et al. Long term surgical outcome and prognostic factors of atypical and malignant meningiomas. *Sci Rep.* 2016;6:35743.

24. Franceschi E, Frappaz D, Rudà R, et al; EURACAN Domain 10. Rare primary central nervous system tumors in adults: an overview. *Front Oncol.* 2020;10:996.

25. Lassman AB, Cloughesy TF. Early results from the CODEL trial for anaplastic oligodendrogliomas: is temozolomide futile? *Neuro Oncol.* 2021;23(3):347–349.

Leukemias

Michael J. Slade

32

GENERAL PRINCIPLES

Leukemia is the result of somatically acquired genetic mutations leading to the dysregulation and clonal expansion of myeloid and/or lymphoid progenitor cells. The accumulation of neoplastic cells, both in the bone marrow and in the peripheral tissues, can manifest with a wide range of signs and symptoms, including cytopenias (and their associated complications), elevation of the total WBC count, dysfunction of involved organs, and constitutional symptoms. The diagnosis is typically suspected based on an abnormal complete blood count (CBC) and peripheral smear and confirmed by subsequent workup. Leukemias are generally subdivided into acute and chronic diseases, with markedly different prognoses, workups, treatments, and possibilities of cure.

Acute Leukemias

Patients with acute leukemias are often symptomatic at presentation, either due to profound anemia or infectious complications. Acute leukemias are the result of abnormal clonal proliferation of mutated progenitor cells. The mutations cause a block in the maturation process, leading to an accumulation of immature cells. The expansion of the abnormal clone leads to suppression of the other elements in the marrow, often producing clinical bone marrow failure and making the patient gravely ill. The clinical course of untreated acute leukemia is usually brief, with patients succumbing within days to weeks from the complications of marrow failure. Any patient with a suspected acute leukemia should be hospitalized for expedited workup and treatment initiation, even if they are currently clinically stable.

Acute Myeloid Leukemia

GENERAL PRINCIPLES

Definition

Acute myeloid leukemia (AML) is characterized by the presence of immature cells (blasts) expressing myeloid markers accumulating in the peripheral blood or bone marrow.[1] In general, AML is a disease of aging and reflects the gradual accumulation of deleterious mutations, deletions, and translocations among hematopoietic cells leading to enhanced proliferation and survival.

Classification

The old classification of AML is the French–American–British (FAB) system, which identifies nine subtypes of AML based on morphology and surface protein expression and attempts to group the subtypes of AML by myeloid lineage and the degree of differentiation (Table 32-1). Multiple systems have been proposed since and three competing classification systems were updated in 2022, the Word Health Organization (WHO),

TABLE 32-1	**ACUTE MYELOGENOUS LEUKEMIA, FAB CLASSIFICATION**		
Subtype	Name	Frequency (%)	Peroxidase/SB/NE[a]
M0	Myeloblastic with minimal differentiation	<5	–/–/–
M1	Myeloblastic without maturation	20	+/+/–
M2	Myeloblastic with maturation	25	+/+/–
M3	Promyelocytic (APL)	10	+/+/–
M4	Myelomonocytic	20	+/+/+
M4Eo	Myelomonocytic with abnormal eosinophils	5–10	+/+/+
M5	Monocytic	20	–/–/+
M6	Erythroleukemia	5	+/+/–
M7	Megakaryoblastic	<5	–/–/+

[a]Myeloperoxidase, Sudan black (SB), and nonspecific esterase (NE) stains.
Data from DeVita VT, Hellman S, Rosenberg S. *Cancer: Principles and Practice of Oncology*. 6th ed. Lippincott Williams & Wilkins; 2001.

International Consensus Classification (ICC), and European LeukemiaNet (ELN) classifications.[1–3] While the discussion of the details of these three systems is beyond the scope of this chapter, it is worthwhile to note all recent classification systems have shifted away from a morphologic and/or phenotype classification and towards a molecular classification of the disease. AML subtypes are now chiefly defined by translation/inversions (i.e., t(8;21), inv(16)), mutations (i.e., TP53, CEBPA), or recurrent cytogenetic changes (i.e., del(7), del(5q)). Consequently, cytogenetic studies and mutational analysis with a next-generation sequencing-based panel at diagnosis are crucial, as they determine diagnosis, treatment, and prognosis (Table 32-2). Data show similar outcomes in patients with AML (>20% blasts) and patients with MDS-IB2 (10–19% blasts).[4] There is currently no consensus on an exact threshold for the diagnosis of AML, but some centers will diagnose AML in patients with appropriate clinical and genetic features with a blast count of >10%, depending on the classification used.

Epidemiology

AML is the most common acute leukemia in adults and accounts for ~80% of cases.[5] The majority (75%) are de novo, though ~20% evolve from a prior hematologic neoplasm (secondary AML) and ~5% occur after prior treatment with radiation or chemotherapy (treatment-related AML). In US, the incidence has been stable for the last 50 years at ~3–5 cases per 100,000.[6] In contrast, AML accounts for <10% of acute leukemias in children under 10 years of age. In adults, the median age at diagnosis is 68 years of age. The incidence increases with age, with 1.3 and 12.2 cases per 100,000 for those under and over 65 years of age, respectively, and a lifetime risk of ~1%. The male-to-female ratio is about 5:3.[7]

Risk Factors

Radiation, previous chemotherapy with alkylating agents or topoisomerase inhibitors, myelodysplasia, myeloproliferative disorders, aplastic anemia, and exposure to benzene are known risk factors for the development of AML. Higher risk for AML is seen in people

TABLE 32-2	CYTOGENETIC ABNORMALITIES IN ACUTE MYELOID LEUKEMIA AND ASSOCIATED PROGNOSIS	
Risk Group	Cytogenetic Findings	Preferred Consolidation Strategy
Favorable	t(15;17); PML-RARα t(8;21); RUNX1-RUNX1T1 inv(16); CBFB-MYH11 Normal cytogenetics with NPM1 mutation without FLT3-ITD bZIP in-frame CEBPA mutation	Chemotherapy
Intermediate	FLT3-ITD with wild-type or mutated NPM1 (normal karyotype) Wild-type NPM1 without FLT3-ITD (normal karyotype) t(9;11)(p21.3;q23.3)/MLLT3::KMT2A Cytogenetic abnormalities not classified as favorable or adverse	Chemotherapy OR allogeneic transplant
Unfavorable	Complex karyotype (defined as ≥3 abnormalities, excluding the favorable-risk cytogenetics) inv(3); RPN1-EVI1 t(6;9); DEK-NUP214 t(9;22)(q34.1;q11.2)/BCR::ABL1 t(8;16)(p11;p13)/KAT6A::CREBBP t(3q26.2;v)/MECOM(EVI1)-rearranged t(v;11); MLL-rearranged −5 or del(5q), −7; −17/abn(17p) Mutated TP53, ASXL1, BCOR, EZH2, RUNX1, SF3B1, SRSF2, STAG2, U2AF1, or ZRSR2	Allogeneic transplant in first remission

Data from Döhner H, Wei AH, Appelbaum FR, et al. Diagnosis and management of AML in adults: 2022 ELN recommendations from an international expert panel. *Blood.* 2022;140(12): 1345–1377.

with Down (particularly AML-M7), Turner, and Klinefelter syndromes. However, despite these recognized risk factors, no antecedent exposures are identified in most cases.

DIAGNOSIS
Clinical Presentation
Marked cytopenias from leukemic infiltration of the marrow result in diverse presentations including fatigue, pallor, and dyspnea on exertion from anemia, hemorrhage from thrombocytopenia, and fevers and infection from neutropenia. Extramedullary tissue invasion by leukemic cells (most commonly with AML-M5) may result in hepatomegaly, splenomegaly, lymphadenopathy, rashes (leukemia cutis), gingival hypertrophy, CNS dysfunction and cranial neuropathies, intestinal involvement, lytic bone lesions, or even establishment of infiltrative masses (i.e., myeloid sarcomas). With myeloblast counts >50,000, **leukostasis** may occur, resulting in dyspnea from pulmonary infiltrates or CNS

dysfunction (ranging from somnolence to cerebral ischemia). **Spontaneous tumor lysis syndrome** may cause hyperuricemia, hyperphosphatemia, hypocalcemia, or hyperkalemia, and renal failure.[8]

Diagnostic Testing

Workup should include the following.

- **CBC.** Pancytopenia or leukocytosis may be present.
- **Coagulation profile.** International normalized ratio (INR), prothrombin time, partial thromboplastin time, D-dimer, and fibrinogen to look for disseminated intravascular coagulation (DIC).
- **Electrolytes.** Tumor lysis may cause hyperkalemia, hypocalcemia, hyperphosphatemia, or hyperuricemia.
- **Lactate dehydrogenase** (LDH).
- **Peripheral smear.** Leukemic myeloblasts on Wright–Giemsa stain of the peripheral blood and bone marrow aspirate demonstrate large nuclei with scant cytoplasm.
- **Lumbar puncture.** This should be done if neurologic symptoms are present.
- **Bone marrow aspirate and biopsy**, evaluated for the following:
  ○ Morphology and histochemical staining
  ○ Flow cytometry, to distinguish myeloid from lymphoid leukemia and to determine the subtype of AML. While surface markers can be highly variable, myeloblasts generally express surface markers associated with immature hematopoietic cells, including CD33, CD34, CD117, and CD13.
  ○ Cytogenetics and FISH, to aid in risk stratification and assist in selection of therapy.
  ○ Molecular studies, to identify abnormalities in specific genes that inform prognosis (FLT3, NPM1, TP53, CEBPA, or MDS-associated mutations) or determine eligibility for therapy (FLT3, IDH1/2).

TREATMENT

Intensive treatment is divided into two phases: **induction** and **consolidation**.[8] The goal is to achieve remission, defined as <5% blasts in the bone marrow and recovery of peripheral blood counts. Additional assays using flow cytometry or sequencing-based approaches are increasingly used to determine measurable residual disease (MRD) negativity after therapy, which is associated with improved outcomes.

Induction chemotherapy traditionally consists of 7 days of cytarabine (Ara-C) and 3 days of anthracycline (daunorubicin or idarubicin; "7+3" regimen). Fit patients with therapy-related AML (tAML) or AML with myelodysplasia-related changes are treated with a liposomal formulation of daunorubicin and cytarabine, which has been shown to be beneficial in this population.[9] In addition, either midostaurin or quizartinib in patients with FLT3 abnormalities, and gemtuzumab ozogamicin in patients with favorable risk, CD33+ disease can be added to the induction regimen. Complete remission can be obtained in ~70–80% of patients <60 years of age and in ~50% of older patients. Patients are generally admitted to the hospital during induction for nearly a month, require frequent blood and platelet transfusions, and often have febrile neutropenia.

Consolidation therapy is essential to prevent relapse and is guided by cytogenetic and molecular studies, age, and patient comorbidities. Therapeutic options include allogeneic bone marrow transplantation (refer to chapter on allogeneic transplant for further details), further chemotherapy with high-dose cytarabine (HiDAC), or other regimens. HiDAC is efficacious as definitive therapy for those with core-binding factor leukemia and serves as a bridge to transplant in patients undergoing allogeneic transplant. HiDAC toxicity increases in patients over 60 years of age due to a higher incidence of cerebellar ataxia (>30% in patients ≥60 years of age). Consequently, dose reductions are commonly employed. It should be noted, though, that in general, evidence regarding the therapeutic benefit of consolidation therapy in older adults is limited. In patients unable to tolerate consolidation therapy and without plans for allogeneic transplant, maintenance therapy with oral azacitidine may be beneficial.[10]

For patient unable to tolerate intensive induction, multiple approaches for **lower-intensity therapy** have been developed, including reduced-dose chemotherapy, hypomethylating agents, and targeted inhibitors in patients with FLT3, IDH1, or IDH2 mutations. Reduced-intensity therapy is not curative, and the goal is to prevent complications, minimize toxicities, and prolong life. The most commonly used therapy in older or unfit adults is the combination of hypomethylating agents (decitabine or azacitidine) with the BCL2 inhibitor venetoclax, which leads to a higher remission rate (37% vs. 18%) and prolongs survival (15 vs. 10 months) compared to hypomethylating agents alone.[11]

In the case of **relapse**, fit patients may either undergo intensive reinduction or receive hypomethylating agents with venetoclax, with a plan for allogeneic hematopoietic cell transplant if remission is achieved. Approximately 30–50% of patients with relapsed AML can achieve a second remission with intensive therapy. Unfit or older patients not eligible for intensive approaches may be evaluated for targeted agents, low-dose chemotherapy, or treated with the best supportive care.

COMPLICATIONS

Leukostasis may cause symptoms that require emergent cytoreduction with hydroxyurea and/or leukapheresis. Tumor lysis syndrome, fever, and neutropenia are all concerns as well. Cytopenias should be supported with transfusions, coagulopathy should be corrected, and febrile episodes should be treated promptly with antibiotics while cultures are pending. Prospective trials have identified 10,000/μL as a relatively safe transfusion threshold for platelets during inpatient induction chemotherapy.[12]

PROGNOSIS

The overall prognosis for AML depends heavily on age and performance status at diagnosis, which determines eligibility for intensive induction and allogeneic hematopoietic transplantation. Survival statistics are particularly grim in adults aged >70 years, with an estimated 5-year survival of <5% versus ~50–60% in patients aged <40 years.[13] The genomic risk features integrated into the ELN 2022 risk classification also stratify patients by outcomes among adverse (5-year survival: 15%), intermediate (34%), and favorable risk groups.[14] Notably, adverse genomic and clinical features (i.e., secondary or treatment-related AML) are more common in older adults, and untangling these factors is challenging. There is also growing interest in dynamically reclassifying risk for patients based on depth of response after induction or allogeneic transplant via MRD testing and multiple ongoing trials are examining these approaches.

Acute Promyelocytic Leukemia

GENERAL PRINCIPLES

Definition

Acute promyelocytic leukemia (APL) has historically been classified as the M3 subtype of AML (Table 32-1). However, it has now been recognized as a disease entity with distinct genomic, clinical, and prognostic features and deserves separate discussion. APL is fundamentally defined by the presence of a gene translocation between the retinoic acid receptor alpha (RARA) locus on the long arm of chromosome 17 and the tumor suppressor PML locus on the long arm of chromosome 15 (t(15;17)(q22;q12)), leading to a fusion *PML:RARA* gene product. The fusion protein blocks the normal retinoic acid-induced differentiation in early myeloid progenitors, leading to maturation arrest and accumulation of immature forms. While t(15;17) is the classic translocation associated with APL, rare variants involving the RARA gene and other partners (PLZF, NPM, NuMA) have been reported.[3]

Epidemiology

Estimates of APL incidence vary widely, with ~5–20% of cases of AML falling into the M3 subtype. Approximately 750 new cases per year are diagnosed in the United States. APL is unusual within the spectrum of myeloid disease in terms of age of onset: incidence peaks in the third decade of life and remains steady through the fifth before gradually declining.

Risk Factors

No association with gender or ethnic background has been established and there are no known risk factors, though APL can be observed after prior cancer treatment with topoisomerase-II inhibitors and ionizing radiation (secondary APL). Unlike secondary AML, secondary APL has equivalent outcomes to *de novo* disease.

DIAGNOSIS

Clinical Presentation

Patients with APL often present with signs and symptoms related to pancytopenia, including fatigue, easy bruising, and infectious complications. However, a unique feature of APL is severe bleeding secondary to DIC. Any patient with suspected AML presenting in DIC should be treated empirically with all-trans retinoic acid (ATRA) pending confirmation of diagnosis and further workup.[15]

Diagnostic Testing

Workup should include the following.

- **CBC.** Pancytopenia is usually present. Significant leukocytosis is unusual and associated with high-risk disease.
- **Coagulation profile.** INR, prothrombin time, partial thromboplastin time, D-dimer, and fibrinogen to look for DIC.
- **Electrolytes.** Tumor lysis may cause hyperkalemia, hypocalcemia, hyperphosphatemia, or hyperuricemia.
- **Lactate dehydrogenase** (LDH).
- **Peripheral smear.** Two variants of APL are recognized: the hypergranular variant (75% of cases) and microgranular variant (25%). The former is associated with the classic finding of Auer rods (eosinophilic needlelike inclusions), while the latter has no evident granules on light microscopy and a bilobed nucleus.
- **Peripheral blood fluorescent in situ hybridization (FISH) for t(15;17).** FISH reliably detects PML-RAR translocation in peripheral blood and should be ordered promptly if there is any delay in performing a bone marrow biopsy at presentation.
- **Bone marrow aspirate and biopsy**, evaluated for the following:
  - Morphology and histochemical staining.
  - Flow cytometry, to distinguish myeloid from lymphoid leukemia and to confirm the subtype of AML. APL cells typically do not express HLA-DR, which can help distinguish them from other subtypes of AML.
  - Cytogenetics, which should confirm presence of t(15;17). In patients with high clinical suspicion for APL and negative t(15;17) testing, additional testing for uncommon rearrangements of the RARA locus is available.

○ Molecular studies are less important in APL (vs. AML and ALL) but are generally still obtained to confirm the diagnosis and identify any related mutations.

TREATMENT

In patients with clinical or pathologic features suggestive of promyelocytic leukemia, therapy with **all-trans retinoic acid** (ATRA) should be initiated immediately without awaiting cytogenetic confirmation of the diagnosis. For patients with **low/intermediate-risk** disease (i.e., those with a total white blood count ≤10,000 at presentation), ATRA combined with **arsenic trioxide** (ATO) yields similar rates of complete remission and an improved safety profile compared to ATRA and chemotherapy, and is now the standard of care.[16] In **high-risk APL** (defined as those who present with a white blood cell count >10,000), the addition of a cytoreducing agent (preferably gemtuzumab ozogamicin, though anthracyclines are also used) to ATRA and ATO treatment is considered. Following achievement of a hematologic remission, patients proceed to consolidation therapy, which commonly overlaps courses of ATO and ATRA per the LeCocco regimen.[16] Maintenance therapy with ATRA is generally not employed in patients who achieve an MRD-negative remission by reverse transcription polymerase chain reaction (RT-PCR) testing for the PML/RAR-α transcript.

Relapse occurs in 5–10% of patients with APL and in ~20–30% of those with **high-risk APL**. ATO is the treatment of choice for most patients with **relapsed APL**, following initial therapy with ATRA and chemotherapy. Second complete remission can be obtained in 85–88% of patients. If an MRD-negative second remission is obtained, consolidation with an autologous hematopoietic cell transplantation (HCT) is recommended, though allogeneic HCT can be used in certain circumstances. If PCR negativity is not obtained, allogeneic HCT is the favored treatment.

COMPLICATIONS

The most feared complication of APL is **coagulopathy**, which accounts for 5–10% of patients with newly diagnosed APL who die during induction. Prompt initiation of treatment with ATRA when APL is suspected (or even considered) is vital to prevent life-threatening hemorrhagic complications and patients should be monitored closely for abnormal coagulation studies or clinical bleeding, which should be treated aggressively with supportive measures. Given the young age of onset and the high cure rate with modern regimens, treatment-related mortality for coagulopathic complications is devastating and requires vigilance.

A second distinctive complication of APL is **differentiation syndrome**, which was previously only observed with ATRA therapy but has now been well characterized in patients with IDH1/2 mutated AML undergoing therapy with IDH inhibitors. Differentiation syndrome occurs when a high number of malignant blasts rapidly undergo differentiation, leading to leukocytosis and release of preinflammatory cytokines accompanied by symptoms of systemic inflammation including fever, tachypnea, tachycardia, and vascular leak syndrome. It can occur either early (the first week) or late (beyond the third week) after initiation of ATRA. Differentiation syndrome can be rapidly fatal if left untreated and is a principal reason for admission of patients with APL during induction. The treatment for differentiation syndrome is steroids (dexamethasone 10 mg every 12 hours) and temporary discontinuation of ATRA/ATO in severe cases.

PROGNOSIS

The natural history of untreated APL is rapid and uniformly fatal clinical progression, with death from bleeding complications within a month. However, with the advent of ATRA-based regimens, APL has the best prognosis of any subtype of AML, with a long-term survival rate of over 90%. APL risk is subdivided into two categories based on WBC (threshold: 10,000/μL). In patients receiving ATRA-based treatment, low-risk disease is associated with a 5-year PFS of 87% versus 81% in high-risk disease.[17]

Acute Lymphoblastic Leukemia

GENERAL PRINCIPLES

Definition

Acute lymphoblastic leukemia (ALL) results from the abnormal proliferation of a lymphoid hematopoietic progenitor cell. It accounts for 80% of childhood leukemias and 20% of adult acute leukemias. The median age at diagnosis is 13 years old, with 39% of cases diagnosed in patients older than 20 years. People with Down syndrome are at a higher risk for developing ALL. The following sections focus on adult ALL, which has a worse prognosis than childhood ALL.

Classification

The broad classification of ALL is based on morphologic (FAB system) and immunophenotypic information (Table 32-3). Similar to AML, modern classification systems have emphasized genomic features, which are often associated with presentation, treatment, and prognosis.[1]

- **The Philadelphia chromosome: t(9;22)(a34;q11); BCR::ABL1:** the most frequent rearrangement in adult ALL and has historically been associated with a poor prognosis, though data from the modern era of tyrosine kinase inhibitors (TKIs) is less clear. It is present in 20–30% of adult and 2–5% of childhood cases. The incidence of t(9;22) increases with age and is present in 40–50% of patients older than 60 years. **Ph-like B-ALL**, which has a transcriptional profile similar to Ph+ ALL but lacks t(9;22) has been recognized and is associated with poor outcomes.
- **t(v;11q23); KMT2A-rearranged:** associated with a poor prognosis, seen in infants <1 year old and adults.
- **t(12;21)(p12;q22) ETV6::RUNX1:** associated with a good prognosis; this is the most common rearrangement seen in children and rarely seen in adults (3–4%). Similar to Ph-like B-ALL, a **ETV6::RUNX1-like** B-ALL has been recognized.
- **t(1;19)(q23;p13.3) TCF3::PBX1:** occurs chiefly in pediatric ALL. Previously associated with poor prognosis, but now considered favorable risk with modern regimens. The

TABLE 32-3	ACUTE LYMPHOBLASTIC LEUKEMIA, IMMUNOTYPE, AND FAB CLASSIFICATION		
Immunotype	Frequency (%)	FAB Subtype	Staining
Pre–B-cell	75	L1, L2	+TdT, +CALLA, B-cell markers (CD19, CD20)
T-cell	20	L1, L2	+TdT, −CALLA, +acid phosphatase, +T-cell markers (CD2, CD7, CD5)
B-cell	5	L3	−TdT, +surface IgG

TdT, terminal deoxynucleotidyl transferase; CALLA, common acute lymphoblastic leukemia antigen.

fusion of TCF3 with HLF on chromosome 19 (i.e., **t(17;19)**) has also been described and is associated with even worse outcomes.

- **t(5;14)(q31.1;q32.1) IGH::IL3:** associated with eosinophilia due to overexpression of IL3. Unclear prognosis due to rarity.
- **iAMP21:** defined by the presence of five or more copies of RUNX1 secondary to amplification of chromosome 21. Traditionally associated with poor prognosis.
- **Hyperdiploidy:** associated with a good prognosis.
- **Hypodiploidy:** associated with a poor prognosis.

DIAGNOSIS

Clinical Presentation

The clinical phenotype of ALL is highly heterogeneous and can, in some cases, present as lymph node involvement and/or splenomegaly with little to no circulating blasts or marrow involvement (termed lymphoblastic lymphoma or LBL). The leukemic form of the disease has a clinical presentation similar to AML, though extramedullary involvement and CNS disease are much more common. Patients generally present with malaise, fatigue, dyspnea, and bone pain. Patients also typically have signs of marrow failure such as bleeding, bruising, fever, and infection. In up to 10% of patients, the CNS may be involved at presentation, manifesting as headache and/or cranial nerve palsies. Leukostasis may also be present. Hepatosplenomegaly and lymphadenopathy can also be seen. ALL can be associated with an anterior mediastinal mass (in T-cell subtypes) or large abdominal lymph nodes (in B-cell subtypes). Involvement of the testicles can be observed in male patients and should be evaluated by physical exam even in asymptomatic patients.

Diagnostic Testing

Basic workup is similar to that for AML. A **peripheral smear** will usually demonstrate the presence of circulating blasts. **Bone marrow** will be hypercellular. Cytoplasmic granules and Auer rods should be absent. However, it can be extremely difficult to diagnose ALL on clinical and morphologic grounds alone. Immunophenotyping is often necessary to distinguish ALL from AML.

TREATMENT

The treatment of adult patients with ALL is extremely complex and should be performed at specialized centers with expertise in acute leukemias and access to allogeneic transplantation. Generally, therapy can be divided broadly into **intensive therapy** for fit patients and **reduced intensity therapy** for unfit and/or older patients, as well as treatment approaches for Philadelphia chromosome positive (Ph+) versus negative (Ph–) ALL.

- In fit patients, multiagent **induction chemotherapy** is the standard of care. Hyper-CVAD (cyclophosphamide, vincristine, dexamethasone, and doxorubicin alternating with high-dose methotrexate and cytarabine with incorporated intrathecal therapy) is one of the most commonly used regimens in adult patients.[18] These multiagent protocols carry the burden of profound myelosuppression, and patients are generally admitted for the first cycle of treatment to be monitored for infectious and cytopenic complications. For patients with CD20-positive ALL, the addition of rituximab should be considered, as it has been associated with improved outcomes and has limited additive toxicity.[19] In younger patients (age 15–39) with Ph– ALL, there is accumulating evidence of improved outcomes with pediatric-inspired regimens containing asparaginase, which is commonly used in the treatment of children with ALL but is poorly tolerated in older and middle-aged adults.[20] In older (age >65 years) or unfit patients, treatment remains beneficial and is generally built from a backbone of corticosteroids, vincristine, and other agents (anthracyclines, methotrexate, cytarabine) depending on overall fitness level. Increasingly, the CD19-CD3 bispecific T-cell engager blinatumomab is integrated into consolidation therapy for patients with B-ALL.[21] Extended **maintenance treatment** postinduction and consolidation is generally recommended for either 2 (males) or 3 (female) years.

- In fit patients with **Ph+ ALL, the** BCR-ABL TKIs imatinib, dasatinib, or ponatinib are added to a backbone of intensive, multiagent chemotherapy (most commonly Hyper-CVAD).[22] In patients achieving rapid MRD negativity by RT-PCR, allogeneic transplant may be deferred and patients should continue maintenance for up to 2–3 years postinduction.[23] For unfit patients, there is increasing interest in **chemotherapy-free regimens,** including the combination of TKI and steroids for induction and blinatumomab for consolidation.[24]

- **CNS prophylaxis** is an important component of therapy for ALL, regardless of intensity, as the disease has a higher incidence of relapse CNS. Patients should be evaluated for CNS involvement at diagnosis with a diagnostic and therapeutic lumbar puncture. Regimens typically consist of intrathecal methotrexate and cytarabine.

- **Relapse**, unfortunately, is common in adult ALL. Standard salvage chemotherapy regimens have limited efficacy, with second complete remission achieved in ~30–70% of patients. For B-ALL, targeted therapy is preferred, with common agents including blinatumomab, the anti-CD22 antibody-drug conjugate inotuzumab ozogamicin or chimeric antigen receptor (CAR) T-cell therapies tisagenlecleucel (age <26) or brexucabtagene autoleucel.[25–27] Salvage options for patients with T-ALL are limited and include nelarabine.[28,29] Fit patients who achieve a second CR should proceed to allogeneic cell transplant if eligible, as this is the only curative therapy in the setting of relapsed disease.

MONITORING/FOLLOW-UP

Relapse in ALL is thought to result from residual leukemic cells that remain following the achievement of a complete remission but are below the limits of detection using morphologic assessment. It is this subclinical level of residual leukemia that is referred to as **minimal residual disease (MRD)**. Increasingly, MRD testing via flow cytometry or real-time quantitative PCR-based assays is being employed to detect evidence of residual ALL and define remission in a more accurate manner. Ph+ ALL can be monitored with similar assays to chronic myeloid leukemia (CML), though notably the p190 (vs. p210) transcript is more common. Further clinical studies are needed to determine the utility of long-term MRD surveillance after completion of therapy.[30]

PROGNOSIS

Although 60–90% of patients can expect to undergo a complete remission with induction chemotherapy, the majority of patients will relapse. Patients who are younger and have good prognostic indicators have a cure rate of 50–70%. Those who are older and have poor prognostic indicators have a cure rate of only 10–30%. Adverse risk factors are summarized in Table 32-4.

Chronic Leukemias

In contrast to acute leukemias, which generally have a fulminant presentation and are characterized by the presence of immature appearing cells in the peripheral blood, chronic leukemias are often diagnosed incidentally or in the setting of subacute symptoms. They are generally characterized by the presence of elevated blood counts dominated by mature or maturing cells that can be morphologically normal but functionally atypical. Another hallmark of chronic leukemias is their ability to transform into more aggressive variants,

TABLE 32-4	ADVERSE PROGNOSTIC FACTORS IN ADULT ACUTE LYMPHOBLASTIC LEUKEMIA (ALL)
Clinical Risk Factors	**Genetic Risk Factors**
Age (<1 or ≥10 y)	Near-haploid (24–31 chromosomes) or low hypodiploid (32–39 chromosomes) karyotypes
Male sex	BCR-ABL1 rearrangement; t(9;22) (q34;q11)
Black or Hispanic race/ethnicity	TCF3-PBX1 rearrangement; t(1;19) (q23;p13)
High WBC at diagnosis (B-ALL: >50,000 cells/μL, T-ALL: >100,000 cells/μL)	Rearrangements involving MLL (KMT2A) with any partner
Persistent measurable residual disease (timepoint and threshold vary by age, disease characteristics, and treatment)	Philadelphia chromosome-like ALL: frequently involves rearrangements in CRLF2, JAK2, or ABL-kinase genes.
CNS involvement at diagnosis	Rearrangements involving MEF2D
Diagnosis of T-ALL	

Adapted from Malard F, Mohty M. Acute lymphoblastic leukemia. *Lancet*. 2020;395:1146–1162.

including Richter transformation (chronic lymphocytic leukemia [CLL]), myeloid blast crisis (CML), and lymphoid blast crisis (CML and, uncommonly, CLL). Chronic leukemias are generally considered to be incurable apart from an allogeneic hematopoietic cell transplant, though this thinking has recently been challenged in the case of CML. Consequently, the management of these diseases is focused on control of the disease, reduction of side effects, and avoidance of toxicities.

Chronic Myeloid Leukemia

GENERAL PRINCIPLES

Epidemiology

CML accounts for 14% of all leukemias and 20% of adult leukemias, with an annual incidence of 1.6 cases per 100,000 adults. The median age at presentation is 65. Since the advent of the tyrosine kinase inhibitor (TKI), imatinib, the annual mortality has decreased from 1% to 2% and the life expectancy of a patient diagnosed with CML who receives TKI approaches normal for age-adjusted controls, leading to dramatic increase in the prevalence of CML.

Etiology

The etiology is unclear; no correlation with monozygotic twins, geography, ethnicity, or economic status has been observed. However, a significantly higher incidence of CML has been noted in survivors of the atomic blasts at Nagasaki and Hiroshima, in radiologists, and in patients treated with radiation to the spine for ankylosing spondylitis.

Pathophysiology

- CML is associated with the fusion of two genes: BCR (on chromosome 22) and ABL1 (on chromosome 9) resulting in the classical BCR-ABL1 fusion gene. This abnormal fusion typically results from a reciprocal translocation between chromosomes 9 and 22, t(9;22)(q34;q11), that gives rise to an abnormal chromosome 22 called the Philadelphia (Ph) chromosome. The BCR-ABL1 fusion gene results in the formation of a unique gene product, the BCR-ABL1 fusion protein. This fusion protein results in the constitutive activation of the ABL1 tyrosine kinase and is implicated in the pathogenesis of CML.[31]

- Blast phase CML is characterized by **cytogenetic evolution** in ~70% of patients. The most common chromosomal abnormalities are trisomy 8 (30–40%), additional Ph chromosome (20–30%), and isochromosome 17 (15–20%). Point mutations in p53 are also seen (20–30%) as well as amplification of c-Myc (20%), and, less commonly, mutations and deletions of RAS, Rb, or p16. As with de novo AML, complex cytogenetics is associated with decreased response rates and survival.

- Traditionally, CML has been described as a **triphasic process**, with **chronic, accelerated**, and **blast** phases. The most recent update of the WHO classification eliminated **accelerated** phase and now CML is managed as a **biphasic disease**.[1]

  o Most patients present in **chronic phase**, characterized by an asymptomatic accumulation of differentiated myeloid cells in the bone marrow, spleen, and peripheral blood. Rising blast count, basophilia, and cytopenias have traditionally been considered hallmarks of transition to more aggressive disease, but accumulation of cytogenetic changes and TKI resistance mutations are the most relevant predictors of outcomes in the TKI era.

  o The **blast phase CML** requires >20% blasts in the bone marrow or peripheral blood and can be either myeloid (70%) or lymphoid (30%). In the 2 years after initial diagnosis of CML, 5–15% of untreated patients will enter blast crisis. In subsequent years, the annual rate of progression increases from 20% to 25%, with progression commonly occurring between 3 and 6 years after diagnosis.

DIAGNOSIS

Clinical Presentation

In most patients, CML is diagnosed incidentally on routine blood work. Symptoms can result from anemia and splenomegaly (fatigue, early satiety, and sensation of abdominal fullness) but may also include weight loss, bleeding, and bruising in advanced disease.

Diagnostic Testing

- **Blood smear** shows leukocytosis with a myeloid shift. In contrast to cases of acute leukemia, in which an arrest in maturation is the rule, **granulocytes at all stages of maturation** are observed (i.e., a "full house"). Anemia and thrombocytosis are common, while basophilia (>7%) occurs in only 10–15% of patients.

- The diagnosis is confirmed by the detection of the **Ph chromosome t(9;22) (q34.1;q11.21)**. Translocation detection can be performed by either FISH or RT-PCR. If diagnosis is made by FISH, it is important to send RT-PCR testing to determine the specific breakpoint for treatment monitoring. p210 is the most common fusion protein (95%), followed by p190 and, more rarely, p230. In 5% of patients, a BCR-ABL fusion can be detected without classic Ph chromosomal cytogenetics, and rarely translocations can involve three or more chromosomes.

TREATMENT

Chronic-Phase Chronic Myeloid Leukemia

All patients with newly diagnosed CML in chronic phase should be treated with **tyrosine kinase inhibitors (TKIs)** as initial therapy. The only exception is pregnancy, where the safety of TKIs is not well established.

- Four **BCR-ABL tyrosine kinase inhibitors (TKIs)** are approved as frontline treatment of chronic phase CML: imatinib, dasatinib, nilotinib, and bosutinib. All four agents are ATP-binding pocket TKIs which, at nanomolar concentrations, bind to the inactive conformation of the BCR-ABL ATP-binding pocket and result in competitive inhibition of BCR-ABL and growth inhibition of BCR-ABL-positive bone marrow progenitor cells. While second-generation TKIs (dasatinib, nilotinib, bosutinib) TKIs lead to deeper, more rapid remissions than imatinib, no difference in survival has been demonstrated between first- and second-generation agents, and choice of initial therapy is based on toxicity, medication interactions, cost to patient, and treatment goals.[32-34] After initiation of treatment, therapy is guided by molecular response, with the goal of reaching deep molecular response (<0.1% BCR-ABL1 transcripts on the International Scale) by 12 months after treatment initiation. Response to TKI treatment is nearly universal and patients who fail to respond to treatment should be carefully assessed for treatment adherence and medication interactions.
- **Toxicity** of TKIs can be substantial. Cytopenias, particularly during treatment initiation, are common and can require dose holds and supportive measures. Skin rash and myalgias also occur frequently and can lead to treatment discontinuation in some patients. However, each TKI also has its unique side effect profile that can help guide therapy.
  - Imatinib has been associated with muscle cramps, edema, nausea, hypophosphatemia, congestive heart failure, and hepatotoxicity and may be avoided in patients with prior gastrointestinal or renal issues.
  - Dasatinib has been associated with pleural and pericardial effusions, pulmonary hypertension, and QT prolongation, as well as platelet inhibition leading to serious bleeding events. It may be avoided in patients with significant prior pulmonary or cardiac disease.
  - Nilotinib has been associated with severe QT prolongation, worsening hypertension, cardiac and vascular events, metabolic and electrolyte abnormalities, and hepatotoxicity. It may be avoided in patients with significant prior cardiac, metabolic, or hepatic disease.
  - Bosutinib has been associated with multiple gastrointestinal toxicities, including diarrhea and gastrointestinal bleeding, as well as abnormal liver function tests. It may be avoided in patients with significant hepatic or gastrointestinal disease.
- The standard recommended duration of TKI therapy is indefinite treatment. However, achieving a **treatment-free remission (TFR)** can be an important **treatment goal** for some patients, especially women desiring pregnancy.[35] Second-generation TKIs are recommended for patients desiring to attempt a TFR due to their association with deeper response. Guidance for treatment response prior to TFR varies, but most trials have a 4–5 log reduction (i.e., MR4–MR5) in BCR-ABL1 transcripts maintained for 1–2 years. Patients in TFR are monitored closely for rising transcript levels and TKIs are restarted if MMR is lost. Even in this select population, ~50% of patients will require TKI reinitiation after attempting a TFR.
- Patients with **relapsed or refractory disease** that remains in **chronic phase** should be carefully assessed for treatment adherence and medication interactions, particularly the use of proton pump inhibitors or other acid-suppressing medications. In patients with good treatment adherence, BCR-ABL1 kinase domain mutation analysis is recommended to determine resistance mutations, which guide subsequent therapy. Unless contraindicated on the basis of mutation testing, switching to a second-generation TKI not previously employed is a reasonable approach. The third-generation TKI ponatinib is also approved as treatment for second line and beyond and is the only ATP-binding pocket TKI that is effective against the T315I mutation but is associated with substantial cardiovascular toxicity.[36] In addition, the non–ATP-binding pocket inhibitor asciminib was recently approved as third-line therapy and can also be effective in T315I mutated disease.[37]

Accelerated and Blast-Phase Chronic Myeloid Leukemia

- As advances are made in the treatment of CML, fewer patients (~7% at 5 years) are progressing to accelerated phase or blast crisis. In addition, 10–15% of patients will initially present in accelerated phase or blast crisis. In general, an attempt is made to achieve a deeper molecular remission and pursue allogeneic HCT after an initial response in eligible patients.
- Treatment of blast phase (BP)-CML remains a challenge, with survival of only 2–4 months in nonresponders. Typical AML induction chemotherapy is used for BP-CML with myeloid features and ALL induction chemotherapy for lymphoid features, with the incorporation of TKIs into induction and consolidation. Patients not eligible for transplant should receive maintenance TKI therapy post-remission. Patients who achieve remissions prior to transplant have reasonably good outcomes, with a 3-year overall survival of ~50%.[38] The use of TKI maintenance posttransplant is controversial but is often given for at least 2 years if well tolerated.

MONITORING/FOLLOW-UP

Follow-up during initial treatment requires CBC monthly, as well as peripheral BCR-ABL qPCR every 3 months until major molecular remission is achieved and then every 3–6 months. Patients attempting TFR should be monitored monthly for 3 months, bimonthly for 6 months, and then quarterly. Rising BCR-ABL transcripts should be quickly reevaluated, and treatment altered accordingly. A bone marrow examination should be performed if a patient has evidence of disease progression.

Chronic Lymphocytic Leukemia

GENERAL PRINCIPLES

CLL is characterized by the progressive accumulation of monoclonal, functionally incompetent lymphocytes. Patients with CLL commonly develop complications associated with loss of effective hematopoiesis and intrinsic immune dysfunction, which can result in the development of autoimmune disorders or recurrent infections.

Classification

CLL has multiple classification systems, including the Rai and Binet staging systems, which are based on anatomic and laboratory parameters. These staging systems were developed to reflect the prognosis and aid in the initiation of treatment (Table 32-5). Molecular and cytogenetic markers have become increasingly useful for prognostication.

Epidemiology

CLL is the most common form of leukemia in adults, accounting for 25–30% of adult leukemia in Western countries. The median age at presentation is 70 years, and the disease is rarely diagnosed in patients <30 years of age. Nearly 5% of elderly individuals have a premalignant form of the disease called monoclonal B-cell lymphocytosis (MBL), which progresses to CLL at the rate of ~1–2% per year. Approximately 20,000 new cases are diagnosed every year in the US, with a slight predominance in male versus female patients (1.5:1) and a higher incidence in Caucasian (vs. Black or Asian) patients in the US.

Pathophysiology

CLL is an accumulation of malignant, immunologically incompetent B-cell lymphocytes with mature morphology and surface markers. The malignant cells of CLL express high

TABLE 32-5 CHRONIC LYMPHOCYTIC LEUKEMIA STAGING AND MOLECULAR PROGNOSTICS

Rai	Binet
Stage 0: lymphocytosis	Stage A: lymphocytosis
Stage 1: lymphadenopathy	Stage B: lymphadenopathy in >3 areas
Stage 2: splenomegaly	Stage C: Hgb <10 g/dL or platelets
Stage 3: Hgb <11 g/dL	<100,000/μL
Stage 4: platelets <100,000/μL	
High-risk markers	*Good-risk cytogenetics*
Elevated β-2-microglobulin, LDH	Deletion 13q
CD38+ in >30% lymphocytes	*High-risk cytogenetics*
ZAP-70+ in >20% lymphocytes	14q rearrangement
Unmutated IgVH	11q rearrangement
	Deletion 17p
Low risk: overall survival, 7–10 y	*High risk:* overall survival, 2–5 y
Rai 0–1	Rai 3–4
Binet A	Binet C
Deletion 13q	Molecular or cytogenetic changes noted
Doubling time >12 mo	Doubling time <12 mo

Hgb, hemoglobin; LDH, lactate dehydrogenase.

levels of the antiapoptotic protein, BCL-2, and express common B-cell antigens CD19, CD20, and CD23. Of note, CD5 antigen, a T-cell antigen, is found in nearly all cases of CLL. CLL is considered to be a biologically equivalent leukemic presentation of small lymphocytic lymphoma (SLL), which resides within the lymph nodes. A positive Coombs test is a common finding (35% of patients), though hemolytic anemia only develops in ~10% of patients during the course of their disease. Immune thrombocytopenia is also seen and occurs in 2–3% of patients.[39] **Richter transformation**, which is a malignant transformation to diffuse large B-cell lymphoma has been variously estimated to occur in 2–5% of patients.[40]

Risk Factors

Patients with a history of **immunodeficiency syndromes** have an increased risk of CLL. There are no clear environmental or occupational risk factors that predispose to CLL, and patients who are exposed to radiation do not appear to have an increased frequency of CLL.

DIAGNOSIS
Clinical Presentation

Many patients are referred for workup due to asymptomatic CBC abnormalities. However, chronic fatigue is a common initial complaint. With bone marrow involvement, patients may develop severe fatigue, anemia, bruising, weight loss, fever, and symptoms related to organ progression. On physical examination, splenomegaly, hepatomegaly, and lymphadenopathy can be present. With advancing immunodeficiency, herpes zoster infections, *Pneumocystis jirovecii* pneumonia, and bacterial infections become more frequent.

Diagnostic Criteria

The diagnosis of CLL per the CLL international working group can be made based on peripheral blood flow cytometry and requires an absolute lymphocyte count (ALC) of

TABLE 32-6 IMMUNOPHENOTYPIC FEATURES OF MALIGNANT CONDITIONS AFFECTING MATURE B LYMPHOCYTES

Disorder	Common Immunophenotype
CLL	DR+, CD19+, CD20+, CD5+, CD22−, CD23+, CD10−, weak sIg
Prolymphocytic leukemia	DR+, CD19+, CD20+, CD5−, CD22+, CD23−, CD10−, bright sIg
Mantle cell lymphoma	DR+, CD19+, CD20+, CD5+, CD22+, CD23−, CD10−, moderate sIg
Follicular lymphoma	DR+, CD19+, CD20+, CD5−, CD22+, CD23−, CD10+, bright sIg
Hairy cell leukemia	DR+, CD19+, CD20+, CD5−, CD22+, CD23−, CD25+, CD10−, CD11c+, CD103+, CD123+, bright sIg
Variant HCL	DR+, CD19+, CD20+, CD5−, CD22+, CD23−, CD25−, CD10−, CD11c+, CD103+, CD123−, bright sIg

CLL, chronic lymphocytic leukemia; sIg, surface immunoglobulin.

>5,000/µL for >3 months with a typical morphology and a typical immunophenotype (light chain restriction, CD5$^+$, CD23$^+$, CD10$^-$, CD19$^+$, CD20^{+dim}, CyclinD1$^-$, CD43‡) (Table 32-6). Patients with evidence of clonal B-cells and ALC <5,000/µL are diagnosed with MBL unless they have cytopenias due to extensive marrow involvement or evidence of extramedullary involvement (i.e., nodal, splenic, or soft tissue disease), which consistent with SLL.

Differential Diagnosis

Benign causes of nonmalignant lymphocytosis must be excluded, including Epstein–Barr virus mononucleosis, chronic infections, autoimmune diseases, drug and allergic reactions, thyrotoxicosis, adrenal insufficiency, and post splenectomy. Other indolent leukemias/lymphomas must also be excluded based on cell surface markers and cell morphology (Table 32-6).

Diagnostic Testing

A **CBC with differential** reveals an **absolute lymphocytosis**. A blood smear should show mature lymphocytes. The **classic smudge cell** is common but nonspecific. Anemia and/or thrombocytopenia may be present from bone marrow infiltration or from an autoimmune phenomenon. It is important to assess renal and hepatic function, LDH, uric acid, beta-2-microglobulin, Coombs antiglobulin, serum protein electrophoresis, and quantitative immunoglobulins. CT scans of the chest, abdomen, and pelvis are indicated based on clinical symptoms and prior to embarking on treatment but are not recommended for asymptomatic patients with early-stage disease. Patients with CLL typically have at least 30% lymphocytes in the bone marrow. A bone marrow biopsy is not required for the diagnosis of CLL or SLL, which is frequently rendered through peripheral blood flow cytometry or lymph node biopsy. Cytogenetic studies should be obtained for **del(17p)**, **del(11q)**, **del(13q)**, **IgVH (immunoglobulin heavy chain variable region) gene rearrangements**, along with flow cytometry for CD38, as these have been shown to have prognostic significance.[41]

TREATMENT

- CLL is an incurable but indolent malignancy and early treatment for asymptomatic patients do not improve outcomes. The median survival for early-stage patients (Rai <3, Binet A/B) is over 10 years even in the absence of treatment and approximately one-third of patients diagnosed with CLL will die of other causes without requiring treatment. It is not necessary to initiate therapy early in the course of CLL. The **need for therapy** is guided by the presence of "active disease" by the International Workshop on CLL criteria, which include massive (>6 cm below costal margin) or symptomatic splenomegaly, massive (>10 cm in long axis) or symptomatic LAD, organ compromise due to extrinsic compression by tumor, rapidly rising ALC (doubling in 6 months or >50% rise in 2 months), evidence of progressive marrow failure (Hgb <10 g/dL, platelet count <100,000 per μL) or constitutional symptoms including fever (>2 weeks duration), weight loss (>10% of body mass in 6 months), fatigue (ECOG ≥2 with ADL interference), and night sweats (>1 month with no infection), or development of autoimmune cytopenia not responsive to corticosteroids. A subset of physicians will also initiate treatment for extreme ALC elevation (>200,000 cells/μL), recurrent infections, or constitutional symptoms not meeting the iwCLL criteria, though this is not considered standard practice.
- The **frontline treatment** for symptomatic CLL has evolved substantially over the last decade, though no single preferred option currently exists.[42] Standard treatment is either indefinite therapy with a Bruton tyrosine kinase (BTK) inhibitor or time-limited therapy with the BCL2 inhibitor venetoclax in combination with an anti-CD20 antibody. In patients undergoing treatment with a BTK inhibitor, next-generation BTK inhibitors (acalabrutinib, zanubrutinib) may be preferred due to more favorable toxicity profiles, though no difference in treatment efficacy has been demonstrated. Therapy is selected based on toxicity profile, life expectancy, and patient preference. Response rates with both therapeutic approaches are excellent and ongoing trials are investigating novel combination and monitoring strategies, though none are currently in clinical practice. While chemoimmunotherapy with fludarabine, cyclophosphamide, and rituximab was previously considered in select patients with favorable risk cytogenetics, it is no longer used due to the risk of secondary MDS.
- The choice of therapy for **refractory and relapsed disease** is based on the initial agents used, with a strong preference to switch classes (i.e., BCL2 inhibitors are used if the initial therapy was BTK inhibitors and vice versa). In patients receiving time-limited therapy who progress after multiple years of treatment, retreatment with the same agent can be considered. In patients who progress on both BTK and BCL2 inhibitors, phosphoinositide 3′-kinase (PI3K) inhibitors (idelalisib and duvelisib) are FDA approved but can be associated with significant toxicities. The non-covalent BTK inhibitor pirtobrutinib can be effective in patients with the C481 mutation and may be effective in patients progressing on other BTK inhibitors.[43]
- Allogeneic bone marrow transplantations can be used in young, fit patients who have progressed on both BTK and BCL2 inhibitors and are not eligible for clinical trials. CAR T-cells are under investigation for CLL but are not currently FDA approved.

COMPLICATIONS

- **Autoimmune hemolytic anemia (AIHA) and autoimmune thrombocytopenia** occur more frequently in advanced-stage patients and those with unmutated IgVH. Initial treatment is standard therapy for AIHA and autoimmune thrombocytopenia processes, with prednisone or equivalent glucocorticoid at a dose of 1 mg/kg/d, tapered after control of blood counts. Local irradiation or splenectomy can control the effects of hypersplenism. However, clone-directed therapy is warranted in patients who do not respond to standard immunosuppression.

- **Infection** can result from hypogammaglobulinemia, T-cell dysfunction, and decreased phagocytic function. Hypogammaglobulinemic patients should not receive prophylactic intravenous immunoglobulin (IVIg, but those with recurrent infections can be treated with IVIg (400 mg/kg IV, every 3–4 weeks, goal IgG trough, ~500 mg/dL), which reduces minor and moderate but not serious bacterial infection rates and does not alter overall survival.
- **Cardiac complications** are common in patients receiving BTK inhibitors, especially ibrutinib, which is associated with worsening hypertension (78%) and atrial fibrillation (13%) and worsening heart failure, arrhythmias, and sudden cardiac death (all <5%). Newer BTK inhibitors (zanubrutinib, acalabrutinib) have a significantly reduced risk of cardiac toxicities but patients with prior cardiac history receiving any BTK inhibitor should be carefully monitored.

PROGNOSIS

Prognosis in CLL is highly variable, with some patients experiencing rapid progression and clinical deterioration despite treatment and dying within a few years of diagnosis and some experiencing an indolent clinical course with no treatment required for over 10 years. The median survival for CLL is currently 10 years, though this may not reflect the outcomes in patients in the age of novel therapies (i.e., BTK and BCL2 inhibitors).

Hairy Cell Leukemia

GENERAL PRINCIPLES

Hairy cell leukemia (HCL) is an uncommon chronic B-cell lymphoproliferative disorder named for the prominent irregular cytoplasmic projections of the malignant cells. It accounts for 2–3% of all leukemias and occurs in men >55 years of age.[44]

PATHOPHYSIOLOGY

HCL is thought to arise from a late-activated, memory B-cell which acquires a mutation in the BRAF gene (V600E) leading to constitutive activation and malignant transformation. Activation of BRAF leads to upregulation of the RAF-MEK-ERK pathway, which enhances cell survival and, to a lesser degree, increases proliferation. Risk factors for this disease are unclear, though ionizing radiation and exposure to pesticides have been associated with an increased risk.

DIAGNOSIS

Clinical Presentation

Most patients present with malaise, fatigue, and symptoms related to cytopenias or splenomegaly, though ~25% of patients are asymptomatic at presentation. On physical examination, splenomegaly and hepatomegaly are evident in 95% and 40%, respectively. With more advanced disease, worsening pancytopenia may lead to bleeding or recurrent infections (bacterial, viral, fungal, or atypical mycobacterial).

Diagnostic Testing

A **peripheral smear** and **bone marrow** reveal the **pathognomonic mononuclear cells**. These cells have characteristic irregular hair-like projections around the border of the cytoplasm. CBC frequently shows anemia and thrombocytopenia and, less frequently, granulocytopenia.

TABLE 32-7	THERAPEUTIC OPTIONS FOR HAIRY CELL LEUKEMIA
Therapy	**Comment**
Cladribine	First-line agent, 7-d IV infusion with >90% response rate. Alternative outpatient treatment schedules may be equally effective.
Pentostatin	Given for 3–6 mo with >75% response rate.
Rituximab	May be used as a single agent with limited efficacy (24% response rate) or in combination with purine analogs
BRAF inhibitors	High response rates for vemurafenib (96%), dabrafenib (86%), and combination dabrafenib/trametinib (89%)
Splenectomy	Achieves a 75% response rate

Although bone marrow aspiration is frequently unsuccessful, secondary to underlying reticulin fibrosis, the biopsy may show the characteristic hairy cells. Hairy cells exhibit a mature B-cell phenotype and are light chain restricted but may express one or more heavy chains. Hairy cells strongly express pan-B-cell antigens including CD19, CD20, and CD22. They usually lack expression of CD5, CD10, CD21, and CD23 but characteristically express **CD11c, CD103, CD25**, CD123, cyclin D1, and annexin A1. HCL is differentiated from CLL, lymphomas, and monocytic leukemia based on the characteristic cell morphology and immune phenotype. The above immunophenotype and the presence of a BRAF V600E mutation is a useful marker to differentiate HCL from "variant" HCL, a related but distinct entity, which often has MAP2K1 mutations and does not express CD25 or CD123.

TREATMENT

Similar to CLL and indolent lymphomas, there is no evidence that early treatment improves outcomes, and many patients can be observed for years without treatment. The decision to treat is based on the development of cytopenias (hemoglobin, <10 g/dL, absolute neutrophil count, <1,000/µL; platelets, <100,000/µL), symptomatic splenomegaly/lymphadenopathy and/or constitutional symptoms. Several treatment options are available (Table 32-7). Typically, the purine analogs **cladribine or pentostatin** is used as frontline therapy and can be reused at relapse in patients with good first remissions (>2 years). Occasionally, splenectomy can be employed in patients with symptoms related to splenomegaly. Rituximab or BRAF inhibitors (vemurafenib or dabrafenib) are often used for patients with poor response or early relapse to frontline therapy.

OUTCOME/PROGNOSIS

Before treatment, median survival was between 5 and 10 years. Survival has markedly improved with current therapies, as most untreated and pretreated patients have excellent response rates to cladribine or pentostatin (85–97%), with 4-year survival rates of up to 96%.[45]

REFERENCES

1. Alaggio R, Amador C, Anagnostopoulos I, et al. The 5th edition of the World Health Organization classification of haematolymphoid tumours: lymphoid neoplasms. *Leukemia.* 2022;36(7):1720–1748.
2. Döhner H, Wei AH, Appelbaum FR, et al. Diagnosis and management of AML in adults: 2022 recommendations from an international expert panel on behalf of the ELN. *Blood.* 2022;140(12):1345–1377.

3. Arber DA, Orazi A, Hasserjian RP, et al. International consensus classification of myeloid neoplasms and acute leukemias: integrating morphologic, clinical, and genomic data. *Blood.* 2022;140(11): 1200–1228.

4. Estey E, Hasserjian RP, Döhner H. Distinguishing AML from MDS: a fixed blast percentage may no longer be optimal. *Blood.* 2022;139(3):323–332.

5. Siegel RL, Miller KD, Jemal A. Cancer statistics, 2015. *CA Cancer J Clin.* 2015;65:5–29.

6. Dores GM, Devesa SS, Curtis RE, Linet MS, Morton LM. Acute leukemia incidence and patient survival among children and adults in the United States, 2001–2007. *Blood.* 2012;119:34–43.

7. Siegel R, Naishadham D, Jemal A. Cancer statistics, 2012. *CA Cancer J Clin.* 2012;62:10–29.

8. DiNardo CD, Wei AH. How I treat acute myeloid leukemia in the era of new drugs. *Blood.* 2020; 135(2):85–96.

9. Krauss AC, Gao X, Li L, et al. FDA approval summary: (daunorubicin and cytarabine) liposome for injection for the treatment of adults with high-risk acute myeloid leukemia. *Clin Cancer Res.* 2019;25(9):2685–2690.

10. Wei AH, Döhner H, Pocock C, et al. Oral azacitidine maintenance therapy for acute myeloid leukemia in first remission. *N Engl J Med.* 2020;383(26):2526–2537.

11. DiNardo CD, Jonas BA, Pullarkat V, et al. Azacitidine and Venetoclax in previously untreated acute myeloid leukemia. *N Engl J Med.* 2020;383:617–629.

12. Stanworth SJ, Estcourt LJ, Powter G, et al. A no-prophylaxis platelet-transfusion strategy for hematologic cancers. *N Engl J Med.* 2013;368(19):1771–1780.

13. Shah A, Andersson TM-L, Rachet B, Björkholm M, Lambert PC. Survival and cure of acute myeloid leukaemia in England, 1971–2006: a population–based study. *Br J Haematol.* 2013;162(4): 509–516.

14. Rausch C, Rothenberg-Thurley M, Dufour A, et al. Validation and refinement of the 2022 European LeukemiaNet genetic risk stratification of acute myeloid leukemia. *Leukemia.* 2023;37(6):1234–1244.

15. Sanz MA, Fenaux P, Tallman MS, et al. Management of acute promyelocytic leukemia: updated recommendations from an expert panel of the European LeukemiaNet. *Blood.* 2019;133(15):1630–1643.

16. Lo-Coco F, Avvisati G, Vignetti M, et al. Retinoic acid and arsenic trioxide for acute promyelocytic leukemia. *N Engl J Med.* 2013;369(2):111–121.

17. Abaza Y, Kantarjian H, Garcia-Manero G, et al. Long-term outcome of acute promyelocytic leukemia treated with all-trans-retinoic acid, arsenic trioxide, and gemtuzumab. *Blood.* 2017;129(10): 1275–1283.

18. Kantarjian HM, O'Brien S, Smith TL, et al. Results of treatment with hyper-CVAD, a dose-intensive regimen, in adult acute lymphocytic leukemia. *J Clin Oncol.* 2000;18(3):547–561.

19. Maury S, Chevret S, Thomas X, et al. Rituximab in B-lineage adult acute lymphoblastic leukemia. *N Engl J Med.* 2016;375(11):1044–1053.

20. Wang AY, Muffly LS, Stock W. Philadelphia chromosome–negative b-cell acute lymphoblastic leukemia in adolescents and young adults. *JCO Oncol Pract.* 2020;16(5):231–238.

21. Litzow MR, Sun Z, Paietta E, et al. Consolidation therapy with blinatumomab improves overall survival in newly diagnosed adult patients with b-lineage acute lymphoblastic leukemia in measurable residual disease negative remission: results from the ECOG-ACRIN E1910 randomized phase III national cooperative clinical trials network trial. *Blood.* 2022;140:LBA–1.

22. Ravandi F. How I treat Philadelphia chromosome–positive acute lymphoblastic leukemia. *Blood.* 2019;133(2):130–136.

23. Ghobadi A, Slade M, Kantarjian H, et al. The role of allogeneic transplant for adult Ph+ ALL in CR1 with complete molecular remission: a retrospective analysis. *Blood.* 2022;140(20):2101–2112.

24. Foà R, Bassan R, Vitale A, et al. Dasatinib–Blinatumomab for ph-positive acute lymphoblastic leukemia in adults. *N Engl J Med.* 2020;383(17):1613–1623.

25. Maude SL, Laetsch TW, Buechner J, et al. Tisagenlecleucel in children and young adults with B-cell lymphoblastic leukemia. *N Engl J Med.* 2018;378(5):439–448.

26. Kantarjian H, Stein A, Gökbuget N, et al. TOWER: blinatumomab versus chemotherapy for advanced acute lymphoblastic leukemia. *N Engl J Med.* 2017;376(9):836–847.

27. Kantarjian HM, DeAngelo DJ, Stelljes M, et al. Inotuzumab ozogamicin versus standard of care in relapsed or refractory acute lymphoblastic leukemia: final report and long-term survival follow-up from the randomized, phase 3 INO-VATE study. *Cancer.* 2019;125(14):2474–2487.

28. Cohen MH, Johnson JR, Massie T, et al. Approval summary: nelarabine for the treatment of T-cell lymphoblastic leukemia/lymphoma. *Clin Cancer Res.* 2006;12(18):5329–5335.

29. Litzow MR, Ferrando AA. How I treat t-cell acute lymphoblastic leukemia in adults. *Blood.* 2015; 126(7):833–841.

30. Saygin C, Cannova J, Stock W, Muffly L. Measurable residual disease in acute lymphoblastic leukemia: methods and clinical context in adult patients. *Haematologica.* 2022;107(12):2783–2793.

31. Faderl S, Talpaz M, Estrov Z, O'Brien S, Kurzrock R, Kantarjian HM. The biology of chronic myeloid leukemia. *N Engl J Med.* 1999;341(3):164–172.

32. Kantarjian H, Shah NP, Hochhaus A, et al. Dasatinib versus imatinib in newly diagnosed chronic-phase chronic myeloid leukemia. *N Engl J Med.* 2010;362(24):2260–2270.

33. Kantarjian HM, Hughes TP, Larson RA, et al. Long-term outcomes with frontline nilotinib versus imatinib in newly diagnosed chronic myeloid leukemia in chronic phase: ENESTnd 10-year analysis. *Leukemia.* 2021;35(2):440–453.

34. Cortes JE, Gambacorti-Passerini C, Deininger MW, et al. bosutinib versus imatinib for newly diagnosed chronic myeloid leukemia: results from the randomized BFORE trial. *J Clin Oncol.* 2018; 36(3):231–237.

35. Atallah E, Schiffer CA, Radich JP, et al. Assessment of outcomes after stopping tyrosine kinase inhibitors among patients with chronic myeloid leukemia: a nonrandomized clinical trial. *JAMA Oncol.* 2021;7:42–50.

36. Cortes J, Apperley J, Lomaia E, et al. Ponatinib dose-ranging study in chronic-phase chronic myeloid leukemia: a randomized, open-label phase 2 clinical trial. *Blood.* 2021;138(21):2042–2050.

37. Rea D, Mauro MJ, Boquimpani C, et al. A phase 3, open-label, randomized study of asciminib, a STAMP Inhibitor, vs Bosutinib in CML after ≥2 prior TKIs. *Blood.* 2021;138(21):2031–2041.

38. Radujkovic A, Dietrich S, Blok H-J, et al. Allogeneic stem cell transplantation for blast crisis chronic myeloid leukemia in the era of tyrosine kinase inhibitors: a retrospective study by the EBMT chronic malignancies working party. *Biol Blood Marrow Transplant.* 2019;25(10):2008–2016.

39. Diehl LF, Ketchum LH. Autoimmune disease and chronic lymphocytic leukemia: autoimmune hemolytic anemia, pure red cell aplasia, and autoimmune thrombocytopenia. *Semin Oncol.* 1998;25:80–97.

40. Tsimberidou A-M, Keating MJ. Richter syndrome: biology, incidence, and therapeutic strategies. *Cancer.* 2005;103(2):216–228.

41. Döhner H, Stilgenbauer S, Benner A, et al. Genomic aberrations and survival in chronic lymphocytic leukemia. *N Engl J Med.* 2000;343(26):1910–1916.

42. Brem EA, O'Brien S. Frontline management of CLL in 2021. *JCO Oncol Pract.* 2022;18(2):109–113.

43. Mato AR, Woyach JA, Brown JR, et al. Pirtobrutinib after a covalent BTK inhibitor in chronic lymphocytic leukemia. *N Engl J Med.* 2023;389:33–44.

44. Grever MR, Abdel-Wahab O, Andritsos LA, et al. Consensus guidelines for the diagnosis and management of patients with classic hairy cell leukemia. *Blood.* 2017;129:553–560.

45. Grever MR. How I treat hairy cell leukemia. *Blood.* 2010;115:21–28.

Lymphoma

33

Ryan Day

GENERAL PRINCIPLES

Lymphomas are clonal lymphoproliferative malignancies. They are highly diverse, with over 70 subtypes in the current WHO classification.[1] Distinctions between lymphoma subtypes, and in some cases, even nonmalignant processes, can be challenging, and pathology review by a trained hematopathologist is key to an accurate diagnosis. Lymphomas are traditionally divided into two morphologic groups, Hodgkin lymphoma (HL) and non-Hodgkin lymphoma (NHL), a classification schema that obscures significant molecular and clinical heterogeneity. In adults, most lymphomas are derived from mature B-cells. Less commonly, adult lymphomas are derived from T-cells, B-cell progenitors, and very rarely from natural killer (NK) cells.

Some risk factors are shared across many lymphomas. B- and T-cells undergo significant genomic stresses related to the genetic rearrangements and somatic mutations required for a broad immunologic repertoire, and rearrangements involving immune genes are common lymphoma drivers. Tonic antigenic stimulation in the setting of chronic infection or autoimmunity increases lymphoma risk, and some viral infections, including Epstein–Barr virus (EBV) and human T-lymphotropic virus (HTLV) 1/2, are directly linked to lymphomagenesis. HIV infection increases lymphoma risk predominantly through impaired immune surveillance, and the risk of developing lymphoma is inversely correlated with CD4 count. Other forms of immunosuppression can also increase lymphoma risk.

Lymphoma treatment is rapidly evolving with the advent of therapies targeted against particular mutations, pathways, or surface markers, including small molecule inhibitors, antibody–drug conjugates (ADCs), bispecific antibodies, and chimeric antigen receptor T (CAR-T) cells. Choosing an appropriate therapy requires careful consideration of both patient- and disease-specific factors. The SARS-CoV-2 pandemic demonstrated that lymphoma patients have decreased vaccination response and increased risk of infection and poor outcomes in the setting of a novel pathogen, and the depth and duration of immune suppression of a treatment regimen is an important contemporary consideration. The full complexities of lymphoma treatment are beyond the scope of this chapter, which will instead focus on an overview of the most common types of lymphoma.

Hodgkin Lymphoma

BACKGROUND AND EPIDEMIOLOGY

HL is a B-cell lymphoma with 8,000–9,000 diagnoses per year in the US. Ninety-five percent of HL cases are classical Hodgkin lymphoma (cHL), which has a bimodal age distribution, with peaks around 30 and after age 50. Nodular lymphocyte predominant Hodgkin lymphoma (NLPHL) accounts for the remaining 5% of HL cases, and has a median age of diagnosis of 30–40. HL is characterized by large dysplastic cells that constitute a minority of tumor volume. The malignant Reed–Sternberg (RS) cells of cHL are large and often multinucleated cells with a characteristic "owl's eye" appearance that exists in a background of mixed nonneoplastic inflammatory cells and fibrosis. cHL has several morphologic subtypes including nodular sclerosis, mixed cellularity, lymphocyte-deplete, and lymphocyte-rich forms, however, these subtypes do not currently impact treatment decisions or prognosis. The malignant cells of NLPHL are large dysplastic cells with a distinctive "popcorn" morphology. Based on molecular features, clinical history, and preferred treatment regimens, NLPHL is probably better classified as an indolent B-cell NHL but is still listed as a subtype of HL in the current WHO classification.

CLINICAL PRESENTATION

cHL most commonly presents as asymptomatic lymph node enlargement. The most common sites of disease are cervical, supraclavicular, and mediastinal lymph nodes, though older patients may present with a heavy burden of abdominal disease. cHL almost always spreads along contiguous lymphatic regions. In patients with significant disease bulk, focal symptoms related to involved lymph node regions can occur, such as dysphagia, chest pain, cough, shortness of breath, and abdominal pain/distention. Extranodal disease occurs in approximately 10% of patients, with common sites being bone, bone marrow, and lung. Systemic B symptoms, including fever, drenching night sweats, and weight loss ($\geq$10% of baseline body weight over 6 months), occur in about one-third of patients and are more common in advanced-stage disease. Pruritus occurs in 20–30% of patients but is not considered a B symptom. Alcohol-associated lymph node pain is rare but relatively pathognomonic for cHL. NLPHL most commonly presents as asymptomatic axillary, cervical, or retroperitoneal lymphadenopathy; mediastinal involvement is rare, and disease spread can be noncontiguous.

DIAGNOSIS AND STAGING

Physical exam should focus on lymph nodes and abdominal exam for hepatosplenomegaly. Fine needle aspiration is insufficient for diagnosis since neoplastic cells comprise a minority of tumor volume and involvement can be heterogeneous, and a core needle biopsy or excisional biopsy is usually required for diagnosis. In addition to characteristic morphologies, cHL and NLPHL have distinct IHC surface phenotypes. cHL RS cells are $CD15^+$, $CD30^+$, $CD45^-$, $CD20^{dim/-}$, while NLHPL cells are $CD15^-$, $CD30^-$, $CD45^+$, $CD20^+$. In diagnosing cHL, care should be taken to rule out other $CD30^+$ lymphomas, including primary mediastinal B-cell lymphoma and T-cell lymphomas, which have distinct morphologies, immunophenotypes, and treatments. Laboratory studies should include CBC with differential, CMP, LDH, HIV, and hepatitis B/C serologies. For cHL, ESR is required for calculation of the International Prognostic Score (IPS, Table 33-1). Pregnancy testing is also indicated for patients of childbearing potential. A TTE or MUGA

TABLE 33-1	CLASSICAL HODGKIN LYMPHOMA INTERNATIONAL PROGNOSTIC SCORE

Serum albumin <4 g/dL
Hemoglobin <10.5 g/dL
Male sex
Age $\geq$45 y
Stage IV disease
White blood cell count $\geq$15,000/mm^3
Absolute lymphocyte count <600/mm^3 or lymphocytes <8% of white blood cell count

TABLE 33-2	ANN ARBOR STAGING SYSTEM

Stage	Description
I	Single lymph node region, or single extranodal organ/site (IE)
II	2 or more lymph node regions on the same side of the diaphragm, or localized involvement of a single extranodal organ/site and its regional lymph nodes (IIE)
III	Lymph node regions on both sides of the diaphragm
IV	Involvement of one or more extranodal sites or isolated extranodal involvement with distant nodal involvement
Modifiers	
A	No systemic symptoms
B	Unexplained fevers >38°C, drenching night sweats, or weight loss >10% of baseline body weight within 6 mo prior to diagnosis
E	Denotes extranodal involvement of a single extranodal site in stage I–III disease

should be obtained since treatment regimens incorporate anthracyclines, and PFTs should be obtained for cHL patients planned for bleomycin. Positron emission tomography–computed tomography (PET-CT) is the preferred imaging modality for both cHL and NLPHL, and it is essential for contemporary risk-adapted cHL therapies.[2–4] Anemia in cHL can be secondary to lymphomatous bone marrow involvement but is more commonly due to chronic inflammation. PET-CT is highly sensitive for detection of bone marrow involvement. Bone marrow biopsy is not required in most cases but should be considered if a patient has thrombocytopenia or neutropenia without confirmed bone marrow disease on PET-CT. Staging is based on the Ann Arbor staging system (Table 33-2). Stage I–II cHL is often divided into "favorable" and "unfavorable" risk groups. Precise definitions vary among groups, but in general, more than three nodal sites, bulky disease (≥7–10 cm), large mediastinal mass (mass > one-third intrathoracic diameter), B symptoms, or elevated ESR (≥30–50 mm/hr) are higher-risk features. For advanced-stage cHL patients (stage III–IV), the IPS (Table 33-1) is used for prognostic stratification.

CLASSICAL HODGKIN LYMPHOMA TREATMENT

cHL is highly curable with 90% long-term survival in limited-stage disease. Current regimens for limited-stage disease are built on the ABVD backbone (doxorubicin, bleomycin, vinblastine, and dacarbazine), with consolidation radiation therapy used in select cases. Febrile neutropenia is rare in cHL with the ABVD regimen, and treatment should not be dose-reduced or delayed due to uncomplicated neutropenia irrespective of grade. Growth factors are generally avoided in patients receiving bleomycin due to increased risk of pulmonary toxicity. Bleomycin should also not be administered to patients at high risk of pulmonary injury, including those with other pulmonary comorbidities, smokers, or those over the age of 50–60.

Because of high cure rates and generally young patient population, minimizing long-term toxicities related to chemotherapy and radiation is an important treatment goal in cHL, and de-escalation strategies to minimize exposure to radiation and bleomycin have been explored in both early- and advanced-stage diseases. Multiple trials have shown that therapy de-escalation in patients with favorable response on PET-CT (Table 33-3) after two cycles of ABVD minimally affects PFS and does not compromise overall survival.[2,3] In

TABLE 33-3 MODIFIED LUGANO/DEAUVILLE SCALE

Score	Description
1	No uptake
2	Uptake ≤ mediastinum
3	Uptake > mediastinum but ≤ liver
4	Uptake moderately higher than liver
5	Uptake markedly higher than liver, or new lesions
NE	Not evaluable
X	New areas of uptake not likely to be related to lymphoma

stage I/II nonbulky disease, current standard of care is two cycles of ABVD, followed by PET-CT. Patients with a good response, defined as a Deauville score of 1–2, can then be treated with one to two cycles of ABVD; involved-node radiation therapy (INRT) can be considered in patients who are at higher risk of complications from additional chemotherapy and have disease in favorable radiation fields, such cervical lymph nodes. For patients with bulky/unfavorable stage I/II disease with a Deauville 1–3 PET-CT after two cycles of ABVD, treatment can be completed with four cycles of AVD,[4] or two cycles of ABVD + INRT if the patient is a good candidate for radiation therapy. PFS with chemotherapy-alone approaches is generally slightly lower than chemotherapy + radiation therapy approaches, but OS is similar since most patients respond well to salvage therapy, and the long-term side effects of mediastinal radiation make chemotherapy-only options reasonable for many early-stage patients.

The current standard of care for patients with stage III/IV cHL is evolving. In the RATHL study, patients with stage III/IV cHL with a Deauville 1–3 PET-CT after two cycles ABVD were de-escalated to four additional cycles of AVD.[4] There was no difference in OS compared to those who received four additional cycles of ABVD, and the PFS difference was not significant. An alternative regimen is AAVD, built on the ABVD backbone but replacing bleomycin with brentuximab vedotin (BV, brand name Adcetris), an anti-CD30 antibody conjugated via a cleavable linker to the tubulin inhibitor monomethyl auristatin E. In the ESCHELON-1 trial, AAVD × 6 had superior PFS and OS to ABVD × 6 in stage III/IV disease (OS HR 0.59, CI 0.40–0.88, P = .009, 6-year OS 93.9% for AAVD vs. 89.4% for ABVD).[5] In subgroup analyses, patients that benefited the most included IPS ≥4, age <60, and males. AAVD carries a different toxicity profile, including increased neuropathy and a requirement for growth factor use due to increased risk of neutropenic fever, and ABVD may still remain appropriate for some patients. For patients over the age of 60 at higher risk of treatment-related complications, a phase 2 study evaluating sequential BV and AVD showed good outcomes, with 84% 2-year PFS and 93% 2-year OS.[6]

Amplification of a region of chromosome 9p containing the T-cell checkpoint genes PD-L1 and PD-L2 is common in cHL, and checkpoint inhibitors have been shown to be efficacious in relapsed cHL.[7,8] Recently presented data using a regimen of the anti-PD-1 antibody nivolumab with AVD ×6 showed superior PFS to AAVD ×6 in stage III/IV cHL (1-year PFS 94%, 95% CI 91–96% for nivolumab + AVD vs. 86%, 95% CI 82–90% for AAVD); OS data is immature. The regimen has not yet received approval in the United States but may become a new standard of care.

Management of patients with positive interim PET-CT after 2 cycles of ABVD is highly context-specific, and multidisciplinary consultation may be helpful. PET-CT-avidity does not always reflect active disease, and biopsy confirmation of refractory disease before changing therapies is appropriate. For patients with partial response to ABVD × 2, options can include continuation of therapies outlined above for patients with some response at all disease foci, addition of consolidative radiation therapy for focal residual disease, or transition to the more intensive regimen of escalated BEACOPP. For patients with frankly progressive disease or relapsed disease, multiple active salvage therapies are available. PD-1 checkpoint inhibitor + chemotherapy regimens are highly active and include pembrolizumab-GVD[7] and nivolumab-ICE; if BV was not used in the front-line setting, BV in combination with nivolumab or ICE is also highly active.[8] Single-agent BV can be considered in patients not fit for more intensive therapy or checkpoint inhibitor therapy. For patients who respond to salvage chemotherapy, autologous transplant with curative intent is standard of care, and high-risk patients (such as those with disease progression within 12 months of initial therapy or extranodal involvement at the time of relapse) have PFS benefit with maintenance BV.[9] Options for patients in the third or later line of therapy include additional chemotherapy (ICE, GVD, GemOx, bendamustine-based regimens, and other regimens), everolimus, and lenalidomide.

CLASSICAL HODGKIN LYMPHOMA FOLLOW-UP

End-of-treatment PET-CT should be used to document complete metabolic response. Standard follow-up includes H&P, CBC, CMP, and ESR every 3–6 months for years 1–2, biannually for year 3, and annually for years 4 and 5. Imaging with CT neck/C/A/P can be considered up to every 6 months for the first 2 years postremission but is of limited utility in detecting early relapses.

For patients who received chest/neck irradiation, long-term toxicities include thyroid dysfunction, cardiovascular disease, and secondary malignancies, especially breast cancer. Patients should receive annual thyroid function tests, biannual lipid and fasting glucose testing, and q10 year stress tests and carotid ultrasounds. Annual breast cancer screening should be initiated in women 8 years after completion of therapy or at age 40, whichever occurs first, including annual mammograms and breast MRI for women who received chest irradiation before the age of 30. Long-term toxicities related to chemotherapy can include neuropathy (especially in patients treated with BV), pulmonary fibrosis in patients treated with bleomycin, and secondary MDS/AML. Infertility occurs in 10% or less of patients treated with ABVD but is of special concern given the younger patient population.

NLPHL TREATMENT AND FOLLOW-UP

Most NLPHL patients present with stage I disease, and patients with highly localized disease in a favorable radiation field can be cured with involved field radiation therapy (IFRT).[10] For patients with stage II–IV disease, watchful waiting may be appropriate in patients with low-volume asymptomatic disease. For patients with treatment indications, R-CHOP (rituximab, cyclophosphamide, doxorubicin, vincristine, and prednisone) and R-CVP (rituximab, vincristine, and prednisone) have been shown to be effective regimens, with ORR around 100% and 5-year PFS 80–90%. Single-agent rituximab also has an ORR of around 100% and low toxicity. While long-term relapse risk is increased compared to chemotherapy-containing regimens, single-agent rituximab is a reasonable option for patients with low tumor bulk, especially those at risk of chemotherapy complications. However, the risk of transformation to aggressive lymphoma appears to be increased in patients with splenic/mesenteric lymph node involvement treated with rituximab alone, and treatment with a chemotherapy-containing regimen is favored for these patients or those with concern for occult transformation, such as patients with an isolated high-SUV focus or B symptoms. Late recurrences are common in NLPHL, and many patients are followed indefinitely with periodic imaging.

Non-Hodgkin Lymphoma

BACKGROUND AND EPIDEMIOLOGY

NHL is the most common lymphoma in adults, with 70,000–80,000 cases diagnosed annually in the United States. They encompass a diverse variety of lymphomas with distinct molecular features and clinical behavior, and with rare exceptions are diseases of older adults. About 85–90% are B-cell–derived. Most of the remaining NHL arise from T-cells, while NK-cell lymphomas are rare. NHL is clinically subdivided into aggressive and indolent lymphomas. Aggressive lymphomas require treatment in days to weeks with multiagent chemoimmunotherapy and are usually treated with curative intent. Indolent lymphomas are generally considered incurable with conventional therapy, and treatment is focused on disease control over long periods of time and minimizing side effects. Many patients with indolent lymphomas do not require upfront treatment, and some patients may never require treatment. There are over 60 types of NHL in the current WHO classification.[1] A full review is beyond the scope of this section, which will instead use the most common variants as prototypes for work-up and management. Other subtypes will be briefly reviewed at the end of the section.

Follicular lymphoma (FL) is the most common indolent lymphoma, with 10,000–15,000 annual diagnoses in the US. It has a median age of presentation around 65 and a median OS of over 15 years in the modern era. FL is believed to arise from germinal center B-cells and is almost universally positive for CD10, a germinal center marker. Over 90% of FL have a t(14;18)(q32;q21) translocation, placing the antiapoptotic gene *BCL2* downstream of the immunoglobulin heavy chain enhancer, driving high levels of BCL2 expression. FL is graded by the number of centroblasts (large, activated, proliferative germinal center B-cells) per high-powered field. Grades 1–3A are managed similarly, while grade 3B, in which centroblasts are present in solid sheets rather than in follicle-like architecture, is a high-grade variant of FL managed like diffuse large B-cell lymphoma (DLBCL).

DLBCL is the most common aggressive B-cell NHL, with 15,000–20,000 annual diagnoses in the US and a median age at presentation of 65. DLBCL may arise *de novo* or from a preexisting indolent lymphoma. Common translocations in DLBCL involve *MYC*, *BCL2*, and/or *BCL6*, often with regulatory regions of the immunoglobulin heavy chain or light chain. High-grade B-cell lymphoma with both *MYC* and *BCL2* or *MYC* and *BCL6* rearrangements is commonly referred to as "double hit" DLBCL and is associated with more aggressive disease. Gene expression profiling has been used to divide DLBCL into germinal center B-cell (GCB) or activated B-cell (ABC) phenotypes, and while gene expression profiling is not routinely done in clinical practice, an IHC algorithm is highly concordant (80–90% concordance). ABC/non-GCB DLCBL is associated with a worse prognosis, but gene expression phenotype is not generally used to select treatment regimens at this time.

CLINICAL PRESENTATION

Indolent lymphomas typically present with painless lymphadenopathy; for patients with significant marrow infiltration, cytopenias may be the presenting complaint. Aggressive lymphomas can present with rapidly enlarging symptomatic lymphadenopathy and about one-third of patients present with B symptoms. Lymphatic spread can be contiguous or with skip lesions. Patients with extranodal involvement may have presenting symptoms related to other disease sites, and patients with CNS involvement may present with neurologic deficits, mental status changes, memory deficits, or seizures.

DIAGNOSIS AND STAGING

Physical exam should focus on lymphatic tissue including lymph nodes, Waldeyer ring, and splenomegaly. FNA may show morphologically abnormal lymphocytes, however, tissue architecture is important for accurate diagnosis, and subtle differences can delineate distinct disease entities. Thus, core or excisional biopsies with flow cytometry and FISH (*MYC, BCL2, BCL6, CCND1*) are preferred for diagnosis. Laboratory studies should include CBC, CMP, LDH, HIV, and hepatitis serologies. Pregnancy testing is indicated for patients with childbearing potential. Beta-2 microglobulin (B2M) can be a useful surrogate for disease burden in mature B-cell NHL, and serum protein electrophoresis, serum-free light chains, and quantitative immunoglobulins may be useful for lymphomas with plasmacytic differentiation. Uric acid and phosphorous should be obtained for aggressive lymphomas at risk for tumor lysis syndrome. Patients planned for anthracycline-containing chemotherapy should undergo a TTE or MUGA. PET-CT is the preferred imaging modality for aggressive B-cell NHL. While PET-CT is also the preferred imaging modality for FL, other indolent B-cell lymphomas have more variable FDG avidity, therefore CT chest/abdomen/pelvis (with neck CT as clinically indicated) may be appropriate unless there is concern for transformation to an aggressive lymphoma. PET-CT is highly predictive of marrow involvement for aggressive B-cell lymphomas, and BM biopsy is not necessary if PET-CT is definitive. Bone marrow biopsy is often necessary for indolent lymphoma to rule out marrow infiltration. CNS work-up including brain MRI and lumbar puncture is warranted for patients with neurologic symptoms or those at high risk for CNS involvement as discussed below.

Disease staging is by the Ann Arbor system (Table 33-2). Numerous clinical risk scores exist for indolent and aggressive lymphoma subtypes, such as the Follicular Lymphoma International Prognostic Index (FLIPI) that incorporates age ≥60, stage III/IV, >4 involved nodal areas, elevated LDH, and Hgb <12 g/dL. The International Prognostic Index (IPI, Table 33-4) is used in DLBCL, and the related CNS-IPI (Table 33-4) is used at the time of presentation to stratify CNS relapse risk.

FOLLICULAR LYMPHOMA TREATMENT

FL is considered largely incurable with modern therapies, though some patients can have long remissions. Patients with highly localized diseases in a favorable radiation field can be cured with local radiation therapy. For patients with more widespread disease, watchful waiting is often appropriate, and ~20% of patients never require treatment. Treatment indications include symptomatic disease, bulky or rapidly enlarging disease, and current or impending end-organ dysfunction.

TABLE 33-4	INTERNATIONAL PROGNOSTIC INDEX AND CNS INTERNATIONAL PROGNOSTIC INDEX
International Prognostic Index	CNS International Prognostic Index
Age >60	Age >60
Ann Arbor stage III or IV	Ann Arbor stage III or IV
Serum LDH > upper limit of normal	Serum LDH > upper limit of normal
ECOG performance stage ≥2	ECOG performance stage ≥2
>1 extranodal site	>1 extranodal site
	Kidney involvement
	Adrenal involvement

In patients with advanced-stage disease requiring treatment, regimen selection is based on disease and patient-specific factors including patient comorbidities, side effect profile, and patient and physician preference. BR (bendamustine and rituximab) × 6 is a well-tolerated and highly effective regimen, with 5-year PFS ~65%[11,12]; in elderly patients or those with comorbidities, four cycles are also reasonable. R-CHOP is also highly effective, with 5-year PFS ~55%,[11,12] but is more toxic and often reserved for patients with more aggressive features (e.g., high SUV or elevated LDH concerning occult transformation, high proliferative index). Single-agent rituximab is active and may be appropriate in some patients, such as those with low disease burden, elderly patients, and patients with significant comorbidities. Maintenance rituximab is associated with superior PFS but not OS,[13] and decision to institute maintenance rituximab should involve risk-benefit calculation. Replacement of rituximab with the alternate anti-CD20 antibody obinutuzumab (O-CHOP or BO) has also been shown to have a PFS but not OS benefit, and choice of CD20 antibody is variable across centers.

Many agents are active in the relapsed setting, though remission duration typically decreases with each line of therapy. Patients with relapse within 24 months of chemoimmunotherapy completion have worse outcomes than those with more prolonged remissions. Some patients will relapse with transformation to DLBCL and are managed as DLBCL. For patients with low-burden asymptomatic FL relapse, watchful waiting is appropriate. For patients requiring treatment, selection of therapy is based on many factors including prior treatment, disease bulk, patient comorbidities, and treatment schedule. Options include single-agent rituximab or obinutuzumab, multiagent chemoimmunotherapy (R-CHOP/O-CHOP or BR/BO), and lenalidomide + rituximab[14] or obinutuzumab. Novel immunotherapies and targeted agents are available in third-line or later relapses. The first-in-class bispecific T-cell engager mosunetuzumab, bridging the B-cell antigen CD20 with the T-cell antigen CD3, had a CR rate of 60% and ORR ~80% in multiply relapsed FL[15] and recently received accelerated approval after two or more lines of therapy. CAR-T cells targeting CD19 (axicabtagene ciloleucel or tisagenlecleucel) are approved after two prior lines of therapy, with CR rates ~70% and ORR >80%.[16,17] It is currently unclear how to sequence cellular therapies given the toxicity profile of these potent agents, the indolent nature of FL, and the older age of many patients with relapsed FL. The oral EZH2 inhibitor tazemetostat has recently been approved for both EZH2 wild-type (~80% of FL) and EZH2 mutant (~20% of FL) disease; while it is most effective in EZH2 mutant disease (ORR 69%), around one-third of EZH wild-type patients respond.[18] PI3K inhibitors used via accelerated approval have been withdrawn from the market due to infectious and inflammatory complications.

DIFFUSE LARGE B-CELL LYMPHOMA TREATMENT

DLBCL is generally treated with curative intent, including in patients with poor performance status if performance status decline is secondary to lymphoma. The preferred treatment for patients with nonbulky stage I/II disease is R-CHOP × 3, followed by an interim PET-CT.[19] Patients with Deauville 1–3 score on interim PET are treated with one additional cycle of R-CHOP, with 4-year PFS of 96%. Patients with partial response (Deauville 4) on interim PET-CT typically receive three additional cycles of R-CHOP. If interim PET-CT is concerning for progressive disease, a biopsy is typically indicated for confirmation; if progressive disease is confirmed, patients are treated for relapsed/refractory disease as below.

The treatment paradigm for patients with bulky stage II or stage III/IV disease is evolving. For years, the standard of care has been R-CHOP × 6 with interim PET-CT after two to four cycles to assess response, with 3-year PFS 56–87%, depending on IPI score. The recently published randomized phase III POLARIX trial[20] evaluated the Pola-R-CHP regimen, in which polatuzumab vedotin, an ADC targeting the B-cell antigen CD79b, replaced vincristine. Pola-R-CHP × 6 was compared against conventional R-CHOP × 6 in advanced-stage DLCBL with IPI ≥2. Pola-R-CHP was shown to have superior EFS (HR 0.73, 95% CI 0.57–0.95, P = .02, 2-year EFS 75.6% vs. 69.4%), trend toward improved CR rate (78.0% vs. 74.0%, P = .16), and fewer patients requiring second-line treatment (22.5% vs. 30.3%); an OS difference was not observed. Side effect profile was overall similar. Some practitioners consider Pola-R-CHP to be the new standard of care for intermediate-to-high-risk DLBCL, while others restrict its use to patients with the most benefit in subgroup analyses, including patients with ABC/non-GCB subtype or IPI ≥3. Longer-term follow-up may clarify the optimal use of this regimen. If a patient is not a candidate for anthracycline-containing therapy due to poor cardiac function, R-CEOP (rituximab, cyclophosphamide, etoposide, vincristine, prednisone) has curative potential, with 5-year and 10-year disease-specific survival of 62% and 58%.[21] R-mini-CHOP is effective in elderly patients (>80) or those with significant comorbidities, with 2-year PFS 47%.[22]

The more intensive regimen DA-R-EPOCH (dose-adjusted infusional doxorubicin, etoposide, and cyclophosphamide, with rituximab and prednisone) has been studied in DLBCL. A phase 2 study showed that DA-R-EPOCH is highly active in *MYC*-rearranged DLBCL, a subtype with worse outcomes than conventional R-CHOP.[23] A phase 3 randomized trial in stage II–IV DLBCL showed no clear benefit to DA-R-EPOCH relative to R-CHOP in DLBCL, and DA-R-EPOCH was associated with increased toxicities.[24] The study was not powered to detect a difference in high-risk subgroups, and some investigators continue to use DA-R-EPOCH in patients with *MYC*-rearranged DLBCL. DA-R-EPOCH is also standard of care in PMBCL as discussed below.

Unlike FL, in the context of DLBCL, there is no PFS benefit with obinutuzumab in place of rituximab, and there is no role for maintenance of rituximab. Consolidative radiation therapy is typically limited to patients with bulky disease or residual disease in a single site amenable to radiation. Patients with testicular involvement should also receive radiation to the contralateral testicle to decrease relapse risk.

Standard therapies for DLBCL are not CNS penetrant, and DLBCL patients with secondary CNS involvement require CNS-directed therapy. Intrathecal methotrexate, cytarabine, and rituximab are effective for patients with leptomeningeal disease but do not have adequate penetration to treat parenchymal CNS disease, which requires systemic high-dose methotrexate in addition to R-CHOP. Whole brain radiation therapy (WBRT) can be associated with significant neurocognitive decline and is usually reserved for relapsed/refractory CNS disease. The role of CNS prophylaxis with intrathecal chemotherapy or systemic CNS-penetrant therapy like high-dose methotrexate or cytarabine is controversial. Patients with the highest risk include those with kidney, adrenal, or testicular involvement, double-hit DLBCL, or elevated CNS IPI (Table 33-4). Multiple retrospective studies have failed to show the benefit of CNS prophylaxis in decreasing the risk of CNS relapse, and the utility of CNS prophylaxis continues to be debated.

DLBCL remains curable in the relapsed setting. Historical treatment has involved salvage chemotherapy followed by autologous transplant in patients with chemosensitive disease, with 5-year DFS of around 50%. Common salvage regimens include R-ICE, R-DHAP, R-ESHAP, and R-GemOx. In recently published trials, anti-CD19 CAR-T cells (axicabtagene ciloleucel, lisocabtagene maraleucel) have superior ORR, CR rate, PFS, and OS compared to salvage chemotherapy followed by autologous transplant in DLBCL patients with primary refractory disease or progression within 1 year of frontline treatment.[17,25] It is unclear at this time which patient subgroups benefit the most from second-line CAR-T, and how to use the response to bridging chemotherapy, if required, to stratify patients. Anti-CD19 CAR-T (axicabtagene ciloleucel, lisocabtagene maraleucel, tisagenlecleucel) are also approved for patients with progressive disease after two or more lines of therapy. Importantly, if chemotherapy is required prior to T-cell collection, bendamustine-containing regimens should be avoided given its T-cell–suppressive properties.

CD20 ×CD3 bispecific T-cell engagers, epcoritamab and glofitamab,[26] have also recently been approved for third and later lines of therapy, including after CAR-T. For patients not appropriate for intensive therapy, other approved regimens include polatuzumab-BR, the Bruton tyrosine kinase (BTK) inhibitor ibrutinib, lenalidomide ± the anti-CD19 antibody tafasitamab, lenalidomide ± rituximab, the nuclear export inhibitor selinexor, and the CD19 ADC loncastuximab tesirine. Choice among agents is driven by side effect profile, patient comorbidities, and treatment schedule.

FOLLOW-UP

For patients with DLBCL, if end-of-treatment PET-CT shows complete metabolic response, recommended follow-up includes H&P with labs every 3–6 months for 5 years, then as indicated. Surveillance imaging after 2 years is not recommended in the absence of clinical indications. For indolent lymphomas, H&P with labs every 3–6 months for 5 years is recommended, then annually as indicated. Surveillance imaging every 6–12 months for up to 2 years is recommended, then no more than annually. Clinicians should be mindful of the risks of cumulative radiation exposure and the incidental detection of clinically insignificant findings, and discontinuation of surveillance imaging is considered reasonable. Long-term complications of therapy include chemotherapy-induced neuropathy, secondary MDS/AML, and anthracycline-induced cardiotoxicity. Rituximab can be associated with delayed-onset (months after completion of therapy) neutropenia of uncertain etiology; bone marrow biopsy is often warranted to rule out a malignant process, but most patients have benign course.

Other Non-Hodgkin Lymphomas

- *High-Grade Transformation*: Approximately 1–3% of indolent B-cell NHL transform to aggressive B-cell NHL annually, typically to DLBCL. Patients generally present with B symptoms, performance status decline, and/or rapidly expanding lymph nodes or extranodal disease. Prognosis is typically poor, and the optimal management remains unclear. Most patients are managed using the DLBCL paradigm outlined above, and enrolled in clinical trials when available.
- *Lymphoblastic Lymphoma*: Lymphoblastic lymphoma is a malignancy arising from immature lymphoid cells, and is more common in the pediatric population than in adults. It is treated similarly to acute lymphoblastic leukemia/lymphoma as outlined in Chapter 32.
- *Burkitt Lymphoma (BL)*: BL is a highly aggressive but curable B-cell lymphoma characterized by MYC overexpression, most commonly via a t(8;14)(q24.1;q32) translocation. There is a male predominance, and heavy abdominal disease burden and extranodal involvement can be present at diagnosis. Biopsy shows a characteristic "starry sky" appearance due to high rates of apoptosis and tingible-body macrophages. BL cells have a doubling time of approximately 24 hours, and BL requires emergent therapy with intensive multiagent chemotherapy such as R-CODOX-M/IVAC, which includes CNS-penetrating therapy. R-hyperCVAD is an alternative used at some centers, and DA-R-EPOCH is effective in older patients (>40 years in the BL context) without CNS involvement. All patients need CNS prophylaxis.
- *Primary Mediastinal B-Cell Lymphoma (PMBCL)*: PMBCL is predominantly a disease of young women, with median age of diagnosis in the mid-30s. Patients typically present with a large mediastinal mass that can cause SVC syndrome or airway compromise. Pathology is similar to DLBCL, but CD30 expression (often weak) is universal. Compartmentalizing fibrosis and CD30 positivity can cause confusion with cHL, but unlike cHL, PMBCL is positive for CD20 and CD45. A phase 2 study of DA-R-EPOCH

showed excellent outcomes without the need for mediastinal radiation,[27] and DA-R-EPOCH is considered by many practitioners to be the standard frontline therapy. Amplification of the PD-L1/PD-L2 region of chromosome 9p is common, and PD-1 checkpoint inhibitors are effective in relapse, as is BV.

- *Gray Zone Lymphoma*: Gray zone lymphoma is a B-cell NHL with morphologic and molecular features overlapping with both DLBCL and cHL. Patients typically present with a bulky mediastinal mass, and there is a male predominance. Neoplastic cells are pleomorphic and sometimes binucleated. Cases with morphologic similarity to cHL are positive for typical B-cell antigens like CD20, CD45, and CD79a, unlike cHL, while cases morphologically similar to DLBCL are often negative for usual B-cell antigens but positive for CD30 and CD15. *MYC* rearrangements and amplifications of 9p can occur. Treatment paradigm is similar to PMBCL.

- *Primary CNS Lymphoma (PCNSL)*: PCNSL is histologically similar to DLBCL, but without sites of systemic disease, and is almost always ABC subtype. Patients present with neurologic symptoms, and diagnosis can be challenging if patients receive steroids prior to biopsy. In addition to PET-CT to rule out systemic DLBCL, a slit-lamp ophthalmic exam is needed to rule out ocular disease. Patients are treated with curative intent with CNS-penetrating therapies including high-dose systemic methotrexate, high-dose cytarabine, and temozolomide. Autologous transplant in first remission, typically with thiotepa-based conditioning, has superior PFS and OS to consolidation with chemotherapy alone. CAR-T, checkpoint inhibitors, ibrutinib, and lenalidomide have activity in the relapsed/refractory setting. WBRT is also effective but can be associated with neurocognitive side effects.

- *Mantle Cell Lymphoma (MCL)*: MCL is a B-cell NHL with a clinical phenotype intermediate between aggressive and indolent disease and is considered incurable with conventional therapy. MCL is characterized by cyclin D1 upregulation, usually via the t(11;14)(q13;q32) translocation, and cyclin D1 can be detected by IHC or FISH. Cells are typically $CD5^+$, $CD20^+$, $CD23^-$; SOX11 is also usually positive. Most patients present with advanced-stage disease, and bone marrow and GI tract involvement at diagnosis are common. Proliferative disease (Ki67 >30%) is a negative prognostic factor, as is TP53 mutation or del(17p). A leukemic variant, often SOX11 negative, can have an indolent clinical history, and watchful waiting is appropriate for some patients. Patients with therapy indications are treated with multiagent chemotherapy. Intensive regimens often incorporate cytarabine, such as R-CHOP alternating with R-DHAP, R-maxiCHOP alternating with high-dose cytarabine, or R-hyperCVAD, with median PFS in the 7–9-year range; R-CHOP alone is less effective. Bendamustine-based regimens including BR and R-BAC (bendamustine, rituximab, and cytarabine) are lower-intensity regimens that are also highly effective. Recently published data show that adding ibrutinib to BR improves PFS but not OS due to significantly increased adverse events. Consolidative autologous transplant in first remission has been shown to improve PFS, and can be considered in appropriate patients. Maintenance rituximab improves both PFS and OS,[28] though the optimal duration of maintenance therapy is controversial. Second-line therapies include regimens incorporating BTK inhibitors, the BCL2 inhibitor venetoclax, lenalidomide, and the proteasome inhibitor bortezomib. Anti-CD19 CAR-T therapy (brexucabtagene autoleucel) is approved in the third line and beyond.

- *Marginal Zone Lymphoma (MZL)*: MZL is an indolent B-cell NHL that can be divided into splenic, nodal, and extranodal subtypes. Within extranodal MZL, mucosa-associated lymphoid tissue (MALT) lymphomas are often triggered by chronic infection/inflammation, with the most common form being gastric MALT lymphoma associated with *Helicobacter pylori* infection. Antibiotic-based *H. pylori* eradication often cures the lymphoma as well, and refractory cases are highly radiosensitive. Splenic MZL can be associated with hepatitis C infection and is highly sensitive to single-agent rituximab. Nodal and non-MALT extranodal MZL are managed similarly to FL.

- *Lymphoplasmacytic Lymphoma (LPL)*: LPL is an indolent lymphoma with plasmacytic differentiation, typically involving the bone marrow, and often with lymph node and splenic involvement.
- *Chronic Lymphocytic Leukemia/Small Lymphocytic Lymphoma (CLL/SLL)*: CLL/SLL is a disease of mature B lymphocytes. It is referred to as CLL if the monoclonal lymphocyte count is $\geq 5 \times 10^9$/L, and SLL if there is nodal or extranodal involvement with a monoclonal lymphocyte count $<5 \times 10^9$/L. Treatment is the same, with the exception that early-stage SLL is potentially curable with radiation therapy. CLL/SLL is discussed in more depth in Chapter 32.
- *Cutaneous T-cell lymphoma (CTCL)*: T-cell lymphomas constitute about 10% of all NHL, with around 7,000 US cases annually. 30–50% of T-cell lymphoma are primary cutaneous T-cell lymphomas, the most common variant of which is mycosis fungoides (MF). MF is a mature T-cell lymphoma that presents as cutaneous patches, plaques, or tumors. Extracutaneous disease involving lymph nodes, spleen, liver, lungs, and blood can occur, while bone marrow involvement is rare. Staging is based on the extent of skin, nodal, visceral organ, and blood involvement. Sézary syndrome is a related entity characterized by erythroderma, lymphadenopathy, and extensive blood involvement. Early-stage disease is indolent, with an essentially normal life span, while patients with advanced disease (tumors, confluent erythema, significant blood involvement) have worse outcomes. For patients with early-stage disease, early aggressive intervention does not improve outcomes, and quality of life is a guiding principle. Initial therapy is skin-directed (topical steroids, topical bexarotene, topical nitrogen mustard, UV therapy). Systemic therapy is added for refractory skin disease, advanced-stage disease, or aggressive features like folliculotropism or large-cell transformation. Sequential single-agent therapies are often used to minimize toxicity. Targeted therapies are well-tolerated and have high response rates, including BV in patients with ≥ 10% CD30 expression, and the anti-CCR4 antibody mogamulizumab. Other options include bexarotene, vorinostat, romidepsin, gemcitabine, pralatrexate, and liposomal doxorubicin. PD-1 checkpoint inhibitors also have activity in later lines of therapy. Allogeneic transplant can be considered in select circumstances.
- *Peripheral T-cell lymphoma (PTCL)*: PTCL is a heterogeneous group of aggressive mature T-cell lymphomas, with around 3,000 cases diagnosed annually. Patients can present with B symptoms and severe illness, and some present with hemophagocytic lymphohistiocytosis. PET-CT is the preferred staging modality, and most cases require bone marrow biopsy to document marrow involvement. Diagnosis can be challenging as surface phenotype can be difficult to distinguish from benign reactive T-cell populations. Sequence-based testing for clonal T-cell receptor rearrangements can clarify unclear cases, but results may not be available before treatment initiation is indicated. The most common subgroups are anaplastic large-cell lymphoma (ALCL), angioimmunoblastic T-cell lymphoma (AITL), and PTCL not otherwise specified (PTCL NOS). ALCL is subdivided into ALK$^+$ and ALK$^-$ groups, based on the presence of *ALK* gene rearrangement.

Historical treatment is with four cycles of CHOP, followed by PET-CT; patients with complete or partial response receive two additional cycles. Based largely on nonrandomized data, autologous transplant in chemosensitive patients may improve 5-year survival from ~25% to 40–50%. The addition of etoposide to CHOP (CHOEP) improves CR rate from ~40–~50%; most of the additional benefit is in patients under the age of 60 with ALK+ ALCL. The ECHELON-2 trial compared BV-CHP to CHOP in CD30$^+$ PTCL patients.[29] BV-CHP improved median 5-year PFS (51.4% vs. 43.0%) and OS (70.1% vs. 61.0%), and ALK$^+$ ALCL patients again had the most benefit. The role of autologous transplant post-BV-CHP is unclear, but subgroup analysis suggests continued benefit, at least in non-ALK$^+$ ALCL subgroups. Studies are ongoing regarding the combination of oral azacitidine + CHOP in AITL. Patients with refractory disease who may be candidate for allogeneic transplants are treated with multiagent chemotherapy. Less intensive options include single-agent BV (if CD30$^+$ and not received in the frontline), bendamustine, gemcitabine, romidepsin, pralatrexate, and belinostat. ALK inhibitors like crizotinib and alectinib have activity in relapsed ALK$^+$ ALCL, and the PI3K inhibitor duvelisib is under study for relapsed PTCL. The role of PD-1 checkpoint inhibitors is also under study; preliminary results suggest activity in some forms of PTCL but acceleration of other forms, and they are not currently approved for use outside of clinical trials.

REFERENCES

1. Swerdlow SH, Campo E, Harris NL, et al., eds *World Health Organization Classification of Tumours of Haematopoietic and Lymphoid Tissues*. Revised 4th ed. IARC; 2017.
2. Radford J, Illidge T, Counsell N, et al. Results of a trial of PET-directed therapy for early-stage Hodgkin's lymphoma. *N Engl J Med*. 2015;372(17):1598–1607.
3. André MPE, Girinsky T, Federico M, et al. Early positron emission tomography response-adapted treatment in stage I and II Hodgkin lymphoma: final results of the randomized EORTC/LYSA/FIL H10 Trial. *J Clin Oncol*. 2017;35(16):1786–1794.
4. Johnson P, Federico M, Kirkwood A, et al. Adapted treatment guided by interim PET-CT scan in advanced Hodgkin's lymphoma. *N Engl J Med*. 2016;374(25):2419–2429.
5. Connors JM, Jurczak W, Straus DJ, et al. Brentuximab vedotin with chemotherapy for stage III or IV Hodgkin's lymphoma. *N Engl J Med*. 2018;378(4):331–344.
6. Evens AM, Advani RH, Helenowski IB, et al. Multicenter phase II study of sequential brentuximab vedotin and doxorubicin, vinblastine, and dacarbazine chemotherapy for older patients with untreated classical Hodgkin lymphoma. *J Clin Oncol*. 2018;36(30):3015–3022.
7. Moskowitz AJ, Shah G, Schöder H, et al. Phase II trial of pembrolizumab plus gemcitabine, vinorelbine, and liposomal doxorubicin as second-line therapy for relapsed or refractory classical Hodgkin lymphoma. *J Clin Oncol*. 2021;39(28):3109–3117.
8. Advani RH, Moskowitz AJ, Bartlett NL, et al. Brentuximab vedotin in combination with nivolumab in relapsed or refractory Hodgkin lymphoma: 3-year study results. *Blood*. 2021;138(6):427–438.
9. Moskowitz CH, Nademanee A, Masszi T, et al; AETHERA Study Group. Brentuximab vedotin as consolidation therapy after autologous stem-cell transplantation in patients with Hodgkin's lymphoma at risk of relapse or progression (AETHERA): a randomised, double-blind, placebo-controlled, phase 3 trial. *Lancet*. 2015;385(9980):1853–1862.
10. Bartlett NL. Treatment of nodular lymphocyte Hodgkin lymphoma: the goldilocks principle. *J Clin Oncol*. 2020;38(7):662–668.
11. Rummel MJ, Niederle N, Maschmeyer G, et al; Study group indolent Lymphomas (StiL). Bendamustine plus rituximab versus CHOP plus rituximab as first-line treatment for patients with indolent and mantle-cell lymphomas: an open-label, multicentre, randomised, phase 3 non-inferiority trial. *Lancet*. 2013;381(9873):1203–1210.
12. Flinn IW, van der Jagt R, Kahl B, et al. First-line treatment of patients with indolent non-Hodgkin lymphoma or mantle-cell lymphoma with bendamustine plus rituximab versus R-CHOP or R-CVP: results of the BRIGHT 5-year follow-up study. *J Clin Oncol*. 2019;37(12):984–991.
13. Bachy E, Seymour JF, Feugier P, et al. Sustained progression-free survival benefit of rituximab maintenance in patients with follicular lymphoma: long-term results of the PRIMA study. *J Clin Oncol*. 2019;37(31):2815–2824.
14. Delfau-Larue M-H, Boulland M-L, Beldi-Ferchiou A, et al. Lenalidomide/rituximab induces high molecular response in untreated follicular lymphoma: LYSA ancillary RELEVANCE study. *Blood Adv*. 2020;4(14):3217–3223.
15. Budde LE, Sehn LH, Matasar M, et al. Safety and efficacy of mosunetuzumab, a bispecific antibody, in patients with relapsed or refractory follicular lymphoma: a single-arm, multicentre, phase 2 study. *Lancet Oncol*. 2022;23(8):1055–1065.
16. Fowler NH, Dickinson M, Dreyling M, et al. Tisagenlecleucel in adult relapsed or refractory follicular lymphoma: the phase 2 ELARA trial. *Nat Med*. 2022;28(2):325–332.
17. Locke FL, Miklos DB, Jacobson CA, et al; All ZUMA-7 Investigators and Contributing Kite Members. Axicabtagene ciloleucel as second-line therapy for large B-cell lymphoma. *N Engl J Med*. 2022;386(7):640–654.
18. Morschhauser F, Tilly H, Chaidos A, et al. Tazemetostat for patients with relapsed or refractory follicular lymphoma: an open-label, single-arm, multicentre, phase 2 trial. *Lancet Oncol*. 2020;21(11):1433–1442.

19. Poeschel V, Held G, Ziepert M, et al; FLYER Trial Investigators; German Lymphoma Alliance. Four versus six cycles of CHOP chemotherapy in combination with six applications of rituximab in patients with aggressive B-cell lymphoma with favourable prognosis (FLYER): a randomised, phase 3, non-inferiority trial. *Lancet.* 2019;394(10216):2271–2281.

20. Tilly H, Morschhauser F, Sehn LH, et al. Polatuzumab vedotin in previously untreated diffuse large b-cell lymphoma. *N Engl J Med.* 2022;386(4):351–363.

21. Moccia AA, Schaff K, Freeman C, et al. Long-term outcomes of R-CEOP show curative potential in patients with DLBCL and a contraindication to anthracyclines. *Blood Adv.* 2021;5(5):1483–1489.

22. Peyrade F, Jardin F, Thieblemont C, et al; Groupe d'Etude des Lymphomes de l'Adulte (GELA) investigators. Attenuated immunochemotherapy regimen (R-miniCHOP) in elderly patients older than 80 years with diffuse large B-cell lymphoma: a multicentre, single-arm, phase 2 trial. *Lancet Oncol.* 2011;12(5):460–468.

23. Dunleavy K, Fanale MA, Abramson JS, et al. Dose-adjusted EPOCH-R (etoposide, prednisone, vincristine, cyclophosphamide, doxorubicin, and rituximab) in untreated aggressive diffuse large B-cell lymphoma with MYC rearrangement: a prospective, multicentre, single-arm phase 2 study. *Lancet Haematol.* 2018;5(12):e609–e617.

24. Bartlett NL, Wilson WH, Jung SH, et al. Dose-adjusted EPOCH-R compared with R-CHOP as frontline therapy for diffuse large B-cell lymphoma: clinical outcomes of the phase III intergroup trial alliance/CALGB 50303. *J Clin Oncol.* 2019;37(21):1790–1799.

25. Abramson JS, Solomon SR, Arnason J, et al. Lisocabtagene maraleucel as second-line therapy for large B-cell lymphoma: primary analysis of the phase 3 TRANSFORM study. *Blood.* 2023; 141(14):1675–1684.

26. Dickinson MJ, Carlo-Stella C, Morschhauser F, et al. Glofitamab for relapsed or refractory diffuse large B-cell lymphoma. *N Engl J Med.* 2022;387(24):2220–2231.

27. Dunleavy K, Pittaluga S, Maeda LS, et al. Dose-adjusted EPOCH-rituximab therapy in primary mediastinal B-cell lymphoma. *N Engl J Med.* 2013;368(15):1408–1416.

28. Martin P, Cohen JB, Wang M, et al. Treatment outcomes and roles of transplantation and maintenance rituximab in patients with previously untreated mantle cell lymphoma: results from large real-world cohorts. *J Clin Oncol.* 2023;41(3):541–554.

29. Horwitz S, O'Connor OA, Pro B, et al. Brentuximab vedotin with chemotherapy for CD30-positive peripheral T-cell lymphoma (ECHELON-2): a global, double-blind, randomised, phase 3 trial. *Lancet.* 2019;393(10168):229–240.

Introduction to Hematopoietic Stem Cell Transplantation

34

Giulia Petrone and Amanda F. Cashen

INTRODUCTION

Hematopoietic stem cell transplantation (HSCT) is a potentially curative therapy for many malignant and nonmalignant hematologic disorders, certain solid tumors, and selected metabolic and autoimmune diseases. HSCT involves the administration of high-dose chemotherapy with or without radiation followed by the infusion of hematopoietic stem and progenitor cells (HSPCs). HSCT is characterized as autologous or allogeneic, depending on whether the stem cells are harvested from the patient or from a donor. The number of HSCT in adult patients continues to steadily increase in the US. Moreover, improvements in supportive care, donor selection, and the introduction of reduced intensity conditioning regimens (RIC) improved transplant outcomes and expanded its use to older patients.[1] This chapter reviews the basic concepts and clinical aspects of both autologous and allogeneic HSCTs.

PATIENT SELECTION AND ELIGIBILITY

Indications for Transplant

Autologous and allogeneic HSCT are used to treat a variety of malignant and nonmalignant disorders (Table 34-1). The most common indication for autologous HSCT is multiple myeloma, while acute leukemia is the main indication for allogeneic HSCT. Early referral for transplant assessment is critical to optimize transplant outcomes. The National Marrow Donor Program (NMDP) and the American Society for Transplantation and Cellular Therapy (ASTCT) have published guidelines with recommended timing for transplant consultation.

- **Multiple myeloma.** Induction with four to six cycles of a three- or four-drug chemotherapy regimen followed by autologous HSCT is the standard of care for newly diagnosed multiple myeloma. Autologous HSCT has been associated with better progression-free survival and overall survival (OS) compared to chemotherapy only, including newer-generation immunomodulatory agents and proteosome inhibitors.
- **Hodgkin lymphoma.** Autologous HSCT is the standard of care in patients with relapsed or refractory disease and confers better outcomes in patients with chemotherapy-sensitive disease.
- **Non-Hodgkin lymphoma (NHL).** Autologous HSCT is indicated for relapsed diffuse large B-cell lymphoma (DLBCL) after the PARMA trial showed improved survival compared to standard chemotherapy. Based on the ZUMA-7[2] and the TRANSFORM[3] studies, patients with primary refractory DLBCL or early relapse (<12 months) are now treated with cellular therapy due to increased complete response rates and better event-free survival compared to salvage chemotherapy followed by autologous HSCT. Indications for autologous HSCT in indolent NHL are less established. Patients with mantle cell lymphoma can benefit from transplant especially if performed early in the disease course. Autologous HSCT is also used in follicular lymphoma patients with early treatment failure or progression within 2 years of initial therapy due to good OS of 70% and low nonrelapse mortality (NRM) of 5–7%. In peripheral T-cell lymphomas,

TABLE 34-1	INDICATIONS FOR HEMATOPOIETIC STEM CELL TRANSPLANT

Autologous Transplant

Plasma cell disorders (multiple myeloma, plasma cell leukemia, light-chain amyloidosis, POEMS syndrome)

Hodgkin and non-Hodgkin lymphoma (diffuse large B-cell lymphoma, primary central nervous system lymphoma, follicular lymphoma, mantle cell lymphoma, T-cell lymphomas)

Acute promyelocytic leukemia

Solid tumors (neuroblastoma, germ cell tumors, Ewing sarcoma)

Autoimmune diseases (multiple sclerosis, systemic sclerosis)

Allogeneic Transplant

Acute and chronic myeloid leukemia

Acute and chronic lymphocytic leukemia

Myelodysplastic and myeloproliferative syndromes

Therapy-related acute myeloid leukemia/myelodysplastic syndrome

Hodgkin and non-Hodgkin lymphoma

Aplastic anemia and other bone marrow failure disorders

Hemoglobinopathies: thalassemia and sickle cell disease

Wiskott–Aldrich syndrome and other immunodeficiency syndromes

Inborn errors of metabolism: Hurler syndrome, adrenoleukodystrophy

---

autologous HSCT is recommended after first complete remission (CR) with OS of 75% in chemotherapy-sensitive patients.

- **Acute myeloid leukemia (AML).** Allogeneic transplant is indicated after CR1 in all eligible patients with intermediate and high-risk AML due to survival benefit compared to consolidation chemotherapy alone (OS 40–60%). Allogeneic HSCT is also indicated in patients with second CR or primary refractory AML, with OS of 30% and 10%, respectively.
- **Acute lymphoblastic leukemia (ALL).** Patients with ALL are stratified into good, intermediate, and poor risk. Good- and intermediate-risk patients are usually treated with chemotherapy, while allogeneic HSCT is reserved for relapse. Allogeneic HSCT is the treatment of choice for poor-risk patients.
- **Myelodysplastic syndrome (MDS).** Allogeneic HSCT is the only curative option for MDS and is indicated for eligible patients with intermediate, high, and very high-risk diseases based on the revised International Prognostic Scoring System.

Patient Eligibility and Pretransplant Evaluation

Transplant eligibility depends on multiple factors, including performance status, concurrent diseases, organ function, and psychosocial assessment. Age alone is not a contraindication, especially with the improvements in supportive care and the introduction of RIC. Patients older than 70 years of age are eligible if appropriately selected. Scoring systems such as the HCT-comorbidity index (HCT-CI) have been developed to estimate the risk of NRM after transplant. Pretransplant evaluation includes collection of a medical history and physical examination to assess performance status (ECOG 0–2 required) and comorbidities, review of initial diagnostic and staging tests including bone marrow (BM) biopsies to confirm the diagnosis, and assess the current disease status, evaluation of baseline organ function such as cardiac function (left ventricular ejection fraction >40% desirable), and pulmonary function (carbon monoxide diffusion in the lung, DLCO, >40% required). Patients undergo testing to evaluate renal and liver function to predict risk of drug toxicity as well as risk of veno-occlusive disease (VOD). Infectious markers including cytomegalovirus (CMV), herpes simplex virus (HSV), HIV, human T-cell lymphoma virus type 1 (HTLV-1), Epstein–Barr virus (EBV), toxoplasmosis, and hepatitis A, B, and C are assessed to decide which patients require disease-specific prophylaxis. Typing of both donor and recipient for HLA antigens and ABO/Rh is necessary for allogeneic HSCT candidates. A psychosocial evaluation is also required to establish the social support needed.

SOURCES OF STEM CELLS

HSPC can be obtained from BM or from peripheral blood (PB) for both autologous and allogenic HSCT. Umbilical cord blood (UCB) is an alternative source of HSPC available for allogenic HSCT.

Bone Marrow

Historically, BM was the main source for HSPC. BM harvest requires multiple aspirations from the iliac crests under regional or general anesthesia and allows the collection of a variable volume of BM. The number of cells necessary depends on the weight of the recipient with a goal of 10–15 mL/kg of recipient weight. BM HSPC can have high hematocrits and require removal of plasma and red blood cells (RBCs) to avoid hemolytic reactions if donor and recipient are ABO/Rh incompatible. BM HSPCs are associated with a modest decreased risk of chronic graft versus host disease (GVHD) and might be preferred in nonmalignant diseases. Specifically, BM HSPC is the preferred graft source for aplastic anemia as it has been associated with better outcomes.

Peripheral Blood

Since the 1990s, mobilized PB HSPCs have become the source of choice because of easier access as well as concern for higher relapse rates associated with BM HSPCs.[4] However, no difference in OS and disease-free survival has been observed in studies that have compared the two graft sources.[5] PB HSPCs have been associated with faster engraftment and a modest increased risk of chronic GVHD (cGVHD) compared to BM HSPCs due to higher amounts of T lymphocytes in the PB.[6] Normally, a small number of HSPCs circulate in the PB but they can be recruited from the BM by administration of hematopoietic growth factors or chemotherapy in a process defined as "stem cell mobilization." Cytokines that are most used for stem cell mobilization are granulocyte colony–stimulating factor (G-CSF or filgrastim) and plerixafor, either alone or in combination. Plerixafor is a CXCR4 antagonist that works by inhibiting the binding of CXCL12 expressed on BM stromal cells to the CXCR4 receptor. This interaction is essential for the homing of HSPCs and its blockage allows mobilization of HSPCs into the blood. Filgrastim and plerixafor are administered to the patient or donor before the collection for up to 4 days. Common side effects of filgrastim are bone pain, myalgia, nausea, headache, and low-grade fevers; a rare side effect is splenic rupture. Plerixafor can cause diarrhea, nausea, and fatigue. Cytotoxic chemotherapy in combination with filgrastim or alone can aid in the mobilization of HSPCs due to the release of large numbers of HSPCs during BM recovery. Cyclophosphamide or other cytotoxic regimens are used in patients undergoing autologous HSCT as a method for stem cell mobilization.

HSPC Harvest

After mobilization, PB CD34+ cells—the population containing HSPC—are collected through apheresis. Only the mononuclear fraction with the HSPCs is retained, while the rest is reinfused into the patient. The collection goal is at least $2–3 \times 10^6$ CD34+ cells/kg per transplant, and ideally, enough stem cells for a second infusion are saved for all patients undergoing allogeneic HSCT and for some autologous indications. For autologous transplants, 2×10^6 CD34+ cells/kg are sufficient but 5×10^6 CD34+ cells/kg increase the chance of early platelet recovery. For allogeneic transplants, the ideal goal is 5×10^6 CD34+ cells/kg but a dose of 3×10^6 CD34+ cells/kg is considered sufficient. In healthy donors, one apheresis session is usually enough to collect the necessary amount of stem cells. Risk factors for suboptimal collection include older age and prior exposure to chemotherapy and/or radiation which are common in patients undergoing autologous HSCT who might require multiple sessions.

Umbilical Cord Blood

UCB is a rapidly available source of HSPC for patients who do not have a matched related or unrelated donor. UCB is the blood present in the umbilical cord and placenta and is collected immediately after birth. It contains 10–20 times fewer HSPCs compared to BM or PB grafts and is mostly used in pediatric patients. Adult patients may require infusion of two different units (double cord allogeneic HSCT) to receive an adequate cell dose, defined as $\geq 2.5 \times 10^7$ CD34+ cells/kg since single UCB units have lower numbers of HSPCs. The advantage of UCB is that it has lower risks of GVHD due to decreased allogeneic reactivity and can be performed despite higher degree of HLA mismatch. The major limitations are slow engraftment with prolonged cytopenia, delayed immune reconstitution with higher risk of post-HSCT infections, increased chance of graft failure, and the unavailability of the donor to collect additional HSPCs in case of graft failure or relapse.

TYPES OF TRANSPLANTS

Autologous HSCT

Autologous HSCT is the most frequently performed transplant in the US, and its main indication is multiple myeloma.[1] The principle of autologous HSCT was based on the observation that the dose-limiting toxicity of many chemotherapeutic treatments is myelosuppression. The infusion of previously harvested HSPC reconstitutes hematopoiesis and allows the administration of high-dose chemotherapy to maximize tumor eradication. Autologous HSCT has fewer complications than allogeneic HSCT, including lack of GVHD and lower risk of infections, so it can be used in older patients. However, the absence of graft-versus-tumor (GVT) effect and the risk of contamination of the graft with cancer cells are associated with higher relapse rates. Attempts have been made to remove or "purge" contaminating tumor cells from the apheresis product using antibody selection, but no studies have shown better outcomes with this technique.

Source of Graft

Mobilized PB HSPC are the preferred source of stem cells for autologous HSCT because of easier collection and faster engraftment. After collection, the graft can be stored by cryopreservation or reinfused. PB HSPC can also be modified by gene editing as a potential treatment for genetic diseases such as hemoglobinopathies.[7]

Syngeneic HSCT

A syngeneic HSCT is a transplant from an identical twin which is similar to an autologous HSCT but has not been associated with improved outcomes. Since syngeneic transplants do not cause GVHD or GVT, they are not preferred over allogeneic HSCTs which rely on GVT effect to reduce relapse risk.

Allogeneic HSCT

Allogeneic HSCT refers to the transplant of a donor's HSPCs to a recipient. Donor and recipient need to be matched for their human leukocyte antigens (HLA) to prevent graft rejection and to minimize immune-mediated damage of host tissue by the graft (GVHD). Like autologous transplants, the conditioning regimen allows eradication of malignant cells or defective host stem cells and eliminates recipient immune cells that can reject the graft. A unique feature of allogeneic HSCT is the potent alloreactivity of donor T lymphocytes and natural killer (NK) cells that recognize and attack foreign tumor cells producing a GVT effect that provides immune surveillance and contributes to the long-lasting clearance of malignant cells. Recent studies show that not only NK cells contribute to GVT, but also their haplotype can be important in reducing relapse rates after allogeneic HSCT.[8]

Source of Graft

Mobilized PB HSPCs are the preferred graft source. In nonmalignant disorders and aplastic anemia, where GVT is not desired, BM grafts are usually preferred due to the decreased likelihood of GVHD.

DONOR SELECTION FOR ALLOGENEIC HSCT

HLA Typing

The most important factor in donor selection is histocompatibility. The major histocompatibility complex (MHC) locus, also called "HLA locus," is located on chromosome 6 and encodes the HLA antigens. HLA genes are highly polymorphic and encode for a variety of different proteins that are expressed on the cell surface and involved in antigen recognition by the immune system. HLA molecules act as alloantigens, potentially triggering immune activation and graft rejection in mismatched patients. HLA molecules are divided into class I (HLA-A, HLA-B, HLA-C) and class II (HLA-DR, HLA-DQ, HLA-DP). HLA typing is performed by high-resolution molecular techniques that use sequence-specific DNA probes to identify HLA alleles. Molecular typing allows very precise HLA matching with improved patient outcomes and has replaced low-resolution serologic testing. Differences identified by molecular typing are called allele mismatches. Besides the HLA antigens, there are other minor histocompatibility antigens that are also involved in alloreactivity. Typing for minor histocompatibility antigens is not necessary, however, mismatches of these minor antigens can trigger both GVHD as well as GVT effect.[9]

HLA Matching

The donor can be either a related family member or an unrelated donor. Donors are classified as matched related donor (MRD), matched unrelated donor (MUD), mismatched unrelated donor (MMUD), and alternative donor sources (haploidentical and cord blood grafts).

Matched Related Donors

A fully matched sibling donor is the preferred graft source as it is associated with improved outcomes and less morbidity, including decreased risk of GVHD. Since HLA genes are tightly clustered on chromosome 6, HLA alleles are inherited as a set, defined as the patient's haplotype. Each sibling has ~25% chance of being HLA-identical if they inherit the same haplotype. Typing of HLA-A, HLA-B, and HLA-DRB1 is sufficient to determine the haplotype (HLA-C is inherited with HLA-B due to their proximity on chromosome 6), and is the minimum requirement when selecting a related donor.[10] Thus, fully matched siblings are 6/6 matches. Despite being the ideal graft, approximately only 30% of patients have a suitable HLA-matched sibling.

Matched Unrelated Donors

To address the need for matched donors, registries of adult volunteers and UCB blood banks have grown worldwide. In the US, the NMDP coordinates unrelated donor transplant searches which require on average up to 4 months. Histocompatibility drives the selection of a suitable donor which is defined as 10/10 match obtained by molecular typing for HLA-A, HLA-B, HLA-C, HLA-DRB1, and HLA-DQB1. Typing of loci HLA-DPB1 and HLA-DRB3/4/5 is usually done as well and is particularly useful if there are multiple available donors. Although it is still controversial if 12/12 matches have better outcomes, mismatches of HLA-DPB1 are associated with higher risk of GVHD.[11] Because of improved typing techniques and increased availability of volunteer donors, the number of MUD transplants is rising. Disadvantages compared to MRD HSCT are the time-consuming and expensive process of finding a suitable donor, the decreased chance of having a second stem cell collection from the same donor in case of graft failure or relapse, and the higher likelihood of mismatch at minor histocompatibility antigens. Moreover, the probability of finding a match is related to how common the patient's HLA haplotype is in the population which is largely dependent on race. The chance of finding an optimal donor is much higher for Caucasian patients of European descent (~75%) compared to Hispanics (~35%), Asians (~30%), and African Americans (~19%).[12]

Mismatched Donors

If there is no suitable matched donor, a single HLA locus mismatched related or unrelated donor (7/8) is considered. Mismatched transplants are associated with increased risk of GVHD, graft failure, and mortality. Some studies suggest that a single mismatch at HLA-B or HLA-C is less deleterious and, specifically, permissive HLA-C mismatches and host-versus-graft-only mismatches may improve outcomes.[10,13]

Haploidentical Donors

Haploidentical donors are mismatched donors at three of the six possible loci (HLA-A, HLA-B, and HLA-DR) that are usually typed in related donors. Every parent shares one haplotype with their children and siblings have ~50% chance of being haploidentical. Thus, haploidentical transplants have been increasing in number and improving the chance of finding a suitable donor regardless of race. The major risks of mismatched transplants are severe GVHD and graft failure but the introduction of posttransplant cyclophosphamide on days +3 and +4 has decreased these complications to rates similar to MRD and MUD with outcomes comparable to fully matched transplants.[14]

UCB Donors

UCB HSCTs require less stringent HLA matching and can be performed with mismatches at two or three HLA antigens. Typing is performed for HLA-A, -B, and -DRB1. Recipient and donor should be a ≥4/6 match, although recent studies suggest that 6/6 matching might be desirable.

Other Factors

Age is an important non–HLA-related factor and donors should be younger than 60 years of age due to better outcomes. If multiple HLA-compatible donors are available, preference is given to younger, CMV-negative (for CMV-negative patients), and ABO-matched male or nulliparous female donors, as there is some evidence for improved clinical outcomes with these grafts. Another factor to consider is the possibility that the recipient may have antibodies against foreign HLA antigens termed donor-specific antibodies (DSAs). DSAs can increase the risk of graft failure so patients should be screened for and, if necessary, treated with desensitization strategies to improve engraftment.

CONDITIONING REGIMENS

Conditioning regimens consist of chemotherapy and/or radiation given the days immediately before the infusion of HSPCs. The purpose is to eradicate lingering malignant cells, make space for the new HSPCs, and, in allogeneic HSCT, immunosuppress the host to

| TABLE 34-2 | COMMON CONDITIONING REGIMENS |

Regimen	Dose
Myeloablative Conditioning	
Allogeneic Regimens	
Cy/TBI	Cyclophosphamide 120 mg/kg + TBI 1,225 cGy + MESNA 120 mg/kg
Bu/Cy	Busulfan 16 mg/kg + Cyclophosphamide 120 mg/kg + MESNA 120 mg/kg
Flu/Bu	Fludarabine 120–150 mg/m^2 + Busulfan 9.6–12.8 mg/kg
Autologous Regimens	
Multiple Myeloma	
High-dose melphalan	Melphalan 200 mg/m^2
Lymphoma	
BEAM	BCNU 450 mg/m^2 + Etoposide 800 mg/m^2 + Ara-C 800 mg/m^2 + Melphalan 140 mg/m^2
Solid Tumors	
MEC	Etoposide 1,200 mg/m^2 + Carboplatinum 1,400 mg/m^2 + Melphalan 140 mg/m^2
Reduced-Intensity Conditioning	
Flu/Bu +/− ATG	Fludarabine 150 mg/m^2 + Busulfan 8 mg/kg + ATG 40 mg/kg
Flu/Mel	Fludarabine 25 mg/m^2 + Melphalan 140 mg/m^2
Nonmyeloablative Conditioning	
Flu/TBI	Fludarabine 60 mg/m^2 + TBI 2 cGy
Flu/Cy	Cyclophosphamide 120 mg/kg + Fludarabine 125 mg/m^2 + MESNA 120 mg/kg
Cy/Thymic RT/ATG	Cyclophosphamide 200 mg/kg + Thymic RT 700 cGy + ATG 45–90 mg/kg + MESNA 200 mg/kg

Ara-C, cytosine arabinose; ATG, antithymocyte globulin; BCNU, 1,3-bis-(2-chloroethyl)-1-nitrosourea; MESNA, (sodium-2)-mercaptoethanesulfonate; RT, radiation therapy; TBI, total-body irradiation.

avoid graft rejection. The choice of a specific regimen depends on the disease treated and on the patient's characteristics. In general, younger patients or patients with active disease are more likely to get higher-intensity conditioning, while older patients or patients with nonmalignant disorders are probably better served with less intense regimens. Specifically, patients with AML and MDS are preferentially treated with myeloablative conditioning regimens (MAC) due to decreased risk of relapse compared to RIC.[15] However, in older patients who are not eligible for MAC, allogeneic HSCT with RIC regimens should still be considered because of survival benefits compared to no transplant. MAC is also favored in AML patients with genomic evidence of minimal residual disease before HSCT due to improved outcomes.[16] Commonly used regimens are listed in Table 34-2.

Myeloablative Conditioning

Per definition, MAC regimens do not allow autologous hematologic recovery. Traditional MAC include myeloablative doses of alkylating agents (cyclophosphamide, busulfan, melphalan) sometimes in association with total-body irradiation (TBI). MAC regimens are frequently used for autologous transplants because the high-dose chemotherapy can control the disease in the absence of GVT effect. Common side effects include mucositis, alopecia, and GI toxicity. Some regimens can also increase the risk of specific complications such as sinusoidal obstruction syndrome of the liver (SOS).

Reduced-Intensity Regimens

Nonmyeloablative regimens cause minimal marrow suppression and do not require stem cell support, while RIC is an intermediate category between MAC and nonmyeloablative regimens. These regimens were designed to reduce the toxicity associated with high-dose therapy and take advantage of the GVT effect to eradicate malignant cells. They are associated with decreased treatment-related mortality but higher relapse rates with comparable rates of acute GVHD (aGVHD) and cGVHD. The advantage of RIC regimens is that older patients and patients with comorbidities can now be considered for HSCT.

HEMATOPOIETIC STEM CELL INFUSION

Once the conditioning regimen is given, stem cells are infused. HSPCs collected for autologous HSCT are cryopreserved in the vapor phase of liquid nitrogen with the cryoprotectant dimethyl sulfoxide (DMSO) while allogeneic grafts are usually infused fresh. Hemolysis of contaminating RBCs can cause renal damage which is prevented by alkalizing the urine with a bicarbonate infusion. Small-volume grafts are usually infused over a 15-minute period, but larger-volume products might require hours. Most side effects during the infusion are due to DMSO or hypersensitivity reactions including nausea, vomiting, unpleasant taste, hypotension, and anaphylaxis.

POSTTRANSPLANT CARE AND COMPLICATIONS

Engraftment

After stem cell infusion, there is a phase of profound myelosuppression. HSPCs are home to the BM and start proliferating in the process of "engraftment." Neutrophil engraftment is defined as an absolute neutrophil count (ANC) >500/mm^3 for 3 consecutive days and typically takes about 2 weeks with HLA-identical PBSC transplants and up to 4 weeks in haploidentical and BM transplants. Administration of colony-stimulating factors, such as G-CSF, accelerates engraftment without improving survival. Platelet engraftment is defined as a platelet count of >20 × 10^3/μL and usually takes longer with a variable recovery time. In allogeneic HSCT, evidence of engraftment is identified by analyzing donor/recipient chimerism either by donor- and recipient-specific short tandem repeats (STRs), or by analyzing the ratio of sex chromosomes using fluorescence in situ hybridization (FISH) probes in sex-mismatched transplants.

Engraftment Syndrome

It is a complication of the first days to weeks after neutrophil recovery and is characterized by a combination of fever, erythematous rash, and noncardiogenic pulmonary edema. Treatment with a short course of corticosteroid is usually effective, especially in patients with significant pulmonary involvement.

Graft Failure

It is the rejection of donor HSPCs and is classified as primary (lack of engraftment with ANC <500/mm^3 by day +28) or secondary (loss of donor HSPCs after initial engraftment). Risk factors for graft failure include HLA mismatch, inadequate conditioning or immunosuppression, low HSPC dose, T-cell depletion of the graft, graft source (more common with UCB or BM), infections, and high titers of DSA. Graft failure can be diagnosed by measuring recipient/donor chimerism and should be distinguished from relapse. Treatment strategies include hematopoietic growth factors, more intensive immunosuppression, donor lymphocyte infusions (DLIs), a second infusion of HSPCs from the original donor, or a second transplant.

Blood Group Incompatibility

Transplantation of ABO incompatible grafts occurs in 30–40% of cases and is classified as major, minor, and bidirectional. Major incompatibility develops when the recipient has ABO antibody against donor RBC antigens (e.g., O recipient, A donor). Minor incompatibility occurs when donor plasma has ABO antibodies against recipient RBC antigens (e.g., A recipient, O donor). Bidirectional mismatch is the presence of both major and minor incompatibility (e.g., donor A, recipient B, or vice versa). Major mismatch can result in immediate or delayed hemolysis, delayed red cell engraftment, or pure red cell aplasia (PRCA). Removal of RBCs from the graft is usually performed in major mismatches, especially from BM grafts, and prevents significant hemolysis. However, recipient ABO antibodies can persist for months and lead to delayed hemolysis or PRCA. If mild hemolysis ensues, transfusion support is sufficient, but more severe reactions might require plasma exchange or rituximab. Minor mismatch can be complicated by immediate hemolysis from the infusion of incompatible plasma which is prevented by removal of plasma from BM grafts (less frequent in PBSC grafts due to collection by apheresis). Another complication is passenger lymphocyte syndrome due to proliferation of lymphocytes in the graft that can cause rapid and massive hemolysis 3–15 days after transplant.

Graft-Versus-Host Disease

GVHD is a complication of allogeneic HSCT caused by alloreactive donor T-cells that recognize recipient antigens. This immune response can be triggered by tissue damage resulting from the conditioning regimen or by infections that further activate donor lymphocytes. The main risk factor for GVHD is major HLA mismatch, however, minor histocompatibility antigens also play an important role. Other risk factors are unrelated or haploidentical donor, a female donor for a male recipient, PBSC grafts, and the intensity of the conditioning regimen. Traditionally, aGVHD and cGVHD were defined by their time of onset but now their diagnosis depends only on the clinical manifestations. Some patients develop an overlap syndrome with classic features of aGVHD along with typical manifestations of cGVHD.

Acute GVHD

aGVHD typically develops 2–42 weeks post-HSCT and it can be classified as persistent, recurrent, or late onset. Usually, aGVHD involves the skin, the liver, and the gastrointestinal (GI) tract. Clinical manifestations vary from a maculopapular rash to severe blistering resembling a burn. Conjugated hyperbilirubinemia due to cholestasis and elevated alkaline phosphatase are signs of liver GVHD. Anorexia, nausea, and vomiting are common features of upper GI involvement, while lower GI symptoms are diarrhea and abdominal cramping. When possible, the diagnosis should be confirmed by biopsy of the affected organ. The severity is graded 1–4 based on the extent of organ involvement according to the Glucksberg criteria. The MAGIC system is a recently developed algorithm that aids in predicting aggressive aGVHD based on symptoms and biopsy results.

aGVHD Prophylaxis

Routine prophylaxis is required due to high morbidity and mortality of aGVHD. The most used regimens combine an antimetabolite agent like methotrexate (MTX) or mycophenolate mofetil (MMF), continued until day +30, and a calcineurin inhibitor, either cyclosporine or tacrolimus, continued until day +100 and then tapered if there are no

GVHD symptoms. Recent studies showed decreased rate of both aGVHD and cGVHD with the addition of antithymocyte globulin (ATG), however, there is concern for higher risk of relapse due to T-cell depletion. Posttransplant high-dose cyclophosphamide (PT-Cy 50 mg/kg on days +3 and +4) was initially studied for haploidentical transplantation and is now used also for MRD and MUD transplants as it showed increased GVHD-free survival compared to traditional regimens. This regimen has dramatically changed mismatched transplants that were limited by high risk of GVHD and is now the preferred regimen for all types of allogeneic HSCTs.[17,18] An alternative method to prevent aGVHD is T-cell depletion by adsorption of lymphocytes or by ATG or other lymphocyte-specific antibodies. However, this is associated with increased risk of graft rejection, relapse, and delayed immune reconstitution. In 2021, Abatacept—a T-cell modulator—was approved in combination with a calcineurin inhibitor and MTX for GVHD prophylaxis.

aGVHD Treatment

First line treatment for aGVHD is corticosteroids.[19] Grade I rashes can be managed with topical steroids. Grade II or higher manifestations are treated with prednisone or methyl-prednisolone 1–2 mg/kg/day tapered gradually. GI symptoms respond to topical steroids including budesonide and beclomethasone. Steroid-refractory patients can be difficult to manage and have a poor prognosis due to recurrent aGVHD, cGVHD, and infections. Ruxolitinib, a JAK1/2 inhibitor, showed promising results in a phase 3 study (overall response 62% compared to 39%) and is approved for steroid-refractory aGVHD.[20]

Chronic GVHD

cGVHD has a poorly understood pathogenesis that revolves around chronic inflammation, loss of self-tolerance, and fibrosis resembling a collagen vascular disease. Clinical manifestations are more heterogeneous than aGVHD and can involve different organs. Risk factors are prior episodes of aGVHD, PSBC grafts, HLA mismatch, and older age of the donor or patient. The National Institutes of Health (NIH) consensus defined the criteria that are used for diagnosis and staging. cGVHD is classified into mild, moderate, or severe disease, depending on the number of affected organs and the amount of functional impairment (graded from 0 to 3). Manifestations of cGVHD resemble autoimmune diseases and commonly involve the skin with different types of rashes such as lichen planus-like or poikiloderma as well as skin thickening. Joints can be affected by stiffness and contractures. Keratoconjunctivitis sicca is a common ocular complication due to lacrimal gland dysfunction causing dry eyes with irritation and pain. GI involvement can lead to malabsorption, unexplained weight loss, esophageal strictures, and dysmotility. Pulmonary fibrosis can result in bronchiolitis obliterans syndrome (BOS) with reduced lung function. Other organs such as the oral mucosa and genitalia can be involved. The diagnosis is usually made clinically by observation of common features but might require histologic confirmation. Of note, while cGVHD—especially with liver or pulmonary involvement—is associated with increased NRM, it is also associated with decreased risk of relapse, perhaps reflecting a GVT effect.

cGVHD Treatment

Since immunosuppression is the mainstay of treatment, if symptoms develop during tapering of the immunosuppressive regimen, increasing the doses might be sufficient. Mild cGVHD can be managed with topical treatment only, while more severe manifestations require systemic corticosteroids. Ibrutinib, a Bruton tyrosine kinase inhibitor, reduces T-cell and B-cell activation and is approved for steroid-refractory cGVHD. In 2021, ruxolitinib was also approved for treatment of cGVHD after failure of one or two prior lines based on a phase 3 study that showed better overall response rate compared to the best available therapy.[21] Most recently, the ROCK2 inhibitor Belumosudil was approved for third-line treatment of cGVHD showing positive responses in patients who failed ibrutinib and ruxolitinib.[22]

Infections

Infections are a frequent complication for all patients receiving a transplant. The risk of infection correlates with the extent of immune impairment and increases in patients who develop GVHD. Autologous HSCT are associated mainly with early bacterial and fungal infections, while allogeneic HSCT can lead to prolonged immunosuppression and late-onset infections due to delayed immune reconstitution. The pre-engraftment period (usually <30 days post-HSCT) is marked by severe neutropenia and mucosal barrier damage from the conditioning regimen and indwelling catheters. Most patients develop neutropenic fevers, presumably from skin and GI organisms, although in most cases pathogens are not isolated. Candida infections, HSV, and varicella zoster virus (VZV) reactivation are also common. The postengraftment phase (days 30–100 post-HSCT) is correlated with impaired cellular and humoral immunity. Invasive *Aspergillus* can cause pneumonia during this period as can Pneumocystis. CMV reactivation can occur and manifests with interstitial pneumonitis, diarrhea, colitis, and retinitis. The late recovery phase (>100 days post-HSCT) is used to describe a variable period of impaired immune function that can last for years, especially in allogeneic HSCT recipients. Patients remain at risk for encapsulated bacterial infection, CMV reactivation, respiratory virus infections, and fungal pneumonia, especially while they are on immune suppression. EBV-related posttransplant lymphoproliferative disease (PTLD) is a possible late complication of prolonged immunosuppression and is managed by withdrawal of the immunosuppressive regimen.

Infection Prophylaxis
Antimicrobial prophylaxis has improved survival in transplant patients.

- **Bacterial prophylaxis.** Fluoroquinolones are used during the pre-engraftment phase and discontinued once the ANC is >500/mm^3.
- **Viral prophylaxis.** HSV and VZV prophylaxis with acyclovir or valacyclovir is used in the early pre-engraftment phase and is continued for 6 months after autologous HSCT and for 12 months or until patients are off immune suppression for allogeneic HSCT. CMV prophylaxis is usually a prerogative of allogeneic HSCT. Prevention of CMV disease is necessary if either the donor or the recipient is CMV positive. One strategy is to monitor CMV replication by PCR and start treatment with ganciclovir when indicated; another option is to give prophylactic letermovir through day 100 after transplant. In patients with CMV infection resistant to ganciclovir, foscarnet or cidofovir can be effective.
- **Fungal prophylaxis.** Fluconazole prophylaxis is used in the pre-engraftment period and is usually given until day 100 post-HSCT. Patients at higher risk of mold infections, such as with prolonged neutropenia or concurrent GVHD requiring immunosuppression, should be covered with mold-active azoles such as voriconazole or posaconazole.
- **Pneumocystis prophylaxis.** Trimethoprim plus sulfamethoxazole (TMP-SMX) twice a week is started in the early pre-engraftment period in all allogeneic HSCT and some autologous HSCT recipients. Prophylaxis is continued until at least 6 months post-HSCT and longer in patients requiring immunosuppression. Alternatives to TMP-SMX are dapsone, atovaquone, or pentamidine.

Gastrointestinal Complications
- **GI toxicity.** Chemotherapy and radiation from the conditioning regimen disrupt the mucosal barriers of the GI tract causing nausea, vomiting, stomatitis, abdominal pain, and diarrhea. High doses of melphalan used for autologous HSCT are associated with severe mucositis which is partially prevented by using ice to cool the oral mucosa throughout the infusion, also defined "cryotherapy."
- **VOD/SOS.** VOD of the liver or hepatic SOS is a complication of the conditioning regimen that can develop within the first 21 days from HSCT and is caused by endothelial

cell injury in hepatic venules, leading to sloughing, venular occlusion, and centrilobular hemorrhagic necrosis. The main risk factor is preexisting liver disease such as prior hepatitis. Other predisposing factors are MAC regimens, especially those with high-dose cyclophosphamide, busulfan, or TBI, treatment with gemtuzumab prior to HSCT, and the use of cyclosporine and MTX for GVHD prophylaxis. The diagnosis is made clinically and requires a bilirubin ≥2 mg/dL with two of the following: painful hepatomegaly, ascites, or weight gain >5% from fluid retention. Some patients require transjugular liver biopsy with portal vein pressure measurement to make the diagnosis. Although spontaneous resolution is seen in most cases, severe VOD can be fatal due to multiorgan failure. Treatment is mainly supportive. Defibrotide is used in severe VOD as it showed improved survival and complete resolution rates at day 100. Low-dose heparin and ursodeoxycholic acid are prophylactic measures that can decrease the incidence of VOD.

Noninfectious Pulmonary Complications

- **Idiopathic pneumonia syndrome (IPS).** It is a noninfectious pneumonitis caused by direct toxicity of the conditioning regimen and it occurs 30–90 days after HSCT. Treatment is supportive but high-dose steroids can also be used.
- **Diffuse alveolar hemorrhage (DAH).** It is also a pneumonitis that occurs in the first weeks after HSCT. If bronchoalveolar lavage (BAL) is performed, it yields blood which is a classic finding. Supportive management and high-dose steroids are the mainstay of treatment.
- **BOS.** It is a chronic obstructive disease that occurs after 3 months from allogeneic HSCT and is a manifestation of lung cGVHD. Symptoms are dry cough and progressive dyspnea. Treatment includes immunosuppression and inhaled steroids.
- **Cryptogenic organizing pneumonia.** It is a chronic restrictive disease that can occur after 3 months from allogeneic HSCT. Manifestations are similar to BOS with dry cough, dyspnea, and fever. Steroids can reverse the lung damage.

Thrombotic Microangiopathy (TMA)

It is a microangiopathic hemolytic anemia that can develop in the first few months after transplant, especially allogeneic HSCT. Calcineurin inhibitors are considered the main risk factor. TMA manifests as renal failure and encephalopathy, but it can also cause severe hemorrhagic diarrhea. Unlike TMA diagnosed in other settings, there is no benefit for plasmapheresis. Supportive care and discontinuation of calcineurin inhibitors/offending agents are the mainstay of therapy. In severe cases, agents such as eculizumab may be considered.

Neurologic Toxicity

- **Posterior reversible encephalopathy syndrome (PRES).** It develops in the early posttransplant period and is more common in allogeneic HSCT. Classic symptoms are confusion, headache, vision changes, and seizures. Calcineurin inhibitors have been associated with PRES and their discontinuation usually resolves the encephalopathy.

Late Complications in Long-Term Survivors

- **Relapse after HSCT.** In patients undergoing autologous HSCTs, relapse is mainly managed by administration of subsequent lines of chemotherapy or, if indicated, cellular therapy. In allogeneic HSCT, withdrawal of immunosuppression is used to boost the GVT effect. DLI is another method to take advantage of the GVT effect. Side effects associated with DLI are aGVHD, cGVHD, and BM aplasia.
- **Secondary malignancies.** The cumulative toxicity of high-dose chemotherapy and radiation results in increased incidence of post-HSCT malignancies. Skin cancer and other solid tumors are frequently associated with TBI. Exposure to alkylating agents can cause

therapy-related AML and MDS. PTLD is a B-cell lymphoma associated with EBV reactivation that is more common with T-cell–depleted grafts.
• **Other complications.** Patients who survive 6 months or more after transplant face complications that require preventative measures. Joint guidelines have been developed with the recommended posttransplant screenings.[23,24] Iron overload is a common complication of frequent transfusions and may require iron chelation therapy. Long-term treatment with corticosteroids predisposes to osteopenia, myopathy, and metabolic abnormalities. Conditioning regimens can result in infertility, hypogonadism, and thyroid dysfunction. HSCT survivors are also at higher risk of renal insufficiency, premature coronary artery disease, depression, and neurocognitive deficits.

CELLULAR THERAPY

Cellular therapy enhances the patient's immune system to recognize and treat hematologic malignancies. Engineered T-cells expressing a chimeric antigen receptor (CAR) construct recognize specific cancer-associated antigens and activate a prolonged immune response.

• **CAR-T.** The CAR construct is a recombinant receptor that activates T-cells in an HLA-independent fashion. To potentiate T-cell activation, second and third generations of CAR-T products containing costimulatory domains have been developed. CAR-T can be autologous or allogeneic, also defined "off the shelf." Autologous CAR-T are manufactured by manipulation of T-cells collected from the patient and genetically modified in a process that may require months. Allogeneic CAR-T are produced from donor-derived T-cells and are readily accessible. Once the CAR-T product is available, the patient receives lymphodepleting chemotherapy and then the cells are infused. CAR-T targeting CD19 for the treatment of ALL was the first to be approved and is now approved for DLBCL after first relapse.[2,3] A CAR-T against the B-cell maturation antigen (BCMA) was recently approved for relapsed/refractory multiple myeloma.[25] Table 34-3 summarizes the approved indications for CAR-T therapy and bispecific agents.
• **Bispecific agents.** These products combine two antibodies, one targeting a cancer-specific antigen, and the second one usually directed against CD3. Approved agents are blinatumomab (CD3 × CD19) for ALL, three different CD3 × CD20 agents used for B-cell lymphomas, and teclistamab (CD3 × BCMA) indicated for multiple myeloma. In 2023, talquetamab, a bispecific agent targeting the G protein–coupled receptor, class C, group 5, member D (GPRC5D) was approved for patients with refractory multiple myeloma, including patients treated with BCMA CAR-T therapy.

TOXICITY OF CELLULAR THERAPY

The unique side effects of cellular therapy are cytokine-release syndrome (CRS) and immune effector cell–associated neurotoxicity syndrome (ICANS). These toxicities are more common after CAR-T therapy compared to other products.

• **CRS.** It is an inflammatory syndrome due to the release of cytokines causing fever, hypotension, hypoxemia and, in severe cases, capillary leak syndrome with multiorgan failure and death. The onset of CRS varies based on the product used but usually, it develops within 2–7 days after infusion. The severity of CRS is stratified from grade 1 to 4 based on the level of supportive treatment required (e.g., supplemental oxygen, vasopressors). Treatment with systemic corticosteroids and tocilizumab, an IL-6 receptor antagonist, is usually started in patients not improving despite supportive care. In severe presentations, siltuximab—an anti–IL-6 antibody—and anakinra—an IL-1 receptor antagonist—have been used with off-label indication.
• **ICANS.** Neurotoxicity associated with CAR-T can manifest as decreased level of consciousness, tremor, dysgraphia, seizures, and aphasia. It is classified by severity (grade 1–4)

TABLE 34-3 APPROVED INDICATIONS FOR CELLULAR THERAPY

Disease	Approved Indication	Type
Acute lymphocytic leukemia	• Primary refractory/resistant • After second relapse	• CD19-directed CAR-T • CD3 × CD19 bispecific T-cell engager
Diffuse large B-cell lymphoma/primary mediastinal B-cell lymphoma	• Primary refractory/resistant • After first relapse • Relapse after autologous HSCT	• CD19-directed CAR-T • CD3 × CD20 bispecific T-cell engager
High-grade B-cell lymphoma, with MYC and BCL2 and/or BCL6 rearrangements	• Primary refractory/resistant • After first relapse • Relapse after autologous HSCT	• CD19-directed CAR-T
Follicular lymphoma	• Transformation to large B-cell lymphoma • Relapsed/refractory (after 2 prior lines)	• CD19-directed CAR-T • CD3 × CD20 bispecific T-cell engager
Mantle cell lymphoma	• Relapsed/refractory	• CD19-directed CAR-T
Multiple myeloma	• Relapsed/refractory (after 3 prior lines)	• BCMA-directed CAR-T • CD3 × BCMA bispecific T-cell engager • CD3 × GPRC5D bispecific T-cell engager
Prostate cancer	• Metastatic castrate resistant	• PAP-GM-CSF–activated CD54+ PBMC

BCMA, B-cell maturation antigen; GM-CSF, granulocyte-macrophage colony-stimulating factor; GPRC5D, G protein–coupled receptor, class C, group 5, member D; PAP, prostatic acid phosphatase; PBMC, peripheral blood mononuclear cells.

and can lead to cerebral edema. The median time of onset is 4 days after infusion of CAR-T. Steroids are the mainstay of management, while tocilizumab is indicated if concurrent CRS is present. Levetiracetam is commonly added for seizure prevention or after the onset of symptoms.

REFERENCES

1. Phelan R, Chen M, Bupp C, et al. Updated trends in hematopoietic cell transplantation in the United States with an additional focus on adolescent and young adult transplantation activity and outcomes. *Transplant Cell Ther.* 2022;28(7):409.e1–409.e10.
2. Locke FL, Miklos DB, Jacobson CA, et al; All ZUMA-7 Investigators and Contributing Kite Members. Axicabtagene ciloleucel as second-line therapy for large B-cell lymphoma. *N Engl J Med.* 2021;386(7):640–654.
3. Kamdar M, Solomon SR, Arnason J, et al; TRANSFORM Investigators. Lisocabtagene maraleucel versus standard of care with salvage chemotherapy followed by autologous stem cell transplantation as second-line treatment in patients with relapsed or refractory large B-cell lymphoma

(TRANSFORM): results from an interim analysis of an open-label, randomised, phase 3 trial. *Lancet.* 2022;399(10343):2294–2308.

4. Bashey A, Zhang MJ, McCurdy SR, et al. Mobilized peripheral blood stem cells versus unstimulated bone marrow as a graft source for T-cell-replete haploidentical donor transplantation using post-transplant cyclophosphamide. *J Clin Oncol.* 2017;35(26):3002–3009.

5. Lee SJ, Logan B, Westervelt P, et al. Comparison of patient-reported outcomes in 5-year survivors who received bone marrow vs peripheral blood unrelated donor transplantation: long-term follow-up of a randomized clinical trial. *JAMA Oncol.* 2016;2(12):1583–1589.

6. Holtick U, Albrecht M, Chemnitz JM, et al. Comparison of bone marrow versus peripheral blood allogeneic hematopoietic stem cell transplantation for hematological malignancies in adults—a systematic review and meta-analysis. *Crit Rev Oncol Hematol.* 2015;94(2):179–188.

7. Frangoul H, Altshuler D, Cappellini MD, et al. CRISPR-cas9 gene editing for sickle cell disease and β-thalassemia. *N Engl J Med.* 2021;384(3):252–260.

8. Weisdorf D, Cooley S, Wang T, et al. KIR B donors improve the outcome for AML patients given reduced intensity conditioning and unrelated donor transplantation. *Blood Adv.* 2020;4(4):740–754.

9. Jadi O, Tang H, Olsen K, et al. Associations of minor histocompatibility antigens with outcomes following allogeneic hematopoietic cell transplantation. *Am J Hematol.* 2023;98(6):940–950.

10. Howard CA, Fernandez-Vina MA, Appelbaum FR, et al. Recommendations for donor human leukocyte antigen assessment and matching for allogeneic stem cell transplantation: consensus opinion of the Blood and Marrow Transplant Clinical Trials Network (BMT CTN). *Biol Blood Marrow Transplant.* 2015;21(1):4–7.

11. Petersdorf EW, Malkki M, O'hUigin C, et al. High HLA-DP expression and graft-versus-host disease. *N Engl J Med.* 2015;373(7):599–609.

12. Gragert L, Eapen M, Williams E, et al. HLA match likelihoods for hematopoietic stem-cell grafts in the U.S. registry. *N Engl J Med.* 2014;371(4):339–348.

13. Fernandez-Viña MA, Wang T, Lee SJ, et al. Identification of a permissible HLA mismatch in hematopoietic stem cell transplantation. *Blood.* 2014;123(8):1270–1278.

14. Grunwald MR, Zhang MJ, Elmariah H, et al. Alternative donor transplantation for myelodysplastic syndromes: haploidentical relative and matched unrelated donors. *Blood Adv.* 2021;5(4):975–983.

15. Scott BL, Pasquini MC, Fei M, et al. Myeloablative versus reduced-intensity conditioning for hematopoietic cell transplantation in acute myelogenous leukemia and myelodysplastic syndromes-long-term follow-up of the BMT CTN 0901 clinical trial. *Transplant Cell Ther.* 2021;27(6):483.e1–483.e6.

16. Hourigan CS, Dillon LW, Gui G, et al. Impact of conditioning intensity of allogeneic transplantation for acute myeloid leukemia with genomic evidence of residual disease. *J Clin Oncol.* 2020; 38(12):1273–1283.

17. Sanz J, Galimard JE, Labopin M, et al; Acute Leukemia Working Party of the European Society for Blood and Marrow Transplantation (EBMT). Post-transplant cyclophosphamide after matched sibling, unrelated and haploidentical donor transplants in patients with acute myeloid leukemia: a comparative study of the ALWP EBMT. *J Hematol Oncol.* 2020;13(1):46.

18. Bolaños-Meade J, Hamadani M, Wu J, et al; BMT CTN 1703 Investigators. Post-transplantation cyclophosphamide-based graft-versus-host disease prophylaxis. *N Engl J Med.* 2023;388(25): 2338–2348.

19. Martin PJ, Rizzo JD, Wingard JR, et al. First- and second-line systemic treatment of acute graft-versus-host disease: recommendations of the American Society of Blood and Marrow Transplantation. *Biol Blood Marrow Transplant.* 2012;18(8):1150–1163.

20. Zeiser R, von Bubnoff N, Butler J, et al; REACH2 Trial Group. Ruxolitinib for glucocorticoid-refractory acute graft-versus-host disease. *N Engl J Med.* 2020;382(19):1800–1810.

21. Zeiser R, Polverelli N, Ram R, et al; REACH3 Investigators. Ruxolitinib for glucocorticoid-refractory chronic graft-versus-host disease. *N Engl J Med.* 2021;385(3):228–238.

22. Cutler C, Lee SJ, Arai S, et al. Belumosudil for chronic graft-versus-host disease after 2 or more prior lines of therapy: the ROCKstar Study. *Blood.* 2021;138(22):2278–2289.

23. Majhail NS, Rizzo JD, Lee SJ, et al. Recommended screening and preventive practices for long-term survivors after hematopoietic cell transplantation. *Biol Blood Marrow Transplant.* 2012;18(3):348–371.

24. Chow EJ, Cushing-Haugen KL, Cheng G-S, et al. Morbidity and mortality differences between hematopoietic cell transplantation survivors and other cancer survivors. *J Clin Oncol.* 2017;35(3):306–313.

25. Munshi NC, Anderson LD Jr, Shah N, et al. Idecabtagene vicleucel in relapsed and refractory multiple myeloma. *N Engl J Med.* 2021;384(8):705–716.

Human Immunodeficiency Virus–Associated Malignancies

35

Thomas A. Odeny

P eople living with HIV are at significantly increased risk of developing a malignancy compared with the general population. Approximately 20% of people with HIV (PWH) will develop a malignancy during their lifetime. Cancer is a leading cause of death in PWH.[1]

HIV is associated with the development of multiple types of cancer and is now also included in the International Agency for Research on Cancer (IARC) classification as a human carcinogen.[2] HIV contributes to the development of cancer through immunosuppression, promoting the tumorigenic effects of coinfection with oncogenic virus such as Epstein–Barr virus (EBV), Kaposi sarcoma herpesvirus (KSHV), human papillomavirus (HPV), and hepatitis B and C viruses. HIV primarily targets CD4+ T-cells, leading to immune dysfunction. This immunosuppression enables oncogenic viruses like EBV, KSHV, and HPV to reactivate and contributes to the development of cancers. For example, in patients with persistent HPV infection, HIV-induced immunosuppression increases the risk of cervical dysplasia and progression to invasive cancer. HIV infection also induces immune dysregulation, causing chronic B-cell stimulation and cytokine activation that contributes to the initiation of malignancies. HIV may also directly transform cells to become malignant, similar to other viral carcinogens, through expression of specific HIV proteins (gp120, Nef, p17, Tat, and reverse transcriptase) that induce oxidative stress.[3] Figure 35-1 shows a summarized timeline of the oncogenic viruses associated with HIV.

The introduction of combination antiretroviral therapy (ART) has resulted in a significant change in the epidemiologic and clinical profile of cancers in PWH by decreasing the mortality associated with opportunistic infections and by improving the longevity of the patients. While overall cancer incidence in PWH has remained unchanged, the incidence of infection-related cancers and the former "AIDS-defining malignancies" (Kaposi sarcoma [KS], invasive cervical cancer, non-Hodgkin lymphoma [NHL]) has declined while the incidence of other cancers has increased.[1] Of note, the terminology "AIDS-defining malignancies" is no longer used because it excludes some cancers for which HIV is a carcinogen (e.g., conjunctival cancer) and many cancers that are more prevalent in PWH (e.g., anal cancer, Hodgkin lymphoma [HL]), and does not reflect advances in lymphoma classification.[4] In the ART era, the burden of cancer in PWH is increasingly influenced by sociodemographic changes, with low- and middle-income countries (LMICs) having higher prevalence of infection-related cancers (Kaposi sarcoma, cervical, liver) and higher-income countries having higher prevalence of cancers that are not directly associated with HIV in particular or infection in general (breast, colon, and prostate).[5]

Immune reconstitution following ART and advances in chemotherapy and supportive care have resulted in improved outcomes of cancers in PWH compared to the pre-ART era.[6] In most cases, the treatment of malignancy in PWH is similar to treatment of the same malignancy in HIV-negative patients. ART is the cornerstone of treating cancer in PWH. Combining ART with chemotherapy, immunotherapy, radiation therapy, or surgery, when indicated, requires careful consideration of when to apply—or depart from—general standards of care. Initiation or continuation of ART among PWH

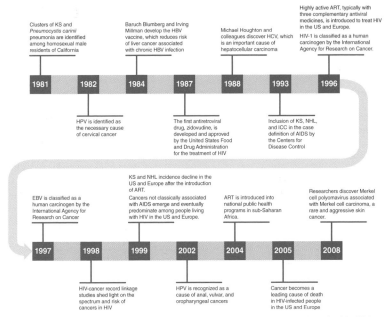

FIGURE 35-1. Summarized timeline of oncogenic viruses associated with HIV.

who have cancer improves cancer treatment outcomes.[7] ART may have a direct effect on the tumor microenvironment (e.g., by reducing expression of immune checkpoints such as PD-L1) that improves functional immunity and results in improved treatment outcomes.[8]

Drug interactions between the chemotherapeutic agents and antiretroviral medications should always be determined and avoided. For example, the older antiretrovirals didanosine, stavudine, and zidovudine are associated with lactic acidosis,[9] and should not be combined with antineoplastic drugs that undergo liver metabolism. Many earlier HIV medicines have toxicities that overlap with cytotoxic chemotherapy. For example, zidovudine, like most cytotoxic chemotherapy, causes bone marrow suppression, with resultant anemia and leucopenia so combined use should be avoided.[10] Similarly, stavudine and didanosine are associated with peripheral neuropathy,[11,12] a well-recognized adverse effect of common cancer drugs such as taxanes, vinca-alkaloids, platinum compounds, as well as the proteasome inhibitor bortezomib. Camptothecins such as irinotecan and topotecan commonly cause diarrhea, as do the protease inhibitors nelfinavir and lopinavir, so those combinations should be avoided. Modern ART regimens that include integrase strand transfer inhibitors are well tolerated and can be used with common cancer therapies.

Also, opportunistic infection prophylaxis should be considered for treatments that involve significant myelosuppression. Importantly, in PWH with cancer and coinfected with hepatitis B virus (HBV), concurrent suppressive therapy is recommended. Fortunately, ART regimens that include tenofovir and lamivudine or emtricitabine are sufficient for suppressing HBV in PWH with cancer. For patients with hepatitis C coinfection, treatment with direct-acting antivirals is recommended.

Kaposi Sarcoma

GENERAL PRINCIPLES

Epidemiology

Restoring immune function in PWH through ART has reduced the prevalence of KS globally. In the US, despite declines in overall incidence of KS, incidence among Black/African Americans has remained stable or increased.[13] Worse, Black/African American people with KS have significantly higher mortality than other groups.[14] In 2020, KS was the leading cause of cancer incidence among men in Malawi, Mozambique, and Uganda, and the leading cause of cancer mortality among men in Mozambique and Uganda.[15,16]

Pathophysiology

KS is caused by KSHV (Kaposi sarcoma–associated herpesvirus), a gamma-herpesvirus, also known as human herpes virus 8 (HHV-8). KSHV also causes primary effusion lymphoma (PEL) and the lymphoproliferative disease KSHV-multicentric Castleman disease (KSHV-MCD).[17,18] KSHV transmission is thought to be predominantly through saliva. Upon infection, KSHV enters a latent state in endothelial cells and B-cells, and therefore infection is lifelong. KS lesions are histologically characterized by neoangiogenesis and proliferating spindle-shaped cells admixed with an inflammatory infiltrate of lymphocytes, plasma cells, and macrophages. The malignant spindle-shaped cells are thought to be derived from KSV-infected circulating endothelial precursors. KSHV and HIV infection act synergistically to produce cytokines, growth factors, antiapoptotic signals, and angiogenic factors that stimulate KS spindle cell growth and create an environment necessary to develop and sustain the tumor.[4]

DIAGNOSIS

Clinical Presentation

The clinical presentation of KS varies from minimal to fulminant disease. The most commonly involved sites are skin, mucous membranes, lymph nodes, gastrointestinal tract, and lungs.

- Cutaneous lesions are typically painless, multifocal, plaque-like or papular, and pinkish to violaceous in color, although they may evolve into nodules and ultimately ulcerate.
- Lymph node involvement can cause lymphedema. Internal disease can present with vague symptoms and can occur in the absence of mucocutaneous manifestations.
- Gastrointestinal involvement is usually asymptomatic but can cause abdominal pain, bleeding, or obstruction.
- Pulmonary involvement by KS may cause interstitial infiltrates or hemorrhagic effusions, resulting in cough, dyspnea, and/or hemoptysis which can be life threatening.

Diagnostic Testing

Diagnosis is established by biopsy and pathology review of suspected lesions. Immunohistochemistry is positive for endothelial markers including CD34 (vascular), podoplanin, LYVE1, and VEGFR3 (lymphatic), as well as KSHV latency-associated nuclear antigen (LANA). Computed tomography (CT) imaging should be obtained as clinically indicated. Bronchoscopy may reveal endobronchial lesions in the setting of normal chest radiograph and should be considered in symptomatic patients. Upper and lower endoscopy should be strongly considered in patients presenting with GI blood loss. Serology for anti–HHV-8 antibodies is not central to the diagnosis.

PROGNOSIS

The AIDS Clinical Trials Group classifies patients with AIDS-related KS into good- and poor-risk groups based on tumor burden (T), CD4 counts (I: CD4 count < or ≥150), and the presence of systemic illness (S). The presence of these factors is denoted by 1 and absence by 0. Compared to patients with T0 disease, those with T1 disease have between 2.4- and 5.2-fold higher risk of death.

TREATMENT

- It is important to note that KS is **not considered a curable malignancy**. The treatment decisions are based on the presence and extent of symptomatic and extracutaneous manifestations.
- Optimization of ART is the first line of therapy. Response rate to ART alone can be seen in 80% of T0 lesions but is unlikely in T1 lesions. In many PWH, however, ART alone is often insufficient to prevent KS progression and development of new cases.[19,20]
- Local therapy is used for bulky lesions or for cosmesis. Also, local therapy is preferred for lesions that are symptomatic (i.e., bleeding, painful) as this may lead to a more rapid resolution of symptoms. Therapeutic options for local treatment include topical alitretinoin, intralesional chemotherapy with vinblastine, radiation therapy, laser therapy, and cryotherapy. Surgical excision of lesions should generally be avoided.
- Individuals with more advanced or progressive diseases are treated with systemic chemotherapy. Indications for systemic chemotherapy include large disease burden, site of disease, rapid disease progression, and organ dysfunction. First-line chemotherapeutic drugs are the liposomal anthracyclines (liposomal doxorubicin [Doxil] and liposomal daunorubicin [Daunoxome]). Overall response rate is ~70% with a median response time of 4 months. Paclitaxel is another approved agent, with reported response rates of 59–71%. Liposomal doxorubicin and paclitaxel have comparable response rates (56% vs. 46%; $P = .49$) and median progression-free survival (79% vs. 78%; $P = .75$) but paclitaxel is associated with significantly more neurotoxicity and alopecia.[21] In LMIC where liposomal doxorubicin may be less available or affordable, paclitaxel is superior to previously used options of oral etoposide and the combination of bleomycin/vincristine.[22] Pomalidomide is an immunomodulatory agent that received accelerated approval in 2020 for KS treatment after failure of ART based on a phase I/II trial showing 67% overall response rate in PWH.[23,24] A larger confirmatory trial by the AIDS Malignancy Consortium is currently underway. Immune checkpoint inhibitors such as pembrolizumab have also been successfully used to treat KS,[25] and confirmatory clinical trials are ongoing. Targeted therapy including VEGF inhibitors, KIT and PDGFR inhibitors, and mTOR inhibitors are being investigated in clinical trials.

HIV-Associated Lymphomas

GENERAL PRINCIPLES

Epidemiology

NHL is the most common hematologic malignancy in PWH. PWH have higher risk of NHL between 11 and 93 times that in the general population.[26,27] In particular, the risk is higher for high-grade NHL such as Burkitt lymphoma and primary central nervous system lymphoma (PCNSL), as well as the rare aggressive subtypes PEL and plasmablastic lymphoma. Although ART has successfully reduced the incidence of NHL,[27] there has been an unexpected surge in occurrence of HL.[28,29] The risk of HL is between 5 and 26 times that in the general population, and is particularly higher among PWH with low CD4 cell counts ranging between 50 and 99.[29]

Pathophysiology

Overall pathogenesis of HIV-related lymphoma is complex. Various pathogenic mechanisms have been suggested, and it is likely resultant of multiple causes acting in concert. Suggested mechanisms include immune dysregulation, HIV-induced immunosuppression, chronic antigenic stimulation, genetic abnormalities, cytokine dysregulation, dendritic cell impairment, and viral infections associated with EBV and KSHV.[30] Of note, lymphoma diagnosis among PWH already receiving ART may be associated with poorer survival outcomes,[31,32] suggesting differences in the pathophysiology and tumor microenvironment between lymphoma occurring in ART-naïve versus ART-exposed PWH.[33] Therefore, although ART is a key part of lymphoma treatment in PWH, duration of ART prior to lymphoma diagnosis and timing of ART initiation may be associated with patient outcomes.[7,33]

Non-Hodgkin Lymphoma

GENERAL PRINCIPLES

Classification and Clinical Presentation

HIV-related NHLs are a heterogeneous group of malignancies. More than 95% of the tumors are derived from B-cells. The majority of HIV-related lymphomas are highly aggressive. Compared to NHL in the general population, HIV-related NHL has a propensity for advanced disease, presence of B symptoms, extranodal disease, leptomeningeal disease, and disease in unusual locations.

- **Diffuse large B-cell lymphoma (DLBCL)** is the most common HIV-related lymphoma. This typically presents with advanced stage with both nodal and extranodal involvement, behaves aggressively, and may have central nervous system (CNS) involvement. It is divided into centroblastic (germinal center B-cell–like) and immunoblastic (activated B-cell–like) subtypes. The immunoblastic subtype is more frequently associated with EBV infection (90%) compared to the centroblastic type (30%). Overexpression of BCL-6, a proto-oncogene product, is usually associated with centroblastic. EBV-positive immunoblastic subtypes typically express the EBV-encoded latent membrane protein-1 as well as CD138.
- **Burkitt lymphoma** accounts for 16–20% of HIV-related lymphoma. It is more common in younger patients and those with CD4 counts >200 μL, usually when there are no other features of immunosuppression. Thirty percent to 50% of HIV-related Burkitt lymphomas are associated with EBV infection. *MYC* activation is involved in all cases.
- **Primary CNS lymphoma (PCNSL)** represents a distinct extranodal presentation of DLBCL. It is usually of the immunoblastic (nongerminal center B-cell–like) type and is associated with severe immunosuppression (CD4 count <50) and universal EBV infection. Its involvement is confined to the craniospinal axis usually without any systemic involvement. B symptoms are rare in PCNSL and clinical features typically depend on the CNS location of the tumor. Most patients (65%) have solitary brain lesions.[34]
- **Primary effusion lymphoma (PEL)** represents <5% of HIV-related lymphomas. Median CD4 count at diagnosis is ~100. It occurs predominately in late stages of disease and carries a poor prognosis. It is universally associated with KSHV infection (100%) and 80% of cases have coinfection with EBV. It is an aggressive tumor and morphologically varies from the immunoblastic to the anaplastic type. By definition it is classified

as a stage IV NHL. An extracavitary variant of PEL can occur outside of effusions. Lymphoma cells are of B-cell origin but do not express B-cell antigens (notably CD20 negative), and express CD138.

- **Plasmablastic lymphoma** is another high-grade, aggressive postgerminal center B-cell lymphoma that typically involves the oral cavity and jaw but has been described in many extranodal sites. It is highly associated with EBV infection (70%) but lacks KSHV infection, unlike PEL. The tumor consists of large plasmablast cells with the morphologic features of B-immunoblasts. Plasmablasts will typically lose B-cell markers (CD20) and will acquire plasma cell markers (CD38, CD138, MUM1/IRF4). Pathologic diagnosis is made by demonstration of large neoplastic cells that resemble B-immunoblasts with the immunophenotype of plasma cells.

DIAGNOSIS

- Since many other HIV-associated diseases, including various infections, can mimic the clinical and imaging features of lymphoma, biopsy is required for diagnosis. The staging workup includes CT of the chest, abdomen, and pelvis, bone marrow evaluation, and FDG-PET imaging. Because CNS involvement is common, MRI of the brain and lumbar puncture for cerebrospinal fluid (CSF) analysis should be considered for all patients with HIV-related lymphoma.
- The workup of a brain mass requires special consideration. CNS imaging cannot reliably differentiate between CNS lymphoma and toxoplasmosis. If brain biopsy is hazardous, PCR for CSF EBV DNA is 80% sensitive and almost 100% specific for PCNSL and, hence, could substitute for a diagnostic biopsy.

TREATMENT

- With the use of ART and anticipated immune restoration, standard-dose chemotherapy with growth factor support is the standard of care in patients with HIV-related NHL. Prophylaxis for opportunistic infections should also be administered. Treatment regimens for all CD20+ HIV-associated NHL should include rituximab as it improves complete response rates, as well as progression-free and overall survival. Concurrent ART with infusional dose-adjusted R-EPOCH (rituximab plus etoposide, prednisone, vincristine, cyclophosphamide, and doxorubicin) is preferred over bolus R-CHOP (rituximab plus cyclophosphamide, doxorubicin, vincristine, and prednisone) in HIV-associated NHL.[35]
- For Burkitt lymphoma in PWH, although the best regimen remains unclear, more aggressive therapy should be considered in patients with adequate functional status. DA-EPOCH-R is generally the best tolerated and is an effective regimen. R-CODOX-M/IVAC (cyclophosphamide, vincristine, doxorubicin, high-dose methotrexate, ifosfamide, etoposide, and cytarabine) and R-Hyper-CVAD (rituximab, hyperfractionated cyclophosphamide, vincristine, doxorubicin, and dexamethasone with alternating cytarabine and methotrexate) have been utilized and have been demonstrated to be effective regimens but are associated with significant toxicity.
- Prophylactic intrathecal methotrexate may be delivered at the time of initial CSF analysis to reduce the risk of leptomeningeal disease, particularly in patients with Burkitt lymphoma, Burkitt-like lymphoma histology, bone marrow, paranasal or paraspinal involvement, or EBV virus coinfection. The utility of CNS prophylaxis in DLBCL is debatable but should be considered in patients with significant extranodal and/or widespread systemic involvement.
- PCNSL is treated with rituximab plus high-dose methotrexate chemotherapy with concurrent ART. Whole-brain radiation therapy is an option for patients who are not eligible for chemotherapy.

- Treatment of PEL and plasmablastic lymphoma are unclear and response rates to CHOP chemotherapy are poor. The general consensus is that more aggressive chemotherapy regimens (DA-EPOCH, Hyper-CVAD, or CODOX-M/IVAC) should be utilized. Daratumumab, an anti-CD38 monoclonal antibody, has been shown to induce clinical responses in cases of refractory PEL.[36,37]
- More recently, pembrolizumab and pomalidomide have shown promising results for EBV-associated NHL in PWH.[38]

PROGNOSIS

HIV-related NHLs are curable, and outcomes have improved greatly in the ART era. Prognosis is dictated by subtype and other prognostic factors. Poor prognostic factors include advanced stage, low CD4 counts (<100), high HIV viral load at diagnosis, older age, elevated lactate dehydrogenase, poor performance status, presence of extranodal disease, prior AIDS-defining illness, and aggressive histology of lymphoma. For all lymphomas, the 2- and 5-year overall survival rates are 53% and 44%, respectively. The 2- and 5-year survival rates by lymphoma subtype are as follows: HL, 72% and 62%, Burkitt lymphoma, 53% and 50%, PCNSL, 24% and 23%, and DLBCL, 56% and 44%.[6]

Hodgkin Lymphoma

Clinical features of HIV-associated HL include a high frequency of B symptoms, advanced-stage disease, a higher incidence of bone marrow involvement, and universal EBV coinfection. Histologic subtypes most often seen are mixed cellularity and lymphocyte depleted. Noncontiguous lymph node spread is more commonly seen. CD4 counts are typically >250 μL. HIV-positive patients typically present with more extensive disease and adverse prognostic features. However, treatment outcomes are similar to matched HIV-negative patients. Treatment includes ART initiated with full-dose chemotherapy. The combination regiment of AAVD (brentuximab vedotin, doxorubicin, vinblastine, and dacarbazine) has shown high response rates (100% complete response, 92% OS) in PWH with advanced stage HL.[39]

Other chemotherapy regimens that have been studied include ABVD (doxorubicin, bleomycin, vinblastine, and dacarbazine), BEACOPP (bleomycin, etoposide, doxorubicin, cyclophosphamide, vincristine, procarbazine, and prednisone), and the Stanford V regimen (doxorubicin, vinblastine, mechlorethamine, etoposide, vincristine, bleomycin, and prednisone), and involved field radiation for initial bulky disease. Salvage chemotherapy studies have not been specifically performed in the HIV population, but relapsed/refractory disease should be managed similarly to HIV-negative patients.[40] Because the risk of neutropenia is higher in PWH receiving treatment for HL than in those without HIV, growth factor support is used when treating HL in PWH using lymphodepleting regimens (e.g., ABVD), unlike in HIV-negative patients where growth factor support is not routinely used or recommended.[41,42] In TB-endemic regions, PET-directed HL therapy may be potentially confounded by presence of nonmalignant causes of lymphadenopathy such as extrapulmonary TB. In such cases, lymph node biopsies for definitive pathologic diagnosis are strongly recommended.

HPV-Associated Cancers

Compared to the general population, PWH have higher prevalence and persistence of HPV infections.[43–47] As a result, the incidence of cancers caused by HPV among PWH is higher than in the general population, even after introduction of ART. These include cervical, anal, vulvar, vaginal, penile, and head and neck cancers. In PWH, infection with more than 1 HPV type is more common which increases their risk for cervical, anal, vulvar, and perianal precancer lesions and cancer. HPV vaccination, which protects against oncogenic high-risk HPV types, is recommended for all individuals with HIV between 9 and 45 years old.

Cervical Cancer

Women with HIV have a sixfold higher risk of cervical cancer. HIV-positive patients with cervical cancer have more intractable disease and have a higher relapse rate compared to those without HIV. Restoring immune function with ART improves treatment outcomes. PWH who have locally advanced cervical cancer and receive ART show comparable 5-year overall survival rates[48] and adverse effects[49,50] to those without HIV following chemoradiation therapy. In fact, among PWH with locally advanced cervical cancer, lack of ART is associated with higher mortality.[51] Cervical cancer screening is recommended for all women 21 years or older.

Anal Cancer

Incidence of anal cancer in the US is rising among both men and women with HIV, and men who have sex with men regardless of HIV status. PWH have >20 times higher risk of anal cancer than people without HIV, and HIV-positive men who have sex with men have 60–80 times higher risk. HPV infection is associated with >90% of anal and rectal squamous cell cancers.

Screening for anal cancer is recommended for PWH aged 35 years or older (symptoms, visual inspection of perianal region, annual digital rectal exam, annual anal Pap testing). Emerging research shows that screening with high-resolution anoscopy and treatment for high-grade squamous intraepithelial lesions (HSIL) in PWH who are 35 years or older significantly reduces the risk of anal cancer.[52] Initiating or continuing ART among PWH diagnosed with anal cancer improves treatment outcomes. Treatment options are the same for people with or without HIV.[53] **Anal cancer in PWH is curable** with concurrent chemotherapy with radiation therapy. The standard of care for locally advanced anal squamous cell cancer is combined chemoradiotherapy with 5-fluorouracil plus mitomycin-C, followed by assessment of treatment response clinically at about 2–3 months (8–12 weeks) after completion of chemoradiotherapy. Whether HIV status is associated with higher toxicity is controversial,[54,55] but long-term outcomes are similar between people with and without HIV.[55]

Other Cancers

Population-based epidemiologic studies have shown an increased risk of several other cancers in PWH, including vulva, vagina, penile, Merkel cell, liver, oral cavity, pharynx, larynx, eye, conjunctiva, lip, squamous cell skin cancer, lung, multiple myeloma, and leukemia. In general, treatment of these cancers in PWH is similar to treatment in people without HIV. Special treatment considerations in PWH will include the presence of coinfections, drug–drug interactions between ART and cancer therapies, and the need for supportive care in PWH, including prophylaxis for infections.

Importantly, PWH should be included in clinical trials without regard to arbitrary CD4 count thresholds as emerging research shows that CD4 counts among those with relapsed/refractory cancers are similar in people with and without HIV.[56] In particular, because immune checkpoint inhibitors have been shown effective for a wide variety of cancers for which PWH are at increased risk, PWH should be included in these trials as evidence shows similar adverse events and survival even among those with low CD4 counts.[57]

Treatment Monitoring for PWH Receiving Cancer Treatment

The World Health Organization (WHO) recommends that viral load is the preferred approach to monitor treatment in PWH receiving ART and that CD4 cell count monitoring is not necessary for PWH who are established on ART.[58] However, some settings (rural or LMIC) may lack capacity to offer routine or efficient viral load testing.[59] In this case, CD4 count and clinical monitoring are recommended by WHO for treatment monitoring. PWH with cancer are likely to have low CD4 counts from cytotoxic cancer therapies.[57] Therefore, support for viral load monitoring should be established in LMIC cancer/HIV clinics in order to more accurately monitor treatment with ART in the setting of concurrent cancer treatment. As point-of-care viral load tests have made viral load monitoring more accessible in LMIC and may be especially beneficial for specific high-risk groups (infants, children, adolescents, pregnant and breastfeeding women, suspected treatment failure),[58] we strongly recommend that PWH with cancer receiving chemotherapy be considered a priority population that could benefit from point-of-care viral load testing.

Immunotherapy and Cellular Therapy

There is a need to limit immunosuppressive cancer treatments such as chemotherapy and radiotherapy in PWH as these may result in worsening CD4 counts that may in turn be associated with increased mortality.[60] Immunotherapy shows promise in harnessing the immune system to combat both HIV and cancer without worsening immunosuppression. PWH have disproportionately higher risk of many cancers for which immune checkpoint inhibitors—a class of cancer immunotherapies—are currently approved. Chronic HIV infection, and in some cases additional viral infections associated with certain cancers (e.g., KS, NHL, cervical cancer, hepatocellular carcinoma), constantly stimulates T-cells and leads to increased expression of immune checkpoints (e.g., PD-1 and CTLA4). This ultimately leads to exhaustion of T-cells.[61-63] Immune checkpoint inhibitors are safe in PWH receiving ART with CD4 counts above 100 cells/uL.[25,64-66] In fact, among patients with advanced cancer enrolled in trials of immune checkpoint inhibitors, PWH have similar baseline CD4 counts as HIV-negative patients, and these low CD4 counts neither increase the risk of treatment-related adverse events nor lower survival after receiving immunotherapy.[57]

REFERENCES

1. Greenberg L, Ryom L, Bakowska E, et al. Trends in cancer incidence in different antiretroviral treatment-eras amongst people with HIV. *Cancers (Basel).* 2023;15(14):3640.
2. Cancer IAfRo. IARC monographs on the identification of carcinogenic hazards to humans. *IARC Monogr Meet.* 2019;124:1–4.
3. Isaguliants M, Bayurova E, Avdoshina D, Kondrashova A, Chiodi F, Palefsky JM. Oncogenic effects of HIV-1 proteins, mechanisms behind. *Cancers (Basel).* 2021;13(2):305.
4. Engels EA, Shiels MS, Barnabas RV, et al. State of the science and future directions for research on HIV and cancer: summary of a joint workshop sponsored by IARC and NCI. *Int J Cancer.* 2024; 154(4):596–606.
5. Bray F, Jemal A, Grey N, Ferlay J, Forman D. Global cancer transitions according to the Human Development Index (2008-2030): a population-based study. *Lancet Oncol.* 2012;13(8):790–801.
6. Gopal S, Patel MR, Yanik EL, et al. Temporal trends in presentation and survival for HIV-associated lymphoma in the antiretroviral therapy era. *J Natl Cancer Inst.* 2013;105(16):1221–1229.

7. Montaño MA, Chagomerana MB, Borok M, Painschab M, Uldrick TS, Ignacio RAB. Impact of antiretroviral therapy on cancer treatment outcomes among people living with HIV in low- and middle-income countries: a systematic review. *Curr HIV/AIDS Rep*. 2021;18(2):105–116.

8. Loharamtaweethong K, Vinyuvat S, Thammasiri J, Chitpakdee S, Supakatitham C, Puripat N. Impact of antiretroviral drugs on PD-L1 expression and copy number gains with clinical outcomes in HIV-positive and -negative locally advanced cervical cancers. *Oncol Lett*. 2019;18(6):5747–5758.

9. Walker UA, Bäuerle J, Laguno M, et al. Depletion of mitochondrial DNA in liver under antiretroviral therapy with didanosine, stavudine, or zalcitabine. *Hepatology*. 2004;39(2):311–317.

10. Yarchoan R, Broder S. Development of antiretroviral therapy for the acquired immunodeficiency syndrome and related disorders. A progress report. *N Engl J Med*. 1987;316(9):557–564.

11. Moyle GJ, Sadler M. Peripheral neuropathy with nucleoside antiretrovirals: risk factors, incidence and management. *Drug Saf*. 1998;19(6):481–494.

12. McGrath CJ, Njoroge J, John-Stewart GC, et al. Increased incidence of symptomatic peripheral neuropathy among adults receiving stavudine- versus zidovudine-based antiretroviral regimens in Kenya. *J Neurovirol*. 2012;18(3):200–204.

13. Royse KE, El Chaer F, Amirian ES, et al. Disparities in Kaposi sarcoma incidence and survival in the United States: 2000–2013. *PLOS One*. 2017;12(8):e0182750.

14. Ragi SD, Moseley I, Ouellette S, Rao B. Epidemiology and survival of Kaposi's sarcoma by race in the united states: a surveillance, epidemiology, and end results database analysis. *Clin Cosmet Investig Dermatol*. 2022;15:1681–1685.

15. Sung H, Ferlay J, Siegel RL, et al. Global cancer statistics 2020: GLOBOCAN estimates of incidence and mortality worldwide for 36 cancers in 185 countries. 2021;71(3):209–249.

16. Horner M-J, Chasimpha S, Spoerri A, et al. High cancer burden among antiretroviral therapy users in Malawi: a record linkage study of observational human immunodeficiency virus cohorts and cancer registry data. *Clin Infect Dis*. 2019;69(5):829–835.

17. Cesarman E, Chang Y, Moore PS, Said JW, Knowles DM. Kaposi's sarcoma–associated herpesvirus-like DNA sequences in AIDS-related body-cavity–based lymphomas. *N Engl J Med*. 1995;332(18):1186–1191.

18. Soulier J, Grollet L, Oksenhendler E, et al. Kaposi's sarcoma-associated herpesvirus-like DNA sequences in multicentric Castleman's disease. *Blood*. 1995;86(4):1276–1280.

19. Bower M, Pria AD, Coyle C, et al. Prospective stage-stratified approach to AIDS-related Kaposi's sarcoma. *J Clin Oncol*. 2014;32(5):409–414.

20. Rohner E, Valeri F, Maskew M, et al. Incidence rate of Kaposi sarcoma in HIV-infected patients on antiretroviral therapy in Southern Africa: a prospective multicohort study. *J Acquir Immune Defic Syndr*. 2014;67(5):547–554.

21. Cianfrocca M, Lee S, Von Roenn J, et al. Randomized trial of paclitaxel versus pegylated liposomal doxorubicin for advanced human immunodeficiency virus-associated Kaposi sarcoma: evidence of symptom palliation from chemotherapy. *Cancer*. 2010;116(16):3969–3977.

22. Krown SE, Moser CB, MacPhail P, et al. Treatment of advanced AIDS-associated Kaposi sarcoma in resource-limited settings: a three-arm, open-label, randomised, non-inferiority trial. *Lancet*. 2020; 395(10231):1195–1207.

23. Polizzotto MN, Uldrick TS, Wyvill KM, et al. Pomalidomide for symptomatic Kaposi's sarcoma in people with and without HIV infection: a Phase I/II study. *J Clin Oncol*. 2016;34(34):4125–4131.

24. Ramaswami R, Polizzotto MN, Lurain K, et al. Safety, activity, and long-term outcomes of pomalidomide in the treatment of Kaposi sarcoma among individuals with or without HIV infection. *Clin Cancer Res*. 2022;28(5):840–850.

25. Uldrick TS, Gonçalves PH, Abdul-Hay M, et al; Cancer Immunotherapy Trials Network (CITN)-12 Study Team. Assessment of the safety of pembrolizumab in patients with HIV and advanced cancer–a phase 1 study. *JAMA Oncol*. 2019;5(9):1332–1339.

26. Maso LD, Polesel J, Serraino D, et al; Cancer and AIDS Registries Linkage (CARL) Study. Pattern of cancer risk in persons with AIDS in Italy in the HAART era. *Br J Cancer*. 2009;100(5):840–847.

27. Hernández-Ramírez RU, Shiels MS, Dubrow R, Engels EA. Cancer risk in HIV-infected people in the USA from 1996 to 2012: a population-based, registry-linkage study. *Lancet HIV*. 2017;4(11): e495–e504.

28. Vaughan J, Perner Y, McAlpine E, Wiggill T. Brief report: HIV-associated Hodgkin lymphoma involving the bone marrow identifies a very high-risk subpopulation in the era of widescale antiretroviral therapy use in Johannesburg, South Africa. *J Acquir Immune Defic Syndr*. 2020;83(4):345–349.

29. Lanoy E, Rosenberg PS, Fily F, et al; FHDH-ANRS CO4. HIV-associated Hodgkin lymphoma during the first months on combination antiretroviral therapy. *Blood*. 2011;118(1):44–49.

30. Carbone A, Vaccher E, Gloghini A. Hematologic cancers in individuals infected by HIV. *Blood.* 2022;139(7):995–1012.

31. Cuellar LE, Anampa-Guzmán A, Holguín AM, et al. Prognostic factors in HIV-positive patients with non-Hodgkin lymphoma: a Peruvian experience. *Infect Agent Cancer.* 2018;13:27.

32. Painschab MS, Kasonkanji E, Zuze T, et al. Mature outcomes and prognostic indices in diffuse large B-cell lymphoma in Malawi: a prospective cohort. *Br J Haematol.* 2019;184(3):364–372.

33. Fedoriw Y, Selitsky S, Montgomery ND, et al. Identifying transcriptional profiles and evaluating prognostic biomarkers of HIV-associated diffuse large B-cell lymphoma from Malawi. *Mod Pathol.* 2020;33(8):1482–1491.

34. Ferreri AJM, Calimeri T, Cwynarski K, et al. Primary central nervous system lymphoma. *Nat Rev Dis Primers.* 2023;9(1):29.

35. Barta SK, Lee JY, Kaplan LD, Noy A, Sparano JA. Pooled analysis of AIDS malignancy consortium trials evaluating rituximab plus CHOP or infusional EPOCH chemotherapy in HIV-associated non-Hodgkin lymphoma. *Cancer.* 2012;118(16):3977–3983.

36. Shrestha P, Astter Y, Davis DA, et al. Daratumumab induces cell-mediated cytotoxicity of primary effusion lymphoma and is active against refractory disease. *Oncoimmunology.* 2023;12(1):2163784.

37. Shah NN, Singavi AK, Harrington A. Daratumumab in primary effusion lymphoma. *N Engl J Med.* 2018;379(7):689–690.

38. Lurain K, Ramaswami R, Mangusan R, et al. Use of pembrolizumab with or without pomalidomide in HIV-associated non-Hodgkin's lymphoma. *J Immunother Cancer.* 2021;9(2):e002097.

39. Rubinstein PG, Moore PC, Bimali M, et al; AIDS Malignancy Consortium; Lymphoma Study Association. Brentuximab vedotin with AVD for stage II–IV HIV-related Hodgkin lymphoma (AMC 085): phase 2 results from an open-label, single arm, multicentre phase 1/2 trial. *Lancet Haematol.* 2023;10(8):e624–e632.

40. Uldrick TS, Little RF. How I treat classical Hodgkin lymphoma in patients infected with human immunodeficiency virus. *Blood.* 2015;125(8):1226–1235; quiz 1355.

41. Cheung MC, Prica A, Graczyk J, Buckstein R, Chan KKW. Granulocyte-colony stimulating factor in secondary prophylaxis for advanced-stage Hodgkin lymphoma treated with ABVD chemotherapy: a cost-effectiveness analysis. *Leuk Lymphoma.* 2016;57(8):1865–1875.

42. Evens AM, Cilley J, Ortiz T, et al. G-CSF is not necessary to maintain over 99% dose-intensity with ABVD in the treatment of Hodgkin lymphoma: low toxicity and excellent outcomes in a 10-year analysis. *Br J Haematol.* 2007;137(6):545–552.

43. Jin Z-Y, Liu X, Ding Y-Y, Zhang Z-F, He N. Cancer risk factors among people living with HIV/AIDS in China: a systematic review and meta-analysis. *Sci Rep.* 2017;7(1):4890.

44. Park LS, Hernández-Ramírez RU, Silverberg MJ, Crothers K, Dubrow R. Prevalence of non-HIV cancer risk factors in persons living with HIV/AIDS: a meta-analysis. *AIDS.* 2016;30(2):273–291.

45. 1993 revised classification system for HIV infection and expanded surveillance case definition for AIDS among adolescents and adults. *MMWR Recomm Rep.* 1992;41(RR-17):1–19.

46. Patel P, Hanson DL, Sullivan PS, et al; Adult and Adolescent Spectrum of Disease Project and HIV Outpatient Study Investigators. Incidence of types of cancer among HIV-infected persons compared with the general population in the United States, 1992–2003. *Ann Intern Med.* 2008;148(10):728–736.

47. Wang C-CJ, Sparano J, Palefsky JM. Human immunodeficiency virus/AIDS, human papillomavirus, and anal cancer. *Surg Oncol Clin N Am.* 2017;26(1):17–31.

48. MacDuffie E, Bvochora-Nsingo M, Chiyapo S, et al. Five-year overall survival following chemoradiation therapy for locally advanced cervical carcinoma in women living with and without HIV infection in Botswana. *Infect Agent Cancer.* 2021;16(1):55.

49. Grover S, Bvochora-Nsingo M, Yeager A, et al. Impact of human immunodeficiency virus infection on survival and acute toxicities from chemoradiation therapy for cervical cancer patients in a limited-resource setting. *Int J Radiat Oncol Biol Phys.* 2018;101(1):201–210.

50. Mdletshe S, Munkupa H, Lishimpi K. Acute toxicity in cervical cancer HIV-positive vs. HIV-negative patients treated by radical chemo-radiation in Zambia. *South Af J Gynaecol Oncol.* 2016; 8(2):37–41.

51. Turdo YQ, Ruffieux Y, Boshomane TMG, et al. Cancer treatment and survival among cervical cancer patients living with or without HIV in South Africa. *Gynecol Oncol Rep.* 2022;43:101069.

52. Palefsky JM, Lee JY, Jay N, et al; ANCHOR Investigators Group. Treatment of anal high-grade squamous intraepithelial lesions to prevent anal cancer. *N Engl J Med.* 2022;386(24):2273–2282.

53. Martin D, Balermpas P, Fokas E, Rödel C, Yildirim M. Are there HIV-specific differences for anal cancer patients treated with standard chemoradiotherapy in the era of combined antiretroviral therapy? *Clin Oncol (R Coll Radiol).* 2017;29(4):248–255.

54. White EC, Khodayari B, Erickson KT, Lien WW, Hwang-Graziano J, Rao AR. Comparison of toxicity and treatment outcomes in HIV-positive versus HIV-negative patients with squamous cell carcinoma of the anal canal. *Am J Clin Oncol.* 2017;40(4):386–392.
55. Bryant AK, Huynh-Le M-P, Simpson DR, Gupta S, Sharabi AB, Murphy JD. Association of HIV Status with outcomes of anal squamous cell carcinoma in the era of highly active antiretroviral therapy. *JAMA Oncol.* 2018;4(1):120–122.
56. Odeny TA, Rosenthal MH, Lurain KA, et al. CD4+ T-cell count eligibility by HIV status among participants receiving immunotherapy for cancer diagnoses. *J Clin Oncol.* 2021;39(Suppl 15):12104–12104.
57. Odeny TA, Lurain K, Strauss J, et al. Effect of CD4+ T cell count on treatment-emergent adverse events among patients with and without HIV receiving immunotherapy for advanced cancer. *J Immunother Cancer.* 2022;10(9):e005128.
58. World Health Organization. *Consolidated Guidelines on HIV Prevention, Testing, Treatment, Service Delivery and Monitoring: Recommendations for A Public Health Approach.* World Health Organization; 2021.
59. Lubega P, Nalugya SJ, Kimuli AN, et al. Adherence to viral load testing guidelines, barriers, and associated factors among persons living with HIV on ART in Southwestern Uganda: a mixed-methods study. *BMC Public Health.* 2022;22(1):1268.
60. Calkins KL, Chander G, Joshu CE, et al. Immune status and associated mortality after cancer treatment among individuals with HIV in the antiretroviral therapy era. *JAMA Oncol.* 2020;6(2):227–235.
61. Lurain K, Ramaswami R, Yarchoan R, Uldrick TS. Anti-PD-1 and Anti-PD-L1 monoclonal antibodies in people living with HIV and cancer. *Curr HIV/AIDS Rep.* 2020;17(5):547–556.
62. Pinato DJ, Kaneko T, D'Alessio A, et al. Integrated phenotyping of the anti-cancer immune response in HIV-associated hepatocellular carcinoma. *JHEP Rep.* 2023;5(7):100741.
63. Khaitan A, Unutmaz D. Revisiting immune exhaustion during HIV infection. *Curr HIV/AIDS Rep.* 2011;8(1):4–11.
64. Gonzalez-Cao M, Morán T, Dalmau J, et al. Assessment of the feasibility and safety of durvalumab for treatment of solid tumors in patients with HIV-1 infection: the phase 2 DURVAST study. *JAMA Oncol.* 2020;6(7):1063–1067.
65. Cook MR, Kim C. Safety and efficacy of immune checkpoint inhibitor therapy in patients with HIV infection and advanced-stage cancer: a systematic review. *JAMA Oncol.* 2019;5(7):1049–1054.
66. Shah NJ, Al-Shbool G, Blackburn M, et al. Safety and efficacy of immune checkpoint inhibitors (ICIs) in cancer patients with HIV, hepatitis B, or hepatitis C viral infection. *J Immunother Cancer.* 2019;7(1):353.

Cancer of Unknown Primary (CUP)

36

Michael D. Bern and Olivia Aranha

GENERAL PRINCIPLES

Definition

Cancers that spread from an unknown primary site distantly are defined as cancer of unknown primary (CUP). After a comprehensive physical exam and diagnostic testing when no anatomic primary site is identified, the cancers are treated based on the subtype and tumor biology. The molecular cancer signature and immunohistochemical profile guide therapy.

Classification Based on Histologic Subtype

Adenocarcinomas: These account for 60–70% of the cancers with an unknown primary. The primary site could be lung, pancreas, stomach, colon, breast, prostate, or liver.

Poorly differentiated carcinoma with or without features of adenocarcinoma: It is the second most common subtype accounting for 30% of the cases. The cancer cell is poorly differentiated making it challenging to determine the cell of origin. The differential diagnosis of these include sarcoma, melanoma, and lymphoma.

Squamous cell carcinoma: These arise from cutaneous epithelium or the inner lining of organs.

Poorly differentiated or undifferentiated malignant neoplasm: It accounts for fewer than 5% of the cases.

Neuroendocrine neoplasm: This type of CUP originates in the neuroendocrine cells in the gastrointestinal system (esophagus, stomach, pancreas, intestine) or lung and is seen in <1% of CUP.

Epidemiology

The incidence of CUP is difficult to estimate due to heterogeneity in diagnostic workup and reporting practices that are influenced by variable definitions of CUP, regional practice variations, and resource availability. Historical data series have estimated that the incidence of CUP accounts for 3–5% of all cancers. However, the incidence of CUP is declining over time, and more recent data suggests that CUP accounts for 1–2% of cancers.[1] The reason for the decline in incidence of CUP is unclear but is likely multifactorial related to widespread adoption of modern imaging techniques including CT and PET scans with higher sensitivity for detecting primary tumors, advancement in identifying the occult cancer with tissue of origin testing using panels of immunohistochemistry (IHC) and genomic profiling assays and declining incidence of certain common primary cancers like smoking-related lung cancer.

Etiology

CUP is a heterogeneous disease with no clear unifying etiology. Epidemiologic studies have linked smoking to an increased risk of CUP, but no unique CUP-specific risk factors have been identified.[2]

Pathophysiology

It is unclear how metastatic disease develops in the absence of a detectable primary tumor in CUP. One theory is that different tumor microenvironments support tumor growth at sites of metastases but suppress tumor growth or induce regression at the site of the primary tumor. Alternatively, some have hypothesized that initiating mutations arise in tissue stem cells that then migrate and form metastases without ever forming a primary tumor.[3] Next-generation sequencing (NGS) has identified the most frequently mutated genes in CUP, which include *TP53, KRAS, CDKN2A, MYC, ARID1A,* and *MCL1*.[4] Additional research is needed to better understand the mechanism of how these genetic alterations lead to CUP.

DIAGNOSIS

Clinical Presentation

The clinical symptoms are varied and depend on the sites of metastases. It can present as unintentional weight loss, poor appetite, a chronic unexplained cough with hoarseness of voice, worsening pain, new palpable lumps, enlarged lymph nodes, altered bowel or bladder habits—diarrhea, constipation, dysuria, increased urinary frequency, fevers of unknown origin, night sweats, bleeding, discharge, and headaches. A thorough physical exam including a pelvic exam in females and prostate evaluation is helpful.

Diagnostic Testing

- **Imaging:** CT Chest, abdomen, and pelvis, mammogram in females is useful in 10–35% of the cases in identifying the primary site.[5]
- **Tumor markers:** CEA, CA 19-9, CA 15-3, CA-125, PSA, chromogranin A are done as part of the initial workup.
- **Pathology:** Obtaining adequate tumor tissue for pathology review is a key first step in identifying the type of CUP.
  - **Light microscopy** identifies morphologic features like glandular differentiation seen in adenocarcinomas. Tumors with poor differentiation and minimal glandular formation are classified as poorly differentiated carcinomas with features of adenocarcinoma. Signet ring features are suggestive of gastric carcinomas and papillary features are associated with ovarian cancer.
  - **Immunohistochemistry:** IHC uses a panel of monoclonal and polyclonal antibodies to various cell components including enzymes, structural components of cells, hormone receptors, oncofetal antigens, and other substances identified by the immunoperoxidase technique. Important staining characteristics of some of the common malignancies are shown in Table 36-1. Pattern of staining of CK20 and CK7 helps define the possible tumor of origin. CK20+, CK7–, and a positive CDX-2 strongly suggest a colorectal primary when taken together with clinical and imaging findings. CK7+/CK20– tumors include lung (adenocarcinoma), biliary tract and pancreas, ovary (nonmucinous), endometrium, thyroid, cervical, and breast cancer. Lung adenocarcinomas are CK7+ and TTF-1 positive. Positive staining for thyroglobulin in concert with TTF-1 is relatively specific for thyroid cancer. Breast carcinomas stain for the estrogen and/or progesterone receptor. They are CK7+ and stain positively for the GATA-binding protein 3 (GATA3). Immunostaining positivity for the renal cell carcinoma marker (RCC-Ma) and paired box gene 8 (PAX8), with a negative CK20 is suggestive of renal cell carcinoma (RCC). CK7+, Wilms tumor (WT-1), and PAX8 positive staining are seen in ovarian adenocarcinomas.
- **Electron microscopy (EM):** EM is helpful, especially in the evaluation of poorly differentiated tumors. Through this modality secretory granules can be seen in neuroendocrine tumors, Weibel–Palade bodies in angiosarcomas, premelanosomes in melanomas and

TABLE 36-1	IMMUNOHISTOCHEMISTRY CHARACTERISTICS OF COMMON TUMORS
Tumor	**Immunoperoxidase Staining**
Carcinoma	CK (CK7 and 20 variable), EMA+
Lymphoma	CLA, EMA(+/−)
Sarcoma	Vimentin, desmin, factor VIII antigen
Melanoma	S-100, HMB-45, Vimentin, NSE
Neuroendocrine	Chromogranin, synaptophysin, CK, EMA, NSE
Germ cell	CK, EMA, β-HCG, AFP
Prostate	PSA, CK7(−), CK20(−), EMA
Breast	CK7(+), CK20(−), EMA, ER, PR, HER2, gross cystic fluid protein 15+
Thyroid	Thyroglobulin (follicular), CK, EMA, calcitonin (medullary)
Colorectal	CK7(−), CK20(+)
Lung cancer	TTF-1(+), Surf-A and Surf-B(+)
Adenocarcinoma of lungs	CK7(+), CK20(−), TTF-1(−)
Other non–small-cell lung cancer	TTF-1(+), chromogranin, NSE
Small-cell lung cancer	
Pancreas	CK7(+), CA 19–9(+)

CK, cytokeratin; EMA, epithelial membrane antigen; CLA, common leukocyte antigen; HMB, human melanoma black; NSE, neuron-specific enolase; ER, estrogen receptor; PR, progesterone receptor; HER2, human epidermal growth factor receptor 2; TTF-1, thyroid transcription factor 1; β-HCG, human chorionic gonadotropin; AFP, alpha feto protein; PSA, prostate-specific antigen.[3,5]

prekeratin filaments, and desmosomes in squamous cell carcinoma. EM is recommended in the evaluation of poorly differentiated neoplasm in young adults when the IHC is inconclusive.

- **Genomic sequencing** and initial testing for programmed cell death ligand 1 (PD-L1) and critical driver mutations such as epidermal growth factor receptor (*EGFR*), the anaplastic lymphoma kinase (*ALK*) fusion oncogene, and other targetable mutations are valuable in selection of a treatment regimen. Comprehensive genomic profiling using an NGS panel may also be able to predict tissue of origin. The detection of somatic gene mutations and germline mutations predicts benefit of systemic therapy including chemotherapy and targeted agents. Microsatellite-high (MSI-H), high tumor mutational burden, and programmed cell death ligand 1 (PD-L1) amplification or overexpression predict benefit of immune checkpoint inhibitors.[6]
- **Molecular cancer classifier assays (MCCAs):** Several MCCAs are available and use either reverse transcriptase polymerase chain reaction (RT-PCR) or gene microarray. The clinical time to receive the results varies from 10 to 14 days. Clinical validation studies show that in 85–95% of the cases, it identifies the tumor of origin in cases of carcinoma unknown primary.[7]
- **Multicancer early detection tests (MCED):** Significant advances have been made recently in MCED tests. These tests screen for multiple malignancies by detecting circulating DNA or proteins shed by tumor cells into the peripheral blood.[8] MCED testing has the potential to detect CUP.[9] However, there is no data at this time showing a mortality benefit with MCED testing to support widespread screening.

TABLE 36-2 GENERAL APPROACH TO MANAGEMENT OF CUP

1. Diagnosis of metastatic cancer with no primary tumor identified on initial evaluation with history and physical exam, laboratory testing, pathologic evaluation, and imaging.
2. Consider additional evaluation for potential primary tumors with PET/CT, mammogram, colonoscopy, EGD, laryngoscopy, bronchoscopy, or further pathologic testing based on the clinical picture.
3. Exclude favorable CUP subsets. If the patient falls into a favorable subset then additional workup and management are subset-specific (see "Special Considerations").
4. Molecular testing with NGS panel and molecular tissue-of-origin testing.
5. Treatment based on molecular tissue-of-origin or with a targeted agent with tissue-agnostic approval if available. Treatment otherwise with empiric chemotherapy regimens.

TREATMENT

Treatment of CUP is focused on identifying a subset of patients with cancers that are curable or highly responsive to specific therapies. Management of patients who fall into this favorable risk subset is outlined separately (see "Special Considerations"). Chemotherapy regimens with broad activity against multiple cancer types are used for cancers that do not fall into this favorable subset.[10] Molecular testing has opened up the possibility of treating CUP based on molecular tissue-of-origin assays or specific actionable mutations, but there is currently little data to support this approach over empiric chemotherapy. Due to overall poor outcomes, clinical trial participation is encouraged. An outline of the general approach to management of CUP is shown in Table 36-2.

- **Empiric chemotherapy.** In patients who do not fall into one of the favorable CUP subsets listed below, management has typically involved empiric treatment with chemotherapy regimens that have activity against multiple tumor types. Numerous chemotherapy regimens have been studied in CUP, but no regimen has been shown to be clearly superior.[11] Preferred treatment options include platinum-containing combination chemotherapy regimens, such as carboplatin-paclitaxel or FOLFOX.
- **Treatment based on molecular tissue-of-origin assays.** As mentioned above, multiple molecular assays are now commercially available to assign a suspected primary tumor for CUP based on gene expression profiling.[12] Two recent randomized trials have failed to show a benefit for treatment tailored to gene expression–based tissue-of-origin compared to empiric chemotherapy for CUP. A phase II trial randomized 130 CUP patients to site-specific treatment based on gene expression profiling or to empiric carboplatin-paclitaxel. This trial found no difference in its primary endpoint of 1-year survival rate.[13] Similarly, the GEFCAPI 04 phase III trial randomized 243 CUP patients to treatment based on gene expression profiling or to gemcitabine-cisplatin and found no difference in its primary endpoint of PFS.[14] However, in the GEFCAPI 04 trial, the most common primary cancer identified was pancreato-biliary cancers (19%), for which gemcitabine-cisplatin has been shown to have activity and which have generally poor outcomes even with site-specific therapies. In addition, due to the small numbers of patients, it is unclear if subsets of CUP patients with predicted primary tumors that have highly active therapies (such as immunotherapy for melanoma) benefitted from these studies. Given the lack of high-quality evidence, the current consensus guidelines do not recommend treatment of CUP based on gene expression profiling. However, because no chemotherapy

regimen has been found to be clearly superior in the treatment of CUP, using gene expression–based tumor-of-origin to guide treatment is a reasonable approach.[10]

- **Treatment with tissue-agnostic targeted therapies.** Molecular profiling of CUP with NGS can identify a subset of patients with genetic alterations that can be targeted with agents that are FDA approved regardless of primary tumor site. Pembrolizumab is approved for dMMR/MSI-H tumors and tumors with high TMB (≥10 mut/Mb) regardless of tissue of origin. Dostarlimab-gxly is similarly approved for dMMR/MSI-H tumors. Larotrectinib and entrectinib can be used to treat tumors with NTRK fusions regardless of tissue of origin and fusion partner.[15] Most recently, selpercatinib has been approved for treatment of tumors with rearranged during transfection (RET) fusions regardless of the primary tumor site.[16]

SPECIAL CONSIDERATIONS

It is important to identify the 10–20% of patients who fall into historically favorable subsets listed below that have specific treatment recommendations.[11,17] These patients are treated either with local therapy or with systemic therapies based on suspected primary tumors and are often excluded from clinical trials of empiric chemotherapy or treatment based on molecular tissue-of-origin assays.

- **Single potentially resectable metastatic lesion.** A subset of patients will have only a single site of metastatic disease identified even after thorough evaluation. These patients should be managed with surgery and/or radiation if feasible to locally treat all clinically apparent diseases.[17] Adjuvant chemotherapy can be added in these patients, but its use should be individualized. Empiric chemotherapy should be considered if the site of metastatic disease is not amenable to local therapy.
- **Extragonadal germ cell tumor in men.** Men with extragonadal germ cell tumors should be treated according to guidelines for testicular cancer even in the absence of an identifiable testicular primary tumor. In addition, young men who present with poorly differentiated carcinoma in a midline distribution involving the retroperitoneum and/or mediastinum can be treated as poor-risk extragonadal germ cell tumors.[17] Additional recommended testing includes circulating tumor markers (beta-hCG and alpha-fetoprotein) and testicular ultrasound. See Chapter 29: Urologic Malignancies for specific treatment regimens.
- **Peritoneal carcinomatosis in women.** Women who present with isolated peritoneal carcinomatosis and histology consistent with ovarian cancer should be treated as stage III ovarian cancer. Additional evaluation should include testing CA-125 level and referral to a gynecologic oncologist to evaluate for potential surgical cytoreduction.[11,17] See Chapter 30: Gynecologic Oncology for additional information.
- **Adenocarcinoma with isolated axillary lymph node involvement in women.** Women with adenocarcinoma involving only the axillary lymph nodes should be treated for a presumed primary breast cancer. Breast examination, mammogram, and breast MRI and/or breast ultrasound if mammogram is negative should be performed to evaluate for an occult primary breast tumor. Biopsy specimens should be evaluated for estrogen receptor, progesterone receptor, and HER2 expression by IHC to guide treatment. These patients are treated according to guidelines for stage II or III (T0, N+, M0) breast cancer. Management should include axillary lymph node dissection (ALND). Local treatment of the ipsilateral breast is also important because a microscopic primary breast tumor can be identified in 72% of patients after mastectomy.[11] Most patients are managed with ALND and ipsilateral modified radical mastectomy, but ALND with whole breast radiation has also been performed.[17] Patients should receive neoadjuvant and/or adjuvant systemic therapy based on ER/PR and HER2 expression. See Chapter 21: Breast Cancer for specific chemotherapy, endocrine therapy, and HER2-directed treatment options.
- **Metastatic adenocarcinoma with elevated PSA in men.** Men with metastatic adenocarcinoma of unknown primary should be evaluated for prostate cancer with either serum

PSA testing or IHC testing for PSA on tumor tissue. Given the high prevalence of prostate cancer and reasonable specificity of PSA testing, patients with significantly elevated PSA levels should be treated as metastatic hormone-sensitive prostate adenocarcinoma.[17] See Chapter 29: Urologic Malignancies for prostate cancer-specific treatment regimens.

- **Squamous cell carcinoma with isolated cervical lymph node involvement.** Patients with squamous cell carcinoma involving only the head and neck lymph nodes should be treated as suspected primary head and neck squamous cell carcinoma.[17] Additional evaluation with dedicated head and neck CT imaging, positron emission tomography-computed tomography (PET/CT), endoscopic evaluation, and testing of biopsy specimens for human papillomavirus (HPV) and Epstein-Barr virus (EBV) is important to determine the extent of disease and can often identify a primary site. If no primary site is identified, then guidelines recommend that HPV-positive tumors should be treated as primary oropharyngeal cancer and EBV-positive tumors should be treated as primary nasopharyngeal cancer. Treatment options for head and neck CUP often involve multimodality therapy including neck dissection and/or radiation with or without chemotherapy that should be determined by a multidisciplinary team. See Chapter 26: Head and Neck Cancer for additional details.

- **Squamous cell carcinoma with isolated inguinal lymph node involvement.** Patients with squamous cell carcinoma of the inguinal lymph nodes should undergo further evaluation with anoscopy and pelvic exam. If additional evaluation does not reveal a primary tumor, then patients should be managed with inguinal lymph node dissection with or without radiation.[17] Adjuvant chemotherapy can be considered in select patients.

- **Neuroendocrine carcinoma.** Well-differentiated neuroendocrine tumors of unknown primary are managed according to the guidelines for well-differentiated gastroenteropancreatic neuroendocrine tumors with treatments such as somatostatin analogs. Treatment options for poorly differentiated neuroendocrine tumors of unknown primary include combination chemotherapy regimens, such as those used for small-cell lung cancer.[11] See Chapter 22: Lung Cancer and Chapter 24: Other GI Malignancies for additional details.

MONITORING/FOLLOW-UP

There are no standard guideline recommendations for monitoring or follow-up of CUP. For patients who fall into a favorable subgroup or are treated based on a molecular tissue-of-origin assay, it is reasonable to follow monitoring guidelines for the suspected primary tumor.

OUTCOME/PROGNOSIS

Outcomes from CUP are highly variable due to the heterogeneous nature of the disease. Overall, CUP is associated with a poor prognosis with a median overall survival of 13 months in the modern era.[18] To aid in clinical decision-making, the MD Anderson Cancer Center recently created a nomogram to estimate survival for the unfavorable subset of CUP patients with a publicly available web-based tool (https://cupnomogram.shinyapps.io/Nomogram/).[19]

REFERENCES

1. Rassy E, Pavlidis N. The currently declining incidence of cancer of unknown primary. *Cancer Epidemiol.* 2019;61:139–141.
2. Hermans KEPE, Kazemzadeh F, Loef C, et al. Risk factors for cancer of unknown primary: a literature review. *BMC Cancer.* 2023;23(1):314.
3. Rassy E, Assi T, Pavlidis N. Exploring the biological hallmarks of cancer of unknown primary: where do we stand today? *Br J Cancer.* 2020;122(8):1124–1132.
4. Ross JS, Wang K, Gay L, et al. Comprehensive genomic profiling of carcinoma of unknown primary site: new routes to targeted therapies. *JAMA Oncol.* 2015;1(1):40–49.

5. Karsell PR, Sheedy PF II, O'Connell MJ. Computed tomography in search of cancer of unknown origin. *JAMA*. 1982;248(3):340–343.

6. Abraham J, Heimberger AB, Marshall J, et al. Machine learning analysis using 77,044 genomic and transcriptomic profiles to accurately predict tumor type. *Transl Oncol*. 2021;14(3):101016.

7. Meiri E, Mueller WC, Rosenwald S, et al. A second-generation microRNA-based assay for diagnosing tumor tissue origin. *Oncologist*. 2012;17(6):801–812.

8. Kisiel JB, Papadopoulos N, Liu MC, Crosby D, Srivastava S, Hawk ET. Multicancer early detection test: preclinical, translational, and clinical evidence-generation plan and provocative questions. *Cancer*. 2022;128(Suppl 4):861–874.

9. Lennon AM, Buchanan AH, Kinde I, et al. Feasibility of blood testing combined with PET-CT to screen for cancer and guide intervention. *Science*. 2020;369(6499):eabb9601.

10. Hainsworth JD, Greco FA. Cancer of unknown primary site: new treatment paradigms in the era of precision medicine. *Am Soc Clin Oncol Educ Book*. 2018;38:20–25.

11. Lee MS, Sanoff HK. Cancer of unknown primary. *BMJ*. 2020;371:m4050.

12. Kato S, Alsafar A, Walavalkar V, Hainsworth J, Kurzrock R. Cancer of unknown primary in the molecular era. *Trends Cancer*. 2021;7(5):465–477.

13. Hayashi H, Kurata T, Takiguchi Y, et al. Randomized phase II trial comparing site-specific treatment based on gene expression profiling with carboplatin and paclitaxel for patients with cancer of unknown primary site. *J Clin Oncol*. 2019;37(7):570–579.

14. Fizazi K, Maillard A, Penel N, et al. LBA15_PR – A phase III trial of empiric chemotherapy with cisplatin and gemcitabine or systemic treatment tailored by molecular gene expression analysis in patients with carcinomas of an unknown primary (CUP) site (GEFCAPI 04). *Ann Oncol*. 2019;30:v851.

15. Lemery S, Fashoyin-Aje L, Marcus L, et al. Development of tissue-agnostic treatments for patients with cancer. *Annu Rev Cancer Biol*. 2022;6(1):147–165.

16. Bhamidipati D, Subbiah V. Impact of tissue-agnostic approvals for patients with gastrointestinal malignancies. *Trends Cancer*. 2023;9(3):237–249.

17. DeVita VT, Rosenberg SA, Lawrence TS. *DeVita, Hellman, and Rosenberg's Cancer*. Wolters Kluwer; 2018.

18. Varghese AM, Arora A, Capanu M, et al. Clinical and molecular characterization of patients with cancer of unknown primary in the modern era. *Ann Oncol*. 2017;28(12):3015–3021.

19. Raghav K, Hwang H, Jácome AA, et al. Development and validation of a novel nomogram for individualized prediction of survival in cancer of unknown primary. *Clin Cancer Res*. 2021;27(12):3414–3421.

Supportive Care in Oncology

37

Oladipo Cole and Angela C. Hirbe

GENERAL PRINCIPLES

Supportive care addresses the physical, mental, and spiritual needs of the cancer patient. Physical symptoms can arise from the cancer itself, the side effects of therapy, medications, or comorbid medical conditions. This chapter focuses on symptom control as an important element of oncology practice, including pain management, nausea and vomiting, mucositis, diarrhea, anorexia, and dyspnea. It also addresses the emotional issues of depression, anxiety, and delirium, and presents an approach to addressing spiritual needs of the cancer patient.

Management by Physical Symptom

Pain Management

GENERAL PRINCIPLES

Pain is a prevalent complaint in cancer patients, occurring in 50–70% of all patients with cancer. More than half of the cancer patients experience moderate to severe pain, and 50–80% of cancer patients are not satisfied with their pain relief. The undertreatment of cancer pain can be attributed to multiple barriers including physician, patient, and societal factors.[1] A physician must remember that each person's pain is different and must be treated as such.

Definition

Pain is always subjective. The International Association for the Study of Pain defines pain as "an unpleasant multidimensional sensory and emotional experience associated with actual or potential tissue damage, or described in relation to such damage." Each individual learns the application of the word through experiences related to injury early in life. Acute pain may be associated with physical signs, including tachycardia, hypertension, hyperventilation, facial grimacing, and verbalizations. However, patients with chronic pain may not exhibit any of these overt physical signs and may not "appear in pain." It is important to remember that pain is always subjective, and the patient's self-reporting is a key element to an accurate pain assessment.

DIAGNOSIS

- The first step in the management of pain depends on a comprehensive pain assessment gathered through history, physical examination, and review of laboratory and radiology studies. Important pain characteristics to elicit from the patient should be descriptions of the pain with regard to *onset, duration, intensity, quality,* and **exacerbating** or **relieving factors**. The physician can use each of these characteristics to identify potential etiologies and institute the appropriate pain management plan.

- Simple tools can reliably aid in the measurement of pain. The most common clinical assessment tools are verbal rating scales and visual analog scales. A verbal rating scale uses words to describe pain such as none, mild, moderate, severe, or excruciating. A visual analog scale uses a line with or without verbal clues or numbers and asks patients to place their pain rating on this scale. The specific scale used to measure pain is less important than the consistent use of a scale over time. For illiterate or pediatric patients, a visual analog scale can be used with pictures to describe the levels of pain as a better pain assessment tool.

TREATMENT

- The World Health Organization (WHO) recommends the use of an analgesic ladder in the approach to the selection of opioids to treat cancer pain.[2-5] Analgesic selection should be guided by the severity of cancer pain. Patients with mild to moderate pain are usually started on acetaminophen or NSAIDs. Patients with moderate to severe pain, or those who had insufficient relief after a trial of acetaminophen or NSAIDs, are treated with an opioid used for moderate pain such as codeine, hydrocodone, dihydrocodeine, and oxycodone. This opioid may be combined with acetaminophen, an NSAID, or an alternative adjuvant drug (tricyclic antidepressant, anticonvulsant, or topical anesthetic). Many of the drugs used for moderate to severe cancer pain are available in US as a combination of the opioid and acetaminophen or aspirin (ASA). The drug can be titrated until the maximum safe dose of acetaminophen (4 g/d) or ASA is reached.
- Patients with severe pain, including those who fail to reach adequate pain relief with drugs from the second step on the WHO ladder, should receive an opioid that is useful in the treatment of severe cancer pain. The drugs useful in the treatment of severe cancer pain include morphine, hydromorphone, fentanyl, oxycodone, and methadone. These opioids may also be combined with acetaminophen, an NSAID, or an adjuvant drug when needed. Patients can experience a variation of analgesia and side effects between the different opioids. A clinician may need to rotate among the various opioids to identify the drugs that have the correct balance between pain control and side effects. These **drugs should be titrated to analgesic effects or intolerable side effects**. There is no maximum dose limitation on the opioid medication itself.
- In the treatment of cancer pain, it is **important to distinguish between acute and chronic pain**, as the goals of treatment are slightly different. Acute pain is a linear event; the pain starts, and, with relief of the offending event, the pain stops. Chronic pain is cyclical in nature, repeating itself over time. For acute pain, the goal of treatment is pain relief. To accomplish pain relief, the drugs administered should have a rapid onset of action, with the desired duration of action (e.g., 2–4 hours). These drugs are given as needed. Common side effects, such as sedation, are usually acceptable and well tolerated by the patient. An example of an acute pain scenario is the patient who falls and suffers a hip fracture at the site of a previous bone metastasis. The patient is treated with short-acting IV narcotics until surgery can be performed to stabilize the fracture.
- **Chronic pain management** has a different focus. The overall goal is pain prevention and the avoidance of undesirable side effects, such as sedation. The analgesic regimen should include long-acting narcotics administered on a regular schedule and should be individualized for the patient based on side effects. Patients with chronic pain also need to have the understanding of how to manage acute exacerbations with short-acting, rapid-onset analgesics, most commonly referred to as breakthrough pain relief. Many cancer patients have chronic pain. Chronic pain is ineffectively managed when the clinician focuses on acute control of the pain in this setting.
- Some types of pain can be treated with procedural approaches in addition to medications. For example, bone pain sometimes responds to radiation therapy, radiofrequency ablation, or vertebroplasty.

Medications

- Opioid therapy can provide effective pain relief to the majority of patients with cancer pain.[2-4] Opioids can be classified as pure agonists or agonist antagonists, based on their interactions with opioid receptors in the body. The drugs that are included in the agonist–antagonist subclass include butorphanol (Stadol), nalbuphine (Nubain), pentazocine (Talwin), and buprenorphine (Buprenex). Drugs in this subclass have a ceiling effect for analgesia and may reverse the effects of pure agonists. For these reasons, use of the mixed agonist–antagonist subclass is not recommended in the treatment of cancer pain.

- When managing chronic pain, it is important to remember that there are wide variations in dose requirements. This variation is not based on the size or age of the patient or the amount of disease present. The analgesic dose required to keep a patient out of pain cannot be predicted, but rather must be determined by educated trial and error. The following are guidelines for opioid use in chronic pain patients.

  - **Start with one drug at the lowest effective dose.** Titrate the drug for pain relief or intolerable side effects. If the patient is unable to tolerate one narcotic due to undesirable side effects, switch to an alternative agent.

  - **Use around-the-clock dosing schedules** to avoid peaks and valleys in serum analgesic levels.

  - Sustained or long-acting release preparations of narcotics are very useful in this population. When converting between modes of administration or drugs, calculate the equianalgesic dosages to avoid undermedicating a patient. See Table 37-1.

  - **Breakthrough pain medications should be the same or a similar drug used for long-acting pain relief.** The minimum effective breakthrough pain medication dose should be equivalent to 12.5% of the patient's total daily narcotic requirements, or 25% of a single bid dose.

  - Keep the regimen as simple as possible. Avoid mixing a variety of analgesic regimens.

  - **Always start an effective bowel regimen when placing a patient on narcotics**, as constipation is a side effect of all narcotics.

  - **Educate the patient and family about dosing and side effects.** Discuss and reassure the patient and family about addiction, tolerance, and physical dependence.

- **Morphine** is the drug of choice for moderate to severe cancer pain. It has a wide range of doses available and flexible methods of delivery. Morphine is available as sustained-release, immediate-release, liquid/sublingual, and parenteral preparations. The sustained-release tablets may be given per rectum or sublingually in patients unable to swallow. **Oxycodone** is available orally as immediate- and sustained-release preparations. **Fentanyl** is available in the parenteral route, as well as the fentanyl (Duragesic) patch for patients unable to swallow or who cannot tolerate morphine or oxycodone. The patches are applied to the chest wall or back and changed every 48–72 hours. The onset of action

TABLE 37-1	EQUIVALENT OPIOID DOSES	
	PO (mg)	SC/IV (mg)
Morphine	30	10
Hydromorphone	7.5	1.5
Methadone	20	10
Codeine	200	NA
Oxycodone	20	NA
Fentanyl	NA	0.05–0.1

NA, not available.

in these long-acting preparations is 12 hours. When starting a patient on long-acting agents, the clinician needs to provide the patient with immediate-relief preparations for use in the interim, until the long-acting narcotic can achieve adequate serum levels for analgesia.

- **Meperidine (Demerol) should be avoided in the treatment of chronic pain.** Meperidine has a very short half-life of 2–3 hours. This is ineffective in the management of chronic pain. Meperidine has a toxic metabolite, normeperidine, which is a weaker analgesic but a potent central nervous system (CNS) stimulant. Normeperidine has a half-life of ≥25–30 hours in the setting of renal failure. This can rapidly lead to accumulation of the drug when used for more than 48–72 hours. CNS toxicity can include irritability, tremors, myoclonus, agitation, and seizures. When CNS toxicity occurs, it is important to stop the drug. Naloxone (Narcan) should not be administered, as the effects of normeperidine are not reversed with naloxone and can precipitate worsening CNS toxicity.

- IM injections should be avoided for the management of cancer pain. The use of IM injections is painful and absorption is unreliable. The onset of action can be 30–60 minutes, and this is not acceptable in the acute pain setting. IV or transmucosal (sublingual or rectal) routes are much more efficacious at getting rapid onset of action in the acute pain setting.

- The perception that the administration of opioid analgesics for chronic pain management causes addiction is prevalent and is a barrier to adequate pain control. Confusion about the differences among addiction, tolerance, and physical dependence is in part responsible.

  ○ **Addiction** is a pattern of drug abuse characterized by drug craving and overwhelming behaviors that are used to obtain a drug.

  ○ **Tolerance** is a state in which escalating doses of opioids are needed to achieve pain control as the drug effectiveness reduces over time. Tolerance occurs with all of the side effects of narcotics, with the exception of constipation. It is important to educate patients and family members that tolerance to many of the common side effects, such as itching or sedation, will develop, and that the drug should not be abruptly discontinued.

  ○ **Physical dependence** is the onset of signs and symptoms of withdrawal with abrupt discontinuation of the opioid. Abrupt withdrawal may result in tachycardia, hypertension, diaphoresis, nausea, vomiting, abdominal pain, psychosis, and hallucinations. This is not the same as addiction. Physical dependence and addiction are not synonymous. When stopping chronic opioid medications, the dose should be reduced in increments of 20% every 2–3 days to avoid the risk of withdrawal symptoms. Finally, it should be remembered that patients experiencing inadequately controlled pain may engage in what appears to be drug-seeking behavior, which is easy to confuse with addiction.

- **Adjuvant analgesics** can be important in the treatment of cancer pain. Adjuvant analgesics include antidepressants, anticonvulsants, corticosteroids, and local anesthetics. Within the antidepressants, tricyclics are the most effective as an adjunctive therapy for neuropathic pain. Common side effects from the tricyclics include orthostatic hypotension, sedation, urinary retention, confusion, and sexual dysfunction. Doses of the tricyclic antidepressants should be started low and titrated for analgesia. Selective norepinephrine reuptake inhibitors (SNRIs) such as duloxetine (Cymbalta) or venlafaxine (Effexor) may be effective as well. Anticonvulsants are also helpful adjunctive therapies in the treatment of neuropathic pain syndromes. These drugs include carbamazepine (Tegretol), phenytoin (Dilantin), gabapentin (Neurontin), and pregabalin (Lyrica). The usual initiating dose of gabapentin is 100 mg tid titrated up to a maximum of 3,600 mg/d. Side effects of these drugs can be self-limiting, including sedation, confusion, and dizziness.

- **Corticosteroids** can be useful in the management of bone metastases, nerve compression, elevated intracranial pressure, and obstruction of a hollow viscus. Local anesthetics such as nerve blocks, lidocaine patches, and eutectic mixture of local anesthetics (EMLA) cream can aid in the treatment of cancer pain. In extreme cases, IV administration of anesthetics can be used in conjunction with IV or intraspinal narcotics to allow the clinician to administer lower doses of narcotics and spare the patient the complications of sedation seen with high doses of narcotics.

- **Bisphosphonates** (pamidronate, zoledronic acid) and calcitonin have been used to treat pain from bony metastases. Clinical trials have failed to demonstrate clear evidence for the ability of bisphosphonates to deliver an analgesic benefit over placebo. Calcitonin provides no benefit in metastatic bone pain over placebo, but some studies suggest that it may reduce the intensity and frequency of neuropathic pain.

Constipation

GENERAL PRINCIPLES

Most constipation in cancer comes from opioid pain management, but the differential diagnosis of constipation is broad.[6,7]

DIAGNOSIS

- Before assuming that all constipation is pain medicine related in the cancer patient, one must remember to consider bowel obstruction, spinal cord compression, hypercalcemia, hypokalemia, diabetes mellitus, hypothyroidism, timing of chemotherapy, uremia, etc., as these must be treated differently. Other possible considerations are different classes of drugs such as antacids, anticholinergics, antidepressants, calcium channel blockers, cholestyramine, clonidine, diuretics, levodopa, NSAIDs, psychotropics, and sympathomimetics.
- During opioid treatment, constipation should be expected. Prophylactic measures should always be initiated with the start of opioid therapy. Constipation occurs with all opioids, and pharmacologic tolerance rarely develops. Symptoms from constipation may become so severe that patients may decide to discontinue pain medications. This is preventable with the use of an aggressive laxative regimen.

TREATMENT

- Dietary interventions are almost never sufficient to prevent constipation.[6] Combinations of agents are often necessary. Clinicians should also avoid the use of bulk-forming agents in the absence of a motility agent, especially in debilitated or anorectic patients. When using these agents, it should be remembered that stool softeners and bulking agents do little to relieve constipation but may make stools more comfortable to pass. Their sole use will only lead to constipation with soft stools, and another agent is necessary for adequate treatment. Also, it should be remembered that the onset of abdominal pain or nausea in a patient taking opioids may be due to unrecognized constipation.
- Laxatives can be classified into three categories: stimulant, osmotic, and detergent agents (Table 37-2). **Stimulant laxatives** irritate the bowel, leading to increased peristaltic activity. **Osmotic laxatives** draw water into the bowel lumen and increase the moisture content of the stool. In addition, they add to overall stool volume. **Detergent laxatives** facilitate the dissolution of fat in water and increase the water content of stool. Laxatives can be titrated to a maximal therapeutic dose. Clinicians should try to simplify the bowel regimen, as this will improve patient compliance. Use of stimulant laxatives such as sennosides/bisacodyl is ideal for preventing opioid-induced constipation.

TABLE 37-2	LAXATIVES
Stimulant laxatives	
Senna	2 tablets bid, titrated to effect (up to 8/d)
Bisacodyl (Dulcolax)	5–15 mg PO or 10 mg PR qhs
Osmotic laxatives	
Lactulose	20 g/30 mL PO every 4–6 h, titrated to effect (or every 2 h in severe constipation)
Sorbitol	30 mL PO every 4–6 h, titrated to effect
Milk of magnesia	15–30 mL/d or twice daily
Magnesium citrate	300-mL bottle per day, bid, scheduled, or prn
Detergent laxatives	
Docusate sodium or calcium	100 mg PO per day or twice daily
Phosphosoda enema	PRN

- **Prokinetic agents** such as metoclopramide (Reglan) can increase peristaltic activity and facilitate stool movement. This agent can be used in combination with other laxative agents. Lubricant stimulants and large-volume enemas can also be used but are not recommended for daily use and prophylaxis of opioid-related constipation. The use of these agents is effective while titrating other laxatives to ensure that the patient is having regular bowel movements.
- Methylnaltrexone is a selective antagonist of the peripheral μ-opioid receptors and can be used to treat opioid-induced constipation that does not respond to other laxatives. The drug has not been shown to affect analgesia or to induce opioid withdrawal. The most common side effects of this medication are mild abdominal pain and flatulence. Lubiprostone is a type 2 chloride channel activator that increases GI fluid secretion. This results in increased tone, enhanced peristalsis, and improvement of both small bowel and colon transit times, which increases overall bowel movement frequency. Care should be taken to ensure that the patient does not have a mechanical obstruction prior to receiving this medication as there is a risk of GI perforation in this setting. Other newer agents include naloxegol, alvimopan, and naldemedine.
- Often patients present with prolonged constipation from narcotics of the order of days to weeks. It is important to identify this immediately and treat it aggressively. One can use enemas or suppositories per rectum, or oral regimens such as lactulose, 20 g every 2 hours, until the bowels move. Patients should be instructed to inform their physician if they do not have a bowel movement within any 48-hour time period while they are on narcotics to avoid potentially life-threatening complications.

Diarrhea

GENERAL PRINCIPLES

Diarrhea can be defined as stools that are looser than normal and that are increased in number over baseline.[6] The definition is based on the frequency, volume, and consistency of stools. In cancer patients, getting up to go to the bathroom multiple times day and night can be exhausting. If persistent, diarrhea can lead to dehydration and electrolyte abnormalities that can lead to the need for a hospital admission.

DIAGNOSIS

Potential causes of diarrhea in the cancer patient can include infections, malabsorption, gastrointestinal bleeding, medications, chemotherapy (particularly 5-FU), radiation to the abdomen or pelvis, and overflow incontinence. It is important to remember that herbals such as ginkgo biloba, ginseng, and licorice may also cause diarrhea.

TREATMENT

- Patients should be instructed on the establishment of normal bowel habits. Any change from the normal baseline should be reported to the physician to avoid severe dehydration or electrolyte imbalances. Patients should be counseled on the avoidance of foods containing lactose or other gas-forming foods that can increase abdominal cramping and pain. Another general approach to diarrhea is to increase the bulk of the stools with the addition of psyllium, bran, or pectin. However, sometimes bulk-forming agents can worsen abdominal cramping and bloating.
- For the medical management of transient or mild diarrhea, the use of attapulgite (Kaopectate) or bismuth salts (Pepto-Bismol) can be useful. Care should be taken to rule out infection by checking *Clostridium difficile* toxin before using antiperistaltic medications in the setting of recent antibiotic use. Potential infectious workup may include checking for fecal leukocytes, ova, and parasites and stool culture. For more persistent and severe diarrhea, agents that slow down peristalsis are more useful, including the following:
  - **Loperamide** (Imodium), 2–4 mg PO every 6 hours (maximum, 8 tablets/d)
  - **Diphenoxylate/atropine** (Lomotil), 2.5–5 mg PO every 6 hours (maximum, 8 tablets/d)
  - **Tincture of opium**, 0.7 mL PO every 4 hours and titrated as needed (Belladonna can be added as an antispasmodic agent.)
  - **Octreotide** (Sandostatin LAR Depot), 10–20 mg IM every 4 weeks
- For persistent, severe secretory diarrhea, the patient should be admitted for parenteral fluid support and the initiation of octreotide.
  - **Octreotide** (Sandostatin), 50–500 µg SC/IV every 8–12 hours. Begin at 50 µg SC/IV, then titrated up to 100 µg per dose every 48 hours to a maximum of 500 µg SC every 8 hours, with titration based on response; may also be given as a continuous IV infusion, 10–80 µg/h.

Nausea and Vomiting

GENERAL PRINCIPLES

Nausea and vomiting are commonly associated with advanced malignancies as a direct result of the disease or as side effects of chemotherapy or other medications.[6,8] There are multiple potential causes of nausea and vomiting in the cancer patient. Different etiologies for nausea and vomiting may require different interventions for control of the symptoms.

DIAGNOSIS

- The three most common forms of chemotherapy-associated nausea are **acute**, which begins within 1–2 hours of chemotherapy; **delayed**, which occurs 24 hours to 5 days after chemotherapy; and **anticipatory**, which is a conditioned response from prior occurrences of chemotherapy.
- A thorough assessment of nausea and vomiting is important to gain an understanding of potential etiologies and to allow for an appropriate choice of antiemetics. A common

mnemonic for potential etiologies is the "11 M's of emesis": metastases, meningeal irritation, movement, mental (anxiety), medications, mucosal irritation, mechanical obstruction, motility, metabolic, microbes, and myocardial (ischemia, congestive heart failure). Identification of the source of nausea and vomiting dictates treatment.

TREATMENT

- For **prevention of chemotherapy-associated acute nausea**, the three classes of drugs with the highest efficacy are corticosteroids (dexamethasone), serotonin ($5\text{-}HT_3$) receptor antagonists (dolasetron, granisetron, ondansetron, palonosetron), and the neurokinin-1 (NK1) receptor antagonist aprepitant (Emend). Treatment recommendations for acute nausea and vomiting are dependent on the emetogenic potential of the chemotherapy.
  - For low-emetogenic therapies, dexamethasone or metoclopramide (a dopamine antagonist) is used. For moderately emetogenic therapies, a $5\text{-}HT_3$ receptor antagonist is combined with dexamethasone.
  - For highly emetogenic chemotherapies, such as platinum-based regimens, aprepitant is combined with a $5\text{-}HT_3$ receptor antagonist and dexamethasone.
  - For delayed nausea, single-agent dexamethasone or dexamethasone plus metoclopramide is recommended. If the combination treatment does not work, aprepitant should be considered.
  - Anticipatory emesis is a conditioned response from prior cycles of chemotherapy. Patients benefit from benzodiazepines and behavioral therapy (hypnosis, desensitization, relaxation, etc.). The best way to prevent anticipatory emesis is good control of acute and delayed emesis in prior cycles of chemotherapy.
- **Nausea and vomiting from a bowel obstruction** can be a challenge to treat, especially when surgery is not an option. **Octreotide** has been shown to effectively inhibit the secretion of fluid into the intestinal lumen and decrease bloating and abdominal pain as well as nausea and vomiting. It may be started by continuous infusion or intermittent SC injection at a dose of 100 μg every 8–12 hours and titrated every 24–48 hours for effect.
- **Dopamine antagonists** are one of the most frequently used antiemetics. These medications have the potential to cause sedation and extrapyramidal symptoms. Medication options include the following:
  - Haloperidol (Haldol), PO, IV, SC
  - Prochlorperazine (Compazine), PO, PR, IV
  - Droperidol (Inapsine), IV
  - Promethazine (Phenergan), PO
  - Perphenazine (Trilafon), PO, IV
  - Trimethobenzamide (Tigan), PO, PR
  - Metoclopramide (Reglan), PO, IV
- **Histamine antagonists** may also cause sedation and can have a beneficial effect in some patients. The antihistamines have the added benefit of anticholinergic properties, which can also be beneficial in patients with dual etiologies of nausea. These drugs include the following:
  - Diphenhydramine (Benadryl), PO, IV
  - Meclizine (Antivert), PO
  - Hydroxyzine (Atarax), PO, IV
- **Scopolamine** is an anticholinergic agent that is useful in treating nausea induced by the vestibular apparatus. It can also be used adjunctively with other antiemetics in empiric therapy. Scopolamine can be given as an IV or SC scheduled or continuous infusion, but it is also conveniently available as a transdermal patch.
- **Serotonin antagonists** have been effective in the treatment of chemotherapy-associated nausea and vomiting. They are also useful for refractory nausea but are typically tried when other medications have failed. The medications available are as follows:

○ Ondansetron (Zofran), PO, IV
○ Granisetron (Kytril), PO, IV
○ Dolasetron (Anzemet), PO, IV
○ Palonosetron (Aloxi), IV
• The NK1 receptor antagonist **aprepitant** (Emend) has become first-line therapy on day 1 for highly emetogenic chemotherapies.
• The use of **dronabinol** (Marinol) and **benzodiazepines** is beneficial in some patients, but the mechanism of action remains unclear. Benzodiazepines (i.e., lorazepam [Ativan] at a 1-mg dose) are often useful in conjunction with other classes of antiemetics and may have a synergistic effect.

Mucositis

GENERAL PRINCIPLES

Mucositis refers to painful inflammation and ulceration of the oral mucosa.[6,9] Mucositis can result from chemotherapy or radiation therapy. Chemotherapeutic agents that are associated commonly with mucositis include bleomycin, cytarabine, doxorubicin, melphalan, methotrexate, etoposide, and 5-FU. Radiation to the head and neck may also cause mucositis. Patient factors that can contribute to worsening symptoms include poor-fitting oral prostheses, periodontal disease, and overall poor oral hygiene. Patients should undergo repair of ill-fitting prostheses, tooth extraction, and repair of periodontal disease before the initiation of chemotherapy. In the event that repair cannot be done before chemotherapy, the physician should make a referral to an oral surgeon once the patient's peripheral blood counts have returned to baseline.

DIAGNOSIS

A **mucositis grading system**, established by the National Cancer Institute, allows the physician to assess mucositis severity in terms of both pain and the patient's ability to continue to eat or drink, graded on a scale from 0–4. A score of 0 is given when there is no evidence of mucositis. When a patient develops nonpainful erythema or ulcers, but is able to eat or drink, a score of 1 is given. A score of 2 is given when there are mildly to moderately painful erythema or ulcers, but the patient is still able to eat or drink without difficulty. This may require intermittent analgesia. Severe erythema, painful ulcers that cause interference with eating and drinking requiring constant analgesia, scores a 3. Finally, a score of 4 is given when the severity of symptoms requires parenteral analgesia and/or nutritional support.

TREATMENT

A standardized approach to the prevention and treatment of mucositis is essential to quality care for the oncology patient. The prophylactic measures usually used include **mouth rinses** with sodium chloride, sodium bicarbonate, chlorhexidine (Peridex), or calcium phosphate (Caphosol). Regimens commonly used for the treatment of mucositis and the associated pain include a **local anesthetic** such as lidocaine, **magnesium-based antacids** (Maalox, Mylanta), **diphenhydramine** (Benadryl), and an **antifungal** such as nystatin (Mycostatin) or Mycelex. These agents are used either alone or at equal concentrations in a mouthwash. The patient can use the mouthwash up to five times per day for relief. In the treatment of severe mucositis, narcotics may need to be used in addition to the agents mentioned earlier. Using 2% morphine mouthwash swish and spit in select patients can be useful, followed by systemic opioids for refractory mucositis.[10]

Anorexia and Cachexia

GENERAL PRINCIPLES

Anorexia and cachexia frequently occur with advanced malignancies and are characterized by a loss of muscle mass and adipose tissue.[11] The increased catabolism of cancer and the anorexia that accompanies it result in increased muscle protein breakdown and lipolysis. These symptoms typically represent progression of disease and are not reversible with parenteral or enteral nutrition. Anorexia and cachexia are significant causes of distress to the patient and their family members.

DIAGNOSIS

Weight loss of more than 5%, decreased appetite, loss of taste and smell, and decreased food intake are the hallmarks of cancer-related anorexia and cachexia. The specific etiologies of these symptoms are not well understood. The clinician should always assess for other potential etiologies underlying the loss of appetite and weight such as dysphagia, odynophagia, infections, and side effects of medications.

TREATMENT

There are several approaches to the general management of anorexia and cachexia.

- Patients should be offered their favorite foods and nutritional supplements if the patients enjoy them. Any **dietary restrictions should be eliminated**. Portion sizes can be reduced, frequency of intake increased, and food should be made to look appetizing. Adjustment of diet in accordance with new taste preference and avoiding food that evokes aversion or has potent odors should be avoided.[12]
- There is a variety of pharmacologic approaches for improving appetite. **Corticosteroids** have an appetite-stimulating effect, as well as effects on the patient's mood and energy level. Dexamethasone (Decadron) at doses of ≤4 mg/d is recommended. Dexamethasone is preferred because of the relative lack of mineralocorticoid effects, but any steroid will be efficacious such as Prednisone 20 mg/d. Steroids are considered only for short-term treatment, as they lose their efficacy over days to weeks. If longer treatment is anticipated, **megestrol** (Megace) has also been shown to improve appetite in cancer patients. There is a large variation in the effective dose of megestrol between individual patients. One should begin with 200 mg PO every 6–8 hours and titrate up to 400–800 mg/d or Megace ES, 650 mg PO daily. The **cannabinoids**, such as dronabinol (Marinol), have been shown to promote weight gain in cancer patients.
- It should be understood that clinical studies have demonstrated no impact on overall survival or improvement in quality of life when anorexia and cachexia are pharmacologically managed. Thus, treatment of anorexia and weight loss is done primarily because anorexia is distressing to the patients and their families.

Dyspnea

GENERAL PRINCIPLES

Dyspnea can be one of the most frightening symptoms to patients and their family members.[13] Some patients with severe tachypnea will not complain of dyspnea, while others who are not tachypneic report severe dyspnea. For the majority of patients, relief of dyspnea can be achieved with simple interventions.

DIAGNOSIS

Respiratory rate, oxygen saturation, and blood gas levels often do not correlate with the patient's subjective report. The clinician must accept the patient's self-report and try to identify and/or correct the underlying etiology of the symptom. In patients with known advanced disease, the burden of investigating the etiology of the dyspnea must be weighed against the limited potential benefit from therapeutic interventions.

TREATMENT

One should first try to identify any obvious treatable cause for dyspnea. For example, volume overload may be able to be managed with low-dose diuretics. Dyspnea caused by pleural effusions may respond to drainage and subsequent pleurex catheter placement. Infections should be treated with antibiotics and bronchospasm with bronchodilators.

There are three widely used medical approaches for symptomatic breathlessness in advanced disease: supplemental oxygen, opioids, and anxiolytics.

- A therapeutic trial of **supplemental oxygen** may be beneficial; it has been suggested that there is a placebo effect in nonhypoxemic patients. In addition, the cool air moving across the patient's face from the supplemental oxygen can have a calming effect and help to relieve the feelings of air hunger. Studies have reported that stimulation of the trigeminal nerve with oxygen can cause a central inhibitory effect and relieve dyspnea. A fan in the room can also help achieve this effect.
- **Opioids** can provide relief in dyspnea without any measurable effect on respiratory rate or blood gas measurements. The precise mechanism by which opioids exert this effect is not known. In an opioid-naïve patient, doses lower than those used to achieve analgesia may be effective. Doses of hydrocodone, 5 mg PO every 4 hours, or codeine, 30 mg PO every 2 hours, can be beneficial in these patients. Other opioids can be useful and administered IV for urgent situations or when the PO route is not available. Patients can be maintained on a fixed schedule of opioid IV every 4–6 hours. An additional dose of a short-acting opioid, equivalent to 25–50% of the amount of baseline opioid, taken every 4 hours can be used hourly for intermittent periods of worsening dyspnea. Sublingual morphine can also be helpful in the terminal dyspneic patient.
- Dyspnea may cause severe anxiety. Some patients with dyspnea may need more effective treatment for their anxiety. **Benzodiazepines** can be used in addition to opioids and other nondrug therapies to reduce dyspnea. The clinician should begin with low doses and titrate for desired effects. Sublingual lorazepam has been shown to be quite effective if there is no IV access.

Anemia

GENERAL PRINCIPLES

Anemia in cancer patients may be due to the effects of their underlying malignancy (particularly when there is bone marrow involvement) and/or treatment. The basic mechanisms involved are decreased erythropoiesis, impaired iron metabolism, and decreased survival time for RBCs. In addition, erythropoietin production may be impaired.

DIAGNOSIS

Diagnosis is made by complete blood count (CBC), with a hemoglobin and hematocrit that are less than normal.

TREATMENT

Current treatment approaches are aimed at treating the underlying malignancy and boosting red cell mass. Transfusions offer only transient effects and have side effects such as transfusion reactions, iron overload, volume overload, and cardiac congestion. It is recommended that transfusions be administered only to those patients who are suffering from symptoms of anemia with hemoglobin <8 g/dL. Recombinant **erythropoietin** has been shown to reduce transfusion requirements and improve outcomes in terms of quality of life and response to treatment. ESAs have also been associated with tumor growth and shorter overall survival.

Emotional Symptom Management

GENERAL PRINCIPLES

Depression occurs in approximately half of the cancer patients, though it is often underdiagnosed and undertreated.[14] Specific problems facing these patients include pain, medication side effects, and changes in functional status.

DIAGNOSIS

Typical features of major depression may be present, such as depressed mood for at least 2 weeks, feelings of guilt or worthlessness, inability to concentrate, decreased energy, preoccupation with death or suicide, anhedonia, and changes in eating or sleeping habits. In cancer patients, one must be aware that drugs such as prednisone, dexamethasone, procarbazine, vincristine, and vinblastine can also cause depression-like symptoms. Loss of appetite, fatigue, or insomnia may be secondary to chemotherapy, the cancer itself, or pain, making it difficult to diagnose depression. Excessive guilt, low self-esteem, the wish to die, and hopelessness are the most diagnostic of depression in the cancer patient. One must be careful to screen for suicidal ideation, as the incidence of suicide is higher in both men and women with cancer.

TREATMENT

- Depression should be screened for and treated in all cancer patients. In addition to counseling by oncologic psychologists, medications can be useful in the treatment of depression.
- **Antidepressants** may require up to 6 weeks before symptoms are alleviated. The selective serotonin reuptake inhibitors (e.g., citalopram, 20–80 mg PO daily), bupropion SR (200–400 mg PO daily), and mirtazapine (usual dosage range 30–45 mg PO daily) are all reasonable first-line agents. (Mirtazapine has sedating effects but may aid those with insomnia; in addition, it may stimulate appetite.) Tricyclic antidepressants have the ability to treat depression and potentiate the effects of opioids on neuropathic pain. Imipramine, amitriptyline, and doxepin are started at 25 mg PO at bedtime, then titrated up to 25–50 mg every 24–48 hours until the desired effect is achieved.

- The **psychostimulants** methylphenidate, dextroamphetamine, and modafinil are an alternative for depressed patients with cancer (e.g., methylphenidate, 5 mg PO at 9:00 a.m. and 12 p.m. daily). They begin to work within a short period of time, provide relief from the sedating effects of opioids, and give the patient improved energy. Tolerance to stimulants can develop, and dosages may have to be adjusted over time.

Anxiety

DIAGNOSIS

The diagnosis and recognition of anxiety can be challenging. Patients often complain of physical and somatic manifestations of anxiety. The patient's subjective level of distress from fear, isolation, estrangement, or other common stressors is often the impetus for treatment.

TREATMENT

Anxiety is usually treated with benzodiazepines, neuroleptics, antihistamines, or nonpharmacologic psychotherapies. Benzodiazepines are first-line therapy for the treatment of anxiety disorders.

- Lorazepam, 0.5–2 mg PO, IV, or IM, every 3–6 hours
- Alprazolam, 0.25–1 mg PO, every 6–8 hours
- Diazepam, 2.5–10 mg PO, PR, IM, or IV every 3–6 hours
- Clonazepam, 1–2 mg PO, every 8–12 hours

Other anxiolytics include the following:

- Haloperidol (0.5–5 mg PO, IV, or SC every 2–12 hours), if there is concern about respiratory depression
- Thioridazine (10–25 mg PO tid), if insomnia and agitation are also present
- Hydroxyzine (25–50 mg every 4–6 hours PO, IV, or SC), which has mild anxiolytic, sedative, and analgesic properties
- Buspirone (10 mg PO tid), a nonbenzodiazepine anxiolytic that is useful in patients with chronic anxiety or anxiety related to adjustment disorders

Nonpharmacologic interventions for anxiety and distress include supportive psychotherapy and behavioral interventions used alone or in combination, relaxation, guided imagery, and hypnosis.

Delirium

GENERAL PRINCIPLES

Delirium is common in advanced cancer and is strongly associated with mortality.[15] The differential diagnosis for delirium in the cancer patient includes dehydration, hypo- and hypernatremia, hypocalcemia, uremia, liver failure, drugs (opiates, radiation, chemotherapeutics, benzodiazepines, tricyclic antidepressants, etc.), brain metastases, paraneoplastic syndrome, and infection.

DIAGNOSIS

One must identify the underlying cause so that supportive therapies can be given. Many scales exist for the diagnosis of delirium, including the Mini Mental Status Exam and Memorial Delirium Assessment Scale, and these should be used to both diagnose and follow delirium.

TREATMENT

If supportive techniques do not work, treatment with neuroleptics or sedative medications can be tried.

- Haloperidol (Haldol), 0.5–1 mg every 1–2 hours PO, IV, or SC is the first drug of choice for treatment of delirium and is usually effective for agitation, paranoia, and fear.
- Zyprexa, 5–10 mg PO, sublingually, is another possible first-line agent, as it can be given under the tongue.
- Lorazepam, 0.5–1 mg PO or IV, plus haloperidol (but not lorazepam alone) can be tried next.
- Chlorpromazine can be used if no response to antipsychotics is observed within 24–48 hours, as it is much more sedating.

Insomnia

DIAGNOSIS

Insomnia, or inability to sleep, is often a result of pain, medications, anxiety, or a mood disorder. Poor sleep can be distressing in the cancer patient, as it can make pain, anxiety, and delirium worse. Proper sleep hygiene and adequate management of pain and other symptoms are beneficial.

TREATMENT

Benzodiazepines (e.g., lorazepam, 0.5–2 mg PO qhs) or antidepressants with sedating effects (e.g., trazodone, 50 mg PO qhs, or amitriptyline, 25–50 mg PO qhs) may be used in conjunction with the nonpharmacologic measures. Newer agents such as zolpidem (Ambien, 5 mg qpm), eszopiclone (Lunesta, 2–3 mg PO qpm), and ramelteon (Rozerem, 8 mg PO qpm) can be tried. One should be careful when treating insomnia in terminally ill patients, as these can be hypnotic drugs. For some patients, improved cognition may be achieved by discontinuing the medications without an effect on insomnia.

Addressing Spiritual Care

- When a person has a malignancy, suffering occurs at many levels.[16] Religion or spiritual belief can be a source of great strength or considerable pain to a patient. Some find new faith during a cancer experience, while others find great turmoil. Spiritual care for the oncology patient can be either uncomfortable for the physician or, if the physician is overzealous, uncomfortable for the patient. Many doctors and nurses are appropriately uneasy when it comes to talking about religion because they fear they might be imposing their religious beliefs on others. The role of the physician is to advocate and try to connect a patient with chaplains, the patient's own religious community, or nonreligious groups that might help to provide solace.

- The role of the **oncologic chaplain** can greatly aid in the spiritual journey of a patient, both as an inpatient and as an outpatient. Chaplains can help identify patients in spiritual distress and address the religious or spiritual issues raised by their illness. Those who have never had strong religious beliefs may not feel an urge to turn to religion, but as trained listeners, chaplains can help patients identify core beliefs, recognize coping skills, and, potentially, help patients to find sources of strength within or beyond themselves.
- Chaplains also help families identify spiritual resources to enhance their coping with the level of distress during a loved one's illness. Often, chaplains are privy to information that may not be provided to the medical professional. This can, with permission, be shared for the benefit of the patient and improvement of care. Therefore, it is appropriate to involve chaplaincy in a patient's care. It is not necessary to ask whether a patient would like a chaplain, as the patient may feel undue pressure based on distorted understandings of a professional chaplain's role. A trained chaplain showing up at the bedside can lead to positive outcomes, even if the patient is enabled to say, "No, thank you" to spiritual care. Chaplains work to help people in crisis find a measure of control in the midst of what can feel like chaos.

REFERENCES

1. Kwon JH. Overcoming barriers in cancer pain management. *J Clin Oncol.* 2014;32:1727–1733.
2. Bonica JJ, Ventafriddi V, Twycross RG, eds. *Cancer Pain.* Vol 1. 2nd ed. Lea & Febiger; 1990.
3. Levy MH. Pharmacologic treatment of cancer pain. *N Engl J Med.* 1996;335(15):1124–1132.
4. Pharo GH, Zhou L. Pharmacologic management of cancer pain. *J Am Osteopath Assoc.* 2005; 105(11 Suppl 5):S21–S28.
5. Sharma S, Hertan L, Jones J. Palliative radiotherapy: current status and future directions. *Semin Oncol.* 2014;41(6):751–763.
6. Ludwig H, Zojer N. Supportive care. *Ann Oncol.* 2007;18(Suppl 1):i37–i44.
7. Candy B, Jones L, Goodman ML, Drake R, Tookman A. Laxatives or methylnaltrexone for the management of constipation in palliative care patients. *Cochrane Database Syst Rev.* 2011;(1):CD003448.
8. Gordon P, LeGrand SB, Walsh D. Nausea and vomiting in advanced cancer. *Eur J Pharmacol.* 2014; 722:187–191.
9. Campos MIDAC, Campos CN, Aarestrup FM, Aarestrup BJ. Oral mucositis in cancer treatment: natural history, prevention and treatment. *Mol Clin Oncol.* 2014;2(3):337–340.
10. Brown TJ, Gupta A. Management of cancer therapy-associated oral mucositis. *JCO Oncol Pract.* 2020;16(3):103–109.
11. Loprinzi CL, Kugler JW, Sloan JA, et al. Randomized comparison of megestrol acetate versus dexamethasone versus fluoxymesterone for the treatment of cancer anorexia/cachexia. *J Clin Oncol.* 1999;17(10):3299–3306.
12. Cotogni P, Stragliotto S, Ossola M, Collo A, Riso S; On Behalf Of The Intersociety Italian Working Group For Nutritional Support In Cancer. The role of nutritional support in cancer patients in palliative care. *Nutrients.* 2021;13(2):306.
13. Ben-Aharon I, Gafter-Gvili A, Leibovici L, Stemmer SM. Interventions for alleviating cancer-related dyspnea: a systematic review and meta-analysis. *Acta Oncol.* 2012;51(8):996–1008.
14. Jaiswal R, Alici Y, Breitbart W. A comprehensive review of palliative care in patients with cancer. *Int Rev Psychiatry.* 2014;26:87–101.
15. Lawlor PG, Bush SH. Delirium in patients with cancer: assessment, impact, mechanisms and management. *Nat Rev Clin Oncol.* 2015;12(2):77–92.
16. Berger J. Identifying spiritual landscapes among oncology patients. *Chaplaincy Today.* 1998;14:15–21.

Oncologic Emergencies

38

Brendan Knapp

P hysicians who treat cancer patients are often called on to evaluate potential oncologic emergencies. To diagnose and appropriately treat an oncologic emergency, a
physician must have a working knowledge of the distinct presentation, appropriate
diagnostic testing, and management of a wide array of complications that are often unique
to cancer patients.

Neutropenic Fever

GENERAL PRINCIPLES

Neutropenic fever is one of the most common complications of chemotherapy. Risk of
infection is slightly increased with neutrophil counts <1,000/μL, markedly increased
with neutrophils <500/μL (severe neutropenia), and highest with neutrophil counts
<100/μL (profound neutropenia). Eighty percent of infections in the neutropenic
patient originate from the patient's own skin or gastrointestinal flora. Long-term vascular access catheters such as a central line are also common sources. The most commonly identified microbes include gram-positive bacteria (*Staphylococcus, Streptococcus*)
and gram-negative aerobes (*Escherichia coli, Klebsiella pneumonia, Enterobacter*), but an
infectious source is identified in only 20–30% of cases.[1]

DEFINITION

Neutropenic fever is defined as a single **temperature >38.3°C** (or a temperature >38.0°C
for more than 1 hour) in patients with an **absolute neutrophil count <500/μL** (or
<1,000/μL that is expected to decrease to <500/μL).[1]

DIAGNOSIS

Clinical Presentation

Signs and symptoms of infection, such as exudate, erythema, and warmth, may not be evident because of the reduced numbers of neutrophils. Physical examination should focus on
the skin, catheter sites, teeth and oropharynx, sinuses, lungs, abdomen, and perianal area.
Digital rectal exam should not be performed due to the potential risk of causing bacterial
translocation.

Diagnostic Testing

Management includes **searching for a source of infection** by obtaining two sets of **blood
cultures**, with one set from any indwelling intravascular catheter. Culture specimens from
other sites of suspected infection should be obtained as clinically indicated, and a chest
x-ray should be performed if respiratory symptoms are present. CT should be performed
on other sites according to clinical features, such as a CT abdomen if concerned for neutropenic enterocolitis.

TREATMENT

Medications

- Antimicrobial therapy should be given immediately, even before test results are available, as patients can die of gram-negative sepsis in a matter of hours after their first fever, despite appearing well at initial presentation.
- **Empiric antimicrobial therapy in neutropenic fever**
  - Initial therapy is antipseudomonal beta-lactam ± aminoglycoside. A single agent such as cefepime (2 g IV every 8 hours in patients with normal renal function) may be used, depending on local sensitivities. A single dose of an aminoglycoside such as gentamicin may be administered regardless of renal function if the patient has signs of septic shock.
  - Agents with activity against methicillin-resistant *Staphylococcus aureus* (e.g., vancomycin or linezolid) should be used in addition to the previously mentioned antibiotics if the patient is hemodynamically unstable, has severe mucositis, is colonized with methicillin-resistant *S. aureus* or cephalosporin-resistant *Streptococci*, has received recent quinolone prophylaxis, or has signs of catheter infection or soft tissue infection.
  - If the patient remains febrile after 4–7 days without a clear source, antifungal coverage should be added. Caspofungin, micafungin, voriconazole, and posaconazole are reasonable choices, depending on the clinical circumstances. Treatment with amphotericin B is usually limited to refractory infections or critically ill patients who have not responded to the above agents.
- The above are only general guidelines. If the patient is penicillin allergic, consider substituting a fourth-generation fluoroquinolone or aztreonam. Aztreonam should not be used as monotherapy in place of a cephalosporin as it lacks gram-positive coverage; therefore aztreonam is typically given in combination with vancomycin.
- Antibacterial choice may vary depending on organisms and resistance patterns in a particular hospital or local community. Always consider other causes of fever in the febrile neutropenic, such as thrombosis or their underlying malignancy.
- Antimicrobials should be continued until the patient has been afebrile for at least two days and the neutrophil count is >500 cells/mm^3 on at least one occasion and is showing a consistently increasing trend.
- The role of colony-stimulating factors in neutropenic fever is controversial, but administration can be considered in critically ill patients.

Other Nonpharmacologic Therapies

In addition to general supportive medical care, other precautions such as visitor screening, hand washing, and proper isolation measures should be maintained during this period.

Epidural Spinal Cord Compression

GENERAL PRINCIPLES

Epidural spinal cord compression (ESCC) occurs in ~5% of cancer patients and is defined by compression of the dural sac and its contents (spinal cord and/or cauda equina) by an extradural tumor mass, with or without resultant symptoms.[2] Early recognition is critical, as delayed diagnosis decreases the likelihood of functional recovery in patients who present with weakness and/or sensory deficits.

ETIOLOGY

Any malignancy can produce epidural compression, with lung, breast, and prostate cancers being the most common, followed by multiple myeloma, lymphoma, and renal cell carcinoma. The thoracic spine is the most common location, followed by the lumbosacral, and then the cervical spine. Compression occurs either by direct extension from metastases in the vertebral bone or by tumor growth through the intervertebral foramina. On occasion, tumors can metastasize directly to the epidural space.

DIAGNOSIS

Clinical Presentation

- **Back pain** is the first symptom in 90% of patients. The pain is generally located midline and is frequently accompanied by referred or radicular pain. The pain, unlike the pain of a herniated disc, may be exacerbated by recumbence and improved by the upright position. It is often worse at night. New or progressive back pain should not be dismissed or attributed to benign etiologies in cancer patients without a thorough evaluation.
- **Weakness and sensory impairment** may follow from hours to months after the onset of pain. Regardless of the spinal compression site, weakness tends to begin in the proximal legs. The weakness can progress to **paraplegia** and occasionally develops abruptly without prior clinical signs. Sensory complaints are very common, and often present prior to onset of weakness. These complaints range from paresthesias to loss of sensation.
- **Autonomic dysfunction**, including impotence and bowel/bladder dysfunction, occurs late and is generally not the sole presenting symptom. Urinary retention is the most common manifestation of autonomic dysfunction.

Diagnostic Testing

- Whole-spine MRI with and without contrast is the best diagnostic test for ESCC and should be obtained as soon as possible after presentation. The entire spine should be imaged because of the high incidence of asymptomatic multilevel disease.
- CT myelography is necessary for patients with contraindications for MRI. CT myelography has similar sensitivity and specificity as MRI, but MRI is noninvasive, safer, and better tolerated.
- One must also consider other causes of spinal cord dysfunction, such as myelopathy, intramedullary metastases, hematoma, and abscess. Lumbar puncture to search for additional causes should not be performed until spinal cord compression is excluded.

TREATMENT

- **Dexamethasone** is indicated in nearly all patients with ESCC, particularly those who are symptomatic. Treatment should begin immediately after the diagnosis is suspected and should not be delayed until the results of imaging studies are available. Dosing is controversial, but a common regimen is a 10 mg IV bolus followed by 4 mg IV every 6 hours.
- All patients should have an immediate **neurosurgical consultation**. Patients should have a baseline assessment, focusing on the oncologic characteristics of the tumor, the mechanical stability, systemic burden of disease, and comorbid conditions.[3] Spinal instability is an independent indication for surgical stabilization. Other situations where surgery should be considered are in patients with relatively radioresistant tumors with high-grade ESCC, and/or those who have symptom progression during or after radiation therapy. Patchell and colleagues (2005) published a pivotal randomized study showing that initial operative treatment benefits a subgroup of patients with ESCC, with improved survival and ambulatory status compared to patients who received radiation alone.[4] Importantly, patients with paraparesis for >48 hours, radiosensitive tumors, and multiple discrete compressive lesions were excluded from this study.
- **Radiation therapy** is also indicated in nearly all patients with ESCC, either in lieu of surgery in those with radiosensitive tumors or after surgery. The most common regimen is 10 fractions of 3 Gy each; shorter courses can be considered in those with limited expected survival.

Malignant Pericardial Effusion and Tamponade

GENERAL PRINCIPLES

- Malignancy is a frequent cause of pericardial disease including pericardial effusion, cardiac tamponade, and pericarditis. An autopsy series of 3,314 patients found that cardiac metastases occur in ~10% of patients dying of cancer,[5] though many of these cases were not clinically significant. Malignant pericardial disease is generally a manifestation of an advanced malignancy.
- The most common malignancies associated with pericardial involvement are lung cancer, breast cancer, and lymphoma.

Pathophysiology

- Some tumors, such as cancers of the esophagus and lung, can involve the pericardium via direct local invasion. Others may invade through the lymphatic system or bloodstream. Tumors in the pericardial space may cause bleeding and create a more rapidly accumulating effusion than in an exudative or transudative process. Pericardial disease may also develop secondary to cancer-directed treatments; common examples include pericarditis due to radiation therapy or pericardial effusions from dasatinib, used in the treatment of chronic myeloid leukemia (CML). Checkpoint inhibitors may rarely cause myopericarditis.

DIAGNOSIS

Clinical Presentation

- Slow-growing effusions may be found incidentally on imaging, or patients may present with subtle nonspecific complaints such as weakness, fatigue, and dyspnea.
- If a large effusion accumulates rapidly, patients can develop **cardiac tamponade** leading to hemodynamic collapse. On evaluation, patients may have signs of hypotension, tachycardia, jugular venous distention, and distant heart tones. Another sign indicative of tamponade is pulsus paradoxus, defined as a decrease in systolic blood pressure >10 mm Hg on inspiration. Importantly, the absence of pulsus paradoxus on exam does not exclude cardiac tamponade.

Differential Diagnosis

- The differential diagnosis of pericardial disease in a patient with malignancy also includes nonmalignant causes, such as hypothyroidism, autoimmune disorders, infection, drug-induced, uremia, and idiopathic pericardial disease.
- Other pathologic entities may present with similar symptoms in the cancer patient.
  - Cardiotoxicity leading to **congestive heart failure** can result from chemotherapy (such as anthracyclines), biologics (such as the monoclonal antibody trastuzumab), or checkpoint inhibitors. 5-Fluorouracil (5-FU), a commonly used antimetabolite, is associated with acute cardiotoxicity that can lead to cardiac arrhythmia, myocardial ischemia, and, rarely, cardiogenic shock. Radiation therapy can also cause cardiomyopathy in the absence of pericardial disease (especially in the setting of mediastinal radiation for non-Hodgkin or Hodgkin lymphoma and left breast radiation for breast cancer). One must always consider other causes of cardiovascular emergencies in the cancer patient, such as coronary artery disease, heart failure, and infectious endocarditis.

Diagnostic Testing

Patients with suspected pericardial disease should have an immediate chest radiograph and ECG.

- On **chest x-ray**, in the presence of a large effusion, the cardiac silhouette is enlarged in a globular, symmetric fashion. Chest x-ray may also reveal signs of pulmonary congestion and/or pleural effusions.
- **ECG** commonly shows sinus tachycardia and may reveal reduced voltage or, with very large effusions, electrical alternans.
- **Transthoracic echocardiography** is the diagnostic test of choice and should be obtained emergently whenever the diagnosis of tamponade is suspected. It will diagnose the effusion and indicate the degree of hemodynamic compromise. Early signs of tamponade on echocardiogram include right atrial and ventricular collapse.
- **CT scan** is also sensitive for diagnosing an effusion. It can detect as little as 50 mL of pericardial fluid and can also identify pericardial thickening and cardiac masses. **MRI** is less commonly used but can also provide direct imaging of the pericardium.

TREATMENT

- With severe hemodynamic compromise, emergent percutaneous **pericardiocentesis** with echocardiographic guidance should be performed. Rapid volume expansion with IV fluids may be used as a temporizing measure to support the patient until echocardiographic guidance is available. The pericardial fluid should be sent for cytology and, if concerned for lymphoma, flow cytometry.
- A pericardial drain or a pericardial window may be necessary. To prevent recurrence, sclerosing agents such as thiotepa are available but are often less effective and have more risks than placing a **surgical pericardial window**. A surgical pericardial window is generally the definitive treatment for a clinically significant pericardial effusion.

Superior Vena Cava Syndrome

GENERAL PRINCIPLES

Definition

Superior vena cava syndrome (SVCS) is the result of **obstruction of blood flow through the SVC**, which can occur by either external compression, tumoral invasion, or thrombus.

Etiology

- **Non–small-cell lung cancer, small-cell lung cancer,** and **lymphoma** are the most common causes (~90%) of SVCS. Other tumors associated with SVCS include breast cancer, germ cell tumors, mesothelioma, and thymic malignancies.[6]
- **Thrombosis of the SVC** in patients with central venous catheters is an increasingly common cause of SVCS. Other nonmalignant causes of SVCS include granulomatous infections, goiter, aortic aneurysms, and fibrosing mediastinitis.

DIAGNOSIS

Clinical Presentation

- Patients typically present with swelling of the neck, face, and upper extremities; swelling may be exacerbated by bending forward. Jugular venous distention, cyanosis, and facial plethora may also be present.
- Shortness of breath, dizziness, and, rarely, obtundation from cerebral edema are possible if the onset is rapid. Very rarely, SVCS can cause laryngeal edema and compromise of the upper airway.

- Vocal cord paralysis and Horner syndrome are also possible if neural structures are invaded. With slowly progressive obstruction, collateral flow has time to develop, and symptoms related to vascular obstruction may be subtle.

Diagnostic Testing
- **Chest radiography** may show a widened superior mediastinum and pleural effusions.
- **CT scan** of the chest with IV contrast is the diagnostic test of choice. CT findings characteristic of SVCS include reduced or absent opacification of central venous structures with prominent collateral venous circulation.
- A diagnosis of the mass should be attempted before treatment is begun if the tissue type of tumor is unknown. Sputum cytology, biopsy of lymph nodes, bronchoscopy, thoracentesis (if a pleural effusion is present), mediastinoscopy, or thoracotomy can be diagnostic. The workup generally progresses first through less-invasive diagnostic testing (e.g., sputum cytology) before more invasive tests are performed (e.g., mediastinoscopy).

TREATMENT

- Supportive measures including anticoagulation if thrombus is present, avoidance of overhydration, and head elevation can be used before definitive management. Glucocorticoids may be useful in steroid-responsive malignancies (e.g., lymphoma) or in the setting of radiation administration for airway obstruction, but otherwise are generally not indicated for SVCS.
- In patients with **life-threatening symptoms** such as respiratory compromise or cerebral edema, **endovascular interventions** such as endovenous stent placement or thrombectomy are indicated.
- In patients without life-threatening symptoms, treatment is individualized. **Radiation therapy** is useful for non–small-cell lung carcinoma and other metastatic solid tumors. **Chemotherapy** is more useful in small-cell lung cancer and lymphoma owing to their exquisite chemosensitivity. Initial **endovenous stenting** may be preferred in tumors that are less sensitive to chemotherapy or radiation.
- SVCS resulting from catheter-related thrombus is treated by anticoagulation and, less frequently, fibrinolysis. Surgical venous bypass and/or resection are used in limited circumstances, including in the setting of thymic or residual germ cell tumors.

Tumor Lysis Syndrome

GENERAL PRINCIPLES

Tumor lysis syndrome (TLS) represents a myriad of metabolic and electrolyte abnormalities that result from the release of intracellular products by rapidly dividing tumor cells prior to therapy or from the lysis of sensitive tumor cells during therapy. TLS usually occurs in the setting of therapy of rapidly growing hematologic malignancies, classically acute lymphoblastic leukemia, and high-grade non-Hodgkin lymphoma (e.g., Burkitt lymphoma). Rarely, TLS has been described after the treatment of solid tumors such as breast and small-cell lung cancer. The size of the tumor, rate of tumor growth, and sensitivity of the tumor cells to chemotherapy predict the risk of development of TLS (Table 38-1).

TABLE 38-1 RISK FACTORS FOR TUMOR LYSIS SYNDROME

Patients at risk for acute tumor lysis syndrome
Tumor type
  High-grade non-Hodgkin lymphoma (e.g., Burkitt lymphoma)
  Acute leukemia (AML or ALL)
  Rapidly growing solid tumors (small-cell lung cancer)
Extent of disease
  Bulky tumors
  Elevated lactate dehydrogenase
  Elevated white blood cell count
Underlying renal dysfunction/oliguria
Elevated pretreatment uric acid

Data from DeVita VT, Lawrence TS, Rosenberg SA, eds. *DeVita, Hellman, and Rosenberg's Cancer: Principles and Practice of Oncology.* 10th ed. Wolters Kluwer Health; 2015:1822–1831.

DIAGNOSIS

Clinical Presentation

TLS is characterized by the following **electrolyte derangements:** hyperuricemia, hyperkalemia, hyperphosphatemia, and hypocalcemia. These electrolyte abnormalities place patients at risk for cardiac arrhythmias and seizures. **Acute renal failure** and uremia can develop from precipitation of uric acid and calcium phosphate crystals in the renal tubules. The Cairo–Bishop definition for TLS is commonly used (Table 38-2).[7]

TREATMENT

The best management of TLS includes identifying patients at risk for TLS and taking preventive measures.

TABLE 38-2 CAIRO–BISHOP DEFINITION OF TUMOR LYSIS SYNDROME

Laboratory tumor lysis syndrome[a]
Uric acid ≥8 mg/dL or 25% increase from baseline
Potassium ≥6 mEq/L or 25% increase from baseline
Phosphorus ≥4.49 mg/dL or 25% increase from baseline
Calcium ≤7 mg/dL or 25% decrease from baseline

Clinical tumor lysis syndrome (Laboratory TLS plus one or more of the following)
Creatinine ≥1.5 times the upper limit of normal (adjusted for age)
Cardiac arrhythmia or sudden death
Seizure

[a]Two or more laboratory changes within 3 d before or 7 d after cytotoxic chemotherapy.
Adapted from Cairo MS, Bishop M. Tumour lysis syndrome: new therapeutic strategies and classification. *Br J Haematol.* 2004;127:3–11.

- **IV hydration** should occur 24–48 hours before initiation of chemotherapy (3 $L/m^2/d$) and during therapy. Consider using IV diuretics to improve urine flow rate if the urine output is <80–100 $mL/m^2/h$. Electrolytes including phosphorus, calcium, and magnesium; uric acid; blood urea nitrogen; and creatinine should be measured up to three times a day in patients at high risk for TLS. **Alkalinization of the urine** to increase uric acid excretion can also be considered in the treatment of hyperuricemia in patients with metabolic acidosis, but it is generally no longer recommended in all-comers.
- **Hyperkalemia** should be treated with standard therapy: glucose and insulin (acutely), potassium lowering agents (e.g., sodium zirconium cyclosilicate), and IV calcium if ECG changes are noted.
- **Hyperuricemia** can be controlled with **allopurinol** (maximum 800 mg/d PO in adults) and/or rasburicase. Uric acid is relatively insoluble and can precipitate in renal tubules, causing acute renal failure. Allopurinol decreases the production of uric acid by inhibiting the enzyme xanthine oxidase, which converts xanthine and hypoxanthine to uric acid. Allopurinol must be dose-reduced in patients with renal failure. Also, allopurinol inhibits the degradation of 6-mercaptopurine and azathioprine, so these drugs must be dose-reduced if the patient is taking allopurinol. Allopurinol does not decrease the amount of uric acid already present. Thus, **one must initiate allopurinol before chemotherapy in patients with preexisting hyperuricemia or in those at high risk for TLS**.
- **Rasburicase** is a recombinant form of the enzyme urate oxidase, which breaks down uric acid to form allantoin. Allantoin is an inactive, soluble metabolite of uric acid and can be renally excreted. Rasburicase is **contraindicated in patients with glucose-6-phosphate dehydrogenase deficiency**, as it can cause hemolysis in this setting. Other side effects of rasburicase include methemoglobinemia and anaphylaxis. The dosing of rasburicase varies; our institution uses an initial 3–6 mg dose, but many institutions use 0.15–0.2 mg/kg for one dose and repeat doses only if hyperuricemia is still present. Rasburicase is now generally the standard of care for pediatric and adult patients with established TLS and may be used in high-risk patients as prophylaxis, particularly those with an elevated pretreatment uric acid.
- **IV calcium should not be administered for hypocalcemia unless the patient is symptomatic or hyperphosphatemia is corrected,** due to the risk of calcium-phosphate deposition. Symptoms of hypocalcemia include muscular (cramps, spasms, and tetany), cardiac (arrhythmias and hypotension), and neurologic (confusion or seizures) abnormalities. In the setting of **hyperphosphatemia**, mild cases may be managed with oral phosphate binders. **Dialysis** may be necessary in patients with poor renal function or metabolic abnormalities not corrected by conservative measures.

Hypercalcemia of Malignancy

GENERAL PRINCIPLES

Hypercalcemia is relatively common and occurs in ~20% of patients with cancer. Malignancies of the lung, breast, head/neck, and kidney, as well as multiple myeloma, are most often associated with hypercalcemia.[8]

Etiology

Most commonly, a tumor causes hypercalcemia by producing ectopic parathyroid hormone-related protein (PTHrP), which stimulates bone resorption via osteoclasts as well as causes renal tubular calcium retention. Less commonly, tumor in bone can have direct osteolytic activity causing release of calcium through local cytokines. Rarely, lymphomas can produce ectopic 1,25-dihydroxyvitamin D to cause hypercalcemia.

DIAGNOSIS

Clinical Presentation

Presenting symptoms are often nonspecific and include fatigue, anorexia, constipation, polydipsia, polyuria, nausea, bone pain, and lethargy. Nephrolithiasis is possible. In severe cases, altered mental status, seizures, and coma can be seen. Hypercalcemia can cause renal parenchymal damage and nephrogenic diabetes insipidus. Hypercalcemia produces a brisk diuresis, and patients are often severely volume depleted.

Diagnostic Testing

Management includes obtaining an **ionized calcium level** (or an albumin level to correct for the hypoalbuminemia that is frequently seen in cancer patients). Serum **intact parathyroid hormone (PTH) levels** should be checked to rule out primary hyperparathyroidism. Intact PTH levels are suppressed in the hypercalcemia of malignancy. PTHrP, 1,25-dihydroxyvitamin D, and 25-hydroxyvitamin D levels should also be obtained. A **serum phosphate level** must be checked, as hypercalcemia often leads to clinically significant hypophosphatemia.

TREATMENT

- Patients are often profoundly volume-depleted with severe hypercalcemia, and the acute treatment of hypercalcemia begins with **IV fluids**. Isotonic saline is started at 200–300 mL/h and decreased after the volume deficit is corrected, with a subsequent goal to maintain a urine output of 100–200 mL/h to aid in calcium excretion. Serum electrolytes, including potassium, phosphate, and magnesium, should be measured every 6–12 hours and corrected accordingly. Oral phosphate repletion is standard if the serum phosphate level is low and the patient has normal renal function, and IV phosphate repletion is generally avoided. **Loop diuretics** may be useful in the setting of renal or heart failure, but otherwise are generally not recommended.
- Other than IV fluids, the mainstay of the treatment of severe hypercalcemia is a **bisphosphonate**. **Zoledronic acid** (4 mg given IV) is most commonly used; other bisphosphonates that may be used include **pamidronate** (60–90 mg IV) and **ibandronate** (2–4 mg IV).
  - Bisphosphonates work by inhibiting bone resorption by osteoclasts. The onset of action of the bisphosphonates is between 2 and 4 days, with a total duration of action lasting between 2 and 4 weeks.
  - Bisphosphonates must be used with caution in patients with underlying renal insufficiency and must be dose reduced in patients with impaired renal function. They generally are avoided in patients with significant renal impairment (creatinine clearance, <30 mL/min). Side effects include flulike symptoms, bone pain, and subsequent hypocalcemia and hypophosphatemia. Rarely, patients treated with bisphosphonates develop osteonecrosis of the jaw.
- **Calcitonin** (4 IU/kg) should be used in patients with severe hypercalcemia and may be administered intramuscularly or subcutaneously every 12 hours; doses can be increased up to 6–8 IU/kg every 6 hours. Nasal application of calcitonin is not efficacious for treatment of hypercalcemia. Calcitonin is relatively nontoxic. It lowers the serum calcium concentration by a maximum of 1–2 mg/dL beginning within 4–6 hours. The **efficacy of calcitonin is limited to the first 48 hours** due to tachyphylaxis. Because of its limited duration of effect, calcitonin is most beneficial in symptomatic patients with calcium >14 mg/L when combined with hydration and bisphosphonates. Calcitonin and hydration provide a rapid reduction in serum calcium concentration, while a bisphosphonate provides a more sustained effect.
- **Glucocorticoids** (e.g., prednisone at an initial dose of 0.5–1 mg/kg/d) may be effective in hypercalcemia due to some hematologic malignancies and myeloma. Steroids can reduce serum calcium levels within 2–5 days.

- **Denosumab** (given 60–120 mg subcutaneously) is a monoclonal antibody to receptor activator of nuclear factor kappa-B ligand (RANKL), and reduces osteoclast activity, limiting bone resorption. It may be used in patients with contraindications to bisphosphonates (including severe renal dysfunction) and in those with refractory hypercalcemia. In addition, **dialysis** is effective if other treatments fail. The definitive treatment of hypercalcemia is successful treatment of the underlying malignancy.

Syndrome of Inappropriate Antidiuresis and Hyponatremia

GENERAL PRINCIPLES

The syndrome of inappropriate secretion of antidiuretic hormone (SIADH) is common among cancer patients. SIADH is due to ectopic ADH production by the tumor and is seen most commonly in small-cell lung cancer, but it can also be seen in many other malignancies including cancers of the head and neck, upper gastrointestinal tract, and genitourinary tract.

Etiology

In addition to SIADH directly related to the malignancy, drugs can also cause inappropriate release of vasopressin or increase its action. Common cancer-related medications implicated in SIADH include cisplatin, vincristine, cyclophosphamide, checkpoint inhibitors, opiates, and certain antiseizure medications. Pulmonary and central nervous system disease may also cause SIADH.[9]

DIAGNOSIS

Clinical Presentation

Patients with SIADH and hyponatremia may present with complaints of anorexia and nausea. With rapid and severe decline in serum sodium concentrations, they may also present with confusion, coma, and seizures. Look for **decreased serum osmolality** (<270 mOsm/L), **urine that is not maximally dilute** (>100 mOsm/L), and **elevated urine sodium** (>20 mEq/L). The diagnosis of SIADH requires the **absence of a hypervolemic state** (manifest by ascites, edema) and **absence of volume contraction**, along with **normal thyroid, renal,** and **adrenal function**.

TREATMENT

- Acute management depends on the chronicity and presence of symptoms. **Fluid restriction** is a mainstay of treatment, with a suggested restriction of <1 L/d. In patients with chronic, asymptomatic, or minimally symptomatic hyponatremia, **oral salt tablets** or **oral urea** may be used to increase the serum sodium. **Loop diuretics** may be added, especially in those with significantly elevated urine osmolarity (e.g., more than twice the serum osmolarity). For chronic hyponatremia, the rate of correction should be <8 mEq/L over a 24-hour period.
- For severe symptomatic hyponatremia, urgent intervention with **hypertonic saline** is indicated. 100 mL of 3% saline may be given to raise the serum sodium by ~2 mEq/L, and doses may be repeated as needed. An initial rate of correction of 4–6 mEq/L over the first 3–4 hours is indicated in those with severe neurologic symptoms but should be limited to 8–10 mEq/L at 24 hours to prevent **osmotic demyelination syndrome** from over-correction.
- **Vasopressin-receptor antagonists** are another option for the treatment of SIADH and produce selective water diuresis without affecting sodium and potassium excretion.

Intravenous **conivaptan** and oral tolvaptan are available and approved for use in patients with hyponatremia due to SIADH. The utility of **tolvaptan** therapy is limited by potential hepatotoxicity, excessive thirst, and cost. It should not be used in patients for more than 30 days and is contraindicated in those with underlying liver disease.[10]

Other Neurologic Emergencies

- **Increased intracerebral pressure and cerebral herniation** (from brain metastases, hemorrhage, venous sinus thrombosis, meningitis, head trauma, infarction, or abscess) may present with severe headaches, cranial nerve palsies, papilledema, bradycardia, and hypertension. Immediate consultation with neurosurgery is recommended. The patient should be stabilized, and maneuvers to lower intracranial pressures such as hyperventilation, head elevation, and IV mannitol and/or dexamethasone should be attempted.
- **Status epilepticus** (from brain metastases, metabolic derangement, or neurotoxicity of cancer therapy). Ensuring an airway as part of the BLS/ACLS algorithm should be the first and foremost concern. Laboratory studies such as glucose, electrolytes, Ca, Mg, serum and urine toxicology screens, serum alcohol level, CBC, urinalysis, and any pertinent medication levels should be obtained. IV benzodiazepines are most commonly used (e.g., 2 mg IV lorazepam), and dosing may be repeated if seizures persist. A loading dose of a longer-acting antiseizure medication should also be given, such as levetiracetam (60 mg/kg, max 4,500 mg), fosphenytoin, or valproate. If the patient does not have IV access, benzodiazepines may be given intramuscularly, intranasally, or per rectum. Neurology consultation is indicated for assistance with antiepileptic choice and dosing.
- **Intracerebral hemorrhage** (from metastatic tumor, thrombocytopenia, or leukostasis). Headache, vomiting, and mental status changes are symptoms of significantly increased intracranial pressure and hemorrhage. Workup includes imaging with a STAT noncontrast head CT scan (MRI if CT is nondiagnostic) and obtaining basic labs and coagulation studies. Therapy largely focuses on maintenance of adequate blood pressure, supportive care, correction of coagulopathy and thrombocytopenia, and neurosurgical consultation.

REFERENCES

1. Freifeld AG, Bow EJ, Sepkowitz KA, et al; Infectious Diseases Society of America. Clinical practice guideline for the use of antimicrobial agents in neutropenic patients with cancer: 2010 update by the Infectious Diseases Society of America. *Clin Infect Dis.* 2011;52(4):e56–e93.
2. Loblaw DA, Perry J, Chambers A, Laperriere NJ. Systematic review of the diagnosis and management of malignant extradural spinal cord compression: the cancer care Ontario Practice Guidelines Initiative's Neuro-Oncology Disease Site Group. *J Clin Oncol.* 2005;23(9):2028–2037.
3. Laufer I, Rubin DG, Lis E, et al. The NOMS framework: approach to the treatment of spinal metastatic tumors. *Oncologist.* 2013;18(6):744–751.
4. Patchell RA, Tibbs PA, Regine WF, et al. Direct decompressive surgical resection in the treatment of spinal cord compression caused by metastatic cancer: a randomised trial. *Lancet.* 2005;366(9486): 643–648.
5. Abraham KP, Reddy V, Gattuso P. Neoplasms metastatic to the heart: review of 3314 consecutive autopsies. *Am J Cardiovasc Pathol.* 1990;3(3):195–198.
6. Wilson LD, Detterbeck FC, Yahalom J. Clinical Practice. Superior vena cava syndrome with malignant causes. *N Engl J Med.* 2007;356(18):1862–1869.
7. Cairo MS, Bishop M. Tumour lysis syndrome: new therapeutic strategies and classification. *Br J Haematol.* 2004;127(1):3–11.
8. Goldner W. Cancer-related hypercalcemia. *J Oncol Pract.* 2016;12(5):426–432.
9. Ellison DH, Berl T. Clinical practice. The syndrome of inappropriate antidiuresis. *N Engl J Med.* 2007;356(20):2064–2072.
10. Torres VE, Chapman AB, Devuyst O, et al; TEMPO 3:4 Trial Investigators. Tolvaptan in patients with autosomal dominant polycystic kidney disease. *N Engl J Med.* 2012;367(25):2407–2418.

Index

Page numbers followed by f refer to figures; page numbers followed by t refer to tables.